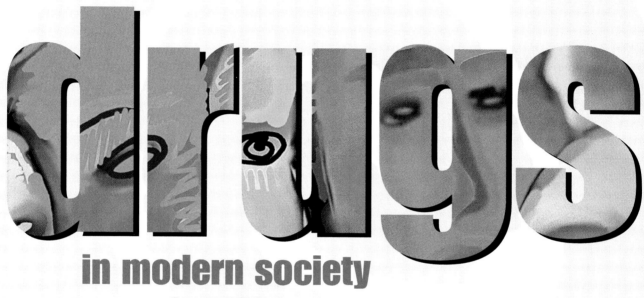

drugs
in modern society
Fourth Edition

Charles R. Carroll
Ball State University

Boston, Massachusetts   Burr Ridge, Illinios   Dubuque, Iowa
Madison, Wisconsin   New York, New York   San Francisco, California   St. Louis, Missouri

WCB/McGraw-Hill

A Division of The **McGraw·Hill** *Companies*

Book Team

Publisher *Bevan O'Callaghan*
Project Editor *Theresa Grutz*
Production Editor *Ann Fuerste*
Proofreading Coordinator *Carrie Barker*
Designer *Jeff Storm*
Art Editor *Miriam Hoffman*
Photo Editor *Rose Deluhery*
Production Manager *Beth Kundert*
Production/Costing Manager *Sherry Padden*
Production/Imaging and Media Development Manager
   Linda Meehan Avenarius
Marketing Manager *Pamela S. Cooper*
Copywriter *Sandy Hyde*

Basal Text *9.8/12 Minion*
Display Type *Univers*
Typesetting System *Macintosh™*
   QuarkXPress™
Paper Stock *50# Mirror Matte*

Vice President of Production and New Media Development *Vickie Putman*
Vice President of Sales and Marketing *Bob McLaughlin*
Vice President of Business Development *Russ Domeyer*
Director of Marketing *John Finn*

Part Openers: **1** © Dave Schaefer/Uniphoto Picture Agency;
2 © Michael Newman/PhotoEdit; **3** © Charles Gupton/Uniphoto
Picture Agency; **4** © Chromosohm Media/The Image Works;
5 © Dion Ogust/The Image Works; **6** © Bob Daemmrich/The Image Works

Cover design by Anna Manhart

Cover image © Diana Ong/SuperStock

Copyedited by Wendy Nelson

Third Reader Ann M. Kelly

contents

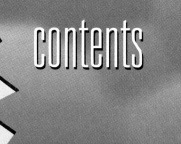

part

Prevention of Alcohol, Tobacco, and Other Drug Problems 313

six

Chapter 13

drug-abuse prevention 315

Chapter 14

alcohol, tobacco, and other drug prevention education 357

boxes

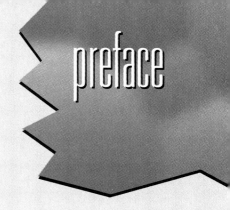

The continuing interest of Americans in the wellness and human potential movements, stress management, holistic health care, natural foods, and physical fitness suggests that people are increasingly concerned about their own health and about preventing health problems. This emphasis on "self-care" and health enhancement and empowerment is, in part, a reaction to the recognized limits of medical care for those already sick or injured. More important, "self-care" and wellness-promoting activities are the result of a growing awareness that one's own lifestyle and personal health habits play critical roles in the development of avoidable diseases and injuries.

According to supportive data for *Healthy People 2000: National Health Promotion and Disease Prevention Objectives,*[1] many of our most pressing health problems are related to the use of alcohol and other drugs, including tobacco. After a ten-year downturn in the use of illegal drugs, recent surveys indicate increasing numbers of young Americans are now abusing marijuana and cocaine. The staggering toll that alcohol and other drug problems exact on society, health, and the economy is growing once again.

Alcohol use itself is now implicated in nearly half of all intentional injuries, such as homicides and suicides. Alcohol-related traffic crashes is one of the leading killers of young Americans. Abuse of alcohol and other drugs significantly increases the risk of transmission of the human immunodeficiency virus (HIV). This can take place directly, through the sharing of contaminated needles, sexual contact with intravenous drug abusers or other drug injectors, or *in utero* infection, or indirectly through adverse effects on immune system functioning and the increased risk of unwanted or unsafe sexual practices.

Tobacco use is responsible for more than one of every five deaths in the United States and is the single most important preventable cause of death and disease in our society. The use of tobacco products is now an acknowledged, major risk factor for diseases of the heart and blood vessels; chronic bronchitis and emphysema; cancers of the lung, larynx, oral cavity, esophagus, pancreas, and bladder; as well as other problems, such as respiratory infections and stomach ulcers.

Some health authorities also relate various lifestyle excesses—faulty nutrition, dangerous driving, unrelenting pressure to achieve, and our overuse of medications—to our national fascination with both legal as well as illegal drugs and both prescribed as well as nonprescribed drugs.

Although the individual's role in promoting health and preventing disease is achieving greater importance, it is recognized that people usually make personal lifestyle choices within a society that glamorizes many hazardous behaviors through advertising and the mass media. Social influences involving peer pressure and the encouragement of risk-taking activities have a tremendous impact, especially on young people. In addition, society continues to support industries that produce unhealthful products, unevenly enacts and enforces laws against behaviors such as driving while intoxicated, and offers somewhat ambiguous messages about those behaviors that are advisable.[2]

1. *Healthy People 2000: National Health Promotion and Disease Prevention Objectives* (Washington, D.C.: U.S. Public Health Service, 1990).

2. Julius B. Richmond, *Healthy people—The surgeon general's report on health promotion and disease prevention* (Washington, D.C.: U.S. Government Printing Office, 1979), p. 17.

Because of these potentially destructive, inaccurate, and often confusing and irrational influences on people, and because of the widespread use and abuse of drugs and medications in America, this text is designed for healthy people—for those who wish to preserve the potential for benefits and minimize the potential for harm that accompany the use of any drug or medicine.

Intended for use in drug education courses for students from a variety of disciplines, *Drugs in Modern Society* provides current, accurate, and documented information about drug substances presented in a scientific and objective manner. Mind-altering or psychoactive drugs are the major focus of this text, but consideration is also given to nonpsychoactives that are frequently misused and to the legal recreational or social drugs infrequently viewed as part of the real drug problem in America.

Drugs in Modern Society explores a variety of drug-related concerns, portrays certain drug-taking behaviors as health-threatening and even life-threatening, and emphasizes the positive benefits of recommended health-promoting actions. However, only you can apply such ideas and interpretations to your own lifestyle. It is hoped that you will be better prepared to make more mature and more responsible decisions regarding drug use and to assist others in making similar decisions affecting their drug-taking behavior.

From a philosophical perspective this book seeks to enhance your freedom of choice in terms of drug use or nonuse. Free choices can be made in consideration of how personal actions affect oneself. However, truly free choices might also concern one's relations with the spirits of other people, ". . . relations involving love, trust, integrity, responsibility, honor, and sacrifice."[3] On occasion, then, such freedom will allow us to do what may not always be best for ourselves. Our freedom of choice will allow us to do what is best for others.

3. Robert D. Russell, "Holistic health," Chapter 1 in *Education in the 80's: Health education.* Robert D. Russell, ed. (Washington, D.C.: National Education Association, 1981), p. 21.

Changes in this Edition

In this revised and updated fourth edition, new or expanded material has been introduced on the following topics: prevalence of alcohol, tobacco, and other drug use; identification of the drug-abusing population; drug-crime relationship; anabolic-androgenic steroids and their dangerous alternatives; widespread overmedication of the elderly; agent-, host-, and environment-related theories on drug abuse and drug dependence; reformulated criteria for substance dependence reflecting the fourth edition of the American Psychiatric Association's Diagnostic and Statistical Manual of Mental Disorders (DSM-IV); gender and ethnic differences in drinking, alcohol abuse, and alcoholism; children of alcoholics; prenatal alcohol exposure; the so-called "French paradox" in relation to alcohol consumption and heart disease; mechanism of impairment observed in alcohol intoxication; endogenous opioids; treatment of narcotic dependent individuals; predictors of tobacco use by young people; increased use of two stimulant drugs—methcathinone (khat or cat) and ephedrine; smoking of toad venom containing a recognized hallucinogenic substance, bufotenine; legislative and law-enforcement efforts as drug-control mechanisms; risk factors for alcohol, tobacco, and other drug problems and promising countermeasures; Employee Assistance Programs and drug testing as responses to alcohol and other drug use in the workplace; alcohol, tobacco, and other drug education as drug abuse prevention programs; and a complete listing of the RADAR (Regional Alcohol and Drug Awareness Resource) Network in the United States.

Organization of the Text

Although each of the 14 chapters is self-contained, this edition is organized into 6 major parts that provide a measure of sequential development and interrelatedness of subjects pertaining to psychoactive drugs and drug-taking behaviors.

Part 1 presents an overview of drug problems in America; an understanding of the persistence of mood modification via drugs despite legal, moral, and social restrictions; and a simplified explanation of drug actions within the human body and of the frequently observed components of drug dependency.

Part 2 examines psychoactive drugs that are collectively referred to as the depressants; those substances that tend to slow the function of the central nervous system. Major consideration is given to alcohol, the nation's number-one drug problem. Additional chapters discuss the narcotics and the sedative-hypnotics.

Part 3 looks at stimulants, the psychoactive drugs that tend to speed up central nervous system function. Primary emphasis is focused on tobacco products, since cigarette smoking is still considered the nation's leading preventable cause of death. A separate chapter considers the ongoing popularity of cocaine use, as well as the amphetamines and caffeine.

Part 4 is concerned with the mind-expanding euphoriants, namely the psychedelics, phencyclidine, and marijuana. The latter drug is a unique and controversial psychoactive, deserving its own rather distinct classification.

Part 5 addresses the less obvious aspects of America's drug problem: the frequent misuse and even abuse of over-the-counter and prescribed medications, many of which are not psychoactive in their effects.

Part 6 offers some new insights into the prevention of alcohol, tobacco, and other drug (ATOD) abuse, and the variety of mechanisms employed to reduce the severity of drug-related problems in a drug-using society. The final chapter will be of primary interest to those developing ATOD prevention education programs in schools, churches, community-health agencies, and businesses and industries. Some instructors will omit this chapter from their assigned readings due to the special nature of planning for educational programs.

Learning Aids

Included in this text are various learning aids that should make your study of drugs and drug-taking behavior more effective and more meaningful. As the reader, you can choose those study aids that seem most valuable for enhancing your knowledge and the adoption of health-promoting and disease-preventing behavior in a drug-using society.

Key Terms

At the beginning of each chapter is a listing of some important terms related to various aspects of drugs, drug-taking behavior, or drug-abuse prevention. These words are defined or described in the chapter and are sometimes used frequently within both that chapter and subsequent chapters of the text.

Chapter Objectives

Also at the beginning of each chapter are several statements that will indicate what the reader can expect to learn or be able to do after mastering the chapter contents. By reading the objectives before studying the chapter, you will identify important sections of the narrative. These can be used as guides in your study.

Chapter Introductions

The opening paragraphs of each chapter provide a brief preview of or commentary on the chapter's contents. After reading these comments, browse through the chapter, paying particular attention to topic headings, illustrations, charts, and boxed material so that you get a feeling for the kinds of ideas and major concepts included in the chapter.

At Issue: Point vs. Counterpoint Boxes

Appearing again in this edition are a series of controversial issues dealing with various drugs, drug use and abuse, and mechanisms for resolving or preventing alcohol and other drug problems. Each "At Issue" box presents both a "point" and a "counterpoint" stance or philosophical position representing extreme viewpoints on a particular topic. As you read each "At Issue" box, decide how you would respond to the various points and counterpoints. You

will encounter a range of beliefs that prove there is no universal agreement on many of the thorny problems and issues that abound in that area of drug use, abuse, and drug dependence. Indeed, the differing viewpoints expressed will serve as the basis of heated debate. But developing a better understanding of the contrasting "points" and "counterpoints" may enable informed individuals to arrive at workable solutions to the numerous dilemmas associated with drug use and abuse.

Chapter Summaries

At the end of each chapter a summary reviews the significant ideas presented in the narrative. A few days after you have read the chapter, you may want to reread this short section. If you discover some terms or major concepts that seem unfamiliar, reread the related portions of the chapter narrative. You may also find it useful to refer once again to both the key terms and chapter objectives at the beginning of the chapter to determine your familiarity with the content of the chapter.

Review Questions and Activities

Appearing at the end of each chapter are several review questions that can be used to check your basic understanding of the major ideas presented in the narrative. The activities are intended to enhance the factual content of the chapter. If you can answer these questions or perform the tasks suggested, you have developed a significant comprehension of the chapter subject matter. If you cannot do this, reread certain sections of the narrative to increase your understanding of the ideas involved.

Glossary

After the last chapter, a glossary compiles drug-related terms with definitions. You may wish to consult this extensive listing for a concise explanation of a particular word or phrase. Sometimes the glossary definition of an important term will provide a more inclusive meaning than the one found in the narrative of a chapter. The glossary can also be a useful guide to the correct spelling of a term or process.

Ancillary Materials

An outstanding ancillary package has been created to meet the needs of instructors. The *Instructor's Manual and Test Item File* was revised by Lynne Durrant of the University of Utah. It contains lecture outlines for each chapter, teaching activities, discussion questions, research topics, essay questions, thought provokers tied to the At Issue boxes, suggested audiovisual aids, and supplemental readings. In addition, more than fifty test questions are included for each chapter.

A **Computerized Test Item File** is available to qualified adopters of the text. MicroTest III is easy to use and allows the instructor to build custom tests and answer keys. MicroTest III is available in Macintosh, DOS, and Windows versions.

The **Brown & Benchmark Drug Transparencies** include more than forty images with an annotated guide. These transparencies will help the instructor present the most important concepts from the book in a visually appealing way.

The AIDS Booklet is updated every six months with the latest information on this devastating disease. It can be packaged free of charge with the textbook.

B&B CourseKits™

B&B CourseKits are course-specific collections of for-sale educational materials custom packaged for maximum convenience and value. B&B CourseKits offer you the flexibility of customizing and combining Brown & Benchmark course materials (B&B CourseKits, Annual Editions®, Taking Sides®, etc.) with your own or other material. Each B&B CourseKit contains two or more instructor-selected items conveniently packaged and priced for your students. For more information on B&B CourseKits, please contact your local Brown & Benchmark representative.

Annual Editions®

Magazines, newspapers, and journals of the public press provide current, first-rate, relevant educational information. If you are interested in exposing your students to a wide range of current, well-balanced, carefully selected articles from some of the most important magazines, newspapers, and journals published today, you may want to consider *Annual Editions: Drugs, Society, & Behavior,* published by the Dushkin Publishing Group, a unit of Brown & Benchmark Publishers. *Annual Editions: Drugs, Society, & Behavior,* is a collection of more than fifty articles on topics related to the latest research and thinking in drugs and society. The currently available edition includes articles that explore such challenging contemporary topics as the impact of public smoking bans, the debate over drug legalization, new research on the physiology of addiction, and the Prozac Culture. *Annual Editions* is updated annually and has a number of helpful features, including a topic guide, an annotated table of contents, and unit overviews. For the professor using *Annual Editions* in the classroom, an Instructor's Resource Guide with Test Questions is available. Consult your Brown & Benchmark Sales Representative for more details.

Taking Sides®

Are you interested in generating classroom discussion and finding a tool to more fully involve your students in their experience of your course? Would you like your students to become more active learners and to develop critical thinking skills? If so, you should examine a new publication from the Dushkin Publishing Group, a unit of Brown & Benchmark Publishers: *Taking Sides: Clashing Views on Controversial Issues in Drugs and Society,* edited by Professor Raymond Goldberg of SUNY College at Cortland. *Taking Sides,* a reader that takes a pro/con approach to issues, is designed to introduce students to controversies in drugs and society. The readings have been selected for their liveliness, currency, and substance, and represent the arguments of leading drug researchers and social commentators and reflect a variety of viewpoints. Seventeen issues are grouped into three parts: Drugs and Public Policy; Researching Tobacco, Caffeine, and Alcohol; and Drug Prevention and Treatment. The issues are self-contained and designed to be used independently. Some example issues are: Should needle exchange programs be promoted? Can caffeine be bad for your health? Is the "disease" of alcoholism a myth?

For the instructor, there is an *Instructor's Manual with Test Questions* and a general guidebook, *Using Taking Sides in the Classroom,* which discusses methods and techniques for integrating the pro/con approach into any classroom setting. Consult your Brown & Benchmark Sales Representative for more details.

CourseMedia™

As educational needs and methods change, Brown & Benchmark adds innovative, contemporary student materials for the computer, audio, and video devices of the 1990s and beyond. These include:

- stand-alone materials,
- study guides,
- software simulations,
- tutorials, and
- exercises.

CourseMedia also includes instructional aids you can use to enhance lectures and discussions, such as:

- videos,
- level I and III videodiscs, and
- CD ROMs.

CourseWorks®

CourseWorks (formerly Kinko's CourseWorks in the United States) is the Brown & Benchmark custom publishing service. With its own printing and distribution facility, CourseWorks gives you the flexibility to add current material to your course at any time. CourseWorks provides you with a unique set of options, including:

- customizing Brown & Benchmark CourseBooks™,
- publishing your own material,
- including any previously published material for which we can secure permissions,
- adding photos,
- performing copy editing, and
- creating custom covers.

acknowledgments

I wish to express my deepest thanks to the many people who have contributed to the evolution of *Drugs in Modern Society*. Without their generous support and assistance, this fourth edition would never have come to fruition.

In particular, I want to acknowledge the valuable contributions of the Center for Substance Abuse Prevention (formerly named the Office for Substance Abuse Prevention), the National Institute on Drug Abuse, the National Institute on Alcohol Abuse and Alcoholism, the U.S. Food and Drug Administration, the U.S. Department of Justice, and the Drug Enforcement Administration for their numerous publications and detailed responses to my unending inquiries. It should be noted that such assistance in no way constitutes any official endorsement of this textbook.

I extend my very special thanks to the following individuals for their significant help in the preparation of specific portions of the manuscript: Margaret Henningson of CompCare Publications; Robert Kirk, formerly of the Distilled Spirits Council of the United States, Inc.; John Langer of the Drug Enforcement Administration, Department of Justice; Dr. Max M. Glatt; the National Council on Alcoholism and Drug Dependence; the Michigan Substance Abuse & Traffic Safety Information Center; Mr. Alex Fundock III of the *Journal of Studies on Alcohol;* and Alcoholics Anonymous World Services, Inc.

In addition, I gratefully acknowledge the expert research assistance provided by the Health Resource Library of Greene Memorial Hospital, Xenia, Ohio; the Medical Library of Ball Memorial Hospital, Muncie, Indiana; and the Science-Health Science Library of Ball State University, Muncie, Indiana.

I also want to recognize the valuable contributions of the following professional colleagues, who reviewed the manuscript and provided many detailed criticisms and ideas for improving the text as it was being developed: Jack Benson, Eastern Washington University; Ronald L. Budig, Illinois State University; Richard Hurley, Brigham Young University, and Chrystyna Kosarchyn, Longwood College.

I want to thank my most effective teachers and consultants in the area of chemical dependence and drug-abuse prevention—those professionals who labor in prevention, therapeutic, and rehabilitation programs, and those precious souls who are in the long process of recovering from their illness.

The members of the editorial and production staffs of Brown & Benchmark Publishers also deserve special recognition for their professional expertise and stimulating assistance.

Finally, I wish to express my heartfelt thanks to my family, who supported, encouraged, and sustained me during this labor of love. Emma and Margaret, you have meant so very much to me!

Charles R. Carroll

Ball State University
Muncie, Indiana

part one

Introduction

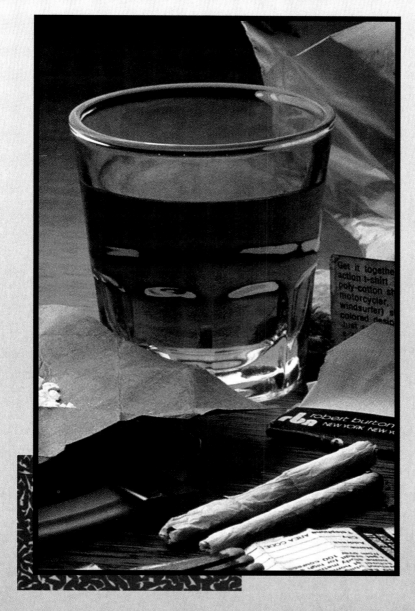

Questions of concern

1. Why do so many people continue to use and abuse psychoactive drugs now that the hazards of such behavior are so well known and publicized?

2. What would our society be like if there were no mind-altering drugs to use or abuse?

3. Why are the consequences of using legal psychoactives so often tolerated or minimized, while the hazards of using illegal drugs are frequently exaggerated?

drinks, and medi

chapter

1

drugs, drinks, and medications

An Introduction

chapter objectives

After you have studied this chapter, you should be able to do the following:

1. Describe the nature of modern drug problems in terms of medical versus social use of drugs, and the use of legally procured drugs versus illegal use of drugs.

2. Define the following terms: *drug, medicine, drug misuse, drug abuse, psychoactive drug, depressant, stimulant, narcotic, psychedelic.*

3. Identify the major types of classes of psychoactive drugs.

4. Explain three different ways of classifying psychoactive drugs.

5. Identify several psychoactive drugs that can be purchased over the counter without a prescription.

6. Discuss the use of psychoactive drugs in relation to their potential for individual and social hazards.

7. Identify several major consequences that may accompany drug-taking behavior, other than the potential for adverse reactions.

8. Distinguish among the following adverse conditions associated with taking psychoactive drugs: toxic reaction, panic, flashback, psychopathology, and drug or chemical dependence.

9. Explain how the following differ from one another: adulterated drugs, look-alikes, and designer drugs.

10. Describe the current psychoactive drug scene in terms of prevalence of use, the drug-abusing population, unanticipated costs, and the nature of the drug-crime relationship.

11. Explain why females are unique regarding use of psychoactive drugs and the potential for adverse consequences associated with using such substances.

12. Differentiate between the use of therapeutic drugs and the use of ergogenic drugs among athletes.

13. Name at least three major types of ergogenic drugs banned by the International Olympic Committee.

14. Describe the potential health threats associated with the use of ergogenic drugs.

15. List five major factors that contribute to the problems of drug misuse and drug abuse among the elderly.

Drug Problems in America

Hard-core use of mind-changing drugs remains firmly entrenched in our society—part of the American way of life that affects both users and nonusers. The news media continue to sensationalize "drug busts" in which law enforcement agents seize imported as well as homegrown marijuana, and raid secret, illegal "speed" labs in suburbia as well as the inner city. School kids learn how to say no to illegal drugs, and some experts now say that treatment and rehabilitation of cocaine abusers would be more effective than law enforcement efforts in reducing the number of cocaine addicts. Meanwhile, Congress funds major health care reforms by increasing cigarette taxes, and public service announcements remind us that "friends don't let friends drive drunk."[1]

In many ways, the national effort to control and prevent the use and abuse of illegal drugs—the "war on drugs"—continues, but in a somewhat subdued, less sensational way. We no longer see those famous "This is your brain on drugs" fried-egg commercials. Some say that the antidrug endeavor is running out of steam. Others claim that illegal drug use and abuse are no longer major national priorities as they appeared to be in the last decade. Despite the expenditure of $10 to $13 billion annually since 1988, it is not always evident that such a war is being won. There are even those who believe that the war on drugs has already been lost.

Although casual, illegal drug use declined over a recent ten-year period and deaths caused by alcohol-related motor vehicle crashes have been reduced significantly, legal and illegal drugs continue to pose a significant threat to the nation. Heavy drug use persists unabated, money laundering proceeds at record levels, and drug-related crime and violence have not declined—they might, in fact, be increasing. And recent studies indicate that our young people, showing signs of being more tolerant toward the use of some illegal substances, are returning to drug abuse.[2] Although the government boasts that drug use has fallen, the variety of intoxicating substances has actually increased, ready to ensnare a new generation.[3]

The United States can certainly be described as a drug-oriented and chemically dependent society. To some extent we have been so in the past, and the future promises more of the same. Not only are millions dependent on the legal "recreational" drugs, alcohol and nicotine, but countless others are addicted to physician-prescribed drugs and the allegedly more dangerous substances distributed everywhere from the salons of the rich and famous to the street corners of the segregated inner cities of our nation—among the poor, the unemployed, and the underclass.[4]

Now that the safety of our airlines, railroads, highways, and merchant marine fleet is threatened by the abuse of alcohol and other drugs, expensive drug detection programs have become standard procedures in the workplace as well as among college, professional, and even some high school athletic teams. Numerous officials, politicians, judges, entertainers, prominent sports figures, and business executives have been exposed, or voluntarily revealed themselves, as cocaine snorters, heroin smokers, alcoholics, tranquilizer dependents, pot puffers, or, more commonly

today, multiple-drug abusers. In many ways, drug abuse and drug dependence have become as American as apple pie.

Drugs and Medicines

All of the mind- and behavior-changing substances mentioned above involve legal, illegal, or potentially harmful chemicals known collectively as *drugs*. Drugs are substances that by their chemical nature can change the way the body functions and the way that people think, feel, and act. Many people incorrectly associate the term *drugs* only with unlawful activities, rebellious youth, and irresponsible thrill-seekers.

On the other hand, *medicines*, which are drugs also, are more frequently perceived as being "good" for people: sick people take medicines to get well. Perhaps we could better determine the goodness or badness of any drug by considering how and why the drug is used and the consequences of using the drug.

While the news media tend to spotlight celebrities, such as River Phoenix and Robin Williams, who become involved with illegal drugs, a major part of our widespread drug problem has nothing to do with cocaine snorters, heroin injectors, pot puffers, or freaked-out users of "angel dust." The "daze of our lives" is just as often the result of people's using pills and capsules that are legally manufactured for use as medicines.

Aided by unprincipled physicians who exchange "no-questions-asked" prescriptions for cash payments, and compounded by our personal efforts of self-medication in a search for pain relief, we often exist with numerous combinations of tranquilizers, cough medicines, and headache remedies in our systems. Though legal and generally approved by society, this form of persistent medical drug use can be very dangerous.

Critics of this supermedicated, tranquilized way of life contend that we are often sedated before birth if our mothers are prescribed antidepressant medication, during birth if they are given painkillers, and at school if our teachers think we have an attention-deficit disorder and we are then placed on Ritalin. Once in the world of work, we are prescribed anti-anxiety drugs to combat tension and painkillers to ease discomfort. If we survive to old age,

we may once again be given antidepressants or even major tranquilizers to make us more subdued, manageable patients.

Drug problems related to such legally prescribed medication were seldom imagined by most people, until physician-prescribed drug dependency adversely affected some famous Americans. Elvis Presley, Elizabeth Taylor, and Michael Jackson have all been victims—to varying degrees—of drug abuse and chemical dependency related to prescription drugs.

Our national drug problems have yet another dimension—the use of legally approved "social" or "recreational" drugs. Until recently, smoking tobacco products and drinking alcoholic beverages were infrequently regarded as drug-taking behaviors. Tobacco cigarettes and cigars, along with alcoholic beverages, have been widely advertised, legally purchased by adults, and socially used by millions of people.

Nevertheless, the nicotine and tars in tobacco, the ethyl alcohol in beers, wines, and distilled spirits, and even the caffeine in coffee, tea, and cola drinks are all drugs. The seriousness of cigarette smoking as a drug-related behavior capable of promoting disease was not widely documented before the *First Surgeon General's Report on Smoking and Health* in 1964. And although many people now acknowledge alcohol as a drug, the nation learned the reality of alcohol abuse when Billy Carter (the brother of one former U.S. president), Betty Ford (the wife of another president), and baseball superstar Mickey Mantle admitted their alcoholism in public.

There is now a growing trend to describe drug dependence, alcoholism, and persistent cigarette smoking as "addictive behaviors." These conditions all involve some form of participation for short-term pleasure or satisfaction at the expense of long-term unfavorable effects. Ever so slowly, it is also being increasingly recognized that chemical dependency is perhaps the most common "disease" encountered by modern medicine, although it is infrequently diagnosed as such.[5]

Drug Use and People Problems

If using drugs and medicines had no long-lasting effects, never impaired physical, mental, social, or spiritual well-being, and always resulted in positive or otherwise health-promoting experiences, there would be no drug problem. But the use of these powerful chemicals, and the less potent chemicals as well, can and does adversely affect humans—from the preborn to the elderly. Drugs and medicines affect people of both sexes and all races, creeds, educational levels, and ethnic and socioeconomic groups. As such, our drug problems basically are "people problems." They involve relationships, self-image, and self-identity. Such problems are based on attitudes and motivations that foster immediate satisfaction of needs and the inability to tolerate pain or frustration. Peer pressure, parent pressure, and the subtle influence of significant others are part of the problem. Living a pressure-filled life of competition, accompanied by the need to succeed at all costs, is also involved, as are conditions of economic deprivation and environmental harshness.

In essence, drug problems lead to many other problems, including

- physical and mental illnesses
- infection with sexually transmitted diseases
- drug addiction or dependency
- adverse reactions and undesired side effects
- premature and sudden deaths
- disrupted family life
- marital discord, often followed by separation or divorce
- aggression
- exploitation of others
- rape
- vandalism and destructive behavior
- impaired performance on the job and in the classroom
- criminal activities that finance an individual's drug supply or "launder" illegal drug profits through financial institutions
- gang-related violence and drug trafficking
- accidents and injuries due to combining drug use with driving or operation of machinery

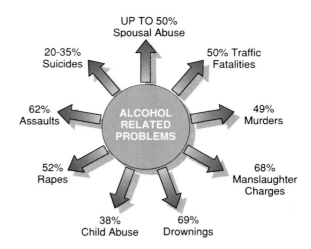

 1.1

Americans have a big problem with alcohol, the number one drug of abuse.

Source: Modified from the Office for Substance Abuse Prevention. Data derived from the National Institute on Alcohol Abuse and Alcoholism.

imprisonment and institutionalization

One drug, alcohol—America's preferred drug of abuse—is associated with several additional problems, as noted in figure 1.1. Such consequences of alcohol and other drug abuse have led George Gallup, Jr., a noted public opinion pollster, to say:

> America does not have a crime problem. America does not have a problem of job absenteeism and low productivity. America does not have a teenage pregnancy problem. America does not have a problem of broken homes and marriages. America has an alcohol and drug problem.[6]

These are just some of the many elements that reveal the comprehensive nature of drug problems. They are often referred to as the symptoms of drug abuse. Moreover, when the nation's number one agricultural crop is alleged to be marijuana (a mood- and behavior-modifying drug), there is little doubt that drug problems exist in America.

There is perhaps a basic issue related to drug abuse and chemical dependency. America's drug problems stem not so much from drugs themselves but from an underlying and widely held belief that such substances can help us face modern life. We act as if having fun, working long and hard, and

coping successfully with the stressors of daily life all depend upon using drugs. Consequently, knowing that no drug produces only positive effects, we should not be surprised that our society has drug problems. We should expect it! Indeed, our society has many drug-related problems.

Basic Definitions

Most topical areas dealing with health promotion and disease prevention have their own special vocabulary of commonly used terms. The drug-problem area is no exception. Therefore, to serve as a foundation for the upcoming chapters in this text, some important terms and concepts are introduced here.

Drug

Any substance that enters the human body and can change either the function or the structure of the human organism is a **drug**. This comprehensive definition of a drug includes practically all foreign materials—even foods, vitamins, plants, snake venom, air pollutants, and pesticides. In chapter 3, a more specific definition of a drug will be provided, although this basic description will not change.

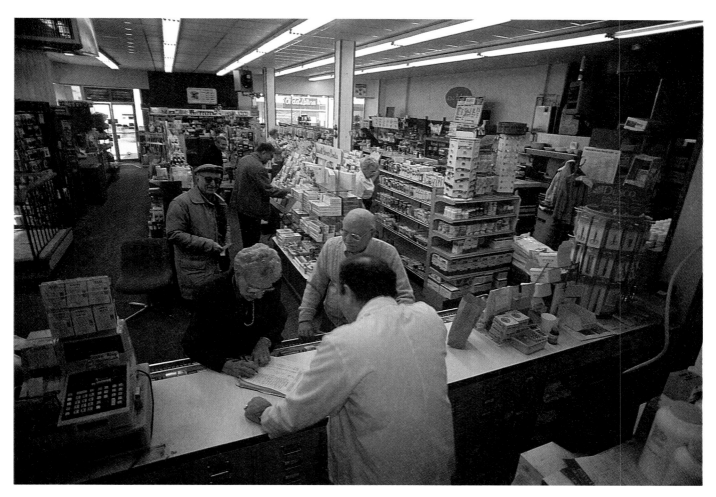

Although over-the-counter drugs are sold in a variety of commercial settings, physician-prescribed medications can be purchased only at a drug store or pharmacy located in a department store, grocery, hospital, or through a mail-order pharmacy service.

© *Larry Mulvehill/The Image Works*

Medicine

Physicians frequently prescribe drugs to treat or prevent illness. However, when drugs are used in the diagnosis, cure, treatment, and prevention of disease, or for the relief of pain or discomfort, the medical profession typically refers to such drug substances as **medicines.**

Many wonders of modern medical practice are based upon **therapeutics,** the use of drugs in treating and preventing disease and in preserving health. Vaccines and toxoids have been effective in the prevention of major communicable diseases such as polio, smallpox, diphtheria, tetanus, and measles. Bacterial infections have been conquered in large measure by antibiotic drugs. Epilepsy and diabetes have been appreciably controlled by Dilantin and insulin, respectively. Anesthetics have provided the patient with a relatively painless experience not only in surgery but also in the dentist's chair. Giant strides have been made in treating the mentally ill with antidepressants and tranquilizers, while AZT may be changing AIDS from a fatal disease to a treatable one.

Prescription drugs, available only by a physician's order, and **over-the-counter** (nonprescription) **drugs** have been very successful in relieving many human ailments when used responsibly. Ideally, drugs should be taken for their intended purposes, according to directions, in the appropriate amount, frequency, strength, or manner, and—in the case of prescribed drugs—under the supervision of a physician.

It should be evident that in order to produce their desired effects, all medicines are composed of drugs, but not all drugs are used as medicines.

Drug Misuse

The unintentional or inappropriate use of prescribed or nonprescribed medicine resulting in the impaired physical, mental, emotional, or social well-being of the user is referred to as **drug misuse.** Some individuals consume drugs in excess of recommended dosages. They double the number of capsules to be taken, or they reduce the standard time interval between doses by one-half. Others take prescribed medications without professional consultation or offer their own medicines to others. For example, a parent might give the remaining portion of a prescribed drug to his or her child because the child's symptoms resemble those of the parent's former ailment. These are all examples of *drug misuse.* Additional drug-misuse practices are listed in box 1.1.

Drug Abuse

Sometimes referred to as substance or chemical abuse, **drug abuse** is the deliberate or unintentional continuous use of mind-changing chemical substances (usually for reasons other than legitimate medical purposes) that results in any degree of physical, mental, emotional, or social impairment of the user, the user's family, or society in general. This comprehensive definition of drug abuse is not based solely on the illegality of the drug that is used, on any specific amount used, time frame of use, or frequency of use. As such, drug abuse does include the unwise use of a legal drug that results in public intoxication or the unsafe operation of a motor vehicle. Many would also consider the use of any legally prohibited drug and the use of any legal drug by underage individuals as additional examples of drug abuse.

In essence, drug abuse involves using illegal as well as legal mind-changing "social" drugs that lead to ill effects and undesirable consequences. It also includes the use of legal medicines by healthy people for social convenience or personal pleasure, and the use of typically nondrug substances, such as gasoline, to produce druglike effects. Since drug abuse has become the focus of public concern and government action, it has been identified almost exclusively with the **psychoactive** (or psychotropic) **drugs** that primarily affect the human mind. See box 1.2 for the danger signals of drug abuse.

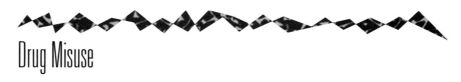

Drug Misuse

Some common examples of drug misuse include these:

Taking prescribed or nonprescribed medicines at the improper time.

Discontinuing the use of a prescribed medicine without consulting one's physician.

Failing to recognize, and then not taking appropriate action regarding, a "side effect" related to a particular drug or medicine.

Taking at the same time duplicate medications prescribed by different physicians.

Combining alcoholic beverages with depressantlike drugs, such as antihistamines, tranquilizers, or sleeping pills.

Stretching the dose of a particular medicine to make it last longer than the originally prescribed period of use.

Failing to inform your present physician of medicines still being taken but prescribed by your former physician.

Continuing to take medication after the original need for such a drug no longer exists.

Saving old medicines for self-treatment at some future time.

Psychoactive Drug

Often described as a psychotropic (mind-affecting) or mind-altering drug, a psychoactive drug is a chemical substance that changes one's thinking, feelings, perceptions, and behavior. These changes are the result of the drug's action on the human brain. Among the psychoactive drugs are those chemicals classified as follows.

Narcotics—The narcotic analgesics, often referred to as opioids, are powerful painkillers and also produce pleasurable feelings and induce sleep.

Depressants—Also known as sedatives, depressants slow down central nervous system function, relax or tranquilize the person, and produce sleep.

Stimulants—These are chemical substances that generally speed up central nervous system function, resulting in alertness and excitability.

Psychedelics—Sometimes known as mind expanders or hallucinogens, these drugs affect a person's perception, awareness, and emotions, and can also cause

hallucinations (completely groundless, false perceptions) as well as illusions (misinterpretations of reality or something imagined).

Marijuana—This intoxicating drug, derived from the hemp plant, can produce both depressant and psychedelic effects.

Inhalants—These are volatile nondrug substances that have druglike effects when inhaled. A few inhalants (specifically, amyl nitrite and nitrous oxide) do have some medical uses.

Many psychoactive drugs already are integrated into the lifestyle of people who daily consume coffee, tea, beer, cola drinks, cocktails, cigarettes, aspirin, and various sleep-enhancing and alertness-promoting preparations. Some of the psychoactive drugs, such as morphine, the barbiturates, and the antidepressants, have legitimate medical uses. However, because all mind-affecting drugs have the ability to modify mood and behavior, they have a high potential not only for misuse but also for abuse in the human quest for pleasure or escape.

box 1.2

Danger Signals of Drug Abuse

Many people take prescribed drugs that affect their moods. Using these drugs wisely is important for physical and emotional health. But sometimes it is difficult to decide when using drugs to handle stress becomes inappropriate. It is important that your use of drugs does not result in catastrophe. Here are some "danger signals" that can help you evaluate your own way of using drugs.

1. Do those close to you often ask about your drug use? Have they noticed any changes in your moods or behavior?

2. Are you defensive if a friend or relative mentions your drug or alcohol use?

3. Are you sometimes embarrassed or frightened by your behavior under the influence of drugs or alcohol?

4. Have you ever gone to see a new doctor because your regular physician would not prescribe the drug you wanted?

5. When you are under pressure or feel anxious, do you automatically take a tranquilizer or drink or both?

6. Do you take drugs more often or for purposes other than those recommended by your doctor?

7. Do you mix drugs and alcohol?

8. Do you drink or take drugs regularly to help you sleep?

9. Do you have to take a pill to get going in the morning?

10. Do you think you have a drug problem?

If you have answered *yes* to a number of these questions, you may be abusing drugs or alcohol. There are places to go for help at the local level. One such place might be a drug-abuse program in your community, listed in the Yellow Pages under "Drug Abuse." Other resources include community crisis centers, telephone hotlines, and the Mental Health Association.

Source: National Institute on Drug Abuse.

People have been attracted to these psychoactive substances because such drugs have been useful in helping individuals cope with and adapt to an everchanging environment. Certainly, smoking, drinking, and taking other drugs can lighten the "load of life"; reduce tensions, anxieties, and frustrations; counteract boredom as well as fatigue; enhance the pleasures of the moment; and, in some instances, provide an escape from the harsh realities of existence. Chemical mood and behavior modifiers have also been employed to enhance self-image, build confidence, gain approval or acceptance, and heal psychological hurts.

Sometimes the use of substances for such personal gratification and temporary adaptation has unanticipated consequences, such as drug dependency, personal and social disorganization, and predisposition to serious and sometimes fatal diseases.

Drug Classifications

It is possible to classify psychoactive drugs—the major focus of this text—in several ways. Such classification allows us to learn the common characteristics of a particular group of drugs.

The first major classification groups specific drugs according to their generalized or localized effects on the brain. This is perhaps the most common way of categorizing drugs, and we will use such a classification generally throughout this text for an analysis of various psychoactive drugs.

Generalized central nervous system depressant effect—Drugs in this category are often referred to as "downers" and have a general effect of slowing down, reducing the function of, or depressing excitable brain tissue. Included in this category are ethyl alcohol, barbiturates, nonbarbiturate sedative-hypnotics, minor tranquilizers (anti-anxiety medications), anesthetics, volatile solvents, and low-dose cannabinoids (marijuana and hashish).

Generalized central nervous system stimulant effect—Sometimes identified as "uppers," the central nervous system stimulants have a

general effect of increasing or speeding up the function of excitable brain tissue. Included in this category are the amphetamines, cocaine, caffeine, and nicotine.

Localized affective or limbic center depressant effect—Included in this category are the antipsychotic drugs (major tranquilizers), the antidepressants, and the antimanic drug lithium, which is used in the treatment of the manic phase of manic-depressive mental illness. These drugs have a localized depressant or modifying effect on the brain's limbic center that controls emotional function. Unlike the central nervous system depressants, the drugs in this category do not slow down the brain's breathing centers.

Psychedelic or hallucinogenic effect—Drugs in this category tend to produce distortion of thought and sensory processes, thereby inducing a psychosis-like state with illusions and hallucinations, often of a visual nature. Lysergic acid diethylamide, mescaline, psilocybin, phencyclidine, and large-dose cannabinoids (marijuana and hashish) are all representative drugs in this group.

Narcotic effect—These drugs, the narcotic analgesics, decrease pain by binding to specific receptors (areas) in certain areas of the brain. In this category are the narcotic-agonists—morphine, heroin, opium, as well as methadone, Darvon, and Demerol—which produce pain relief, euphoria, and depression of breathing. The narcotic antagonists, Naloxone, Naltrexone, and Cyclazocine, which block the effects of the agonists, are also in this drug group. When used alone, the antagonists have few or no drug effects.

A classification of psychoactive drugs commonly purchased over the counter without a prescription reveals the widespread availability of these medications. Such a classification appears in table 1.1. These nonprescription items are used to treat minor symptoms, such as drowsiness and sleeplessness, aches and pains, and the relief of allergic reactions. Of course, alcoholic beverages and tobacco products are bought for a variety of reasons, and are not usually intended for use as medicines.

An additional classification is suggested by the Comprehensive Drug Abuse Prevention and Control Act of 1970, Title II, more commonly known as the **Controlled Substances Act.** This public law enacted by Congress sorts psychoactive drugs (except for ethyl alcohol, nicotine, and caffeine) into five schedules or categories, based on their actual or relative potential for abuse, their likelihood of causing psychic or physiological dependence, and their current acceptability for medical treatment. This classification is shown in box 1.3.

The last drug classification to be considered here may be interpreted as somewhat controversial. Nevertheless, a consideration of both *personal* and *social* hazards associated with drug use, misuse, and abuse is important. When you

table 1.1 Commonly Purchased Over-the-Counter (Nonprescription) Psychoactive Substances

Major Group with Representative Examples	Drug Contents
Alcoholic Beverages	
Beer	Ethyl alcohol, congeners
Wine	Ethyl alcohol, congeners
Distilled spirits	Ethyl alcohol, congeners
Allergy/Cold Relief Medications	
Actifed	Pseudoephedrine hydrochloride
	Triprolidine hydrochloride
Benadryl	Diphenhydramine hydrochloride
Dimetapp Elixir	Brompheniramine maleate
	Phenylpropanolamine hydrochloride
Contac Maximum	Phenylpropanolamine hydrochloride
	Chlorpheniramine maleate
Analgesics (Pain Relievers)	
Advil, Nuprin, Medipren	Ibuprofen
Aleve	Naproxen sodium
Bayer Aspirin, Bufferin	Acetylsalicylic acid
Tylenol, Excedrin	Acetaminophen
Appetite Suppressants	
Acutrim	Phenylpropanolamine hydrochloride
Dexatrim	Phenylpropanolamine hydrochloride
Sleep Aids	
Excedrin PM	Acetaminophen
	Diphenhydramine citrate
Nytol	Diphenhydramine hydrochloride
Sominex	Diphenhydramine hydrochloride
Unisom	Doxylamine succinate
Stimulants	
No Doz	Caffeine
Vivarin	Caffeine
Tobacco Products	
Cigarettes	Nicotine
Cigars	Nicotine
Pipe tobacco	Nicotine
Chewing tobacco	Nicotine
Snuff	Nicotine

consider the potential, inherent hazards of psychological or physical dependence or both, development of tolerance, possibility of irreversible damage to body tissues and disease, likelihood of accidental death or overdose, and predisposition to social dysfunction, recklessness, and self-destructive behavior, you formulate a classification of drugs according to their decreasing personal hazards. An interpretation of one such classification follows:[7]

Very high individual hazard rating: cocaine and amphetamines, ethyl alcohol

Relatively high individual hazard rating: sedative-hypnotics, heroin, volatile inhalants, tobacco cigarettes

Intermediate individual hazard rating: LSD, PCP

Relatively low individual hazard rating: marijuana

It should be noted that cocaine, alcohol, and tobacco cigarettes are all capable of causing serious body-organ or tissue damage. By contrast, there is a somewhat lower potential for heroin either to cause tissue damage or to produce self-destructive behavior. Frequently, heroin users take their narcotic in order to function normally; but often, like coke users and crack smokers, they commit serious crime to finance their drug-taking behavior. Of course, there are always the very real dangers of physical disability or death due to overdose of cocaine and heroin, as noted in figure 1.2. Accidents occurring while a person is under the influence of alcohol, LSD, PCP, and marijuana can also have serious and even fatal outcomes.

In rank-ordering psychoactive drugs according to their inherent *hazard potential to society,* Samuel Irwin originally suggested the following list.[8]

1. Alcohol

2. Sedative-hypnotics

3. Stimulants

4. Heroin

5. Volatile solvents

6. Cigarettes

7. LSD

8. Marijuana

While alcohol is considered here the most potentially hazardous drug to society in terms of its probable misuse and/or abuse and subsequent "harm to others," federal law defines alcohol as legal. However, federal law stipulates that marijuana is illegal even though its potential hazard to society is considered here the lowest of all drugs so ranked in this particular classification. In rank-ordering these drugs, "harm to others" was defined as causing or contributing to social apathy, driving accidents, aggressiveness, and crimes of violence.

Such a classification of drugs is, to be certain, open to criticism and may be described by some as irresponsible or at least controversial. Indeed, law enforcement officials may rank heroin and cocaine as having the greatest adverse effect on society, while social workers may

identify alcohol and health educators might focus on tobacco smoking as the top-ranking social drug problem.

After studying the various drugs described in this text, you may want to rerank the psychoactive drugs for their inherent potential for personal and social hazards. However, such a classification does suggest that legalized drugs are not harmless and that under certain circumstances illegal drug use may have minimal risks to the welfare of both individual drug takers and the society.

Drug Problems: Health-Related Consequences

The benefits generally associated with misusing and abusing drugs are (1) the experience of some physical or psychological pleasure, that is, drug use might make some people feel good or better; and (2) the reduction of a frustrating or stressful condition, that is, drug use might help others feel less frustrated, less stressed, or less painful.

Such benefits should be weighed against the disadvantages, risks, and hazards that often accompany drug-taking behavior. More deaths, illnesses, and disabilities are due to substance abuse than to any other preventable health condition.[9] Of the two million deaths in the United States each year, more than one in four is now related to alcohol abuse, illicit use of psychoactive drugs, or tobacco use. Many such deaths and other related losses could be reduced significantly by changing people's lifestyles and personal behaviors. Several of these conditions will be explored in later chapters of this text. However, of special concern are the following health-related consequences that may represent an immediate problem for many drug takers.

Delay in Seeking Proper Medical Treatment

Frequent unsupervised use of drugs for a health problem may so effectively mask the symptoms of a disorder or disease that the person believes the condition has been controlled or cured. Therefore, the individual

might not seek medical attention early. When such a disorder finally comes to a physician's attention, often little can be done to remedy the problem that has progressed under the protective cover of drugs.

Reduction in Personal Problem-Solving Effectiveness

Using drugs often makes the consumer feel better for a while. However, the underlying causes motivating drug use remain. The ability to utilize other problem-solving techniques, particularly in interpersonal relationships and identity crises, is often impaired. In fact, the techniques may never even be attempted. This is especially true if one is under the influence of certain drugs, such as ethyl alcohol or barbiturates, on a continuing basis.

Experience of Additional Health Problems

The self-administered use of any psychoactive substance makes the drug taker vulnerable to a number of possible and fairly predictable adverse reactions, including these:

1. **Toxic reaction**—A toxic or poisonous reaction accompanies an overdose of any drug. If too much of a chemical substance is taken in at any one time, a temporary condition of intoxication (poisoning) occurs. This is characterized by a disturbance of function in one or more body-support systems. Intoxication with ethyl alcohol, sedatives, opiates, and even PCP can result in death because of the serious depressant effect these drugs have on the breathing center of the central nervous system.

2. **Panic**—First-time users of marijuana, one of the psychedelics, or even a stimulant often develop fears of losing self-control or of having done physical harm to themselves. Afraid of going crazy, the individuals sometimes exhibit uncontrollable behavior.

3. **Flashback**—After repeated use of psychedelics, a drug user may

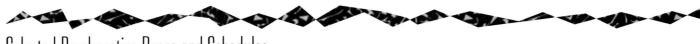

Selected Psychoactive Drugs and Schedules

box 1.3

In schedules II, III, and IV, examples of trademark products appear in parentheses.

Schedule I

Substances with a high potential for abuse and dependence. There is no currently accepted medical use in the United States. (Available for research purposes only.)

Heroin

Psychedelics: LSD, mescaline, peyote, psilocybin, DMT, DED, and amphetamine variants: MDA, MDMA, DMA, PMA, STP, DOM, DOB

Phencyclidine (veterinary drug only) and its analogues: PCE, PCPy, TCP

Methaqualone

Marijuana: in spite of recent studies indicating a variety of potential therapeutic uses; and THC, marijuana's active ingredient

Hashish

Designer drugs

Schedule II

Substances with a high potential for abuse, but such drugs have a currently accepted medical use in the United States, often with severe restriction. Abuse may lead to severe psychological or physical dependence. (Usually available by written prescription only, but in an emergency, oral orders may be given to a dispenser. No refills are permitted.)

Opium

Morphine

Codeine

Hydromorphone (Dilaudid)

Meperidine (Demoral)

Cocaine

Oxycodone (Percodan)

Amphetamines

Methylphenidate (Ritalin)

Barbiturates: amobarbital, pentobarbital, and secobarbital

Dronabinol (Marinol), synthetic delta-9-THC

Nabilone (Cesamet), synthetic cannabinoid

Schedule III

Substances with a potential for abuse less than drugs in Schedules I and II. Such drugs have a currently accepted medical use in the United States. Abuse may lead to moderate or low physical or high psychological dependence. (Available by written or oral prescription; five refills in six months with medical authorization.)

experience a flashback, the undesirable recurrence of a drug's effects with no recent drug intake (consumption) to explain the alteration of one's sense of time and visual illusions and hallucinations. Reaction to such a flashback may range from mild puzzlement and delight to a full-blown panic.

4. **Psychopathology**—A psychopathological condition is the occurrence of one or more severe mental disorders, such as major depression, schizophrenia (thought disorder), or bipolar manic-depression. These disorders can occur in a person having a

substance-abuse problem. Such an individual may be described as a "dually diagnosed" patient—that is, one who has both a mental disorder and a substance-abuse condition. Although there are various forms of this dually diagnosed state, psychoactive substances appear to either unleash or uncover an underlying, preexisting mental disorder or to permanently imbalance the brain's chemistry through years of chronic, toxic effects on the brain of alcohol, other depressants, stimulants, PCP, and even psychedelics.[10] Another form of psychopathology is the organic brain

syndrome resulting from physical changes in the brain, sometimes due to long-term poisonous effects of central nervous system depressants, inhalants, and PCP. This syndrome is manifested by confusion, disorientation, and decreased intellectual functioning.

5. **Drug dependence**—Drug dependence is a maladaptive (faulty or inadequate) pattern of substance use leading to observable and significant impairment or distress. According to the latest edition of the *Diagnostic and Statistical Manual of Mental Disorders* (DSM-IV), at least three

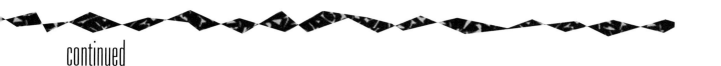

continued

Anabolic steroids, although they are not immediately euphoric in their effect

Derivatives of barbituric acid except those listed in another schedule

Glutethimide (Doriden)

Methyprylon (Noludar)

Nalorphine

Chlorphentermine

Phendimetrazine

Paregoric

Tylenol with codeine #4

Schedule IV

Substances with a low potential for abuse relative to drugs in Schedule III. These drugs have a currently accepted medical use in the United States. Abuse may lead to limited physical or psychological dependence relative to drugs in Schedule III. (Available by written or oral prescription; five refills in six months with medical authorization.)

Barbiturates: barbital, phenobarbital

Chloral hydrate

Ethchlorvynol (Placidyl)

Ethinamate (Valmid)

Meprobamate (Equanil, Miltown)

Propoxyphene (Darvon)

Pentazocine (Talwin-NX)

Benzodiazepine anti-anxiety drugs: (Xanax, Valium, Librium, Ativan, Serax, Dalmane [used as a sleep-promoting sedative], and Tranxene)

Schedule V

Substances with a low potential for abuse relative to drugs in Schedule IV. Such drugs have a currently accepted medical use in the United States and may lead to limited physical dependence or psychological dependence in relation to drugs in Schedule IV. (Availability without prescription depends upon individual state laws.)

Preparations containing limited quantities of certain narcotic drugs used generally for antitussive and antidiarrheal purposes.

Actifed with codeine cough syrup

Lomotil

Parepectolin

Robitussin A-C cough syrup

Triaminic expectorant with codeine

Schedules established by the Controlled Substances Act.
Source: U.S. Drug Enforcement Administration.

---

of the following conditions must be present for substance dependence to be indicated:

- Developing a tolerance for a drug, thus making it necessary to increase the amount of any substance to achieve intoxication or desired effects

- Experiencing typical withdrawal symptoms when use of a drug is stopped or when using the drug to relieve or avoid withdrawal symptoms

- Taking more of a drug, or using it longer, than intended

- Desiring persistently or unsuccessfully attempting to reduce or control substance use

- Spending excessive time getting and taking a drug and recovering from the drug's effects

- Giving up important social, occupational, or recreational activities because of substance use

- Continuing substance use despite knowing that such use likely causes or makes worse a persistent or recurring physical or psychological problem.

Concepts of drug dependency will be discussed in greater detail in chapter 3.

Use of Adulterated Drugs

When individuals buy "street drugs," they do not always get what they bargained for. Drugs may be mixed, or "cut," with cheaper, inferior, or even more hazardous substances. Most frequently, there is no manufacturing control over the actual composition of the illegal pills, powders, and capsules; there is no standard dosage; and there is little concern on the part of drug sellers for the toxicity of their fraudulent products. Such drug tampering or altering is called **adulteration.**

Typically, street drugs are mixed with other chemicals that mimic or even increase another drug's action. Sometimes drugs capable of producing a strong physical dependency are added to marijuana. Such a subtle practice tends to create a steady customer who will eventually need the "hidden drug" in order to function normally.

In many instances, the street drug doesn't even contain the major drug ingredient that the buyer is seeking. Instead, there will likely be entirely different or possibly similar chemical substances in the adulterated product, which is frequently cut with poisons, insecticides, animal tranquilizers, oregano, catnip, milk sugar, or quinine. These items are used to stretch the final product and to increase the seller's profit.

Depending upon what the adulterating substance is, the user stands a high risk of having an unanticipated drug experience or a toxic reaction, and possibly being treated by medical personnel who lack information about the true nature or composition of the consumed drug.

Consumption of Look-Alikes

Nearly twenty years ago, drug takers began to be plagued with so-called **look-alike drugs** that were copies of pharmaceutical amphetamines and other psychoactive drugs. Known as peashooters or turkeys, these drugs usually consisted of 100 percent legal, uncontrolled substances, such as nonprescription stimulants, decongestants, and antihistamines—drugs commonly found in over-the-counter cold remedies. The popularity of these bogus drugs increased initially when physicians reduced the number of prescriptions they wrote for diet pills.

Soon after legal "speed" became available through head shops and mail-order firms, simulations of cocaine and imitations of methaqualone (Quaalude) began to surface in the drug traffic throughout the United States. Consequently, many states outlawed such imitation drugs that were promoted especially for young people. Then, in 1982, the U.S. Food and Drug Administration outlawed the triple combinations of caffeine, phenylpropanolamine, and ephedrine, the most common ingredients of look-alikes at that time.

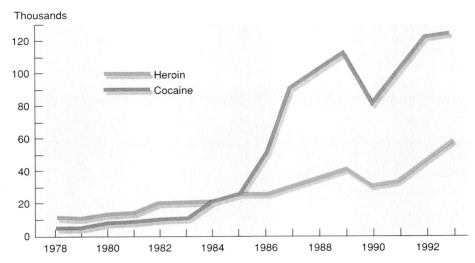

figure 1.2

Cocaine and Heroin Mentions in Drug-Related Emergency Room Episodes, 1988–92. One indicator of the individual hazard rating associated with psychoactive drugs can be derived from statistics collected by the Drug Abuse Warning Network (DAWN). This information base, monitored by the National Institute on Drug Abuse, collects data from hundreds of hospital emergency rooms and medical examiners located in specific metropolitan and rural areas of the United States.

Recently, DAWN reported record levels of cocaine- and heroin-related emergency room visits. Cocaine-related emergencies increased from an estimated 101,200 in 1991 to 119,800 in 1992, with individuals 26 to 34 years old having the highest rate of visits. Between 1988 and 1992, cocaine-related emergencies doubled among those 35 years of age and older, making this age group the fastest growing group seeking medical service at emergency rooms for drug-related health problems. Cocaine users often seek medical assistance for detoxification, unexpected drug reactions, and chronic effects of drug use.

Heroin-related hospital emergencies rose by 34 percent in 1992, from 35,400 in 1991 to 48,000 in 1992. During the same time period, the number of heroin-related emergencies increased for every adult age group, especially those 35 years and older. As was the case for cocaine-related emergencies, the rate of heroin-related emergencies was highest among those aged 26 to 34.

Though not shown in this chart, adverse reactions to marijuana increased 48 percent from 1991 to 1992, to almost 24,000 per year. This recent increase suggests that marijuana use is now making a significant comeback.

Sources: Illustration: Drug Abuse Warning Network, National Institute on Drug Abuse (1988–1991); Substance Abuse and Mental Health Services Administration (1992); Legend: Cocaine Abuse Warning Network, National Institute on Drug Abuse; and Substance Abuse and Mental Health Services Administration.

Today, single-ingredient look-alikes no longer resemble their predecessors in size, shape, or color. The original logos, product codes, and even the action or "punch" of earlier simulations are absent. Although the once-heavy demand for look-alike speed (caffeine-only "body stimulants") and phenylpropanolamine-only "diet pills" has declined sharply, these single-ingredient "pseudopharmaceuticals" are still the drugs of choice among some teenagers.

Extremely profitable to their manufacturers, the first-generation look-alikes were often intended for misrepresentation in street transactions with inexperienced drug users. Such concoctions as legal speed and continuous-action stimulants sometimes caused severe toxic reactions and even death. A particular hazard was an **idiosyncratic response,** a special sensitivity in certain people to a specific chemical substance. In addition, once the dosage of a look-alike was increased significantly, drug users were in peril if they were unknowingly exposed to the genuine psychoactive substance in the future.

Use of High-Tech Designer Drugs

As various states and the federal government moved to forbid the manufacture and sale of look-alikes, unscrupulous "kitchen chemists" introduced the "designer-drug" phenomenon. **Designer drugs** are synthetic substances produced by chemically engineering or altering existing drugs in order to make "act-alike" psychoactives that were initially legal. Modified slightly in terms of molecular structure, the newly designed and manufactured drugs were not initially controlled or regulated by the federal government. However, federal law now makes illegal all such chemical concoctions—even those not yet discovered and not yet produced—with a molecular structure or psychoactive action similar to a presently controlled substance.

The relatively new synthetic designer products typically produce effects that are similar to the "parent," illegal drugs. For instance, synthetic heroin (China White) can be nearly 3,000 times more powerful than traditional heroin and is therefore more hazardous to use. The "synthetic heroin" was analyzed and identified not as an opiate-based narcotic but rather as alpha methyl fentanyl (AMF), an easily concocted chemical variant of a surgical anesthetic. Still another type of synthetic heroin, also sold on the street as China White, proved to be an unwanted chemical contaminant known as MPTP. This accidental product of designer-drug technology causes permanent, progressive brain and nervous system damage and paralysis—typical of Parkinson's disease.

Another designer drug is MDMA, or Ecstasy, a chemical cousin of the psychedelic drug MDA. By chemically changing MDA, the "kitchen chemists" working in secret labs wanted to produce a new drug with the effects of its parent but of shorter duration. Ecstasy became popular because of its ability to neutralize emotional defenses. However, this particular designer drug was severely restricted and permanently placed in Schedule I of controlled drugs in 1988, due to MDMA's potential for causing psychotic experiences and brain damage.

Use of designer drugs presents some major health risks, such as overdose death and degeneration of the nerves. But many of these new concoctions have never been tested before, and their potency and selective action are unknown. Moreover, without any quality control, designer drugs are often sold on the street contaminated with impurities and poisonous by-products.[11]

Nevertheless, the abuse of these high-technology creations will likely continue, because such drugs are relatively inexpensive to produce and pharmacologically superior (more potent) than other illicit drugs.[12] In addition, most designer drugs are still rather difficult to detect in blood and urine samples, due to the drugs' low concentrations in the body's fluids.

New concentrated or varied forms of existing illegal drugs are constantly renamed and then marketed to certain ethnic or income groups. For example, an amphetamine-like substance made from phenylpropanolamine is available as "U4EA" or "Euphoria," known as the "thinking man's cocaine." "Croak" is now sold in some areas of the nation as a prepackaged mixture of "ice" (smokable methamphetamine) and crack, while a mixture of crack cocaine and regular cocaine is also available as croak. A combination of crack and heroin (the old "speedball") is marketed as "moon rock." Taking their cue from Madison Avenue advertisers, some street peddlers have been featuring a newly packaged form of heroin, called "his" or "heroin-in-a-straw." Powdered heroin is tapped into a straw and then the ends are heat-sealed.

As a sign of the innovative 1990s, modern drug abusers themselves are now creating their own versions of designer drugs with unique and esoteric combinations of psychoactive substances. For instance, drug abusers who prefer a "sandwich" get rubber-tipped glass pipes and insert two rocks of crack cocaine with heroin powder between them, and then smoke away. To make a "blunt," some teenagers slice open a cigar and mix marijuana or a marijuana-cocaine combination in with the tobacco. To increase the "punch," sometimes the blunt is dipped in malt liquor to produce a "B-40." And when blunts are filled with marijuana and crack cocaine, they are called "turbos" or "woolly

blunts." To achieve a trancelike state, some young people resort to dissolving gamma hydroxy butyrate (GHB)—an illegal chemical that reduces fat—in water and then mixing in amphetamines to fashion a "Max" cocktail.

Suicide

Currently, suicide is ranked as the eighth leading cause of death in the United States. Although the highest suicide rate is recorded among persons over 65 years of age, the greatest number of suicides occurs among persons 15 to 24 years of age. In this latter age group, self-imposed death is now the second leading cause of mortality among white men.[13] At present, an estimated 10,000 American college students attempt suicide each year, and some 1,000 succeed.

Nearly one-third of all suicides had been drinking before death, and at least 20 percent were intoxicated at the time of death. It is also estimated that up to 15 percent of all single-vehicle traffic accidents have a suicidal intent, with many of those involved having double-indemnity insurance policies.[14] In addition, suicide is one of the more frequent causes of death in long-term heavy drinkers, among whom the rate of suicide is 55 times greater than in the general population.[15]

The association between suicide and the abuse of alcohol and other drugs is further highlighted in data from the **Drug Abuse Warning Network** (DAWN), a large-scale drug-abuse data collection system sponsored by the National Institute on Drug Abuse. DAWN records substances linked with drug-abuse episodes reported by emergency rooms and medical examiners in various metropolitan areas of the United States. According to DAWN, suicide was the drug-use motive in 43 percent of emergency room deaths or admissions involving female patients and in 17 percent of such episodes involving male patients.[16]

The relationship between drug abuse and suicide is rather complex and likely involves at least two basic considerations. First, some authorities believe that certain already depressed people use excessive amounts of alcohol or other drugs, especially narcotics and sedative-hypnotics (including the anti-anxiety minor tranquilizers) as the means or instruments of self-destruction. Second, others emphasize that drugs such as alcohol, cocaine, amphetamines, barbiturates, minor tranquilizers, marijuana, psychedelics, and many nonpsychoactive prescription medicines tend to bring on and intensify psychological depression in individuals who might then develop a fatal despondency that leads to suicide. It is possible that both explanations apply in any analysis of this serious drug-related problem.

The correlation between alcohol and other drugs and suicide attempts is often based on a specific drug's general disinhibition effects and its impairment of the brain's integrative capacity.[17] For instance, an individual under the influence of alcohol has lost control of those psychic-guarding mechanisms that tend to restrain hidden thoughts and basic impulses. And when a person's integrative ability is impaired, memory, concentration, and judgment are lessened and an objective and rational evaluation of any situation is severely limited. Under such psychic and emotional circumstances, suicide may be perceived as the very best solution to an otherwise intolerable condition.

Cocaine and amphetamine abuse is often viewed as contributing to the extreme fatigue and severe depression that follow the use of these two stimulant-type drugs. After prolonged use of cocaine, the state of psychological depression (known as post-cocaine depression) may reach suicidal proportions due to the depletion of a specific chemical messenger (neurotransmitter) from the nerve cells. Suicide has also occurred following the use of those drugs that produce hallucinations. The resulting depression and fears of remaining psychotic may lead to self-destructive behavior.

HIV Infection and AIDS

Today, **HIV infection** and AIDS are listed as the ninth leading cause of death in the United States. Because a particular method of taking certain psychoactive drugs is related to the transmission or spread of **acquired immune deficiency**

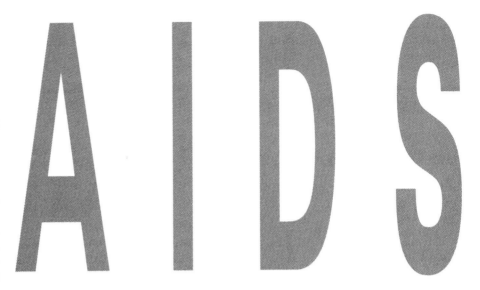

syndrome (AIDS), a consideration of this often fatal, but now treatable, disease is most appropriate. Medical research has proved that the human immunodeficiency virus (HIV) causes AIDS. A serious, life-threatening illness for which there is no present drug prevention or drug cure, AIDS involves a breakdown of the body's own internal defense system that makes the HIV-infected person more likely to develop certain other diseases that cause death. These "opportunistic" illnesses that overwhelm an individual with a compromised (weakened) immune system include Pneumocystis carinii pneumonia (a parasitic infection of the lungs) and Kaposi's sarcoma (a form of cancer of the blood vessel walls visible as blue-violet to brownish skin blotches or bumps).

Although the AIDS-causing virus can be spread from an infected mother to her child perinatally (that is, before, during, and possibly after childbirth through breast-feeding), the major ways of transmitting HIV are through intimate sexual behaviors—involving the exchange of semen, vaginal secretions, or blood—and through exposure to blood and blood products. Nevertheless, all of these ways of spreading the HIV can be associated with the abuse of alcohol and other drugs.

Perhaps the most obvious relationship between drugs and AIDS is that intravenous (IV) drug users—those who inject

illegal drugs directly into their veins—make up the second largest group of people with AIDS in the United States. Currently, female and heterosexual male IV drug abusers account for nearly one-quarter of all diagnosed cases of AIDS in America. Another 6 percent of such cases occur among homosexual or bisexual males who are also IV drug users. A full 30 percent of all AIDS cases are now appearing in people with injection-drug use as the major risk factor. Significantly, these are precisely the people who are most likely to transmit the HIV virus to heterosexual partners.[18]

The most dangerous and rapid way to get or give HIV involves the sharing of "dirty" (blood-contaminated) needles and syringes by IV drug users. Frequently, cotton or other materials used as filters, and containers ("cookers") in which a drug is heated and/or dissolved, are also shared. Blood from a previous user most typically lodges in the tip of the hypodermic needle or in the syringe, but it might also be found in other parts of the injection apparatus, collectively referred to as the "works."

Drug injection, whether intravenous or nonintravenous (as seen in skin-popping of heroin or intramuscular injection of bodybuilding steroids), and transmission of HIV are detailed in the following account, which explains why such drug-taking methods are so hazardous.

At Issue

Are we winning the "war on drugs"?

Point: Yes, indeed! Victory is within our grasp as the insidious fog of drug abuse has begun to lift. Although illicit drug use and the effects of drug abuse are still widely prevalent in society, there is solid evidence that younger people turned against drugs during the last decade. The numbers of illegal drug users, drinkers, and tobacco smokers are much lower now than during the peak levels of the 1970s and early 1980s. Despite the recent upturn in marijuana and heroin use, the facts suggest that we can still win the on-going war on drugs!

Counterpoint: Not by a long shot! We are not only failing to win the war on drugs; we are actually losing this pseudo-war with its bungling efforts focused so greatly on reducing the supply of drugs. Although younger people are saying no to drugs in larger numbers than ever before, the number of Americans 35 years of age and older considered current drug users is now increasing. Both monthly and weekly cocaine users are on the rise, as are drug-related emergency room cases involving cocaine and heroin. If we are winning such a drug war, why is drug abuse concentrating into those social groups—older and inner-city addicts—who can least afford the problems caused by addiction? Moreover, the cocaine supply has not been reduced, despite intense interdiction efforts. As a nation, we are reluctant to deal with the root causes of drug abuse. We have a serious lack of treatment centers, and we are relying more and more on prisons as "holding pens" for repeat drug offenders. Indeed, the majority of federal prisoners are jailed for drug law violations. Is the cost of apprehending, trying, housing, and feeding all these "criminals" really worth the so-called protection to our society? At best, the war on drugs has involved only limited skirmishes, and our strictest interdiction efforts have not prevented the birth of 600,000 drug-affected babies in the past few years. Who says we're winning this war?

During injection, the user may draw his/her own blood into the syringe to mix with the dissolved drug and then inject the blood/drug mixture, a procedure known as "booting." This is done to make sure all traces of the drug are removed from the syringe efficiently. As a result, however, any blood from a prior user which remains in the syringe or in the tip of the needle is injected directly into subsequent users. Traditionally, any cleaning of the syringe or needle involves rinsing them in water or blowing into them. Sterilization equipment is not readily available to users and speed of injection is often paramount in the minds of addicts.[19]

Two factors have been associated consistently with the spread of HIV among intravenous drug users and drug injectors: the frequency of drug injection and the use of "shooting galleries"—places where drug users can rent or borrow injection equipment. Research has also revealed that injecting cocaine alone carries a threefold risk of HIV infection over injecting heroin alone.[20,21] Such a risk is due to the tendency of cocaine users to inject more frequently than heroin users (cocaine is shorter-acting than heroin), to draw more blood into the syringe to mix with the drug prior to injecting than is done with IV use of heroin, and to use the drug more often in "shooting galleries."

Even the crack (cocaine) smoking population contributes to HIV transmission because (1) cocaine, heroin, and other drugs of abuse are occasionally injected along with smoking crack; (2) the rates of prostitution to support drug habits, or the direct exchange of sex for drugs, are high among male and female crack users, often in localities where the "johns" may be former or current IV drug users; (3) the hypersexuality related with cocaine can lead to having multiple sex partners; and (4) the prevalence of syphilis and gonorrhea (sexually transmitted diseases) is high among crack users, perhaps predisposing them to HIV infection.[22]

Another area of concern relating drug abuse to HIV infection and AIDS is the fact that alcohol, cocaine, heroin, volatile nitrites, and possibly marijuana all are likely to interfere with or suppress various components of the normal immune defense mechanism in the human body.[23–25] As a consequence, some drug abusers appear to be predisposed to HIV infection or its consequences.[26,27]

Furthermore, it is believed that the AIDS-causing virus infects and overwhelms an immune system that has been activated, compromised, or challenged in some way. Chemical agents may cause this activation and therefore function as correlated factors (cofactors), but not causal factors, in HIV infection that often progresses to a full-blown case of AIDS.

The last important way in which alcohol and other drugs may affect the spread of HIV and AIDS pertains to the general disinhibition (unblocking) effects of some psychoactive drugs on sexual and risk-taking behaviors.[28] While many believe that alcohol, marijuana, cocaine, and volatile nitrites act as aphrodisiacs—drugs that allegedly increase libido and the enjoyment of sexual behaviors—the use of these chemicals also tends to make people more likely to engage in unwanted and unsafe sexual practices. Without the restraints of conscience, better judgment, propriety, and morality that often serve to control behavior, anything goes—and often does.

The use of alcohol and other drugs not only lowers one's inhibitions, but also tends to impair judgment. "Sex under the influence" (SUI) of drugs prevents an individual from making informed and rational decisions about sexual interaction, partners, behaviors, and especially about preventive and self-protective actions. Moreover, being under the influence of alcohol or some other drug of abuse may lead to a misperception of another's sexual intent, men's sexual violence and exploitation of women, an impairment of women's ability to send and receive verbal and non-verbal cues, and a lessening of a person's ability to resist sexual assault.[29]

SUI can also result in an unwanted pregnancy and the contraction of a sexually transmitted disease, including AIDS. By all accounts, "sex under the influence" can be a very dangerous experience.

The Drug Scene: An Overview

Two of the more reliable, major sources of information about drug use in America are the National Household Survey on Drug Abuse (NHSDA) and the Monitoring the Future (MTF) survey, also known as the High School Senior Survey. The former provides information on drug-use patterns and trends among the American noninstitutionalized household population, while the latter furnishes comparable information on eighth- and tenth-graders and senior high school students, as well as American college students and young adults in their twenties and early thirties who are high school graduates. In addition, the Office of National Drug Control Policy, the Drug Use Forecasting (DUF) program of the National Institute of Justice, and the National Institute on Drug Abuse Epidemiology Work Group also gather valuable statistics on various drug-user groups throughout the United States. Data provided by these agencies are summarized in this section.[30–35]

General Findings: Prevalence of Use

- The use of illegal drugs, alcohol, and cigarettes generally peaked during the late 1970s and declined thereafter.

- Marijuana continues to be the most commonly used illicit drug in the United States, with about 5 million people using this drug weekly. Nevertheless, alcohol is by far the most widely used and abused drug in America, where beers, wines, and distilled spirits are also illegal beverages in every state for people under the age of 21.

- Many Americans, particularly the young, have used illegal drugs. About 46 percent of high school seniors have used an illicit drug at least once by the time they reached their senior year of high school.

- Although most drug takers are infrequent users, more than 75 million persons in the U.S. household population have used illicit drugs at least once.

- Many drug users have used more than one drug; two-thirds of the household population have used either alcohol or illicit drugs in the past year. Moreover, illicit drug use, heavy alcohol consumption, and smoking often occur together. Of nearly 11 million heavy drinkers in the United States, at least one-fourth also currently use illegal drugs. An estimated 12 percent of all American smokers also use illicit drugs.

- Although current rates of illicit drug use have remained stable or increased somewhat in the past few years, these rates of current use are dramatically below those of 1979 for all age groups except for those 35 years and older. Such a shift is apparently linked to the aging of the drug-using population of the 1970s.

- At present, the annual number of Americans using at least one illicit drug is nearly 12 million. Men continue to have a higher rate (7.4 percent) of illicit drug use than women (4.1 percent). Among 18- to 34-year-olds, those who have not completed high school have the highest rate of illicit drug use (15 percent), while college graduates have the lowest rate (just 6 percent). Employment status also correlates with rates of illegal drug use. Nearly 12 percent of unemployed adults are current drug users, while just 6 percent of employed adults currently use illicit drugs.

- The MTF survey recorded important declines through 1991 in rates of use of marijuana, cocaine, amphetamines, and a number of other drugs among American high school students, college students, and young adult high school graduates. However, by the mid 1990s, surveys found evidence of increased use of marijuana, inhalants, hallucinogens, cocaine, and stimulants among eighth-graders. This unexpected increase among the youngest respondents surveyed, coupled with evidence of relaxing attitudes about the harmfulness and acceptability of drug use, has caused great concern among drug control authorities.

- The MTF survey also detected slippage in such attitudes and norms among high school seniors, suggesting increases in use among that population. By the mid 1990s, the use of marijuana, inhalants, stimulants, LSD, and other hallucinogens was up in nearly all grade levels. Both college and young-adult samples also revealed evidence of a reversal, with early increases in marijuana and LSD use.

- Recently, the Office of National Drug Control Policy found that heroin use had increased once again across the nation; "speedballing"—injecting heroin and cocaine intravenously—has become widespread, despite the concern with transmitting the HIV virus, and marijuana use continues to rise.

- Nearly 2.7 million Americans are now classed as hard-core (weekly) drug abusers. These people use the bulk of the nation's $49 billion worth of drugs annually. This estimated figure has not changed

table 1.2

Characteristics of Users by Drug of Abuse as Reported by Treatment Providers, According to Geographical Regions of the Coterminous United States, 1994

	Census Region*	Percentage of Users by Race/Ethnicity			Percentage of Users by Sex	
		African American	White	Hispanic Other	Male	Female
Heroin	1	27%	59%	14%	77%	23%
	2	55%	38%	7%	74%	26%
	3	40%	57%	3%	78%	22%
	4	16%	39%	45%	64%	36%
Cocaine/ Crack	1	41%	49%	10%	78%	22%
	2	62%	33%	5%	61%	39%
	3	39%	56%	5%	69%	31%
	4	14%	62%	24%	74%	26%
Marijuana	1	14%	66%	20%	88%	12%
	2	31%	63%	6%	76%	24%
	3	22%	74%	4%	73%	27%
	4	3%	72%	25%	71%	29%

* Census regions are identified on p. 20.
Source: *Pulse Check: National Trends in Drug Abuse*, Office of National Drug Control Policy, 1994.

much since 1988, despite massive government efforts to control the use and abuse of psychoactive drugs.

The Drug-Abusing Population

- According to the NHSDA, males are more likely than females to have ever used drugs and to have used them in the past month.

- People aged 26 to 34 are the most likely to have ever used drugs, while those 18 to 25 are the most likely to have used drugs in the past month. By 1995, lifetime rates of use will be highest among persons 31 to 39 years old, reflecting the peak drug-using years of the late 1970s.

- Most young people have their first alcoholic drink at 12 or 13 years of age; nearly all first tobacco use begins before high school graduation; and relatively few individuals begin illicit drug use after their mid twenties.

- Whites and African Americans are more likely than Hispanic Americans to have ever used illicit drugs. However, the prevalence of drug use varies across urban and rural areas and regions of the United States (see table 1.2 and the specified "census regions" on the next page).

- Analyses of the MTF survey data indicate higher rates of drug use for whites than for African Americans. Past-year use of most drugs (marijuana, cocaine, hallucinogens, heroin, stimulants, sedatives, tranquilizers, and cigarettes) has been highest among Native Americans.

- MTF data also reveal that alcohol use was highest among whites, slightly higher than among Native Americans. Rates of use were lowest among Asian Americans and almost as low among African Americans.

- An estimated 103 million to 120 million Americans aged 14 years and older (about two-thirds of the

drinking-age population) drink alcoholic beverages at least occasionally. Reflecting a variety of definitions, alcohol dependents (or alcoholics) are estimated to number between 12 million and 18 million people. However, problem drinkers who are not necessarily dependent on alcohol may number several million more Americans.

- The per capita consumption of absolute alcohol is now about 2.25 gallons of ethanol per person per year (see fig. 1.3). But half of all drinkers are "light" drinkers who consume no more than 10 percent of all alcoholic beverages used in the United States. In reality, most of the drinking-age population either abstains or drinks very little.

- Junior and senior high school students consume about 35 percent of all wine coolers sold in the United States and 1.1 billion cans of beer each year, thus making up a relatively small but significant part of

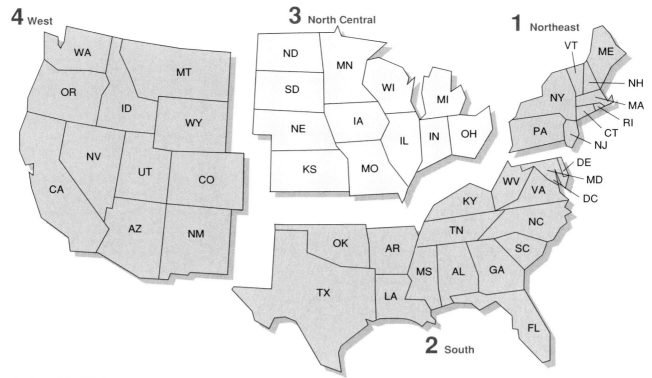

Census Regions of the U.S.A.

Source: National Institute on Alcohol Abuse and Alcoholism and the Alcohol Research Information Service.

the alcohol-consuming population. The rate of "binge drinking" (consumption of five or more drinks in a row at least once in a two-week period) now stands at 14 percent for eighth-graders, 23 percent for tenth-graders, and 28 percent for seniors in high school.

· Daily drinking on most college campuses has declined recently, but many students appear to confine their drinking to weekends, when they tend to drink heavily and with the intention of getting drunk. Binge drinking is reported by 41 percent of college students.

· Today there are between 46 million and 50 million U.S. smokers, who consume an estimated 2,629 cigarettes per person each year. Although some dispute the concept of nicotine addiction, many health authorities believe that most current cigarette smokers are addicted. The uncounted chain-smokers of America display evidence of dependence on their nicotine

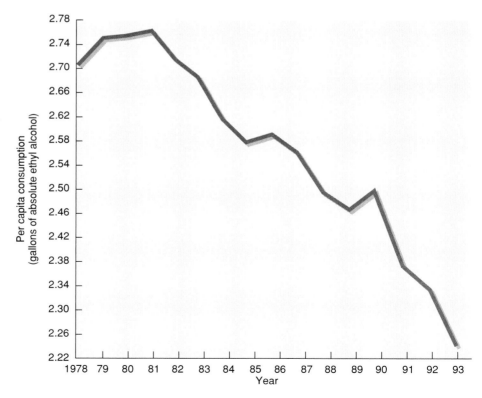

figure 1.3

Recent Pattern of Per Capita Consumption of Pure (absolute) Alcohol in the United States from 1978 through 1993.

Source: National Institute on Alcohol Abuse and Alcoholism and the Alcohol Research Information Service.

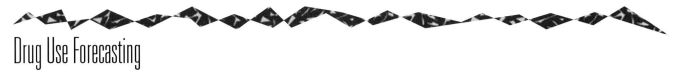

box 1.4

Drug Use Forecasting

The National Institute of Justice established the Drug Use Forecasting (DUF) program in 1987 to measure the extent of drug use by persons charged with criminal behavior in major American cities. The DUF program uses an objective measure—urinalysis results—to determine types and levels of drug use by this segment of the population.

The Institute's program has now grown to include twenty-four sites across the nation, where samples of male arrestees are tested. In twenty-one locations, females are tested. All those who take part in the program do so voluntarily and anonymously.

Overall Drug Use. Recently, the percentage of males testing positive for drug use at any one site ranged from 47 percent (Phoenix) to 78 percent (Philadelphia). For female booked arrestees, the percentage testing positive ranged from 44 percent (San Antonio) to 85 percent (Manhattan). Cocaine was the prevalent drug in the majority of sites—a position it has held since 1988—and in some sites, data have shown an increase in cocaine use.

Multiple Drugs. Male arrestees in San Diego and female arrestees in Manhattan were most likely to test positive for more than one drug—39 percent and 35 percent, respectively. Multiple drug use was also high for male arrestees in Chicago, Philadelphia, and Manhattan, and for female arrestees in San Diego, Philadelphia, Portland, and Los Angeles.

Marijuana. The percentage of male arrestees testing positive for marijuana ranged from 17 percent in Cleveland to 38 percent in Omaha. Female arrestees testing positive for marijuana ranged from 8 percent in New Orleans and Washington, D.C., to 26 percent in Indianapolis.

Opiates (Heroin). Opiate use among male booked arrestees ranged from 1 percent in Ft. Lauderdale to 19 percent in Chicago. Among females, the range of opiate use was from 3 percent in Ft. Lauderdale and Kansas City to 24 percent in Manhattan.

Other Drugs. Amphetamine use remained highest among arrestees in San Diego. Less than 9 percent of male and female arrestees tested positive for PCP. Benzodiazepine (Valium, for example) use ranged from 1 to 14 percent for male arrestees and from 3 to 18 percent for females. Methadone positives were highest for Manhattan arrestees.

Drug Use Trends. Annual trend data from DUF surveys indicate that drug use among arrestees remains at high levels, especially for cocaine. In many sites, cocaine use has shown an increase. Since 1992, marijuana use has also begun to rise. Clearly, drug use continues to be a serious problem in the United States.

Source: Modified from National Institute of Justice, U.S. Department of Justice, 1993.

delivery systems. Many of them claim they want to quit smoking but cannot do so.

· At least one-third of high-school-age youth in the United States continue to smoke or use smokeless tobacco. Nearly 3,000 young people begin smoking for the first time each day.

· At least one-half of all people arrested for major crimes in the United States—including homicide, theft, and assault—were using illegal drugs at the time of their arrest (see box 1.4).

· According to the Center on Addiction and Substance Abuse of Columbia University, one in four mothers on welfare uses illicit drugs (having used drugs at least once in the past year) or drinks alcohol excessively (having drunk five or more drinks in a row two or more times a month). One-half of all mothers on welfare smoke cigarettes.

· Among the youngest parents on Aid to Families with Dependent Children, the rate of addiction and drug abuse is 37 percent.

Some Unanticipated Consequences[36]

· A person dying from alcohol-related causes loses, on the average, 26 years off the normal life span; a person dying from drug-related causes loses over 37 years; and a person dying

from smoking-related causes loses nearly 20 years. The toll among America's minorities is even greater (see box 1.5).

· AIDS among injecting drug users is the fastest growing cause of death among substance abusers.

· Substance abuse drives up health care costs and tends to block any attempt to curb such expenditures. Between 25 and 40 percent of all general hospital patients are there because of complications related to alcoholism.

· The total economic costs of substance abuse on the economy are staggering and amount to an estimated $238 billion each year.

Chemical Dependency and Minorities

box 1.5

Chemical Dependency: Excess Minority Deaths

Alcohol, tobacco, and illicit drug use are factors in about one-quarter of U.S. deaths each year. Data indicate that the portion of minority deaths arising from these causes is even greater than that in the general population. We can gain some insight into the gravity of chemical dependency as a contributing cause of death among minorities by examining the excess incidence and mortality figures for some major causes of death within specific populations. The underlying substance-related cause cannot be implicated in every excess death from these causes. Nonetheless, evidence suggests that curbing the use and abuse of alcohol, drugs, and tobacco could help minorities close the gap in death rates from cirrhosis, heart disease, unintentional injuries, homicide, and cancers of the mouth, esophagus, and lung.

Excess incidence and death rates are the difference between rates actually occurring in the designated populations and those that would have been expected had the group experienced the same age- and sex-specific rates as the nonminority population, which furnish a baseline of 100 percent.

Source: The Secretary's Task Force on Black and Minority Health, U.S. Department of Health and Human Services, Public Health Service, and *Closing the Gap*, a series of fact sheets developed by the Office of Minority Health, U.S. Department of Health and Human Services, 1990.

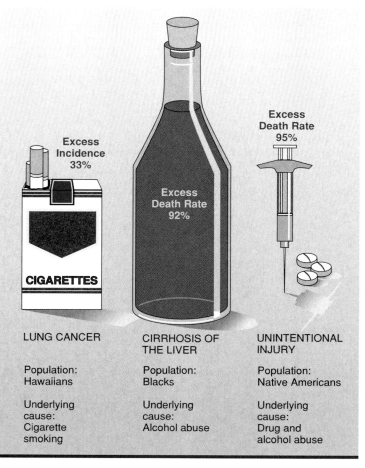

LUNG CANCER

Population: Hawaiians

Underlying cause: Cigarette smoking

CIRRHOSIS OF THE LIVER

Population: Blacks

Underlying cause: Alcohol abuse

UNINTENTIONAL INJURY

Population: Native Americans

Underlying cause: Drug and alcohol abuse

Such a cost includes the expenses of treating substance abusers, the productivity losses caused by premature death and inability to perform usual activities, expenditures related to crime and destruction of property, and other losses.

- The conservatively estimated price tag for alcohol problems is $99 billion annually; the major expenses are related to productivity losses associated with illness and death. Each year, the total bill for illicit drug use is an estimated $67 billion, of which the major expense is crime and law enforcement. And the annual cost of smoking is now thought to be at least $72 billion, most of which is spent on losses due to premature deaths. However, a recent study by the Centers for Disease Control and Prevention claims the yearly medical costs alone now associated with cigarettes are a staggering $50 billion, or about $2 per pack of cigarettes. But many such costs cannot be estimated easily, as noted in table 1.3.

The Drug-Crime Relationship

- Drugs and crimes are problems that are often closely related in rather complex ways. Drug-crime relationships are usually expressed as drug-defined offenses, drug-related offenses, and interactional circumstances, as explained in box 1.6.

- Drug users report greater involvement in crime and are more likely than nonusers to have criminal records.

- Persons with criminal records are much more likely than ones without criminal records to report being drug users.

- Crimes typically rise in number as drug use increases.

- Criminal activity is as much as two to three times higher among frequent users of heroin or cocaine than among irregular users or nonusers.

22   Introduction

1.3 Unspecified Costs to Society of Illegal Drug Use

Categories of Costs			
Criminal Justice Expenditures on Drug-Related Crime	**Health Care Costs**	**Lost Productivity Costs**	**Other Costs to Society**
• Investigating robberies, burglaries, and thefts for drug money and adjudicating and punishing the offenders • Investigating assaults and homicides in the drug business (or by a drug user who has lost control) and adjudicating and punishing the offenders	• Injuries resulting from drug-related child abuse/neglect • Injuries from drug-related accidents • Injuries from drug-related crime • Other medical care for illegal drug users, including volunteer services and outpatient services, such as emergency room visits • Resources used in nonhospital settings	• Lost productivity of drug-related accident victims • Lost productivity of drug-related crime victims • Time away from work and homemaking to care for drug users and their dependents • Drug-related educational problems and school dropouts • Offenders incarcerated for drug-related or drug-defined crimes	• Loss of property values due to drug-related neighborhood crime • Property damaged or destroyed in fires and in workplace and vehicular accidents • Agricultural resources devoted to illegal drug cultivation/production • Toxins introduced into public air and water supplies by drug production • Workplace prevention programs such as drug testing and employee assistance programs • Averting behavior by potential victims of drug-related crime • Pain and suffering costs to illegal drug users and their families and friends

Source: Bureau of Justice Statistics, U.S. Department of Justice.

- An unusually high proportion of people in drug treatment programs report involvement in serious crimes.

- Involvement in crime sometimes precedes drug use, but just as often drug use occurs before involvement in crime. However, frequent use of multiple drugs generally follows involvement in property crime, and its onset may speed up the development of a criminal career.

- Some drugs, particularly alcohol, cocaine, amphetamines, and PCP, increase the likelihood that users will act violently, but this drug-violence relationship is not especially strong, except in the case of alcohol use.

- Frequently, drug users commit violent crimes in order to get money to buy drugs and thereby support their drug use. Nevertheless, drug users support themselves and their drug abuse in various ways, including through gainful employment as well as by receiving some form of public welfare or assistance.

- Violence is common in drug trafficking as a result of disagreements about transactions and because traffickers often seek a competitive advantage over rival dealers through violent means.

- Violence is common in illegal drug distribution, and many homicides are related to drug trafficking.

The Drug Scene: Prospects for the Future

The use of psychoactive drugs and the occurrence of substance abuse and chemical dependency among youth are often used to predict the extent of such problems in the near future. If such a relationship is accurate, then the years ahead will be filled with an abundance of psychoactive drugs and many drug-related problems.

Alcohol and other drug abuse among young Americans is still staggering! Although the situation is not close to being solved, the past several years have witnessed a downturn in the use of most illegal drugs among both high school students and young adults. More American youths are, in fact, choosing

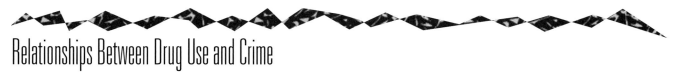

Relationships Between Drug Use and Crime

Drugs and Crime Relationship	Definition	Examples
Drug-defined offenses	Violations of laws prohibiting or regulating the possession, use, distribution, or manufacture of illegal drugs.	Drug possession or use. Marijuana cultivation. Methamphetamine production. Cocaine, heroin, or marijuana sales.
Drug-related offenses	Offenses in which a drug's pharmacologic effects contribute; offenses motivated by the user's need for money to support continued use; and offenses connected with drug distribution itself.	Violent behavior resulting from drug effects. Stealing to get money to buy drugs. Violence against rival drug dealers.
Interactional circumstances	Drug use and crime are common aspects of a deviant lifestyle. The likelihood and frequency of involvement in illegal activity is increased because drug users and offenders are exposed to situations that encourage crime.	A life orientation with an emphasis on short-term goals supported by illegal activities. Opportunities to offend resulting from contacts with offenders and illegal markets. Criminal skills learned from other offenders.

Source: Bureau of Justice Statistics, U.S. Department of Justice.

a drug-free lifestyle today than their counterparts of the past decade. But recent surveys point to alarming tendencies: increased experimentation once again with illegal drugs, and a decline in negative attitudes toward or perceived risks of drug abuse.

Only the future will tell if the recent increase in use of specific illegal drugs is a temporary or permanent trend in our drug-using society. Four uncertain factors in predicting drug use and abuse patterns could play a major role in the drug scene of the future.

One factor in the prediction equation is the *role of parents who were drug users themselves* during the 1960s, 1970s, and 1980s. Will they approve, encourage, discourage, or tolerate the use of marijuana, cocaine, alcohol, or some other drug by their own children?

The second factor relates to *organized, national efforts to reduce the supply and demand of mood-modifying chemicals,* especially the illegal ones. We do not yet know whether U.S.A.-sponsored programs in countries such as Bolivia, Colombia, Mexico, and Thailand will effectively eliminate

or reduce the harvest and production of illegal drugs. And we don't know if educational programs and drug-testing programs to detect use of illegal psychoactives among various population groups in America will be successful in permanently lowering drug abuse or discouraging initial use of illicit drugs. However, we do know that epidemics of drug abuse do not occur spontaneously. Law enforcement officials also know that early recognition of the spiraling stages of drug use can forestall the next likely events in a drug's developing utilization, if appropriate countermeasures are taken at the local community level.[37]

Also to be considered is a third factor, the *number of individuals who will perceive risks of and develop negative attitudes toward drugs.* The more an individual believes in the personally threatening and socially disrupting aspects of drug use, and the more firmly held those negative biases tend to be, the less likely there will be serious drug use by such a person, even if drugs are available and even with various pressures to use drugs. But how long will such negative attitudes and perceptions of

adverse consequences of drug use persist? Will large numbers of young people in the future adopt a new drug of choice—a drug that promises rewards without penalties, a drug without risks?

The last factor in the prediction equation is the *success or failure of the continuing movement to legalize certain or all presently illegal psychoactives.* The battle lines have now been formed between those who believe the war on drugs has already been lost, and those who maintain that present antidrug measures are working and are necessary to achieve alcohol- and drug-free schools and work environments.

It had been predicted that the 1980s revival of conservatism in national politics and traditional values among the general public would have a dampening effect on attitudes and practices regarding alcohol and drug abuse. Indeed, the nation has experienced a ten-year decline in alcohol and other drug abuse, but such a general trend may now be reversing among young people. The national commitment to dealing with problems of drug misuse, substance abuse, and chemical dependency will likely continue and remain substantial. However, it is unlikely that the public desire to end drug problems will ever be realized. As long as the recreational use of alcohol and tobacco products persists among large numbers of Americans, there will probably be serious drug problems in the United States.

Considering demographic data, rising concern for legal liability, the growing influence of nonsmokers, the increasing importance of health promotion and disease prevention, general attitudes of Americans expressed in surveys, and recent actions of both private organizations and governments at local, state, and federal levels, we can make the following predictions about our future drug policies and drug-taking practices:

1. There will likely be additional restrictions placed on tobacco smoking in public and sales to minors, with a further increase in taxes on both tobacco products and alcoholic beverages. Such actions will likely result in a further decline in the use of both legal drugs—nicotine and alcohol.

2. There will likely be periodic increases in the usage of illegal psychoactive drugs, followed by declines in usage after countermeasures are once again implemented.

3. There will likely be a limited tolerance of occasional adult use of currently illicit drugs, particularly marijuana. Such tolerance, however, will not be extended to the workplace or to those under the age of majority or to the public use of illegal drugs.

4. There will likely be no widespread legalization of currently illegal psychoactives, despite federal and state flirtations with changes in present anti-drug-use laws and penalties.

5. There will likely be even stricter laws to curtail driving under the influence of alcohol, marijuana, and other mind-changing drugs and medicines. Further restrictions on the advertising of alcoholic beverages and tobacco products, along with stronger warning messages on beverage alcohol and tobacco containers, are anticipated. Drug-testing programs to discourage illegal drug use among the military, government employees, the workforce in private-sector business and industry, and among student-athletes could lower the demand for illegal psychoactives.

6. There will likely emerge a renewed national commitment to protect young people from exposure to drugs. This effort will be facilitated by a smaller number of young people in the total population, and by better-informed parents who will be enabled to take part in primary- and secondary-prevention activities. Additionally, there will likely be more effective school- and community-based education and intervention programs.

The drug scene will likely be marked by considerable, though evolving, change. Based upon the popularity of psychedelics in the 1960s, the widespread use of marijuana in the 1970s, the cocaine/crack cocaine epidemic of the 1980s, and now the apparent resurgence of both psychedelics and high-purity heroin in the 1990s, it is fairly certain that drug fashions will change, and change again.[38]

Drug Use and Abuse Among Women

Both men and women are psychoactive drug consumers, but females use virtually all types of illicit drugs less frequently than males do.[39] The only major exception to this generalization is in regard to the use of medically prescribed psychotherapeutic drugs (sedatives, tranquilizers, stimulants, and analgesics). Regardless of age, women who reported having used such drugs were more likely than men to have had these drugs prescribed for them by physicians.[40]

In fact, women use nearly twice as many drugs for each class of these medicines as do men. The higher prevalence of drug use by women has been related to

1. a woman's greater likelihood of visiting a physician and, consequently, greater chance of being prescribed a drug for pain, insomnia, anxiety, panic, fatigue, or depression;

2. the excessive and sometimes competing demands characterizing the modern female social roles of career achiever, marriage partner, homemaker, parent, and community organizer, participant, or leader; and

3. the less frequent use of alternative substances, such as alcohol, in coping with emotional stress.

Alarmingly, large numbers of these female drug users are women of child-bearing age. The actual extent of psychoactive drug use during pregnancy is often underestimated, although drug use of any kind during pregnancy is not usually recommended by physicians unless necessary. Studies of pregnant women from all socioeconomic groups reveal that a majority take prescribed medications. Additionally, a majority of the same women also report self-medication, primarily for the relief of anxiety or pain. Nonprescribed drugs detected frequently in pregnant women include aspirin, barbiturate sedatives, and quinine. The magnitude of psychoactive drug use during pregnancy is even more alarming when you consider marijuana and tobacco smoking and the consumption of alcoholic beverages and caffeine.

Although the effects of most psychoactive drugs do not differ greatly between women and men, there is a certain pharmacological uniqueness of the female. Such uniqueness pertains to both her potential role in human reproduction as well as her gender-linked attributes of body size, body content, hormonal fluctuations and the menstrual cycle, and lack of a certain chemical enzyme that helps break down at least one major psychoactive drug in the male.

table 1.4 Drug Use During Pregnancy

Drug	Effect on Fetus	Safe Use of Drug
Alcohol	Increased risk of spontaneous abortion, "fetal alcohol syndrome," and infant addiction; low birth weight, mental retardation, physical deformity, and behavioral problems, including hyperactivity, restlessness, and poor attention span. Especially dangerous during first three months of pregnancy.	Should be avoided.
Amphetamines	Possibility of numerous birth defects resulting in damage to the liver, heart, and brain; abnormal bone and organ development; greater risk of miscarriage, stillbirth, and premature birth; poor coordination after birth.	Only under doctor's supervision.
Aspirin	During last three months of pregnancy, frequent use may cause excessive bleeding at delivery and may prolong pregnancy and labor.	Under doctor's supervision.
Barbiturates	Mothers who take large doses may have babies who are addicted. Babies may have tremors, restlessness, irritability, breathing difficulties, poor coordination, and slow reflexes.	Only under doctor's supervision.
Cocaine	Possible neurological damage, diminished motor abilities, smaller body length, lower birth weight, smaller head circumference; higher risk of kidney disorders, heart problems, seizures and strokes; increased risk of sudden infant death syndrome, and greater likelihood of visual problems, lack of coordinated movements, and developmental retardation with disturbed behavior and possible learning difficulties.	Should be avoided.
Inhalants	Possibility of "fetal solvents syndrome" with physical defects and mental retardation similar to fetal alcohol syndrome; increased likelihood of miscarriage or stillbirth.	Should be avoided.
Marijuana	May cause a variety of congenital birth defects, including a reduction in birth weight and height as demonstrated in human babies; increased tremors and prolonged startles and stares in newborns; possibility of low birth weight, stillbirth, and premature birth; and increased risk of behavioral problems in newborns.	Should be avoided.
Narcotics	Infant addiction, increased risk of miscarriage, early death, HIV infection; slowed growth, possible learning disabilities.	Should be avoided.
Nicotine	Higher risk of miscarriage, premature birth with low-birth-weight babies; increased risk of infant death, slowed growth, bleeding problems in delivery; increased risk of infant heart and lung disease.	Should be avoided.
Psychedelics	High risk of miscarriage; PCP is especially linked with brain and nervous system damage, muscle control problems, deficits in speech and social skills.	Should be avoided.
Tranquilizers	If drug is taken during the first three months of pregnancy, there is the possibility of cleft lip or palate or other congenital malformations; infant addiction, damage to heart and blood vessels, mental retardation.	Avoid if you might become pregnant and during early pregnancy. Use only under doctor's supervision.

Source: Modified from the National Institute on Drug Abuse.

First, a female's offspring will eventually develop from ova that are present in her ovaries from the beginning of her own embryonic life. Therefore, there is the possibility of **mutagenic** (gene toxic) **effects** of drugs on future offspring. Mutagenic effects carry a risk of infertility as well as cancer. Of equal concern is the effect of various drugs on the fetus if the mother takes them during pregnancy; see table 1.4.

While drug-induced congenital abnormalities occur primarily during early pregnancy, some drugs have the potential to affect the growth of the fetus and its postbirth behavioral and mental performance when exposure occurs at later stages of pregnancy. Even after birth, maternally consumed drugs can enter the newborn through milk from the mother's breast.

It should be realized that a pregnant woman's use of a psychoactive drug will result in the transfer of that drug to the fetus. The drug, present in the mother's bloodstream, crosses the placenta where it is then distributed into the fetus and the fetal brain. Such a drug will then accumulate in the fetus to levels that are at least as high as those achieved in the mother. Whether or not the drug will have toxic or adverse effects on the fetus depends in part on the size and frequency of doses that the mother takes.

It is clear that physically and mentally healthy women are far more likely to give birth to healthy babies. Therefore, drug use of any kind should be avoided or strictly supervised by a physician throughout pregnancy and during the nursing period. It is tragic that so few women are aware of their pregnant state until the developing embryo is well into the vulnerable stage of prenatal growth and development.[41,42]

Secondly, other gender-related factors contribute to the pharmacological uniqueness of the female with regard to drugs and their effects in her body. The overall smaller body size, the greater proportion of body fat—in which alcohol is less soluble than in water—and the lower proportion of water in the bodies of women in comparison with men's bodies place females at increased risk of rapid alcohol intoxication. With less body fluid and a lower water content in which to dilute any drug consumed, women may feel the effects of some drugs more rapidly than men do. The changes in hormonal levels during the menstrual cycle also tend to influence the absorption of drugs, that is, the transfer of the drug across the gastrointestinal tract into the bloodstream. Just before menstruation, the absorption of alcohol, for instance, is faster than at other times in the menstrual cycle.

Recent studies suggest that women are more susceptible to the effects of ethyl alcohol, because females have much less of a protective stomach enzyme than do males. This enzyme breaks down some of the alcohol that is consumed before it enters the bloodstream.[43] As a consequence, women tend to absorb more alcohol into their bloodstreams and experience higher blood alcohol levels than do men of similar size and weight who drink equivalent amounts of alcohol.

Another special concern regarding drug use and abuse among women relates to the growing number of female athletes. As more females increase their participation in sports and intensify their competition, their growing success and heightened aspirations have produced a corresponding increase in drug usage.

Women's greater commitment to sports training has been accompanied by the use of chemicals to improve athletic performance, the so-called ergogenic drugs described in the next section. The entry of women athletes into the "power sports" of weight lifting and shot putting, for example, may also have resulted in a role conflict between concepts of traditional femininity and athletic prowess. Smaller, less-powerful females sometimes resolve the conflict by using steroids, despite their masculinizing effects on the female body.

Emphasis on "being thin" and striving for a high percentage of lean muscle mass and a low percentage of body fat have also produced chemical problems for some women. Laxatives, diet pills, diuretics, and amphetamines are often used to control weight and lose body fat. These conditions, in turn, have been related to the epidemic of serious eating disorders, such as anorexia nervosa and bulimia, and to alcohol abuse and alcoholism among women. Some bulimics who consume alcohol apparently cut down on eating and binging.

Drug Use and Abuse Among Athletes

There is nothing new about the use of drugs among athletes. Traditionally, chemical compounds have been employed in treating injuries, alleviating anxiety and nervous conditions, and relieving pain and inflammation sustained in sports competition. Drugs used in this manner are referred to as **therapeutic agents,** and include antibacterial medications, muscle relaxants, anti-inflammatory drugs, and analgesics (painkillers).

Ergogenic Drugs

Certain drugs have also been used not to cure disease or restore health but rather to enhance athletic performance. When used to artificially improve athletic skills or competition, drugs are described as **ergogenic agents.**

Occasionally, some ergogenic drugs are effective. Others appear to work because of the "placebo effect"—the user's strong faith in or expectation of benefit from the substance used. This placebo effect is explained in detail in chapter 3.

Many of the psychoactive ergogenics are potentially hazardous, often causing dramatic changes in behavior, heart failure, strokes, and blood vessel disease. Although their use has been universally condemned, ergogenics still appear to be abused widely in many amateur and professional sporting contests. Some observers believe that certain recent records achieved in national and international sports competition are due to the use of ergogenic drugs.

In reaction to the increasing use of ergogenic drugs, the International Olympic Committee has banned the following substances:

Psychomotor stimulants, including amphetamines and cocaine

Sympathomimetic amines, such as ephedrine and related compounds

Miscellaneous central nervous system stimulants, including amiphenazole, leptazol, and strychnine

Narcotic analgesics, such as codeine, heroin, methadone, and morphine

Anabolic steroids, synthetic male hormones

Stimulants, such as amphetamines and cocaine, have been used to produce alertness, a decreased sense of fatigue, elevated mood, and enhanced confidence, ability to concentrate, muscle coordination, and aggressiveness—all valuable factors in improving athletic performance. Occasionally amphetamines and cocaine are used together by athletes engaged in contact sports, but these drugs might also be used to increase the stamina of runners and cyclists.

Codeine (a widely used painkiller) and the anesthetic drugs are employed to enable injured players to continue competition. The pain-relieving effects of these substances block the warning signals of bodily injury.

Of all these ergogenic substances, the **anabolic-androgenic steroids** (AAS)—originally called anabolic steroids—are the most frequently abused. (*Anabolic* means "building-up of muscle"; *androgenic* means "producing male characteristics"; and steroids are the class of drugs that resemble bodily hormones.) Commonly known as "roids," AAS drugs are synthetic derivatives of testosterone, the major male sex hormone; they are used by both male and female athletes to build lean muscle mass and to improve the strength and mechanical efficiency of skeletal muscles. Many athletes also believe that these drugs enhance aggressiveness, another desirable characteristic in today's competitive sports scene. As a consequence, anabolic steroids are viewed as giving athletes an added advantage in training and in competition.

Restricted originally to world-class power lifters and weight lifters, steroids eventually became available for use in various sports at both the professional and amateur levels. For the past several years, these drugs have been popular among athletes in swimming, track and field, weight lifting, football, and basketball as well as in bodybuilding. However, other groups are also involved in using these "quick fix" forms of self-medication.[44] First are the "fighting elite," the law enforcement officers, firefighters, bar bouncers, and even some construction workers who believe that AAS drugs will give them a competitive edge to "always be on top." The other nonathletes now taking steroids are the "aesthetic users" who simply want to look better and feel better about themselves.

Studies on the prevalence of use indicate that more than three hundred thousand individuals now take AAS drugs each year and that there are more than one million current or former AAS users in this country.[45] Most of the AAS use in the past year has been concentrated among those less than 26 years of age. It is apparent that

AAS use affects a large number of men and women from various racial and age groups across the nation. Furthermore, use has now spread from the Olympic, professional, and college levels of competition to recreational athletes as well as to young students in high schools, junior highs, and even grade schools.

The following items also suggest the magnitude of consumption and the countermeasures to prevent such use.

- Until recently, at least 70 percent of the steroid production in the United States has not been used for legitimate medical purposes. Although a prescription is needed to get these drugs legally, almost no one has needed a prescription to obtain them.

- An estimated $400 million worth of the drugs are bought and sold annually on the "black market."

- Commenting on the frustrating task of discouraging the use of AAS, Dave Redding, former strength coach of the Cleveland Browns, claims that high school kids want to take steroids because they want to be college stars and college kids take them because they want to be professional stars.

- The National Football League now includes steroid testing when testing for drug abuse among its players.

- The National Collegiate Athletic Conference now tests for both anabolic steroids and chemical "masking agents" that are sometimes taken in an attempt to cover up steroid use. Under new drug-testing measures, first-time offenders could lose an entire year's playing eligibility. Players testing positive for steroids a second time will be banned for life from NCAA sports.

- In response to the Anabolic Steroids Control Act of the U.S. Congress, the Drug Enforcement Administration (DEA) placed anabolic steroids on Schedule III of the Controlled Substances Act in

1991. As controlled drugs with high abuse potential, anabolic steroids may not be manufactured, distributed, or dispensed without a registration from the DEA. Special record keeping, inventory, and security procedures now apply to nearly all of the anabolic steroids. Various penalties now apply for violation of the newly established procedures, for instance, any person who gives anabolic steroids to a minor can be sentenced to prison for ten years.

The various anabolic-androgenic steroids can be taken either by mouth or by injection; the latter method is now preferred by most users. Frequently these drugs are used in increasingly higher doses, a practice that is known as "pyramiding." When several different types of steroids, or a combination of different strengths of pills and injectables, are taken jointly or in cycles, the usage pattern is described as "stacking." For instance, about four or five months before competition, dosage levels will be gradually increased to ten to one hundred times greater than recommended therapeutic amounts. Then, to avoid detection, dosage levels are reduced several weeks before the mandatory drug testing for a particular event. Sometimes these drugs are taken in a cyclical manner, with a six- to twelve-week period of use followed by a drug-free period of one to several months.[46]

Despite the alleged benefits of using AAS drugs—greater endurance, increase in lean muscle mass and aggressiveness, enhanced physical appearance, and a decrease in muscle recovery time—the 1994 edition of the *Physicians' Desk Reference* carries this advisory for such drugs: "Anabolic steroids have not been shown to enhance athletic performance."[47] Controlled research on male athletes given steroids has been far from conclusive, with only marginal evidence to support enhanced strength. There is no evidence, however, of an increased capacity for aerobic work.[48] Nevertheless, these AAS drugs probably can increase a woman's strength, since steroids are variations of testosterone, the male sex hormone that has masculinizing effects in the female.

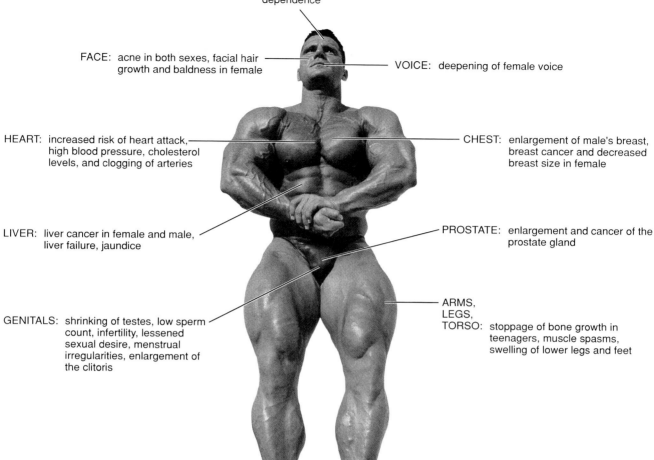

MIND: increased hostility, aggressive behavior, paranoia, depression, anxiety, hallucinations, eating compulsions, psychological dependence

FACE: acne in both sexes, facial hair growth and baldness in female

VOICE: deepening of female voice

HEART: increased risk of heart attack, high blood pressure, cholesterol levels, and clogging of arteries

CHEST: enlargement of male's breast, breast cancer and decreased breast size in female

LIVER: liver cancer in female and male, liver failure, jaundice

PROSTATE: enlargement and cancer of the prostate gland

GENITALS: shrinking of testes, low sperm count, infertility, lessened sexual desire, menstrual irregularities, enlargement of the clitoris

ARMS, LEGS, TORSO: stoppage of bone growth in teenagers, muscle spasms, swelling of lower legs and feet

 1.4

Anabolic-androgenic steroids and their adverse side effects.*
Anavar, Anadrol-50, Testred, Anabolin, Deca-Durabolin, and Testex are some of the more frequently used anabolic-androgenic steroid drugs. Developed originally for patients with muscle problems, these drugs are also used medically to treat certain types of breast cancer, growth problems, arthritis, long-term infections, and anemia. But anabolic steroids can have many undesirable side effects, some of which can be life-threatening, especially with long-term, high-dose use without close medical supervision.

*Sources: Office of Substance Abuse Prevention. 1989. The Fact Is . . . The Use of Steroids in Sports Can Be Dangerous. Rockville, Maryland: National Clearinghouse for Alcohol and Drug Information.

The United States Pharmacopeial Convention, Inc. 1990. Drug Information for the Consumer, 89–90. Mount Vernon, New York: Consumers Union.

Tricker, Ray, O'Neill, Michael, and Cook, David. 1989. "The Incidence of Anabolic Steriod Use Among Competitive Bodybuilders," Journal of Drug Education, Vol. 19, No. 4: 313–325.

Photo © Uniphoto Picture Agency

Although the use of ergogenic drugs often gives athletes an assumed competitive edge against other contestants, their repeated intake carries the risk of potential threats to the health of the drug users themselves. Amphetamine users often find they must resort to sedatives or tranquilizers to facilitate sleep. And painkillers, by masking the body's messages of injury, can lead to crippling damage of the joints.

Anabolic steroids can also have a variety of life-threatening side effects, including higher blood pressure, less favorable blood-fat ratios, higher cholesterol levels, and increased risk of heart attack and liver cancer.

Oral anabolic-androgenic steroids include Anavar, Anadrol-50, Android-F, Testred, and Vigorex, while commonly used injectables include Anabolin, Deca-Durabolin, Decolone, Delatest, Andronate, and Testex. Developed originally for patients with muscle problems, these drugs are also used medically to treat certain types of breast cancer, growth problems, arthritis, long-term infections, and anemia. But anabolic steroids can have many undesirable side effects, some of which can be life threatening, especially with long-term, high-dose use without close medical supervision.

Recently, serious psychiatric risks have been associated with steroid use. Users typically display elation, overestimation of their capacities, irritability, and hyperactivity or recklessness in their driving, spending, or sexual habits. These behaviors are common symptoms of mania—an abnormal state of euphoria beyond normal happiness, joy, and pleasure.[49] Another symptom frequently noticed is the heightened aggressiveness ("roid rage") displayed not only during use, but also as part of the withdrawal process, when steroid use is discontinued rather suddenly. Roid rage can also include major depression, irritability, and antisocial behavior. Evidence now suggests that many long-term steroid users develop a steroid addiction or dependence. Loss of control over the amount of steroids used, preoccupation with

continued use, development of tolerance, and the use of steroids to avoid or control withdrawal symptoms are all part of AAS dependence.[50]

The continuing use of ergogenic drugs is frequently related to fears that one's opponent in athletic competition has already discovered a magical formula that assures superiority and victory. Consequently, the use of performance-enhancing agents becomes a matter of survival. Everyone seems to be doing it. Because of such perceived pressure and prevalence of use, this form of drug abuse is basically coercive rather than an act of free choice. Of course, such continuing drug abuse could also be an addictive behavior, in which persistent use is not exactly an act of free choice either.

Sport fans, however, may also be encouraging this type of drug abuse by expecting total perfection of athletes. Many fans tend to value winning—often at any cost—more than honest competition. They will frequently "boo" the loser and cheer loudly when a player "draws blood" from a competitor. The fans unwittingly create the pressure to win by any means and provide the stimulus to avoid the "shame of losing." In such cases the words of Pogo, a once-popular comic strip character, may be most appropriate: "We have met the enemy, and they is us!"

Of course, there is also an ethical viewpoint regarding the use of ergogenic agents. When athletes use performance-enhancing drugs, they break the code of conduct that governs most sport activities. Involving cheating and lying, this form of drug use violates the spirit of competition by rewarding willingness to cheat or take health risks.[51] These characteristics and attitudes oppose natural ability, skill, and willingness to train intensively—the very qualities a sport is intended to reward.

Dangerous Alternatives to Anabolic-Androgenic Steroids

A number of equally dangerous alternatives to using AAS have been devised to achieve performance-enhancing effects for competitive athletes. First is "blood

doping," the injection of blood, one's own or another's, in an attempt to enhance performance and increase endurance by increasing the total number of red blood cells available for oxygenation. Because this procedure involves blood transfusion, infections and even fatal reactions due to error may occur.

Lately, a synthetic form of the human hormone erythropoietin (Epoetin and Epogen) has been used by some athletes to increase red blood cell production in the human body. Unlike typical blood doping, this synthesized product can be self-injected. Because this drug can lead to increased blood clotting, its use is vigorously discouraged by medical authorities.

Gamma hydroxybutyrate (GHB) and clenbuterol are two additional steroid alternatives. GHB, a common ingredient in many so-called performance enhancers, is a deadly, illegal drug that can cause headaches, nausea, vomiting, diarrhea, seizures, and nervous system disorders. Contrary to popular belief, GHB does not produce a "high" in its users. Clenbuterol, an extremely popular item on the black market, can unexpectedly produce muscle tremors, fast heart rates, headaches, nausea, and chills after eating beef liver containing residues of this drug.[52]

More recently, a synthetic form of human growth hormone (HGH) has been used by some athletes to increase tendon and ligament strength and to avoid bone damage that sometimes occurs with the use of anabolic-androgenic steroids. Potentially adverse effects of this relatively new ergogenic drug include hypothyroidism, heart disease, increased incidence of leukemia, and impaired metabolism of various body chemicals.

Recreational Drugs

Increasing attention has been focused on drug abuse in sports, since college and especially professional athletes have been charged with possession or use of illegal recreational drugs or found to be addicted to some psychoactive substance. In response to charges of scandal as well as efforts to prove their athletes were

1.5 Selected Drugs for Which College Athletes Are Frequently Tested

Anabolic-Androgenic Steroids	Benzodiazepines (Dalmane, Librium, Valium)
Stimulant Drugs	Phenothiazine, chlorpromazine
Amphetamines	
Methamphetamine	**Narcotic Drugs**
Phenmetrazine (Preludin)	Heroin
Cocaine	Morphine
	Codeine
Depressant Drugs	Meperidine (Demerol)
Barbiturates	Hydromorphone (Dilaudid)
Phenobarbital	Methadone
Short-acting barbiturates (Nembutal, Seconal, Amytal)	**THC or Its Metabolites**
Methaqualone	Marijuana
Tranquilizers	Hashish
	Phencyclidine (PCP)

"clean" or not using social drugs, many colleges began NCAA-sponsored drug testing to reduce and hopefully eliminate drug use among students participating in college sports. (See table 1.5.)

Many colleges, especially NCAA Division I schools, now have rather comprehensive drug-testing programs, often in combination with drug education and counseling. Testing is typically accomplished by obtaining urine samples from athletes. After the samples are frozen and divided, they are tested for both separate drug categories and specific drug substances.

In addition to the performance-enhancement use of anabolic-androgenic steroids and amphetamines, the most frequently abused psychoactive drugs by athletes are alcohol, marijuana, and cocaine. Alcohol is, by far, the number one drug of abuse at both the collegiate and the professional level. Despite the frequent association between former professional athletes and the beers they now endorse, drinking beer or any other alcoholic beverage is the surest way to diminish athletic performance.

Even small amounts of alcohol consumed just before or during sport activities will slow down one's physical performance, due to alcohol's depressant effect on the central nervous system. Reaction time, hand-eye coordination, accuracy, balance, and gross motor skills are all adversely affected. With higher blood-alcohol levels, voluntary actions become increasingly clumsy. Other effects of alcohol also tend to undermine physical performance:

1. Though it is a concentrated source of calories, alcohol is an inefficient source of fuel. Since it must first be processed by the liver, alcohol cannot be used directly by the muscles.

2. Even at low to moderate doses, alcohol causes blood vessels within muscles to constrict, while blood vessels at the surface of the skin dilate. Physical performance tends to deteriorate, because blood cannot easily reach the working muscles where it is needed.

3. In the presence of alcohol, the pancreas tends to produce an excessive amount of insulin. When this occurs, a condition known as temporary hypoglycemia (low blood sugar) can develop, which can then result in fatigue during exercise.

4. Moderate to heavy drinking blocks the release from the pituitary gland of ADH, a hormone that regulates the amount of water retained by the kidneys. This action can cause dehydration, marked by extreme thirst and physical weakness.

While there are numerous motivations for drinking alcoholic beverages, athletes, in particular, might view alcohol as a so-called recreational drug that serves their unique needs. Alcohol might function as a reward for a good performance, a quick way to calm down after heated competition, or a convenient cure for the boredom between games or the next competitive event. Sometimes drinking represents nothing more than conformity to the subtle social pressure of other athletes.

Marijuana has no ergogenic value, so its use is primarily related to producing feelings of relaxation after the excessive pressures of competition. Using marijuana prior to sport activities tends to lower blood pressure, blocks normal sweating, and interferes with the ability to follow a moving object from one point to another, a function referred to as tracking ability. Cocaine, which has performance-enhancing properties already described in this section, is a rather expensive and dangerous way of reexperiencing the euphoria of competition or reinforcing one's self-image as an invincible, conquering hero. As a central nervous system stimulant, cocaine can also remove the psychological sting of defeat.

Drug Use and Abuse Among the Elderly

If you want evidence of senior citizens' drug use, inspect the medicine cabinet or bedside table in the homes of your parents and grandparents. And if you happen to have an aged relative confined in a nursing home, inquire about the number of prescribed medications being taken by that individual. You will likely be shocked, as the author was, at the sheer volume of drugs, both prescribed and nonprescribed, taken by the elderly.

Currently, Americans over age 60 comprise nearly 16 percent of the total population. Yet, each year, senior citizens use approximately 30 percent of all prescription drugs and 40 percent of all sleeping pills. About four in ten senior citizens also use five or more prescription drugs at the same time. Even more alarmingly, these older Americans account for 30 percent of all hospitalizations and 51 percent of all deaths from adverse drug reactions.[53]

With the number of senior citizens increasing rapidly, the amount of medicine used by this segment of the population will likely become phenomenal. And the improper use of drugs, misdiagnoses by physicians, and inappropriate dosage levels—already major problems—will also become phenomenal.

Emerging from a national conspiracy of silence and neglect is an epidemic of inappropriate drug prescribing for the elderly.[54] Research has revealed that nearly a quarter of all Americans aged 65 or older are routinely given prescriptions for drugs that they should almost never take and often do not even need. Medication errors among both noninstitutionalized patients as well as those in health care facilities have become extremely high; some physicians and drug companies have used elderly patients as test subjects for drug experiments without obtaining informed consent from the affected individuals; and adverse drug interactions are routinely seen in hospitals as well as in nonsupervised settings.[55] All of these conditions are part of the "mismedication" of older Americans.

While the wise use of medications can be very beneficial for older people, a number of factors related particularly to the elderly contribute to the increased potential for drug misuse, abuse, and numerous drug interactions with serious and undesirable side effects.[56,57]

1. *Aging is accompanied by normal changes in the body that actually make adverse drug reactions more likely.* Older adults typically weigh less and have a smaller amount of water and a larger proportion of fat than younger adults. These changes affect the amount of a drug needed per pound of body weight or body water to be safe and effective, the dilution of a drug after it enters the body, and the duration of drug action. In addition, many older adults experience an increased sensitivity to many drugs and decreased abilities to maintain blood pressure and compensate for changes in temperature.

 table 1.6 **Common Medication Errors Experienced by the Elderly**

Failure to take medicines at the right time	Inability to maintain an adequate supply of medicine
Difficulty in remembering to take medicines	Difficulty reading the label and understanding directions
Trouble opening the bottle, jar, or container	Taking a greater or smaller dosage than specified in the directions
Difficulty separating or breaking tablets	Inability to distinguish between medicines that look alike
Problems encountered with mixing or preparing medication	

Other commonly anticipated changes include reduced kidney and liver function, a weakened heart, lowered effectiveness of the immune system, and loss of intestinal flexibility. Such alterations make the elderly more likely to need drug therapy, but the same changes also tend to influence the effect any drug will have within the body. The results of these changes are too often an increased drug effect leading to a toxic (poisonous) condition or a decreased drug effect that fails to relieve the illness.

2. *The occurrence of the pharmaceutical revolution in conjunction with the decline of the extended family.* Without family support or consolation, the elderly are increasingly placed on chemical tranquilizers, antidepressants, and sedatives to combat their depression, loneliness, and isolation.

3. *Changes in sleep patterns that often lead to drug dependency.* Confronted with the inability to sleep as well as when they were young, many older people are prescribed sleeping pills containing depressant drugs, hypnotics, and tranquilizers. If such medication is stopped, these people often experience increased wakefulness and nightmares, which are sufficient to motivate continued usage of the drugs.

4. *Many physicians overprescribe psychoactive drugs for the elderly.* Encouraged by the promotional practices of pharmaceutical companies, physicians have tended to increase their reliance on drugs as their primary method of treatment. This is especially true regarding the emotional life and sleeping pattern of older patients. This situation allegedly has occurred without a similar increase in the pharmacological training of physicians regarding geriatric patients.

5. *Mismanagement of medicines is a common problem among the aged.* It is not unusual for older people to be taking three or more drugs—often prescribed by two or more physicians—at the same time. This pattern of taking multiple drugs concurrently is known as **polydrug use.** Because of self-medication, any number of drugs purchased over the counter may also be used simultaneously. Multiple drug use makes it difficult for many people to remember whether or not they have taken a particular drug. Inability to distinguish between colored medicines, impaired vision that prevents reading label instructions, and decreased ability to hear or understand directions all combine to precipitate numerous **medication errors**—decreasing or increasing recommended dosage, improper timing of medicine intake, sharing drugs with relatives and friends, omission of dosage, or stopping drug use altogether due to lack of funds or merely feeling better (see table 1.6). Inappropriate prescribing is a particular problem

with at least twenty medications, including antidepressants, arthritis drugs, antihypertensives for controlling high blood pressure, blood thinners, dementia treatments, diabetes drugs, muscle relaxants, pain relievers, sleeping aids, and tranquilizers for the control of anxiety. These are among the more frequently prescribed medicines for the elderly.

Evidently there is a greater need for drug education both for the elderly and their physicians. There appears to be an equal need to become aware of nondrug alternatives to the health problems of the aged, especially problems now solved by sleeping pills and tranquilizers. Until the overmedication syndrome is reversed in treating and caring for the elderly, one might conclude logically that older Americans themselves are more abused than are their drugs.

While the misuse of pain-relieving medicines, minor tranquilizers, barbiturates and other sleep-inducing drugs, and numerous over-the-counter medications is common and a growing problem for the elderly, most senior citizens at present have little involvement with illegal psychoactive substances. Although this situation may change in the future, the major drug problems of the elderly center around alcohol and the legal pharmaceuticals, often used in combination.

There are numerous motivations for using and abusing alcohol, the drug of choice among the elderly. Many seniors tend to slide almost inadvertently into alcohol abuse. After years of abstinence or non-problematic drinking, some elderly persons begin drinking in a search for relief from boredom, physical pain, emotional stress, loneliness, isolation, or loss. These situations characterize late-onset alcohol abuse or dependence, which accounts for almost one-third of older problem drinkers. The other two-thirds of elderly alcohol abusers display what is known as early-onset alcohol abuse or dependence, the continuation of lifelong problem drinking.

Unlike alcohol abuse in younger age groups, several unique factors tend to complicate the detection, diagnosis, and treatment of alcohol problems in the elderly. These include the following:[58,59]

1. The ability of the elderly to hide or deny their drinking problem. This situation applies especially to the more than 8 million Americans over 65 years of age who live alone—over a quarter of the total senior citizen population.

2. The elderly are frequently unaware they have a drinking problem, particularly if they are affected by chronic aches, pains, and other physical and psychological complaints. Quite often, the elderly suffer from symptoms that they as well as their own physicians do not associate with their use of alcoholic beverages. Many indications of physical, psychological, and social deterioration associated with alcoholism are attributed falsely to the "natural aging process" or to Alzheimer's disease.

3. Families and physicians are unable or unwilling to recognize alcohol abuse among the elderly. In some instances, children encourage their aging parents to use alcohol so as to promote sleep and alleviate aches and pains, while physicians mistakenly assume their elderly patients are too old to have a drinking problem.

Chapter Summary

1. American drug problems involve the use of legal medications, illegal drugs, and the recreational or social use of drugs intended for medical purposes. Legal drugs, such as alcohol and the nicotine in cigarettes, also contribute to current drug problems.

2. A drug is a substance that can change the structure or function of the body, while a medicine is a drug used in diagnosis, care, treatment, or prevention of disease.

3. Drug misuse involves the unintentional or inappropriate use of prescribed or nonprescribed medicine, whereas drug abuse is the deliberate use of chemical substances for reasons other than their intended medical purposes, resulting in personal or social impairment.

4. Psychoactive drugs change thought, feelings, perceptions, and behavior, and are specified as narcotics, depressants, stimulants, psychedelics, and inhalants.

5. Psychoactive drugs may be classified by their general or localized effects on the central nervous system, by their relative degree of medical usefulness and abuse potential, and by their potential for causing personal and social dangers.

6. Drug problems related to the use of psychoactive substances include delay in proper medical treatment, reduction in problem-solving effectiveness, experience of adverse reactions, the use of adulterated drugs, the consumption of fake drugs and potent "designer drugs," and increased risk of suicide and infection with HIV, the virus that causes AIDS.

7. Adverse reactions or conditions associated with psychoactive drug use are toxic reactions, panic, flashback, psychopathology, and drug dependence.

8. Although the use of illegal drugs, alcohol, and cigarettes generally peaked in the late 1970s, more than 75 million Americans have used at least one illegal drug in their lifetimes. Alcohol is by far the most widely abused drug in the nation, but marijuana is still the most commonly used illegal drug. The use of psychoactive drugs varies according to gender and race/ethnicity, and across urban and rural areas of the United States.

9. Premature deaths, health care costs, loss of productivity, and expenses related to crime and destruction of property are among the unanticipated consequences of

psychoactive substance abuse. One other disturbing consequence of our current illegal drug problem is criminal activity, which typically rises as drug use increases. Although complex, drug-crime relationships are expressed as drug-defined and drug-related offenses, and as interactional circumstances.

10. Women tend to use more psychoactive drugs than do men. However, females possess a pharmacological uniqueness regarding psychoactive drugs, a uniqueness related to human reproduction potential, and gender-linked attributes of body weight and size, amount of body fat and water, hormonal changes during the menstrual cycle, and the lack of a stomach enzyme that breaks down alcohol in men.

11. During pregnancy, psychoactive drug use by mothers may contribute to a variety of congenital birth defects among their offspring. Nicotine, cocaine, marijuana, and alcohol should be avoided, and aspirin, tranquilizers, barbiturates, and amphetamines should be taken during pregnancy only under medical supervision.

12. Ergogenic aids, drugs used to artificially improve athletic competition, include stimulants, painkillers, and anabolic-androgenic steroids.

13. The continued use of ergogenic drugs can result in serious health problems for athletes, including drug dependence, liver and kidney damage, and crippling injuries.

14. Mismanagement of medicines leading to numerous medication errors is common among the elderly, who take more than 25 percent of all medicines and yet account for only 16 percent of the total U.S. population.

15. Overmedication of the elderly is usually related to prescribed sleeping pills, hypnotics, and tranquilizers, while adverse reactions are linked to several nonpsychoactive medicines: cardiovascular drugs, anticonvulsants, and certain antibiotics.

Review Questions and Activities

1. Explain how illegal chemical substances, legally produced medicines, and legal social drugs all contribute to the current drug problem in America.

2. Distinguish between the following terms: *drug* and *medicine*; *drug misuse* and *drug abuse*.

3. List several examples of therapeutic drugs.

4. Identify five major classes of psychoactive drugs.

5. Survey class members to determine their use of psychoactive drugs purchased over the counter (OTC) without a prescription. Do any of these OTC medicines have common drug ingredients? (Ask class members to copy down the drugs listed on the label.)

6. Classify each of the following psychoactive drugs according to their *effects* on the central nervous system, their *ability to be purchased without a prescription,* the *provisions of the Controlled Substances Act,* and their potential for individual and social harm: beverage alcohol, nicotine in cigarettes, heroin, cocaine, marijuana, amphetamine, and LSD.

7. Identify the major health-related consequences often associated with drug-taking behavior.

8. Define each of the following terms in relation to psychoactive drug use:

toxic reaction, panic, flashback, psychopathology, and *drug dependence.*

9. How do adulterated drugs differ from "look-alikes"?

10. Describe the current drug scene in terms of prevalence of use, the drug-abusing population, unanticipated consequences of substance abuse, and the drug-crime relationship.

11. Explain the unique potential problems associated with use of psychoactive drugs among women.

12. Name several specific adverse effects that psychoactive drugs may have on the developing embryo or fetus.

13. What is the difference between a therapeutic drug and an ergogenic drug?

14. Identify three major types of ergogenic drugs often used by athletes.

15. Discuss the potential hazards associated with the use of ergogenics, especially the anabolic-androgenic steroids.

16. In what ways might sport fans be contributing to the continuing practice of doping?

17. Relate the following factors to drug misuse and abuse among the elderly: (a) normal aging processes; (b) decline of the extended family; (c) changes in sleep patterns; (d) physician reliance on drug therapy; and (e) polydrug use.

References

1. "New Prevention Program Provides What Has Been Missing in Traditional Programs," *Bottom Line on Alcohol in Society* 15, no. 2 (summer 1994): 5–16.
2. Office of National Drug Control Policy, *National Drug Control Strategy: Reclaiming Our Communities from Drugs and Violence,*

vol. 9 (Washington, D.C.: Office of National Drug Control Policy, Executive Office of the President, 1994).

3. Jill Smolowe, "Choose Your Poison," *Time*, 26 July 1993, 56–57.

4. Preface to "Political Pharmacology: Thinking about Drugs," *Daedalus* 121, no. 3 (summer 1992): vi.

5. Harold Doweiko, *Concepts of Chemical Dependency*, 2d ed. (Pacific Grove, Calif: Brooks/Cole, 1993), 4–5.

6. George Gallup, Jr., as quoted in *Prevention Plus II: Tools for Creating and Sustaining Drug-Free Communities*, Office for Substance Abuse Prevention, DHHS Pub. No. (ADM) 89-1649 (Washington, D.C.: Government Printing Office), 2.

7. Samuel Irwin, *Drugs of Abuse: An Introduction to Their Actions and Potential Hazards*, 8th rev. ed. (Phoenix: Do It Now Foundation, 1989), 29–33.

8. Irwin, *Drugs of Abuse*, 32.

9. Institute for Health Policy, Brandeis University, *Substance Abuse: The Nation's Number One Health Problem*, vol. 8 (Princeton, N.J.: Robert Wood Johnson Foundation, 1993).

10. Darryl Inaba and William Cohen, *Uppers, Downers, All Arounders*, 2d ed. (Ashland, Ore.: CNS Productions, 1993), 322–24.

11. M. M. Kirsch, *Designer Drugs*, vol. 4 (Minneapolis: CompCare, 1986).

12. Ronald H. Ng, "Laboratory Consultant," *Clinical Chemistry News* 15, no. 7 (July 1989): 25.

13. U.S. Public Health Service, *Healthy People 2000: National Health Promotion and Disease Prevention Objectives*, Summary Report (Boston: Jones & Bartlett, 1992), 17. Reprinted from DHHS Publication No. (PHS) 91-50213.

14. Sidney Cohen, *The Substance Abuse Problem. Vol. 2: New Issues for the 1980s* (New York: Haworth Press, 1985), 113.

15. Gail Gleason Milgram and the Editors of Consumer Reports Books, *The Facts about Drinking* (Mount Vernon, N.Y.: Consumers Union, 1990), 57.

16. National Institute on Drug Abuse, *Annual Data 1988* (Washington, D.C.: U.S. Government Printing Office, 1989), iii, 14.

17. Jean Kinney and Gwen Leaton, *Loosening the Grip* (St. Louis: Times Mirror/Mosby College Publishing, 1991), 340–41.

18. Institute of Medicine, National Academy of Sciences, *Confronting AIDS: Update 1988* (Washington, D.C.: National Academy Press, 1988), 84.

19. Don des Jarlais and Dana E. Hunt, "AIDS and Intravenous Drug Use," *National Institute of Justice AIDS Bulletin*, February 1988, 2.

20. Richard E. Chaisson and others, "Cocaine Use and HIV Infection in Intravenous Drug Uses

in San Francisco," *Journal of the American Medical Association* 261, no. 4 (27 January 1989): 561–65.

21. Dale D. Chitwood and others, "HIV Seropositivity of Needles from Shooting Galleries in South Florida," *American Journal of Public Health* 80, no. 2 (February 1990): 150–52.

22. Nicholas Freudenberg, *Preventing AIDS: A Guide to Effective Education for the Prevention of HIV Infection* (Washington, D.C.: American Public Health Association, 1990), 130.

23. Barry Stimmel and the Editors of Consumer Reports Books, *The Facts about Drug Use: Coping with Drugs and Alcohol in Your Family, at Work, in Your Community* (New York: Haworth Medical Press, 1993), 271–73.

24. National Institute on Alcohol Abuse and Alcoholism, "Alcohol and AIDS," *Alcohol Alert* no. 15, PH 311 (January 1992): 1–4.

25. Omar Bagasra, Balla Kajdacsy, Harold Lischner, and Roger Pomerantz, "Alcohol Intake Increases Human Immunodeficiency Virus Type I Replication in Human Peripheral Blood Mononuclear Cells," *Journal of Infectious Diseases* 167, no. 4 (April 1993): 789–97.

26. Donald I. Abrams, "The Nature of AIDS," in *Acquired Immune Deficiency Syndrome and Chemical Dependency* (Washington, D.C.: U.S. Government Printing Office, 1988), 3–14.

27. Rob Roy MacGregor, "Alcohol and the Immune System," in *Acquired Immune Deficiency and Chemical Dependency* (Washington, D.C.: U.S. Government Printing Office, 1988), 31–41.

28. "Alcohol's Connection to AIDS under Research," *Substance Abuse Report* 20, no. 24 (1 December 1989): 7.

29. Antonia Abbey, *Sex and Substance Abuse: What Are the Links?* draft copy, Module 1 in Project Direction (the National Collegiate Substance Abuse Prevention Initiative) (Muncie, Ind.: Eta Sigma Gamma, 1990), 3–5.

30. National Institute on Drug Abuse, *National Household Survey on Drug Abuse: Highlights 1993* (Washington, D.C.: U.S. Government Printing Office, 1994).

31. Lloyd Johnston, Patrick O'Malley, and Jerold Bachman, *National Survey Results on Drug Use from the Monitoring the Future Study, 1975–1992. Vol. 1: Secondary School Students* (1993 update, 31 January 1994, for the National Institute on Drug Abuse) (Washington, D.C.: U.S. Government Printing Office, 1993). 1994 update recorded in *Substance Abuse Report* 26, no. 1 (1 January 1995): 1–2.

32. Lloyd Johnston, Patrick O'Malley, and Jerold Bachman, *National Survey Results on Drug Use from the Monitoring the Future Study, 1975–1992. Vol. 2: College Students and Young

Adults*, prepared for the National Institute on Drug Abuse (Washington, D.C.: U.S. Government Printing Office, 1993).

33. Office of National Drug Control Policy, *National Drug Control Strategy: Reclaiming Our Communities from Drugs and Violence* (Washington, D.C.: Office of National Drug Control Policy, Executive Office of the President, 1994).

34. Donna Hunt and the Office of National Drug Control Policy, *Pulse Check: National Trends in Drug Abuse* (Washington, D.C.: U.S. Government Printing Office, 1994).

35. Institute for Health Policy, Brandeis University, *Substance Abuse*.

36. Ibid., 16–31.

37. Marcia Chaiken, "Can Drug Epidemics Be Anticipated?" *National Institute of Justice Journal* no. 226 (April 1993): 23–30.

38. Sidney Cohen, "Drug Abuse: The Coming Years," in *The Substance Abuse Problem*, 263.

39. Except where indicated otherwise, material in this section has been derived substantially from various publications of the National Institute on Drug Abuse.

40. Jacqueline Horton, "Addictive Behaviors," in *The Women's Health Book*, ed. Jacqueline Horton (Washington, D.C.: Jacobs Institute of Women's Health and Elsevier, 1992), 79.

41. Ira J. Chasnoff and others, "Temporal Patterns of Cocaine Use in Pregnancy: Perinatal Outcomes," *Journal of the American Medical Association* 261, no. 12 (24–31 March 1989): 1741–44.

42. Diana Petitti and Charlotte Coleman, "Cocaine and the Risk of Low Birth Weight," *American Journal of Public Health* 80, no. 1 (January 1990): 25–28.

43. Mario Frezza and others, "High Blood Alcohol Levels in Women: The Role of Decreased Gastric Alcohol Dehydrogenase Activity and First-Pass Metabolism," *New England Journal of Medicine* 322, no. 2 (11 January 1990): 95–99.

44. Corinne Groark, "When Pumping Up Can Lead to Serious Health Problems and Side Effects," *Employee Assistance: Solutions to the Problems* 4, no. 4 (November 1991): 8.

45. Charles Yesalis, Nancy Kennedy, Adrea Kopstein, and Michael Bahrke, "Anabolic-Androgenic Steroid Use in the United States," *Journal of the American Medical Association* 270, no. 10 (8 September 1993): 1217–21.

46. Stimmel and others, *The Facts about Drug Use*, 293.

47. *Physicians' Desk Reference*, 48th ed. (Montvale, N.J.: Medical Economics Data Production Company, 1994), 2350.

48. Stimmel and others, *The Facts about Drug Use*, 295.

49. Harrison Pope and David Katz, "What Are the Psychiatric Risks of Anabolic Steroids?" *Harvard Mental Health Letter* 7, no. 10 (April 1991): 8.

50. Doweiko, *Concepts of Chemical Dependency*, 171–72.

51. Thomas Murray, "Human Growth Hormone in Sports: No," *Physician and Sports Medicine* 14, no. 5 (May 1986): 29.

52. Raja Mishra, "Steroids and Sports Are a Losing Proposition," *FDA Consumer* 25, no. 7 (September 1991): 25–27.

53. Hank Tweed, *Drugs and Alcohol: A Guide for Older People* (Tempe, Ariz.: D.I.N. Publications, 1991), 1–2.

54. Sharon Willcox, David Himmelstein, and Steffie Woodhandler, "Inappropriate Drug Prescribing for the Community-Dwelling Elderly," *Journal of the American Medical Association* 272, no. 4 (27 July 1994): 292–96.

55. David Schneider, "The Pharmacology of Aging," in *Frontiers in Therapeutic Drug Monitoring and Clinical Toxicology* [Special issue], *Clinical Chemistry News* (June 1992): 22–26.

56. "Alcohol and the Elderly: A Growing Concern for Families and Health Care Professionals," *Street Pharmacologist* 8, no. 4 (April 1985): 1.

57. "Nine Reasons Why Older Adults Are More Likely to Get Adverse Drug Reactions Than Younger Adults," *Public Citizen Health Research Group Health Letter* 6, no. 11 (November 1990): 5–6.

58. G. Maddox, L. Robins, and N. Rosenberg, eds., *Nature and Extent of Alcohol Problems among the Elderly,* National Institute on Alcohol Abuse and Alcoholism Research Monograph 14 (Washington, D.C.: U.S. Government Printing Office, 1984).

59. National Institute on Alcohol Abuse and Alcoholism, *Alcohol and Health,* Eighth Special Report to the U.S. Congress (Rockville, Md.: Public Health Service, National Institutes of Health, 1994), 23–24.

chapter

2

the allure of drugs

Mood Modification

Addiction Cycle
Agent-Related Etiology
Aphrodisiac
Coping
Decreased Awareness
Demographics
Drug-Abuse Epidemic
Drug Reinforcer
Enabling Factors
Endemic Drug Use
Environment-Related Etiology
Etiology
Genetic Predisposition
Host-Related Etiology
Increased Awareness
Modeling
Mood Modification
Multifactorial Theory
Peer-Group Influence
Predisposing Factors
Reinforcing Factors
Risk Factor
Social Drug
Youth Rebellion

chapter objectives

After you have studied this chapter you should be able to do the following:

1. Discuss the origins of drug-taking behavior in terms of personal mood modification.

2. Distinguish between increased awareness and decreased awareness in relation to use of drugs.

3. Explain how young people are "taught to use and abuse drugs" by adults.

4. Distinguish between youth rebellion and pursuit of recreation as factors motivating drug abuse among young people.

5. Analyze drug-taking behavior according to predisposing, enabling, and reinforcing factors.

6. Explain why adolescents are particularly susceptible to the beginning of drug-taking behavior.

7. Describe the role of basic curiosity in the initial use of psychoactive drugs.

8. Discuss the role of psychoactive drug use in the process of coping and adjusting to stress.

9. Identify the basic steps in the addiction cycle.

10. Explain drug use as a possible reflection of preexisting personality difficulties.

11. Distinguish between factors of availability and accessibility as they pertain to enabling drug use and abuse.

12. Identify two pharmacological effects of addicting drugs that foster the continuation of drug abuse.

13. Explain the role of drug reinforcers in the pleasure-motivated use of psychoactive drugs.

14. Identify at least five functional aspects of psychoactive-drug-taking behavior.

15. Explain how the following factors could influence drug use: the changing composition of a nation's population; the women's movement; adverse economic conditions; and an emphasis on a natural lifestyle.

16. Describe the influence of the peer group on the use of psychoactive drugs.

17. Identify two possible effects of media drug advertising on the use and abuse of psychoactive substances.

18. Define the term *parental modeling* as it relates to drug-taking behavior.

19. Compare three characteristics of family life that often contribute to drug abuse with those that apparently minimize problems of drug abuse among children.

20. Compare and contrast agent-related, host-related, and environment-related etiological factors in drug abuse and drug dependence.

21. Relate the term *multifactorial theory* to drug abuse and drug dependence.

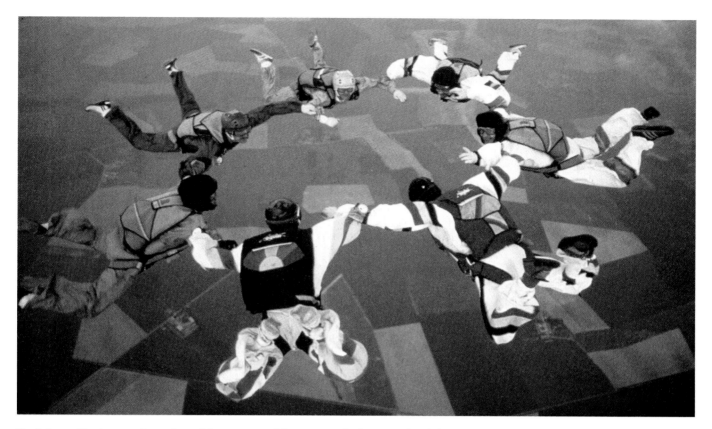

Skydiving, making love, praying and exercising are some of the ways people change or alter their consciousness. Psychoactive drugs also offer an easy and relatively quick way to achieve such a goal, but this form of "flying high" can be potentially more dangerous.

© G. Savage/Vantstadt/Photo Researchers, Inc.

Origins of Drug-Taking Behavior

Most behavioral scientists agree that there is no single explanation for drug-taking behavior, although many theories that focus on just one cause have been proposed. While any drug is usually taken or used for some immediate benefit or advantage, it is quite likely that a combination of several predisposing factors contribute to the use of legal "recreational" drugs as well as to the use of illegal and nonmedical use of psychoactive substances.

Drug-taking behavior that persists despite numerous adverse consequences to both individuals and society has also confused researchers for many years. Today there are various educated guesses to explain the continuing use and abuse of mind-altering chemicals that appear to produce many problems. Nevertheless,

there is considerable agreement that the factors responsible for beginning nonmedical use of drugs are often quite different from those that produce extended use.[1] Whatever initiates substance abuse might not be the basis for perpetuating substance abuse.

Mood Modification

Perhaps the primary reason many people seek out and take psychoactive drugs is to change their conscious experience.[2] Typically, they want to feel better, or just different. One researcher contends that this desire for intoxication—being influenced by a drug's effects—is an acquired motivation similar to the basic drives of hunger, thirst, and even sex.[3]

Although there are many ways to change or alter consciousness—praying, exercising, dancing, making love, and skydiving are just a few—psychoactive drugs

provide an easy and relatively quick way to achieve this goal. This changed consciousness is typically described as **mood modification** consisting of some alteration in thinking, feeling, or behaving. Mood modification is often associated with altered states of consciousness "marked by feelings of euphoria, lightness, self-transcendence, concentration, and energy."[4] There is little wonder that mood modification is one function of psychoactive drugs that many people regard highly.

Some experts claim that drug use and abuse originate in the historical search for pleasure and relief from pain in a harsh environment. Certain drugs serve as popular and readily available agents for temporarily achieving **increased awareness,** a form of psychic stimulation allowing for variations in thought processes, ideas, and even behaviors.[5] From these altered perceptions comes the impetus for progress, innovation, and social advancement.

However, still others increasingly view the abuse of alcohol and other drugs as having deep social roots. The abuse of these psychoactive substances originates, along with compulsive gambling, sexual dysfunctions, chronic insomnia, and depression, in the human's alienation from a society that constantly seeks to beat down individuality and nonconformity.[6] It is possible, then, that drug-taking behavior represents an effort at adjusting to a variety of environmental challenges, often ending in **decreased awareness.** This state or condition of decreased awareness represents an escape from reality and a desire for total narcosis. Here, too, drugs are convenient agents for changing mood and behavior—to feel less pain, to get relief, to feel nothing.

Social Definition of Drug Abuse

America's drug problems are also related to socially defined attitudes, values, and behavioral norms regarding drugs and their perceived usefulness. For example, in America there is no widely held, consistent agreement on the acceptability or unacceptability of drug usage. While millions of people engage in legal mood modification by drinking, smoking, and pill taking, many others—including these same drug users—adamantly oppose the nonmedical use of illegal drugs. Apparently, approved or "appropriate" drug use is still more closely related "to how a drug is obtained and the purpose for which it is used rather than to its effects."[7]

Before 1960, much of the illegal and nonmedical use of drugs was thought to occur among criminals, the urban poor, and nonwhites. These population groups were considered to be dangerous and a threat to the social and moral order. Law enforcement was preoccupied with catching and punishing individual drug takers.

When illegal drug use spread to white, middle- and upper-class youths in the early 1960s, the public definition of "appropriate" drug use was altered slightly and temporarily to reluctantly embrace marijuana. Major law-enforcement efforts were undertaken to curb the new "soft" drugs (nonnarcotic stimulants, depressants, and

Is intoxication a basic human need?

Point:
The human pursuit of intoxication (i.e., drug-induced altered consciousness) is a universal drive as basic as hunger and thirst. In fact, people of all ages throughout history have enjoyed altering their consciousness, both naturally and chemically, just as little children like to spin around until they are dizzy and disoriented. Some respected scientists believe that humans have a natural need to change their awareness from time to time, in response to a harsh or boring environment, or in an effort to decrease feelings of fatigue, tension, and anxiety. Just as important, intoxication can enhance or enliven our experiences and vitalize our own perceptions. Intoxication can also be a unifying symbol, a temporary condition encouraging solidarity and social relationships with fellow drug users. Indeed, the desired effects of taking mind-changing drugs can be an exhilarating experience with new and unique psychic characteristics.

Counterpoint:
To describe intoxication as a desirable and basic human need is both ridiculous and tragic. Such a concept runs counter to the traditions of Western civilization that emphasize the importance of human reasoning, decision-making ability, and the wisdom of maintaining rational control over human behavior. To become intoxicated with drugs impairs these distinctly human abilities. Moreover, there is not a single anticipated effect of intoxication that cannot be achieved through natural highs, including meditation and prayer. Major religions of the world oppose intoxication and drunkenness, because such conditions of impairment interfere with the creator-creature relationship. Moreover, there is also potential danger that any drug used continuously to achieve intoxication for whatever reason will impede psychological and spiritual growth and possibly result in drug dependence.

hallucinogens). Several states even undertook to decriminalize the possession of relatively small amounts of marijuana for private use. Federal government efforts at drug-abuse prevention were redirected from the drug takers to the drug producers and drug pushers. Evidently, another factor that has an impact on the public's definition of "appropriate" drug use is the *type of person who uses drugs.*[8]

Such unusual perceptions and interpretations of various drugs, how they are obtained, why they are used, and who uses them are reflected in various social applications: contradictory and unenforceable drug laws, ambiguous messages subtly conveyed about the desirability of altered states of consciousness, and the toleration of social disorganization resulting from legalized drug use.

Perhaps an underlying issue that society must face is whether or not there is such a thing as responsible drug use as distinguished from irresponsible use, and how such responsible use should be defined. Even if this issue and other related ones are ever resolved, the origin of drug problems will likely be found to be as much in the collectively held attitudes and values of society as in the individual drug takers or their psychoactive chemicals.

A Drug for Every Ailment

Although drug taking has typically been associated with a rebellion of youth against authority, drug usage is more accurately an imitation of adult behavior. Repeatedly, young people see adults treating their own symptoms, using liquor, coffee, tobacco, and various medicines to change their own moods, to be comforted, and to escape from pain or other irritations. Thus, the achievement of instant relief through medication and the promises of a happy, painless solution to every problem are not creations of the youth culture. The older generation has set an example with its overflowing medicine cabinets, the suggestion that for every ailment there is a drug to cure it, and the basic denial of anxiety, worry, and depression as normal feelings. In effect, suffering and pain have lost their cultural significance. With pain now being so easy to kill, it appears quite rational to flee from it rather than face it, even at the cost of addiction.[9]

In a true sense, the adult "teachers" have been most effective; the young "students" have learned their lessons well. Increasingly, and with few exceptions, both groups subscribe to the idea that existence without drugs is impossible. Such devoted reliance upon chemical mood modification may be a symptom of an attempt to will what cannot be willed—sleep, rapid reading, simultaneous orgasm, creativity, spontaneity, and the enjoyment of old age. Too often we turn to external things such as drugs to solve, even if only temporarily, a myriad of internal problems; this is a frightening commentary on our materialistic culture.

Also contributing to this growing reliance on drugs are the technology of the pharmaceutical industry, the subtle compliance of medical practitioners, and the often unreasonable expectations of many patients. Modern drug therapy is now characterized by the new "wonder drugs" introduced each year, a vast increase in drug promotion through advertising to both physicians and patients, and the tendency of both the public and the medical profession to rely on medication for nearly every physical and mental problem. Indeed, the modern physician's role is to get the right drug to the right patient in time for the medicine to do some good.[10] And in many cases it is not uncommon for sophisticated patients to request and even demand specific drugs from their physicians.

Rebellion Against the Establishment Versus Recreational Use

When drug taking was no longer confined to the ghetto, the existing drug problem became a **drug-abuse epidemic,** a sudden increase in the use of illegal drugs. Beginning in the 1960s, drug use among middle-class youth was viewed typically as a "chemical cop-out." Parents were outraged when their children engaged in illegal and health-endangering activities. But the concern and reaction stemmed perhaps as much from the older generation's realization that its children were challenging and even repudiating values cherished by the so-called establishment.[11] Organized religion, patriotism, the sanctity of marriage and premarital chastity, the accumulation of wealth, and the right and competence of parents, schools, and government to lead and make decisions all became the targets of those holding a defiant, authority-resistant, "in-your-face" philosophy.

While drug use may have symbolized a **youth rebellion,** it was not just a rejection of parental values. The rebellion was a generational process over independence, a common confrontation between parent and child. Adolescents, perceiving adults to be living sterile, pointless, and insignificant lives, sought to be as unlike their parents as possible. This they achieved through the hallucinogenic, mind-expanding drugs in their search for new levels of consciousness, understanding, self-analysis, and communication. Illegal drug use was also an attempt to test parental tolerance, concern, and maybe even interest.

It is unlikely that rebellion against and alienation from parents and authority alone can explain the continued use of illegal and recreational drugs at present. Surely the country does not have so many millions of rebels who smoke pot and guzzle booze merely to project a social message of rebellion or indifference. It is fairly certain that much of the drug usage today is motivated by self-indulgence, a desire to feel better, an attempt to escape from boredom or routine,

and perceived social pressure. In essence, our so-called recreational drug use is precisely just that—the pursuit of recreation in a "let's party" atmosphere.

Using and Abusing Drugs: A Behavioral Analysis

Why individuals use drugs and abuse chemical substances remains somewhat a mystery. Those who study drug-taking behavior suggest that complex physical, psychological, and social factors interact to convert nonusers into users and experimental users into frequent abusers. One model proposed recently to explore health behaviors considers **predisposing, enabling,** and **reinforcing factors.**[12] Such a model will be used in this chapter to analyze various internal and external forces, motivations, attitudes, demographic variables, and influences of individuals and institutions in the use and abuse of psychoactive drugs (see box 2.1).

Predisposing Factors in the Use and Abuse of Drugs

The factors in this category collectively contribute to drug-taking behavior and include the existing knowledge base of individuals, their beliefs, attitudes, and those human characteristics that make them particularly susceptible or inclined in advance to use and abuse drugs.

Demographics and Sociocultural Influences

Demographics Demographics are distinct social characteristics and vital statistics of human populations. They provide a unique insight into various predisposing forces that appear to determine or strongly influence the use or nonuse of alcohol and other drugs. Specific demographics, based on studies of large populations of Americans, are listed below:[13–15]

> *Age and gender.* Younger people drink and use drugs more often than older people do. Males typically

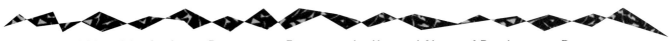

box 2.1

A Conceptual Model for Analyzing Determining Factors in the Use and Abuse of Psychoactive Drugs

Predisposing Influences (Susceptibility)	Enabling Influences (Facilitation)	Reinforcing Influences (Encouragement)
Attitudes about drugs and the "quick fix"	Availability of drugs	Mood modification, increased awareness and unawareness
Demographics and sociocultural influences		
Adolescence	Accessibility to drugs	Experience of pleasure
Myths about drugs	Ineffective legal deterrence	Drugs help to accomplish tasks
Personality and coping	Lack of social controls	Social and peer-group pressure
Unique psychological characteristics	Inability to say "no" to experimentation	Advertising and media programming about drug taking
Social changes and conflicts	Effects of addicting drugs: withdrawal, depression, and mental impairment	Family dynamics
Heredity	Actions of the "enabler"	Influence of modeling
Family: psychological aspects	Family interference with treatment of drug abuser	

The three basic categories of determinants (predisposing, enabling, and reinforcing) should not be viewed as separate or discrete influences in the use and abuse of psychoactive drugs. Rather, they might be considered more appropriately as interdependent, interconnected, and even supplementary. As such, the three categories actually portray drug-taking behavior as the result of many diverse and interrelated factors that initiate and perpetuate drug use and drug abuse. Can you identify additional factors in each category?

drink more often than women at any age level, and men are much more likely than women to abuse psychoactive drugs.

Family structure. Single and divorced people tend to drink more heavily, all things being equal, than married people; marital instability does not always lead to increased usage, due to a sharp drop in short-term income.

Income. The more affluent individuals, in terms of real family income, typically drink more than the less affluent.

Education. Education tends to lower the likelihood that a person would use drugs. College-educated people might be expected to have a lower incidence of substance abuse, yet individuals who finish any educational program—eighth grade, high school, or college—have lower rates of alcoholism than "noncompleters" who begin the next level of education but drop out before finishing the program.

Occupation. Construction workers have the highest prevalence of active substance-abuse disorders, followed by carpenters, auto mechanics, and transportation workers. Retail salespersons, farm workers, precision metal workers, groundskeepers, machine operators, janitors, store clerks, and waiters and waitresses all have higher than average drug-use prevalence rates. The highest rates of alcoholism are also observed among skilled and unskilled laborers. By contrast, health care workers (especially nurses and physicians) have the lowest prevalence of substance abuse, while the lowest rates of alcoholism are among managers and professionals.

Employment. About 6 percent of employed adults (18 years of age and older) currently use drugs, compared with nearly 12 percent of the unemployed. However, since so many more people have jobs, about 71 percent of current drug users are employed.

Race. Nationally, about 74 percent of all drug users are white, 13 percent are African American, and 10 percent are Hispanic American. Nevertheless, the percentage of African Americans (6.8 percent) who use drugs is about the same as for Hispanic Americans (6.2 percent) and whites (5.5 percent).

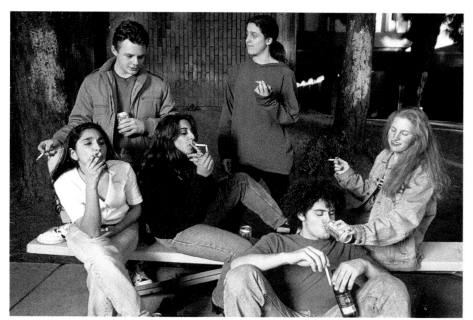

If you look carefully, you can detect two of the so-called "gateway drugs" being used by these young people. The traditional entry substances to drug-taking behavior are being used at increasingly younger ages, often beginning during middle school.

© Michael Newman/PhotoEdit

Sociocultural Influences

Whether youth-oriented television, movies, and concerts influence group and individual drug-taking behavior or merely reflect current practices, there is a growing impression that the "drug culture" is staging a strong return.[16] After more than ten years in which illegal psychoactive drugs were portrayed as demons, musical groups, television programs, movies, and even fashion apparel have recreated a popular culture that once again glorifies and promotes the use of psychoactive drugs, especially marijuana.

Because of such recent developments, the activities of the National Organization for the Reform of Marijuana Laws (NORML) have also increased, and despite a television advertising ban on tobacco products, scenes of cigarette smoking have actually increased in programming. Whether they are the forerunners of a "new age of drugs" or just a temporary reversal in the long-term trend of declining drug use, these current pro-drug happenings are not evidence of a successful "war on drugs."

Adolescence

Since individuals are not born as drug users, and nonmedical use of chemical substances during infancy and early childhood is still considered abnormal, the initial experimentation and subsequent, more regular patterns of drug use typically occur during adolescence. Moreover, the traditional entry substances to drug taking continue to be tobacco, alcohol, and marijuana—the so-called gateway drugs. However, the increasing popularity of "crack" cocaine has led to that drug's becoming a gateway drug, especially in impoverished urban communities.

Tobacco use usually begins by age 16.[17] Almost all first use occurs before graduation from high school. By contrast, most students are between 12 and 13 years old when they take their first alcoholic drink.[18] It is now apparent that the period of greatest risk for beginning the use of tobacco and alcohol is during early adolescence, often when children are entering junior high school. For too many youths, the use of alcohol and other drugs actually begins during the elementary school years.

Because experimentation with numerous chemical substances is commonly reported and experienced among adolescents, some authorities now believe that limited drug use is a "normal part" of growing up. For some, early experimental drug use is equated with "coming of age in America," a rite of passage marking one's entry into adulthood and departure from childhood.

Indeed, a recent study confirms the idea that drug experimentation can be a normal adolescent development and need not lead to long-term catastrophic consequences. Adolescents who had engaged in some drug experimentation were rated as the best adjusted; frequent users were maladjusted and marked by interpersonal alienation, poor impulse control, and evident emotional distress. By contrast, 18-year-old adolescents who had never experimented with any drug were described as anxious, emotionally constricted, and lacking in social skills.[19]

However, other research has demonstrated that the younger persons are when they first use a drug, including alcohol (outside the context of medical treatment and/or limited family or religious rituals), the more likely they are to have alcohol and other drug problems. Consequently, those who first use beverage alcohol in a peer setting at ages 12 to 13 are far more likely to have drug problems with alcohol than are young people who first use alcohol at age 21.[20]

The teen and preteen years are times of exploring new ideas, fast learning, and risk taking.[21] Young people exhibit an excessive drive in their pursuit of new and novel sensations and stimulation. Experimenting with an expanded range of behaviors and lifestyles is often viewed as part of the natural process of separating from parents and developing a sense of independence and personal identity. At the same time, adolescents tend to develop an increased sense of concern with their own appearance and abilities—described as "adolescent egocentrism." These two conditions make teenagers especially vulnerable to the influences of peer groups.

Young people often accept dares to try the untried, including mind-altering drugs if available. They are known for

table 2.1 Possible Risk Factors in the Use of Drugs Among Youth, According to Six Categories
(Not all factors listed have been consistently found to be risk factors)

Ecological Environment

Poverty Living in an economically depressed area with • high unemployment • inadequate housing • poor schools • inadequate health and social services	• high prevalence of crime • high prevalence of illegal drug use Minority status involving • racial discrimination • culture devalued in American society • differing generational levels of assimilation	• cultural and language barriers to getting adequate health care and other social services • low educational levels • low achievement expectations from society

Family Environment

Alcohol and other drug dependency of parent(s) Parental abuse and neglect of children Antisocial, sexually deviant, or mentally ill parents High levels of family stress, including financial strain Large, overcrowded family	Unemployed or underemployed parents Parents with little education Socially isolated parents Single female parent without family/other support Family instability High level of marital and family conflict and/or family violence	Parental absenteeism due to separation, divorce, or death Lack of family rituals Inadequate parenting and low parent/child contact Frequent family moves

Constitutional Vulnerability of the Child

Child of an alcohol or other drug abuser Less than 2 years between the child and its older/younger siblings	Birth defects, including possible neurological and neurochemical dysfunctions Neuropsychological vulnerabilities	Physically handicapped Physical or mental health problems Learning disability

Early Behavior Problems

Aggressiveness combined with shyness Aggressiveness Decreased social inhibition Emotional problems Inability to express feelings appropriately	Hypersensitivity Hyperactivity Inability to cope with stress Problems with relationships Cognitive problems	Low self-esteem Difficult temperament Personality characteristics of ego under-control; rapid tempo, inability to delay gratification, overreacting

Adolescent Problems

School failure and dropout At risk of dropping out Delinquency Violent acts	Gateway drug use Other drug use and abuse Early unprotected sexual activity Teenage pregnancy/teen parenthood	Unemployed or underemployed At risk of being unemployed Mental health problems Suicidal

Negative Adolescent Behavior and Experiences

Lack of bonding to society (family, school, and community) Rebelliousness and nonconformity Resistance to authority Strong need for independence	Cultural alienation Fragile ego Feelings of failure Present versus future orientation Hopelessness	Lack of self-confidence Low self-esteem Inability to form positive close relationships Vulnerability to negative peer pressure

Source: From the Office of Substance Abuse Prevention, U.S. Department of Health and Human Services.

their willingness to take risks; they have not yet mastered control over their impulses. Oriented to the here and now, many adolescents do not delay for very long the immediate satisfaction of needs or the resolution of frustration. Simply stated, many teenagers cannot tolerate frustration. The emphasis is on having fun now, not on the probable or possible future consequences related to using chemical substances. When confronted with the possibility of adverse effects due to using nonmedical drugs, adolescents tend to be underconcerned with such effects and overestimate their ability to avoid harmful, destructive patterns of drug and alcohol use. They are, after all, "ten feet tall and bullet-proof," as the saying goes. They may also begin to see the evident contradictions and inconsistencies in the arguments of parents and other authority figures who counsel against the use of mood-modifying substances.

In an attempt to prevent alcohol and other drug use among young people, possible risk factors have been studied for many years. **Risk factors** are conditions or characteristics that, when present, increase the probability of psychoactive drug use, although the presence of any one risk factor does not mean that drug use will, in fact, take place.

A recent study of possible risk factors, listed in table 2.1, showed that

1. early alcohol use was associated with early use of marijuana and with early cocaine use; and

2. delinquency—including running away from home, school truancy, fighting and violence, and theft—was significantly associated with the use of marijuana, the use of cocaine, and the use of both those drugs over time.[22]

Furthermore, this study concluded that poverty and inner-city residence are not, by themselves, risk factors for drug use by children. Of the many risk factors examined, researchers eventually concluded that no single factor or set of factors has been found to explain drug use. In all likelihood, drug use develops from the interaction of multiple risk factors and numerous combinations of risk factors that occur.

Curiosity

The thirst for new experiences has attracted more than just teenagers into the arena of drug use, sometimes with unexpected results. Nevertheless, the potential for partaking in the novel, the possibility for untried delights, and the promise of profound and unpredictable effects have lured many thousands to explore the world of the inner self—the uncharted wilderness of the psyche. Curiosity has been quite sufficient to entice some individuals into drug experimentation.

The much-publicized gurus and entertainment stars, aided by sensational media accounts of drug happenings and the lyrics of "acid" and "heavy-metal" rock, have raised the hopes and aspirations of many with the psychedelic gospel of salvation. In essence, curiosity feeds on the media's portrayal of both legal and illegal nonmedical drug use as an important part of becoming and staying popular, increasing one's sex appeal, and having a good time.

Of course, the prevalence of myths serves to heighten the allure of drugs, and makes the temptation to use mood modifiers almost irresistible. According to tradition and convenience more than fact, getting high is the greatest accomplishment, real men hold their liquor, cocaine makes a person sexy or sexier, chewing tobacco makes for better athletic performance, and a "downer drug" will solve all of life's problems. Natural curiosity and widely held myths are important elements in the initiation of drug use.

Personality and Coping

Coping is a term for various methods or techniques used to adjust—to accommodate to the demands of stress and daily living without being overwhelmed. One's general pattern of coping behaviors is known as one's *personality.*

Psychoactive drugs, especially alcohol, tobacco, and marijuana, are often used as a coping method in dealing with problems of personal identity, self-esteem, boredom, family discord, academic pressures, and chronic depression. In some instances, drug abuse is related to asserting independence or more simply a self-indulgent desire for well-being. In fact, various pills, booze, tobacco, and pot appear to resolve these stress-generating problems, at least temporarily. Mood modifiers, therefore, are convenient tools in the search for relief, escape, love, security, and power.

One of the dangers associated with any drug taken for coping purposes is that its prolonged use tends to undermine self-esteem and personal power. Temporary feelings of enhanced power, confidence, security, and even creativity are assigned to the drug rather than to the self. As the drug is credited for its beneficial effects, drug takers tend to confirm their own personal deficiencies and thereby prolong their dependence on chemicals. Now the drug takers are less powerful than the drug, and their feelings of personal adequacy plunge even lower. This situation results in more drug taking in an attempt to resolve personal inadequacy.

Such a scenario is described as the **addiction cycle.**[23] Elements of this cycle have been identified as follows.

1. Psychoactive drug use tends to eliminate pain and reduces personal awareness during a period of drug intoxication.

2. While escaping from the pain of uncomfortable feelings about self or the environment, the drug taker is less able to pay attention to problems or to deal with them constructively.

3. Without alcohol, barbiturates, tranquilizers, heroin, or other narcotics—frequent objects of addictions—the drug abuser experiences mental pain when thinking about his or her life.

4. The reduced self-regard, the personal disapproval, and the lowered self-esteem are sufficient to generate further use of drugs.

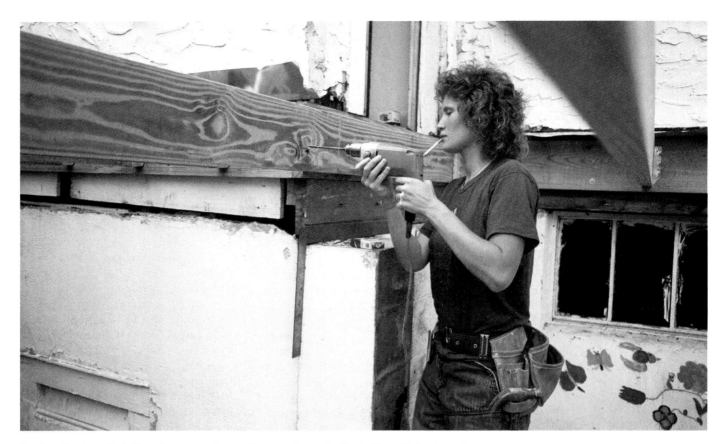

Psychoactive drugs, including tobacco, are often used as a coping method in dealing with the demands of daily living and high-stress jobs. Sometimes, such use leads to involvement in the addiction cycle.
© *Richard Hutchings/PhotoEdit*

Now the addiction cycle has been completed, but the individual is less able to deal with interpersonal, professional, or existential problems.

The addiction cycle suggests that a drug-dependent individual is addicted not to any particular drug, but to the effects a drug produces for a given person in specific circumstances.[24] Furthermore, this concept indicates that drug dependence is just as likely to occur with a "presentable" middle-class person as it is with a "ghetto resident."

Although the foregoing discussion has dealt with drug use in the search for personal and social adjustment, research also reveals that drug use may be a symptom of preexisting personality difficulties. In comparison with those who are not preoccupied with drugs, "consistent" or "convinced" drug users often display high novelty-seeking tendencies, high risk-taking behavior, and little or no need for praise or approval. Such individuals tend to be impulsive. They like to try exciting and dangerous things, and do not worry about the consequences of their high-risk behavior. Moreover, personality factors such as rebelliousness, orientation toward independence, low self-concept, alienation, and a high tolerance of deviance have also been related to drug use, especially among youth.[25]

Despite extensive studies linking various personality traits to a predisposition for heavy alcohol and other drug use as well as for addiction, no general "addictive personality" seems to exist.[26] Each addiction and each drug-use problem is different from the next; each individual's personality and drug-using circumstances differ from the next person's. Long-term surveys of drug use in normal populations further suggest that personality factors indicative of maladjustment usually precede the use of marijuana and other illegal drugs. Delinquent and deviant activities, as well as attitudes and values favorable to defiance, also occur before involvement with illicit drugs.

Escape to the inner self is one response of people who feel estranged from society and close friends. Surrounded by ugliness, confusion, and people who cannot be trusted or believed, the person undertakes a search for beauty, meaning, and truth—a search for God within. Self-encounter, with its intensity of feelings and emotions, is highly prized. Drugs might provide the ticket for such an adventure. The promised rewards are self-knowledge and experience of one's inner being.

An orientation to the here and now sometimes follows an exaggerated emphasis on the self as supreme and all-important. Without a meaningful past and unwilling to plan for an unknown and uncontrollable future, the modern person tends to focus on the here and now. Deferring gratification and working for some distant reward become counter-productive. The immediate experience is cherished; it is the only thing that matters; it is the only thing that can be grasped and held on to. The now experience is the hallmark of the now generation. Hedonism has ascended its throne. Enjoy yourself; it is later than you think! Have your pleasure; pay for it later! Maybe, if you are lucky, there will not be a later!

Changes and Conflicts in Society

It is true that the use of drugs has been related to their availability. Futurists predict persistent drug use in the next twenty years as the proliferation of new medications continues and the reservoir of misused and abused drugs expands with the aid of innovative designer drugs, adulterated substances, diverted pharmaceuticals, and the latest concoctions of "kitchen chemists."

The epidemic use of drugs has evolved into a type of **endemic drug use,** a situation in which a significant yet declining number of people engage in semitolerated forms of drug-taking behavior on a continuing basis. As such, endemic use of alcohol and other drugs will not likely disappear in America, where it has become something of a tradition.[27]

However, as with most social phenomena, drug use will likely persist, decline, or even increase as a consequence of several notable and predisposing forces:[28]

1. *The changing composition of the nation's population.* With fewer young people in proportion to the growing numbers of the elderly, the drug-abuse potential may actually decline while drug misuse and medication errors increase, as noted in chapter 1.

2. *The women's movement.* Females are adopting more behaviors previously defined as masculine. As women smoke more cigarettes and drink more alcoholic beverages, their incidence of lung cancer and alcoholism accelerates. With equality in the realm of socially approved drug use has come the gender-equal penalty of disease.

3. *The possibility of adverse economic conditions.* Declines in economic conditions carry the potential for future epidemics of drug abuse. Although the most recent epidemic began in the relative economic affluence of the 1960s, the upsurge of drug usage coincided with the social protest of the Vietnam War era. Will new economic depressions precipitate another increase in illicit drug use? If large numbers of individuals feel alienated from the greater society, because of unemployment and its consequences of depersonalization and dehumanization, they may seek comfort in psychoactive chemicals.

4. *The new emphasis on natural and healthful lifestyles.* As more individuals engage in health-promoting and disease-preventing activities, rates of drug misuse and abuse will likely decline. Fewer drugs will be consumed as negative attitudes toward them emerge.

Analysts also cite numerous changes and conflicts in society as contributing factors in the illegal and nonmedical use of drugs. The most frequently mentioned are these:

The irrelevancy of the past, with its structure, order, and controlling institutions of neighborhood, community, and church in an ever more transient society

Changes in family life, with less emphasis on permanence of relationship, marital fidelity, or the modeling, discipline, counseling, and educational functions of parenting

Confusion of appropriate adult roles, responsibilities, and value systems, coupled with the extension of the social and economic dependence of adolescence

Decline of the "work ethic," the need to achieve, the belief in self-restraint, accompanied by increased leisure time

Commercial messages of advertisers that tend to promote a theme of self-indulgence, not only for over-the-counter drugs but for all products in general

The gradual loss of privacy, the sense of community, and the ability to influence the social institutions, especially bureaucracy

An increase in permissiveness, normlessness, and individualism manifest in the philosophy of freedom to do "one's own thing"

Environmental deprivations, including poor housing, high rates of disease, and inadequate nutrition and education

Loss of confidence in and a growing disrespect for law among large segments of the population

Success increasingly measured in material terms, but for many the lack of opportunity for achieving success by legitimate means

Proliferation of superficial relationships and the ascent of rationality at the expense of human feelings and the life of emotions

Confronted by a confusing future, certain to be marked by more change and conflict, individuals respond to such crises with a variety of adjustive responses. Common options include constructive or destructive rebellion, regression and personality disorders, passive acceptance or passive withdrawal, and preoccupation with the experience of the present. Drug taking both accompanies and sometimes facilitates such responses. Predictably, psychoactive substances will remain available for various reasons—to promote social interactions, stimulate artistic creativity, enhance physical performance, treat illnesses, relieve pain, escape from boredom and stress, function in religious ceremonies, alter human moods, heighten pleasure, and satisfy the human needs to relax, delude, arouse, destroy, and fantasize.[29]

Heredity

Although genetic transmission is not considered a predisposing factor in the initiation of using psychoactive drugs, heredity is now thought to play a significant role in alcoholism, one of many drug dependencies and clearly a form of substance abuse.[30],[31] Recently, researchers established an association between a "dopamine receptor gene" and alcoholism.[32] While this initial association has not yet been supported by other research, such a finding indicates that an abnormality in a specific gene may cause susceptibility to at least one subtype of alcoholism. Although surprisingly strong, this genetic linkage has not been proven as causing alcoholism itself. Nevertheless, the development of alcoholism is not just a case of genetics versus the environment; it is definitely one of genetics *and* the environment.[33]

Precisely how **genetic predisposition** combines with environmental influences in the development of alcoholism has not yet been completely determined. The leading explanations center around specific variations in nerve cell or membrane function, sensitivity to alcohol's effects, and brain-wave patterns. Such inherited variations likely result in a neurochemical vulnerability to alcoholism.

While evidence of a genetic component in alcoholism has now been established, there is no direct indication so far that heredity is also a contributing factor in other forms of psychoactive drug abuse. However, genetics may be a determining factor in individual responsiveness to specific mood modifiers and other drugs as well. Such hereditary influences could explain why some people are more sensitive than other people to drug effects, and therefore more susceptible to certain drug dependencies.

There is also the possibility that some common genetic defect—perhaps a neurochemical deficiency—will be found to be the basis for all drug dependencies. If such a susceptibility is indeed inherited, then the absence of the basic neurochemical defect might suggest that some resistance to drug dependence is inherited too.

Enabling Factors in the Use and Abuse of Drugs

In this second category are those factors that enable, facilitate, or make possible drug-taking behavior and substance abuse.

Common enabling forces include the availability of both legal and illegal psychoactives, accessibility to various mood modifiers, actions of community and government agencies, and various skills or lack thereof possessed by the potential drug user or drug abuser.

Availability

It is often claimed that without drugs there would be no drug use or abuse. Certainly the presence of psychoactive drugs is an important enabling factor that allows people to engage in drug-taking behavior and sustain certain consequences of that behavior. For instance, while there is no evidence in the United States that a greater number of outlets selling beverage alcohol causes new drinking, several studies now indicate that a lower minimum drinking age does lead to greater accident and fatality rates among young people who have been drinking and driving.[34]

Despite a decade of decline in the casual use of psychoactive chemicals, mood- and behavior-modifying drugs are still plentiful and widely available to a broad cross section of society. Each year billions of gallons of beverage alcohol, billions of tobacco cigarettes, and at least three billion doses of illegal drugs are consumed for nonmedical reasons. And each year American drug problems remain at epidemic levels. Many people now believe that whenever the nonmedical use of mind-changing drugs in any society becomes significant, there will likely be significant drug problems.

Accessibility

Until thirty-five years ago, most persons, including the young, could easily obtain just three major psychoactive substances: alcohol, tobacco products, and intoxicating inhalants, such as gasoline and airplane glue. Numerous other legal and illegal mood modifiers were available, but use of such drugs was confined generally to small population subgroups. Young people did not usually have money to buy illegal drugs; strict parental supervision did not permit or allow drug usage, though beer drinking and cigarette smoking were often tolerated if not approved; and fear of getting caught by police officials was somewhat higher than today. In brief, most

people, especially the young, could not obtain illegal drugs even if they were available. Moreover, they did not feel a need to obtain such mind-altering substances.

Growing up safely and soberly is not quite so simple at present in America. Affluence has made expensive drugs obtainable, and expanded production and distribution have made them more affordable. If part- or full-time jobs are not adequate to finance the acquisition of drugs, then both young and old beg, borrow, pawn, steal, rob, or engage in some other criminal activity to get what they want or need. Liberated by more permissive parents and the automobile, teenagers are freed to seek out drugs—if "drug pushers" don't deliver in the neighborhood or at school.

Social and Institutional Deficiencies

Among the more subtle enabling factors in drug-taking behavior and substance abuse are the inadequacy of legal deterrence and the absence of drug-use standards or guides. Many people perceive the prohibitions and penalties associated with illegal drug use as largely ineffective. Getting caught is no longer viewed quite so negatively or as shameful; rather, it is commonly seen as an unfair intrusion into the private pursuit of happiness. The person who gets caught is merely unlucky and unfortunate. In fact, there is a relatively low risk of getting caught violating most drug-use laws today.

In addition, few guidelines have been adopted to bring social controls to drug-taking behavior. There appears to be continuing fear of doing cocaine, especially crack cocaine, but marijuana, smoked and snorted heroin, and LSD have resurfaced as drugs of choice, largely because their methods of use are considered safe ways to avoid transmission of the AIDS virus. Regarding alcohol, there is only a slowly evolving consensus about the meaning of reduced-risk use. Guidelines that discourage heavy consumption of alcohol, reject intoxication, and promote the social use of alcohol (rather binge drinking to get drunk) have attracted only a minority of all youthful drinkers.

Those who promote "responsible usage" of illegal drugs—responsible decisions and actions that could reduce many of the unwanted consequences of taking psychoactives—are criticized for encouraging general use of alcohol and other drugs or, at least, unlawful behavior. The prevailing attitude among the general public is that the individuals who use illegal psychoactives deserve all the difficulties they experience, and that they should be punished for criminal activity. Such a belief actually fosters many problems that usually accompany substance abuse—such as the need to build more jails and prisons in which to incarcerate drug offenders, thus raising taxes, and the higher level of HIV transmission that results when needle exchange programs are prohibited.

Personal and Professional Deficiencies

As research revealed the general ineffectiveness of drug education programs, it became apparent that most young people started using drugs because they had never acquired skills for dealing with peer pressure or feelings of personal and social insecurity. Children often feel that personal value and significance are measured by group conformity, which frequently includes taking drugs. Just as important, however, is the inadequacy of most people, especially children and teenagers, to say no to behavior they don't really want to engage in. Thus, young people are practically defenseless when interaction with psychoactive drugs becomes possible. They have no skills for resisting or avoiding drugs or achieving self-confidence without drugs. They just can't say no to drugs.

A little-discussed enabling factor that contributes to drug abuse is inadequate physician training and care of patients. Many who experience long-lasting pain, stress, or tension, as well as many "hidden" or undiscovered alcoholics, are treated with psychoactive therapeutic medications, particularly anti-anxiety medications and sedative-hypnotics. Without proper medical diagnosis and careful treatment management skills, physicians sometimes unwittingly promote chronic drug dependencies in their own patients.

Peculiar Effects of Drugs

Not to be overlooked as a decisive factor in the continuing use of specific psychoactive chemicals is the pharmacology (effects or actions) of drugs themselves. Drug users often persist in the use/abuse cycle because withdrawal symptoms and after-use depression are too severe to endure. Drugs are taken to avoid the drastic changes in physical functioning and behavior experienced in alcohol withdrawal, to feel normal again in heroin withdrawal, and to escape the post-high depression found in cocaine addicts deprived of their drug supply.

Others who are mentally impaired by the effects of drugs such as alcohol can no longer evaluate the seriousness of their problem-producing drinking behavior. They continue to drink because they no longer have control over the drug. Now the drug controls the user, and the substance abuse persists.

Enabling Process

In nearly every case of drug abuse, including alcoholism, the drug-dependent individual has a supporting cast of actors and actresses—essentials in most stage plays and theatrical performances. However, in this real-life drama, the supporting cast assumes the role of an *enabler*, who effectively protects the dependent person from the natural and logical consequences of drug abuse and thereby contributes to a worsening of the disease.

Usually, enabling behavior is well-intentioned, sincere, and motivated by a sense of love and loyalty. Fear, shame, and desire for family self-preservation are other motivations behind enabling. Through the enabling process, the many physical, social, occupational, and economic problems that tend to plague the dependent and his or her family are postponed, at least temporarily. But by softening the impact of these problems, and by preventing the occurrence of life crises that might lead the dependent into treatment, the enabler actually prolongs the disease of drug dependency.[35]

The enabler can be anyone who has a relationship with the dependent, such as child, parent, fellow worker, friend, neighbor, lover, or roommate. Even physicians, police, and judges sometimes function as enablers. Most frequently, though, the dependent's spouse is the primary enabler.

Enabling practices are many and varied, and they include "covering up" for the dependent's mistakes or negligence; making excuses; lying to protect the dependent; apologizing repeatedly for the dependent's erratic and sometimes bizarre behavior; and gradually taking over the dependent's responsibilities within the family. Additional enabling behaviors focus on denying that drug abuse is really a problem; avoiding situations and conflicts that might cause the dependent to use drugs again; minimizing the seriousness of the problems associated with the dependent's drug usage; rationalizing drug use so as to excuse the dependent's inappropriate behavior; attempting to control the amount of drug consumed; waiting and hoping that the drug problem will go away; and refusing to talk about drug use and abuse.[36]

While these enabling actions may seem irrational and illogical, the enabler most often perceives them as survival tactics. Such activities are rarely labeled as choices or alternatives; enablers often have no alternatives as they view the deteriorating condition of the dependent, the relationship with the dependent, or the family of the dependent. But by their own survival practices, enablers make possible, or facilitate, the continuing use and abuse of drugs. They reduce the likelihood of intervention by someone or some agency; they thereby postpone the dependent's entry into a treatment and rehabilitation program.

Reinforcing Factors in the Use and Abuse of Drugs

The third category of determinants having an impact on drug-taking behavior and substance abuse is the *reinforcing factors*. Among these are influences that generally encourage the continuation of drug use once it has begun, although they may in some instances be influential in initiating drug use. Specific reinforcing factors are the experience of pleasure or relief of pain resulting from using drugs (as noted in table 2.2); the realization of other beneficial functions of drug usage; the importance of peers in drug-taking behavior; and the impact of media advertising on the nonmedical use of psychoactive chemicals.

2.2 Perceived Desirable and Other Effects, Duration of Effects, and the Drug Enforcement Administration's View of Risk of Dependence of Selected Illegal Psychoactive Drugs

| Drug Type | Short-Term Effects | | Duration of Acute Effects | DEA View of Risk of Dependence |
	Desired	Other		
Heroin	• Euphoria • Pain reduction	• Respiratory depression • Nausea • Drowsiness	• 3 to 6 hours	• Physical—high • Psychological—high
Cocaine	• Excitement • Euphoria • Increased alertness, wakefulness	• Increased blood pressure • Increased respiratory rate • Nausea • Cold sweats • Twitching • Headache	• 1 to 2 hours	• Physical—possible • Psychological—high
Crack Cocaine	• Same as cocaine • More rapid high than cocaine	• Same as cocaine	• About 5 minutes	• Same as cocaine
Marijuana	• Euphoria • Relaxation	• Accelerated heartbeat • Impairment of perception, judgment, fine motor skills, and memory	• 2 to 4 hours	• Physical—unknown • Psychological—moderate
Amphetamines	• Euphoria • Excitement • Increased alertness, wakefulness	• Increased blood pressure • Increased pulse rate • Insomnia • Loss of appetite	• 2 to 4 hours	• Physical—possible • Psychological—high
LSD	• Illusions and hallucinations • Excitement • Euphoria	• Poor perception of time and distance • Acute anxiety, restlessness, sleeplessness • Sometimes depression	• 8 to 12 hours	• Physical—none • Psychological—unknown

Source: Modified from the National Institute on Drug Abuse.

Another factor in drug use and abuse, the influence of the family, is usually described as a reinforcing determinant. However, in a concluding section of this chapter, we will examine the role of the family as predisposing and enabling, as well as reinforcing, drug-taking behavior and substance abuse.

Pleasure

According to one theory of learning, behavior is controlled by its consequences. Therefore, an activity followed by a positive event will be strengthened or maintained, while an activity followed by an unpleasant event will be weakened or eliminated.[37] This learning theory (operant conditioning) can also be used to help explain why people use drugs on a continuing basis.

Those consequences that strengthen or maintain drug-taking behavior are referred to as *reinforcers*. When a so-called positive stimulus, such as feeling good or getting high, is added to a marijuana-smoking situation, and when the pleasure and enjoyment serve to maintain the "pot-puffing," the condition is described as *positive reinforcement*. And when a so-called negative stimulus, such as reduction of tension or pain, is removed from an alcohol-drinking situation, but the relief experienced also maintains the drinking behavior, the condition is referred to as *negative reinforcement*. Thus, the consequences of drug-taking can function as either positive or negative reinforcers, both of which serve to maintain or increase the likelihood of repeated drug use.

While negative reinforcers are often described as contributing to "relief or escape drinking," too few people seem willing to associate enjoyment, euphoria, and delights—the essence of pleasure—with drug taking. This is certainly the case with adolescent drug use. Perhaps many adults assume that young people already have more than their fair share of pleasure. Why should they need more? And yet the pleasurable effects associated with psychoactive drug use are certainly potent **drug reinforcers** of drug-taking behavior among both young people and adults. The short-term effects of drugs produced soon after taking them will increase the likelihood of their repeated use, provided the experience is rewarding either personally or socially or both.

The varieties of drug-derived fun or pleasure are many. There can be experiences of inner peace, tranquility, joyous delight, relaxation, serenity; kaleidoscopic perceptions; surges of exhilaration; and heightened and prolonged physical sensations. The universality of these pleasurable appeals has been acknowledged throughout history as a general explanation for most nonmedical drug use.

For any behavior, the more rapidly a reward or pleasant experience follows the particular activity, and the more often such behavior is rewarded, the stronger the learning or habit becomes. And the use of psychoactive drugs is no exception to this general rule. If a drug is injected or inhaled, the reinforcement occurs rapidly, leading to the development of a strong habit. On the other hand, if the drug is short-acting and must be used frequently each day, there are many occasions for reinforcement or learning of drug-taking behavior. If the drug used is also one that

causes physical dependence, the motivation for repeated use is established firmly in the fear of experiencing the discomfort of withdrawal.[38] Originally taken to experience pleasure, the drug is now used to avoid pain, a powerful motivating force.

Functional Aspects of Using Drugs

Sometimes overlooked as reinforcing and rewarding the persistent use of psychoactives is the fact that these chemicals can help people to accomplish certain tasks perceived as desirable. For instance, amphetamines can help students to stay awake all night to cram for a test. Stimulants have also been used to extend the performance of truck drivers and improve the physical ability and reaction time of athletes. Painkillers have been most effective in reducing the discomfort of injury and disease. Sedatives help people to achieve a drug-assisted sleep. Tranquilizers calm the anxious person.

Those who seek to improve their sexual performance and enjoyment have often resorted to certain psychoactive drugs for their alleged **aphrodisiac** effects. Cocaine and Ecstasy are chemical substances often believed to be endowed with such hoped-for powers. Alcohol has long been valued as a "sexual enhancer." As Ogden Nash once observed: "Candy is dandy but liquor is quicker." In practice, however, most people find that Shakespeare's reference to alcohol is more accurate: alcohol provokes and unprovokes lust; alcohol provokes the desire, but it takes away the performance. Too much alcohol actually prevents a male's erection and a female's orgasmic response.

Presently, there is no scientific evidence supporting the belief that marijuana has any physical aphrodisiac effect. Recent studies suggest that among some males there is a temporary but definite lowering of the male sex hormone in the blood following use of marijuana. A loss of sexual interest is likely. But due to marijuana's effect on one's memory, sense of time, and attention span, some marijuana smokers believe that it increases one's sexual enjoyment. Of course, the socially communicated and strongly held belief in such a positive sexual effect is likely to have psychological substantiation. The placebo effect—believing that something will happen—is most powerful when supported by myth.

Of course, the passivity of certain drug experiences may help others avoid the potential embarrassment of an unwanted or undesirable sexual encounter, or even the necessity of any sexual activity.

LSD and other psychedelic drugs have also been used to search for greater insight, personal understanding, awareness of subconscious thoughts, and creativity—evidence of mind expansion. Some people have turned to drugs to forget the past and escape the present temporarily, to keep going, to keep from going crazy, or to keep from committing suicide. Still other alcoholics and drug addicts seem to be attracted to their psychoactives because of who they are and what their personalities find attractive and comforting. Drugs offer the troubled abuser a temporary refuge, a way of organizing his or her defective, lonely, and frightening life.[39] In this sense, drugs make whole the minds, hearts, and bodies of broken people, at least until the drugs lose their ability to give addicts a feeling of being put back into one piece again.

Social and Peer-Group Aspects

It is probable that the more popular psychoactive chemicals—alcohol, tobacco cigarettes, and marijuana—are used both initially and continually thereafter as **social drugs.** As such, they are vehicles that help people better enjoy the company of others. While the adoption and repeated use of mood modifiers are related to their ability to enrich social intercourse, their distribution to others is often a form of social exchange, a learning phenomenon, or a rite of passage.

In recreational or social settings, the power of **peer-group influence** is considerable among friends and acquaintances. This is particularly true for adolescents and young adults who have doubts about their own identity and are concerned with affiliation. Often they willingly conform to group norms and participate in activities chosen by their peers. For lonely and emotionally isolated young people in need of belonging to something or someone, the only thing they have to do is smoke, drink, or take other drugs. Thus, drug-using groups are easy to join. Drug taking becomes symbolic of group identification. Coparticipation in an activity that is both secret and illegal often fosters a bond of conspiracy that further cements such interrelationships and enables the continuation of alcohol and other drug abuse.

There is now widespread agreement that association with alcohol- and other drug-using peers during adolescence is one of the strongest predictors of adolescent alcohol and other drug use.[40] The influence of peers is especially powerful for beginning the use of tobacco cigarettes and marijuana. When friendship and friendship groups revolve around the use of mind-changing drugs, however, nonusing peers do not generally fit in. In fact, alcohol- and other drug-using peers are usually intolerant of or uninterested in pursuing friendships with nonusing peers.[41]

While communal use of drugs sometimes unites and promotes social exchange, it also accomplishes another function for youths—isolation of the group from the world of reality. Drugs can also serve to protect and insulate youths from adults, a function also performed sometimes by the unintelligible language of slang terms.

Recognizing peer-group influence in the promotion of illegal drugs, observers often compare the spread of drugs from person to person as a form of communicable disease. Thus, we now have a new interpretation of the traditional social diseases.

Advertising and Media Programming

The promised benefits of taking drugs are familiar. They include a change in pace or mood, relief from tension and boredom, a pickup to combat fatigue, the promotion of sleep, or just plain fun. Such benefits also are frequently cited in the appeals of television commercials, as is well known even by preschoolers. Such beliefs are also portrayed on television and in motion pictures where characters drink alcoholic beverages more frequently than people in real-life situations do. A typical American adolescent is exposed to approximately three thousand acts of drinking per year through television alone, according to the federal Office of Substance Abuse Prevention. These repeated exposures to the modeled behavior of athletes and former athletes, rock stars, television celebrities, and other attractive people are likely to result in behavioral change, if social learning theory is valid. Advertisers are banking on it!

Advertising The invitation to drug use comes not only where over-the-counter psychoactives, beers, and wines are touted, but also in newspapers and magazines and on outdoor billboards, where distilled spirits and tobacco products are advertised widely. Presently, the distilled spirits industry voluntarily withholds advertising of "hard" liquors on commercial television (but not from cable television), and the tobacco industry is restricted by law from promoting cigarettes and smokeless tobacco on TV.

Because of the likely influence of advertising on young and impressionable people, health authorities have proposed a ban on all television beer ads. Others have advocated the total prohibition of all media advertising of alcoholic beverages. Supporters of such restrictions are particularly concerned about the inappropriate portrayal of drinking while driving or pregnant. The underlying messages of the alcohol advertising are (1) that use of these products is risk-free and (2) that alcoholic beverages are normal and essential parts of social events. In other words, you can't have a good time unless you drink, and if you drink, you can always have a good time!

Product advertising is often defended as the voice of free choice and the only way manufacturers can win consumers away from competing brands. But as critics maintain, the advertising of beverage alcohol also tends to

glamorize alcohol use and give a one-sided view without providing information about the likely, adverse consequences, such as combining alcoholic beverages with auto racing

associate drinking alcoholic beverages, especially beer, with various professional sports teams and former well-known athletes, supposedly conveying approval of consumption by important role models

recruit new first-time drinkers—including young people—by making sweeter drinks (fruit-flavored wine coolers) that will be more acceptable and pleasing from the very first sip, and by the clever use of lovable "party animals" as the focus of the commercials

target "powerless people," such as minorities, women, and people of color (such as African Americans and Hispanic Americans) by promising them power, sexual attractiveness, and achievement

attract underage college males to beer consumption by encouraging "drinking marathons" during spring break, and by advocating "sure-fire ways to scam babes" through various drinking practices

convey the message that drinking is the key to fun and sexual success

In the face of declining sales to an ever-declining market of domestic smokers, cigarette makers also advertise widely in the print media, but not on television. Some national and regional sporting events are also supported by manufacturers of tobacco products. Not content with emphasizing traditional themes of success, romance, adventure, or just having fun, at least one major cigarette maker has subtly encouraged sexism and law-breaking.[42] Not only did this example of advertising encourage male violence—a possible prelude to rape—through "smooth moves" (grabbing a women out of the water, dragging her back to the shore, the more she kicks and screams, the better); the same ad implicitly tells underage boys how they can get free cigarettes by having friends redeem coupons that came with the ad. In addition, the same ad also advises "breaking the ice by offering her a cigarette."

Although a causal link between drug advertising and drug abuse has not been established with any degree of certainty, it is assumed that such ads do influence the heavier use of drugs among the general public. Apparently, the billions of dollars spent each year by alcohol and tobacco manufacturers to promote their products is certain proof that they believe advertising is a cost-effective method of attracting customers. There is now a consensus that massive and persistent advertising for over-the-counter drugs has taught both young and older Americans that pills and potions are the answer to just about every health problem—real or imagined.

One observer, who defines addiction basically as a need for something that gives the feeling of completeness, raises a further condemnation of advertising: We are smart enough not to believe in the ridiculous claims of individual ads, but can we escape their underlying message that only by buying or taking something into our bodies can we be made whole and healthy? Do we have any reasonable complaint about the amount of addiction in society when we teach it every day through sponsored ads in the mass media?[43] Nothing fulfills our love for the quick fix better than drugs—legal as well as illegal.

Television Programming and Movie Scripts

Surveys of television programs indicate that the average young person will be exposed to thousands of drinking episodes annually, and an increasing number of cigarette-smoking instances, through television. Critics of such gratuitous advertising contend that the frequency of alcohol and cigarette use in television programs exaggerates the prevalence of drinking and smoking in the real population and conveys the impression that everyone is either "bending the elbow" or "lighting up." In these instances, television is purveying norms that do not reflect American drinking and smoking practices.

Many of the circumstances in which drinking is portrayed on television deliver other messages that are also incomplete and basically inaccurate. Too often, drink-

ing is pictured as consequence free. As described by the Office for Substance Abuse Prevention, it is not uncommon for a television or movie hero to "put a few drinks away" and then rush off in a sports car. No questions asked and no harm done. In addition, television and movie characters frequently use alcohol to reduce tension in uncomfortable or frustrating situations. As a consequence, young people learn the value of "relief drinking"—that alcohol can lessen pain or discomfort.

What viewers do not learn is the fact that, in the long run, such relief drinking lessens neither discomfort and unhappiness nor frustration. Screenwriters tend to have greater artistic leeway and they are more likely to depict characters who use illegal drugs in a casual and, once again, risk-free manner.

The Family's Influence on Drug Abuse

Initially, drug abuse appears to be a problem of adolescence. As already indicated, psychoactive chemicals are often employed in coping with the process of growing up and achieving personal identity and autonomy.

It is common knowledge that children of smokers tend to smoke themselves. If parents drink and take pills to

escape personal problems, to feel better, or to have a "good time," their children may grow up to believe that mood modification is the appropriate solution to disappointments and other forms of stress. This relationship between parental drug-taking behavior and that of their children is referred to as **modeling.**

Although an adolescent's first use of legal alcohol and cigarettes and illegal marijuana is mainly a social phenomenon with heavy peer-group influence, research demonstrates a striking relationship between parent-child interaction and the use of *other illegal drugs*. It is concluded that more serious drug involvement is predominantly a family affair, but not necessarily based on parental modeling.[44]

According to research, the typical family with an adolescent drug abuser is one in which one parent is intensely involved with the abuser, while the other is more punitive, distant, and/or absent. Usually, the overinvolved, indulgent, overprotective parent is of the opposite sex of the abuser.

The drug-abusing offspring may serve a function for the parents, either as a channel for their communication or as a disrupter whose distracting behavior keeps their own fights from materializing. On the other hand, the drug abuser may assume a "sick" state in order to position himself, like a child, as the focus of the parents' attention.

Selected Theories on Drug Abuse and Drug Dependence

box 2.3

Agent-Related Theories and Etiological Factors

The term *agent* refers to the psychoactive drug.

According to the *disease model of chemical dependence,* the major theory under this category, the drug itself causes drug abuse and drug dependence. Taking enough drugs for a long enough time will eventually lead to psychological dependence, tolerance, and physical dependence evidenced by withdrawal symptoms.

Specific psychoactive drugs cause specific long-lasting effects in the body that in turn cause or lead to drug addiction or drug dependence. While many people drink alcoholic beverages supposedly to relieve depression, in reality alcohol as well as

heroin can cause serious depression. Although people use cocaine and amphetamines to feel stimulated, these particular drugs can induce mania in people with the mental problem known as manic-depression, a bipolar (having two extremes) disorder.

At the cellular level, there is a change or adaptation within the nerve cells and other body cells and organs in response to the toxic effects of psychoactive drugs. Such changes then lead to alterations in drug metabolism, sensitivity to a drug's effects, and eventually to tolerance and physical dependence with a variety of withdrawal symptoms.

Host-Related Theories and Etiological Factors

The term *host* refers to the person who takes the drug. Within that individual, there is some predisposition or unusual condition that makes that person particularly susceptible to the effects of a psychoactive drug, including drug abuse and/or drug dependence.

Foremost in this category is the *genetic theory,* which proposes either a specific "alcoholism gene" or other "drug-specific gene" that places an individual at increased risk for inheriting a psychoactive substance-abuse or dependence disorder. Another interpretation of the genetic theory is that an individual inherits not one or more specific dependency-producing genes, but, rather, certain genetic factors that combine with a heavy-drug-using environment, which in turn produces a greater chance or risk of taking large amounts of any particular drug.[‡] These genetic factors may include the absence of any inherited biochemical protection from drug dependence, an exaggerated and sometimes opposite response to a particular drug, an abnormal brain-wave pattern that disables a person from correctly identifying certain stimuli or recognizing the effects of a certain drug, and alteration of specific brain chemicals or neurotransmitters.

A general *biological theory* suggests that some genetically determined or even noninherited biophysical or biochemical condition exists that forms the basis of drug dependency. Such factors may include a faulty enzyme system that results in altered metabolism and the production of a commonly addictive compound at the cellular level, an imbalance of endocrine gland functioning, and a shortage or depletion of morphine-like brain chemicals known as endorphins.

A comprehensive *psychological theory* advances the importance of drug use and drug abuse as learned behaviors based on the stimulus-response mechanism. For some people, due in part to genetic influences, specific drugs may be differentially reinforcing (that is, function as either positive or negative reinforcers). Others may have developed unique reactions to stress, unreasonable expectations about a drug's ability to have positive effects, or limited coping skills that impel them to use drugs to reduce or eliminate pain, anxiety, helplessness, and even shame. Despite the failure to identify common personality characteristics for all drug abusers and drug-dependent individuals, some investigators still characterize such people as disorganized, problem-prone, undercontrolled,

---

The onset of adolescence, with its threat of losing the teenager to outsiders, initiates parental panic. Then, the family becomes stuck at this developmental stage. A chronic, repetitive process sets in, centered on the individuation, growing up, and leaving of the "identified" patient. In order for the family to maintain its "perceived" stability, all members conspire to keep the drug abuser in a dependent, incompetent role.

Thus, drug taking serves the dual function of simultaneously letting the offspring be distant, independent, and individuated, while at the same time making him or her dependent, in need of money

and sustenance, and loyal to the family. In such cases, one of the most effective means of maintaining family homeostasis is to interfere with the drug-abuser's treatment.

A cluster of distinguishing factors for drug-abusing families appears to include the following:

1. A higher incidence of multigenerational chemical dependency—especially alcohol among males

2. A greater prevalence of other addictionlike behaviors, such as gambling and watching television continuously

3. More primitive and direct expressions of conflict, with open alliances between the drug abuser and the overinvolved parent

4. The existence of a peer group or subculture to which the drug abuser retreats following family conflict

5. Mothers who display "symbiotic" child-rearing practices further into the life of the offspring than do mothers of "normal" children

6. A preponderance of death themes and premature, unexpected, or untimely deaths within the family

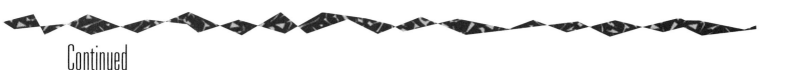

Continued

impulsive, and sensation-seeking. Some personality types, especially the antisocial and the borderline, appear to be highly susceptible to drug dependence.

The last major host-related theory, the *psychiatric disorders theory,* suggests that severe mental illness causes drug abuse and drug dependence. People with such mental problems use and abuse drugs for purposes of self-medication. However, impaired

judgment may make such individuals more susceptible to substance abuse. It is well known that anxious and panicked individuals will self-medicate with sedative drugs, impulsive people sometimes use opioids, and the depressed resort to stimulant use. With or without a preexisting psychiatric disorder, people will use various drugs in order to feel normal again and to avoid real or imagined pain—physical as well as psychological.

Environment-Related Theories and Etiological Factors

The term *environment* refers to the sociocultural setting and all the external circumstances and interrelational settings in which a psychoactive drug is used.

In this category is *social learning theory* again, but the emphasis here is on the modeling influences of parents and even peers, who sometimes teach or convey the idea that drug abuse is an acceptable way of solving problems or an expected and rewarded behavior. Some authorities firmly believe that addicted parents cannot help but teach addiction to their children. Individuals often learn that they are not held responsible for their behaviors while intoxicated, or that drinking and drugging are appropriate ways of coping with environmental stressors.

According to the *cultural theory,* some groups not only approve of huge consumption of alcoholic beverages as proof of maturity or manhood or having been accepted into a particular group or occupation, but also subtly encourage relief drinking as a common way to deal with anxiety. Both practices are conducive to problem drinking and alcohol dependence. Other aspects of this theory emphasize the absence of clear guidelines for low-risk use of certain psychoactive drugs as well as the lack of socially acceptable

alternatives to drinking and drugging as ways of relieving tension and boredom. Many drug problems result from these cultural deficiencies and the ambivalence sometimes associated with using alcohol and perhaps marijuana.

Another major explanation, the *environmental stress theory,* suggests that negative life events, such as the death of a loved one, prolonged unemployment, financial loss, or dysfunctional or violent family life, all contribute to stress. Though induced in the external environment, the stress is internalized and results in changes in specific brain chemicals or neurotransmitters. Such changes thus make the affected person more susceptible to drug abuse and drug dependence.

Because some individuals lack opportunities, abilities, or hope of achieving some goal or ideal, they may develop serious feelings of despair or even depression. The *alienation theory* states that deprived people, living in the midst of affluence or some other favorable circumstance but unable to participate in, or disabled from participating in, such desirable conditions, feel estranged from the greater society and turn to alcohol and other drugs for consolation.

‡Marc A. Schuckit, "A Clinical Model of Genetic Influences in Alcohol Dependence," *Journal of Studies on Alcohol* 55 (1994): 5–17.

While other factors—environmental, physiological, economic, conditional, and genetic, for example—probably play a critical role in the origin of drug abuse, the importance of the family in the genesis of drug problems should not be minimized.

Theories on Drug Abuse and Drug Dependence

The foregoing observations, concepts, and descriptions have provided some insight into the causes, or **etiology,** of alcohol and other drug use and abuse. Numerous etiological factors have been examined within a

framework of predisposing, enabling, and reinforcing determinants. However, many scientists and drug-abuse therapists are not quite satisfied that they really know why people continue to use drugs in ways that are often personally and socially destructive. Consequently, researchers have formulated various models and theories that explain, wholly or in part, the underlying causes of drug abuse and drug dependence, sometimes referred to as addiction. These numerous theories (educated speculations) are presented in box 2.3.

Notice that the several theories are categorized under three major public health headings or models, each representing an important though contrasting class

of etiological factors. The first heading deals with the so-called *agent,* in this case the psychoactive drug. According to this agent-based model, abuse and dependence have an **agent-related etiology:** psychoactive drugs themselves cause drug abuse and drug dependence or addiction. Often known as the disease model of chemical dependence, the basics of this particular theory propose that most everyone who takes one or more psychoactive drugs long enough and in large enough amounts will likely develop drug abuse and/or drug dependence.

In the second major category are theories of **host-related etiology,** which explain drug abuse and drug dependence as the result of some predisposition or unusual condition within the so-called *host,* that is, the person who takes the drug. Whether it is genetics (genetic theory), or faulty metabolism of drugs (biological theory), or failure to have learned appropriate coping skills or having learned addictive behaviors (psychological theory), or the development of a psychiatric disorder, something within the individual makes that person especially vulnerable to drug abuse and/or drug dependence.

The last major category is identified as **environment-related etiology,** including those etiological factors operating in the drug taker's external circumstances, experiences, and interrelational settings. Factors external to the drug taker and other than the drug itself are considered as impelling the individual into drug abuse and eventually drug dependence. Some of the theories identified in this category are social learning theory (with its emphasis on modeling influences), sociocultural theory, and environmental stress theory (which views individuals as seeking escape from the harshness of their surroundings through mood-changing drugs).

In each of the three categories, some theories focus on specific causative factors or forces. However, many authorities now believe that two or more factors from two or more categories interact in rather complex ways to result in drug abuse and drug dependence. It is probable that both heredity and environment combine in some as yet undefined way in a psychologically unique and susceptible individual who uses a psychoactive drug in a particular social setting. And from such an intricate combination the conditions of drug abuse and drug dependence develop. Such combination theories are sometimes called **multifactorial** or multifaceted—having many possible causative or contributing factors.

Chapter Summary

1. Drug-taking behavior is likely the result of many interrelated factors. Moreover, a consensus exists that the influences that initiate nonmedical use of drugs are usually quite different from those that produce extended drug abuse.

2. Mood modification (change in consciousness) is probably the primary reason people take psychoactive drugs. In fact, drug use often originates in the search for pleasure or relief from pain.

3. Youth often take drugs in imitation of adults, many of whom are convinced that an appropriate drug treatment exists for every ailment.

4. Youth rebellion, often viewed as a contributing factor in the drug-abuse epidemic of the 1960s, was both a rejection of traditional values and a generational conflict between parents and children. By contrast, much of today's drug abuse is likely motivated by the pursuit of recreation and the pleasure principle.

5. An analysis of drug-taking behavior reveals a framework of predisposing influences (that make the individual susceptible), enabling influences (that facilitate initial use and abuse), and reinforcing influences (that encourage continuing drug use and abuse).

6. Predisposing factors in drug-taking behavior include demographics, sociocultural factors, and aspects of adolescence, including experimentation, egocentrism, risk taking, and impulsivity. Low self-esteem and social confidence, the need for peer approval, and the tendency to overestimate the ability to avoid destructive drug use also predispose the adolescent to use of drugs.

7. Basic curiosity about the new and novel, and the widespread prevalence of myths about the desirability of using drugs, predispose people to initiating drug use.

8. Use of psychoactive drugs often reflects basic personality factors and represents attempts to cope with problems of personal identity, self-esteem, boredom, and assertion of independence.

9. A unique and somewhat controversial concept is that of the "addiction cycle," in which a drug-dependent individual is addicted more to the effects of a particular drug than to the drug or chemical itself. For instance, when taking drugs to cope with stress, the user credits the drug for its beneficial effects. However, in doing so, the drug taker confirms his or her own inadequacy and lack of independence and power.

10. Epidemic (sudden increase) and endemic (widespread prevalence over a continuing time period) drug use are influenced by changes in the national population, the women's liberation movement, adverse economic conditions, and numerous alterations and conflicts in American society.

11. Enabling factors in drug taking include the widespread availability of psychoactives; accessibility of mood modifiers made possible by affluence and parental permissiveness; ineffectiveness of legal deterrence; and lack of social controls, including guidelines for responsible use of drugs. Additional enablers are the lack of defensive skills in saying no to drugs; the mismanagement of patients by physicians; the pharmacology of addicting (dependency-producing) drugs; and the actions of enablers.

12. Reinforcing factors in drug use and abuse are the experience of pleasure, the fact that psychoactive drugs often help people accomplish tasks perceived as desirable, the influence of peer groups, and the impact of drug advertising in the media and television programming.

13. The family's influence in the use and abuse of drugs can be viewed as predisposing, enabling, and also reinforcing. Of importance are parental modeling and the nature of parent-child interactions. The typical family with a teenage drug abuser has one parent intensely involved with the abuser, while the other is more punitive, distant, and/or absent. The drug-abusing child serves as a

communication channel for the parents or as a disrupter of family stability. On the other hand, the drug abuser may seek a "sick state" in order to focus parental interest on himself or herself.

14. Theories of drug abuse and drug dependence are considered under three major classifications: those that are related to the agent (the drug itself), those that are related to the host (the drug taker), and those that are related to the environment (the sociocultural setting). While these theories provide differing explanations, some authorities now suggest a multifactorial approach to the etiology of drug abuse and drug dependence.

Review Questions and Activities

1. Define the term *mood modification*.

2. Distinguish between the concepts of increased awareness and decreased awareness.

3. Explain how socially defined attitudes, values, and behaviors concerning drugs influence the current drug problem.

4. What are some possible effects on individuals and society due to the widely held belief that an effective drug exists for every ailment?

5. Discuss the importance of adult drug-taking behavior, youthful rebellion against the establishment, and the pursuit of recreation and pleasure in the occurrence of drug abuse in young people.

6. Distinguish among the following terms related to drug-taking behavior: *predisposing factors, enabling factors,* and *reinforcing factors.*

7. Why does experimental use of psychoactive drugs so often occur during the adolescent stage of human development?

8. Explain how psychoactive drugs used as coping mechanisms can result in decreased self-esteem and diminished feelings of personal power.

9. What psychological characteristics commonly describe the individual likely to become preoccupied with drugs?

10. What changes and/or conflicts in society are currently operating to influence the usage of psychoactive drugs in America?

11. How do the factors of availability and accessibility enable or facilitate drug use and abuse?

12. In what specific ways do the effects of addicting drugs contribute to the continuing use and abuse of psychoactive substances?

13. In what ways are psychoactive drugs reinforcers of drug-taking behavior?

14. Explain how some of the functional uses of psychoactive drugs could lead to serious difficulties.

15. In what specific psychological aspects are young people often vulnerable to the power of peer-group influence in the recreational use of drugs?

16. Survey television, radio, and newsprint media for three days and record the number, type, and relative appeal of drug-related commercials. What message or messages are being conveyed in these commercials about drug use?

17. Discuss the potential role of family life in the origin of drug-abuse problems.

18. Using the major factors under the categories of predisposing, enabling, and reinforcing determinants, rank-order the causes of or influences on drug use and abuse from the most important to the least important. Compare your rank-ordered list with those of other class members and discuss similarities and differences in the lists.

19. What major factors are used in box 2.3 to categorize various theories on drug abuse and drug dependence? Which major category of etiological factors appears to be the most significant causative force?

References

1. Sidney Cohen, "Substance Abuse: Initiation and Perpetuation," in *Substance Abuse Problems* (New York: Haworth Press, 1985), 219–23.

2. Andrew Weil and Winifred Rosen, *From Chocolate to Morphine,* rev. ed. (Boston: Houghton Mifflin, 1993), 14.

3. Ronald K. Siegel, *Intoxication: Life in Pursuit of Artificial Paradise* (New York: E. P. Dutton, 1989), 10, 207–27, 313.

4. Weil and Rosen, *From Chocolate to Morphine,* 15.

5. Morris E. Chafetz, *Liquor: The Servant of Man* (Boston: Little, Brown, 1965), 150–74.

6. Joel Fort, as profiled in Edwin Kiester, Jr., "The Man from Help," *Human Behavior* (August 1973): 56.

7. Frank R. Scarpitti and Susan K. Datesman, "Introduction," in *Drugs and the Youth Culture,* ed. F. R. Scarpitti and S. K. Datesman (Beverly Hills, Calif.: Sage, 1980), 10.

8. Ibid.

9. Ivan Illich, "Medical Nemesis," in *The Nation's Health,* ed. P. Lee, N. Brown, and I. Red (San Francisco: Boyd & Fraser, 1981), 78.

10. Mark S. Gold, with Michael Boyette, *Wonder Drugs: How They Work* (New York: Simon & Schuster, 1987), 18.

11. Goerge M. Carstairs, "A Land of Lotus-Eaters?" *American Journal of Psychiatry* 125 (May 1969): 1578.

12. Lawrence W. Green and others, *Health Education Planning: A Diagnostic Approach* (Palo Alto, Calif.: Mayfield, 1980), 68–76.

13. "Who Uses What: Drug Use by Occupation," *Substance Abuse Report* 24, no. 8 (15 April 1993): 4.

14. Andrew Treno, Robert Parker, and Harold Holder. "Understanding U.S. Alcohol Consumption with Social and Economic Factors: A Multivariate Series Analysis, 1950–1986," *Journal of Studies on Alcohol* 54, no. 2 (1993): 146–56.

15. Kathleen Bucholz, "Alcohol Abuse and Dependence from a Psychiatric Perspective, *Alcohol Health and Research World* 16, no. 2 (1992): 197–208.

16. John Leland, "Just Say Maybe," *Newsweek,* 1 November 1993, 51–54.

17. Office on Smoking and Health, *Preventing Tobacco Use among Young People: A Report of the Surgeon General—At a Glance* (Atlanta: Centers for Disease Control and Prevention, 1994), 1.

18. Office of the Inspector General, *Youth and Alcohol: A National Survey (Drinking Habits, Access, Attitudes, and Knowledge)* (Washington, D.C.: Department of Health and Human Services and the National Clearinghouse for Alcohol and Drug Information, 1991), 4.

19. Jonathan Shedler and Jack Block, "Adolescent Drug Use and Psychological Health," *American Psychologist* 45, no. 5 (May 1990): 612–30.

20. Robert Dupont, ed., *Stopping Alcohol and Other Drug Use before It Starts: The Future of Prevention,* Office for Substance Abuse Prevention Monograph No. 1, DHHS Publication No. ADM–89–1645 (Washington, D.C.: U.S. Government Printing Office, 1989), 3.

21. Rebecca Razavi, "Risk Taking in Children and Adolescents," *ADAMHA News* 15, no. 3 (May 1989): 9.

22. U.S. General Accounting Office, *Drug Use among Youth: No Simple Answers to Guide Prevention* (Washington, D.C.: U.S. General Accounting Office, 1993), 4, 10, 30.

23. Stanton Peele, *How Much Is Too Much* (Englewood Cliffs, N.J.: Prentice-Hall, 1981), 2–4.

24. Stanton Peele, *The Addiction Experience* (Center City, Minn.: Hazelden Foundation, 1980), 5.

25. Bureau of Justice Statistics, *Drugs, Crime, and the Justice System* (Washington, D.C.: U.S. Government Printing Office, 1992), 22.

26. "Is There an Addictive Personality" *University of California at Berkeley Wellness Letter* 6, no. 9 (June 1990): 1–2.

27. Felicity Barringer, "Youthful Drinking Persists: With Teens and Alcohol, It's Just Say When," *New York Times,* 23 June 1991, 1, 4.

28. Louise G. Richards, "The Epidemiology of Youthful Drug Use," in *Drugs and the Youth Culture,* ed. F. Scarpitti and S. Datesman (Beverly Hills, Calif.: Sage, 1980), 55.

29. Harvey B. Milkman and Stanley G. Sunderwirth, *Craving for Ecstasy: The Consciousness and Chemistry of Escape* (Lexington, Mass.: Lexington Books, 1987), 18.

30. George Vaillant, *The Natural History of Alcoholism* (Cambridge: Harvard University Press, 1983), 63–71.

31. National Institute on Alcohol Abuse and Alcoholism, *Alcohol and Health: The Eights Special Report to the U.S. Congress* (Rockville, Md.: National Institutes of Health, Public Health Service, 1993), 61–83.

32. Kenneth Blum and others, "Allelic Association of Human Dopamine D2 Receptor Gene in Alcoholism," *Journal of the American Medical Association* 263, no. 15 (18 April 1990): 2055–60.

33. Ting-Kai Li and Jane C. Lockmuller, "Why Are Some People More Susceptible to Alcoholism?" *Alcoholism Health and Research World* 13, no. 4 (1989): 310–15.

34. Steve Olson, with Dean Gerstein, *Alcohol in America: Taking Action to Prevent Abuse* (Washington, D.C.: National Academy Press, 1985), 40–41.

35. Al Mooney, Arlene Eisenberg, and Howard Eisenberg, *The Recovery Book* (New York: Workman, 1992), 501.

36. Louis Krupnick and Elizabeth Krupnick, *From Despair to Decision* (Minneapolis: CompCare, 1985), 24.

37. Michael Lewis and Jane Lockmuller, "Alcohol Reinforcement: Complex Determinant of Drinking," *Alcohol Health and Research World* 14, no. 2 (1990): 98–104.

38. J. Jaffe, R. Petersen, and R. Hodgson, *Addictions: Issues and Answers* (New York: Harper & Row, 1980), 18.

39. Benjamin Stein, "The Lure of Drugs: They 'Organize' an Addict's Life," *Newsday,* 4 December 1988, 6.

40. Helene White, Marsha Bates, and Valerie Johnson, Learning to Drink: Familial, Peer, and Media Influences," in *Society, Culture, and Drinking Patterns Reexamined* (New Brunswick, N.J.: Rutgers Center of Alcohol Studies, 1991), 177–97.

41. Office of Substance Abuse Prevention, *Prevention Plus II: Tools for Creating and Sustaining Drug-Free Communities* (Washington, D.C.: U.S. Government Printing Office, 1989), 26.

42. "Camel Ad: Is Male Violence a 'Smooth Move'?" *Public Citizen Health Research Group Health Letter* 5, no. 8 (August 1989): 11–12.

43. Philip Slater, "Society's Pressure Causes Drug Dependency," in *Opposing Viewpoints: Chemical Dependency,* ed. Claudia B. Debner (St. Paul: Greenhaven Press, 1985), 25.

44. Material in this section is derived substantially from publications of the National Institute on Drug Abuse.

chapter

3

pharmacology

Drug Actions and Interactions

chapter objectives

After you have studied this chapter, you should be able to do the following:

1. Define the following terms: *pharmacology, drug, pharmacodynamics, therapeutics, toxicology, metabolism, drug receptor, neuron, electrochemical transmission of nerve impulses, drug interaction, drug dependence, placebo.*

2. Describe four major methods of drug administration.

3. Describe the basic patterns of drug distribution within the body.

4. Explain the significance of the blood-brain barrier in relation to psychoactive drugs.

5. Discuss the various processes involved in the elimination of drugs from the body.

6. Explain drug activity in terms of the drug-receptor interaction.

7. Name six different ways or actions by which drugs can change cell function.

8. Explain how factors of dose, age, body weight, gender, time, disease, and emotional states could affect drug actions.

9. Describe the general organization of the nervous system in terms of major functions and structures.

10. Distinguish between the central nervous system and the peripheral nervous system with its major subdivisions.

11. Compare the general functions of the sympathetic and parasympathetic divisions of the autonomic nervous system.

12. Explain in detail the various processes involved in continuing a nerve impulse from one neuron to another.

13. Name several neurotransmitters.

14. Identify several parts of the human brain that are affected either directly or indirectly by psychoactive drugs.

15. Relate several recreational psychoactives and several prescribed medications with specific effects on human sexual function.

16. Identify and briefly discuss the effects of three different drugs on each of the following body systems: cardiovascular-renal, endocrine, gastrointestinal, and respiratory.

17. Discuss the major aspects of chemotherapy in the control of diseases.

18. Distinguish among the following terms: *physical dependence, psychological dependence, tolerance,* and *withdrawal sickness.*

19. Identify several criteria established by the American Psychiatric Association by which to describe a drug-dependent individual.

20. Describe addiction or drug dependence as a process.

21. Explain how each of the following conditions differ from one another: tachyphylaxis, kindling, cross-tolerance, and cross-dependence.

22. Explain four major categories of drug interactions.

23. Identify four factors thought to be responsible for the placebo effect.

Pharmacology

In their search for sustaining foods, prehistoric humans undoubtedly introduced a wide assortment of substances into their bodies. These people sought nourishment, but occasionally they also experienced drowsiness and sleep, intense pleasures, reduction of pain, and sometimes even poisoning and sudden death. While modern Americans may be somewhat more sophisticated about their food intake, many still desire some of the changes in thinking, feeling, and behavior achieved almost accidentally by their ancient counterparts.

With advances in scientific investigation, researchers eventually sought to determine the relation between substances taken into the body and the resulting changes in body function and behavior. Such endeavors have given rise to the scientific discipline of pharmacology.

The branch of science that deals with the interaction of chemical agents with living organisms is known as **pharmacology.**[1] Traditionally, the major concern of pharmacology has been the study of drugs intended for medicinal use, such as drugs used to diagnose (specify or determine via examination), prevent, treat, or cure disease. Even when such chemicals were misused and abused, sometimes for recreational purposes rather than for treating disease, the standard description of a drug was considered adequate. However, with the introduction of oral contraceptives in the mid 1950s, pharmacologists had to revise their definition of a drug. The "Pill" was not used in the diagnosis, prevention, treatment, or cure of disease—unless pregnancy was to be considered a disease.

Consequently, pharmacologists have revised their definition of drugs to include *any substance that in small amounts produces significant changes in a person's body, mind, or both.*[2] This newer definition seems more appropriate now, especially with the increased use of recreational drugs, street drugs, and designer drugs, many of which never had any intended medical use.

The science of pharmacology has given rise to three major subdivisions now recognized as special areas of study and practice:

1. *Pharmacodynamics*—the study of where and how drugs act in the body, and how drugs are changed by the body.

2. *Therapeutics*—the use of drugs in treating disease. When drugs are used specifically to destroy or weaken invading organisms, the treatment is referred to as **chemotherapy.**

3. *Toxicology*—the study of poisons and the treatment of drug poisoning, including intoxication, resulting from the presence of harmful chemicals in the body.

How Drugs Enter the Body

In order for a drug to have any more than a superficial effect, like antacids in the stomach or antidandruff shampoos on the scalp, the chemical agent must enter the blood-vascular system. It must be absorbed or transported from the site of administration into the bloodstream, and then distributed by the blood throughout the body to various tissues and fluids. The manner in which the drug is introduced (the route of administration) is an important factor in determining how fast the drug acts, how long its effects will be sustained, the intensity of the drug's action, and the degree of localization of the drug's action.[3]

Although drugs can be administered in several ways, they are usually given or taken *orally* (by mouth), *parenterally* (by injection), or by *inhalation* (breathing in through one's nose). Other means of introducing drugs into the body are by way of absorption across the mucous membranes of the rectum and vagina, across the skin barrier (transdermally), and by surgical implantation.

Most commonly, drugs in capsule, tablet or caplet, pill, or liquid form enter the body by way of the mouth. From the mouth, the solid or liquid drug passes into the stomach and eventually into the intestine, where most of the chemicals are absorbed (transferred) into the bloodstream. Oral administration is convenient, permits self-medication, and avoids the physical and psychological discomforts of injection. However, this route of administration is not ideal for all drugs. Absorption is sometimes slowed by the presence of food in the stomach and the excessive movement of the gastrointestinal tract.

Less commonly, drugs can be given *rectally,* that is, through the rectum, the terminal end of the digestive tract. This method is particularly advantageous if the person is unconscious, has difficulty in swallowing, or is vomiting. However, drugs administered rectally in the form of a suppository or even an enema may be incompletely and irregularly absorbed.

The term *parenteral* describes the administration of drugs, such as antibiotics, insulin, and anticlotting medicine, into the bloodstream directly or indirectly by **injection,** without having to be absorbed through the digestive tract. This can be accomplished by *intravenous injection* (known as an IV or "mainlining," in which a drug is inserted directly into a vein); *intramuscular injection* or IM (directly into muscle tissue); or *subcutaneous injection* or "skin-popping" (just beneath the skin's surface). On rare occasions, drugs may be injected directly into the peritoneal or visceral cavity of the body as well as into the cerebrospinal fluid. Each of the more common routes of drug administration has its distinct advantages and disadvantages, as noted below.[4]

Administration of drugs by injection

1. produces a more rapid response than can be obtained by oral or rectal administration.

2. achieves more accurate dosage, since drug destruction in the digestive tract is avoided.

3. bypasses the unpredictable absorption processes occurring in the stomach and intestine.

4. provides insufficient time, in comparison with orally administered drugs, to counteract unexpected drug reactions or accidental overdose. Once given, an injection cannot be recalled.

5. requires sterile conditions in order to avoid infectious diseases caused by bacteria and viruses that can damage the liver, heart, and other body organs.

6. presents a potentially painful situation for the drug taker, and a life-threatening situation if the virus that causes acquired immune deficiency syndrome (AIDS) is transmitted by using shared, blood-contaminated needles for intravenous injection.

Certain drugs in mist form can be administered by **inhalation,** in which chemicals are absorbed into the blood by passing through the lungs. Volatile anesthetic gases, paint thinner and gasoline vapors, nonvolatile aerosols, tobacco and marijuana smoke, and the smoke of freebased and "crack" cocaine can pass through the thin membranes of the lungs' air sacs and readily enter the bloodstream.

Inhalation of drugs produces an extremely rapid effect, because chemicals absorbed into the blood from the lungs go directly to the brain and bypass the heart in their initial distribution. As a consequence, volatile gases are the preferred form of anesthetics since their blood levels can be controlled with great precision. This control of dosage is also a major advantage of breathing in drug vapors and drug smoke. Other than volatile gases, the major disadvantage of inhalation is the potential for irritation of and damage to lung tissue.

A variation of inhalation is known as *snorting,* the intranasal administration of drugs. In this route of entry, a water-soluble drug such as cocaine is snorted or sniffed, being absorbed through the moist mucous membranes that line the nasal passages. The drug enters the blood vessels near the surface lining.

While most psychoactive drugs are administered by mouth, rectum, injection,

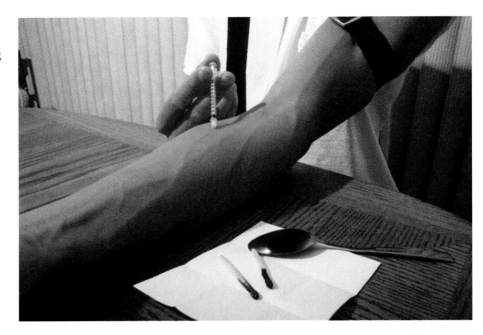

Shooting up heroin. This picture demonstrates the parenteral administration of drugs in which a solution of a chemical substance (heroin) is injected into the bloodstream. The drug abuser is engaging in intravenous injection, a form of parenteral drug use commonly known as "mainlining."
© Tony Freeman/PhotoEdit

or inhaling, the future of drug use could be changed dramatically by the development and approval of a relatively new drug form. During the last decade, the U.S. Food and Drug Administration authorized use of a rate-controlled, transdermal drug system—a method by which a drug is absorbed through the skin. Worn on the skin's surface behind the ear or on the arm or chest as small disks or patches, the drug is absorbed directly into the bloodstream at programmed rates.

Each small patch of the transdermal system is composed of four layers, or membranes, that serve as a backing container, a drug reservoir, a rate-of-release controller, and an adhesive that holds the "circle of drug" to the skin. Although the first drugs to be dispensed in transdermal patches were used to alleviate motion sickness and angina pectoris, we might yet be assured, using this method, of continuous mood modification in the future.

Another recently devised method of drug administration has arrived after extensive research: nasal sprays that promote the absorption of certain medicines through the mucosa of the nasal cavity (directly into the blood vessels of the nostrils).

Drug Distribution and Elimination

After a drug has been absorbed into the bloodstream, it is widely *distributed* throughout the body. Such dispersal, however, reflects the physical and chemical nature of the drug and its ability to spread or pass through various membranes—cell walls, capillaries, the brain, and the placenta.

This selective ability of a particular drug to spread from areas of high concentration to areas of low concentration is known as its **solubility,** that is, its condition or quality of being dissolved in body tissue.[5] Some drugs are more soluble in body fats, while others are more easily dissolved in water. Because most cell membranes contain several fat layers, drugs that are soluble in fat can pass through the membranes rapidly. All psychoactive drugs are soluble in fat, though some dissolve faster than others.[6]

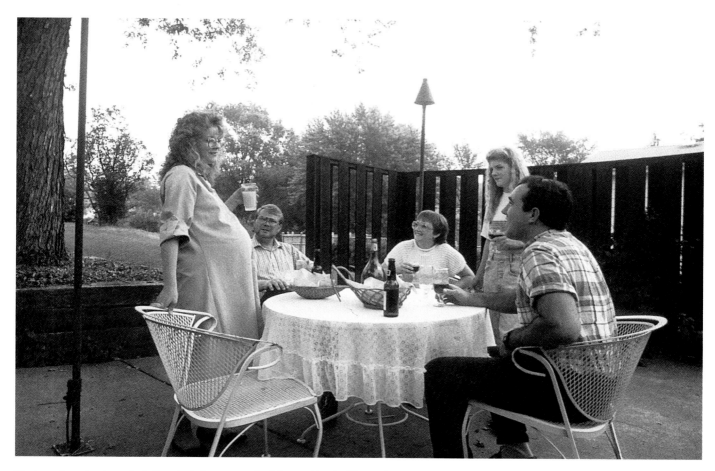

Most psychoactive drugs, including alcohol, can cross the "placental barrier." Recognizing this fact, the pregnant woman in this photo is being good to her baby before it is born by drinking non-alcoholic beverages during her pregnancy.

© James L. Shaffer

Four basic *patterns of drug distribution* have been identified:[7]

1. Some drugs, including blood-plasma substitutes, remain largely within the bloodstream.

2. Other compounds, such as ethyl alcohol and certain sulfa drugs, become almost uniformly distributed throughout each and every body cell.

3. Most drugs are unevenly distributed in the body in accordance with their solubility and differential ability to penetrate different membranes of the body.

4. Very few drugs actually concentrate in one or more body tissues or organs that may not even be the sites of drug action.

It should be noted that although *psychoactive drugs* affect mood and behavior—functions controlled by the nervous system—most of these chemicals will be found outside the brain at any given time, even during states of drug intoxication and poisoning.

The Blood-Brain Barrier

To have a psychoactive effect, a drug must be able to leave the tiny blood vessels (capillaries) supplying the brain and enter the nearby nerve cells. Because of the unique, tightly fused cell wall structure of the capillaries in the brain—unlike those in other body parts—a selective resistance to movement effectively prevents certain substances from entering brain tissue. This "resistance to the passage of some substances through the brain's capillary walls"—based on drug solubility—is known as the **blood-brain barrier.**[8]

Fat-soluble drugs, such as the general anesthetics, and water-soluble molecules easily cross the blood-brain barrier, as do those drugs already identified as having a psychoactive effect. Heroin actually crosses the barrier more easily than morphine, due to heroin's greater fat solubility. Though acting as a protector of the brain against certain toxic substances, the blood-brain barrier is neither absolute nor invariable.[9]

Certain disease states modify the permeability of the blood-brain barrier, allowing the entry of penicillin during periods of brain inflammation and trauma. Ordinarily, this common antibiotic cannot easily cross the barrier.

Metabolism and Excretion

As drugs are circulated throughout the body, they undergo processes of *metabolism* and *excretion*, both of which are responsible for the *elimination* of the drugs and the termination of drug action.

The complex chemical changes that alter drugs and convert them to substances that can be eliminated from the body are known collectively as **metabolism.** A special system of enzymes that function mainly in the liver cells carries out these metabolic reactions. Thus, the liver is a vital body organ that transforms fat-soluble substances to more water-soluble compounds and changes poisonous chemicals to less toxic metabolism by-products. Such liver functions are referred to as *biotransformation.*

When the recently biotransformed substances are carried by the blood to the *kidneys,* the metabolized drug by-products are *excreted,* or eliminated from the body in the urine. Consequently the kidneys, with their filtering action, are the major route of eliminating biotransformed and toxic substances from the human body. This action of the kidneys helps maintain the body's chemical **homeostasis,** that internal state of constancy or equilibrium necessary for normal functioning.

Although most drugs are excreted by the kidneys, small amounts will also be eliminated via several minor pathways of excretion. These routes include sweat, saliva, gastric secretions, bile, feces, mother's milk, and the lungs. Though several psychoactive substances are absorbed through the lungs, including nicotine, marijuana, and cocaine, only the highly volatile drugs such as anesthetic gases are excreted through the lungs.

Drug Actions

Although there are technical distinctions between drug actions and drug effects, this brief description will employ these terms interchangeably.

Drug actions are the result of a chemical interaction with some part of the human organism. In general, drugs replace body chemicals that are deficient, act against bacteria and other disease-causing agents, or interfere with cellular function. In this text, two major pharmacological

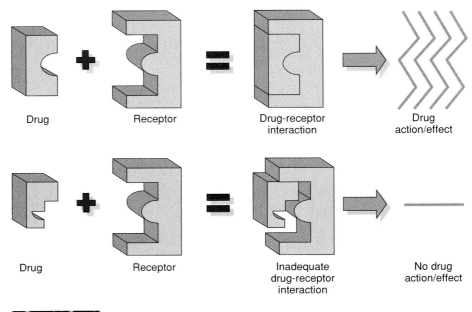

figure 3.1

The drug-receptor interaction.

actions will be described: (1) those resulting from the use of *structurally nonspecific drugs;* and (2) those associated with *structurally specific drugs.*

A structurally nonspecific drug action results when a particular chemical substance is given or applied in a relatively large dose that forms a thin layer over an entire area of body cells. Examples of such a drug are the anesthetic gases, ethyl alcohol, and antiseptic preparations. An antiseptic, for instance, acts in a nonspecific way on all human cells encountered, as well as on all bacterial cells in a human wound. The antiseptic effectively kills or retards microbial growth.

On the other hand, structurally specific drugs produce effects based upon their unique chemical structure. The interaction between such drug molecules and human cells involves very small, highly specific areas called *receptors.*

According to major theories of drug activity, *receptors* or receptor substances are thought to be localized portions on the surface of or within a particular cell, such as the cellular membrane, enzymes, and nucleic acids. It is further presumed that a particular drug must interact with or attach itself to the appropriate receptor in a body cell before any change in cell function occurs.

The **drug-receptor interaction** is often compared with a "lock-and-key" mechanism as illustrated in figure 3.1. According to this concept, the better-fitting drug molecule bonded with the appropriate receptor produces the more desirable effect or action. If the drug binds inadequately to the drug receptor, there is no drug action or effect.

The body's own natural chemicals, called *neurotransmitters*—discussed later in this chapter—also bind to these receptor sites and initiate a particular response in the cell. If a drug binds to the same site, adds to the effects of the body's own neurotransmitters, and enhances cell response, the drug is referred to as an *agonist.* However, if a drug prevents the body's own natural chemicals from binding to its receptor, and as a consequence blocks a particular cell response, the drug is then identified as an *antagonist.*[10]

In general, drugs change cell function by one or more of the following specific methods.[11]

1. **Stimulation**—an increase in the rate of functional activity. Cocaine, caffeine, amphetamines, and methylphenidate (Ritalin) tend to speed up central nervous system function.

2. **Depression**—a reduction in the rate of functional activity. Ethyl alcohol, narcotics, sedative-hypnotics, and tranquilizers slow down or depress the function of the central nervous system. Low doses of marijuana may also have a depressant effect.

3. *Blocking*—an obstruction that effectively prevents a particular action or response. This action is probably the consequence of depression. Antihistamine drugs block typical allergic reactions.

   Another form of blocking, known as *inhibition,* is the likely method of changing cell function by using a psychedelic drug. By interfering with or inhibiting the normal function of certain chemicals manufactured in the brain, LSD permits the brain to be assaulted by an excessive amount of sensory input. One result of this "sensory overload" is visual hallucinations; another is bizarre behavior related to gross distortion of thought and sensory processes—evidence of the psychedelic effect. At high-dose levels, marijuana sometimes acts as a psychedelic drug, too.

4. *Replacement*—the provision of a substitute or equivalent substance to restore an optimal condition. The administration of insulin to diabetics is an example of replacement therapy.

5. *Killing or inactivating organisms*—the destruction or prevention of the growth of disease-causing organisms. Antibiotics kill bacteria by interfering with the manufacture of bacterial cell walls.

6. *Irritation*—the abnormal excitation of some body part or function. This action may be an exaggerated form of stimulation. Laxatives irritate the large intestine to initiate defecation.

Factors Influencing Drug Actions

In addition to the route of administration, drug distribution throughout the body, and processes of drug metabolism and elimination, the following factors should also be noted as influencing drug responses.

Dose-Response Relationship

The quantity or amount of drug that is taken at any particular time is called the **dose** or dosage. In some instances, the greater the dose, the greater the drug effect or response. However, for other drugs, an increase in dosage beyond the level needed to produce a given response will have little or no effect.

The *threshold dose,* or minimal dose, is the smallest amount of a given drug capable of producing a detectable response. Less than such an amount is known as a *subthreshold dose,* which fails to produce a detectable response. However, drugs are also said to have a *maximum effect,* the greatest response produced by a specific drug, regardless of the dose administered.

Because of the considerable variation among drugs and the differing responses by individuals to the same dosage of the same drug, the term *median effective dose* is used to express such variability. Abbreviated as ED_{50}, the median effective dose describes the dosage required to produce a specific response in 50 percent of test subjects. If the response to a particular dose is death, the dosage is identified as the *lethal dose.* That amount of drug that will be fatal for 50 percent of test subjects is then called the *median lethal dose,* or LD_{50}.

In this consideration of dosage, it should be noted that even though all drugs are potential poisons when given in sufficient amounts, even the most deadly poisons are usually nontoxic (nonpoisonous) when given at extremely low dose levels.

When psychoactives or any other drugs are used in the treatment of illness,[12] the dosage must be sufficient to produce a beneficial response without causing adverse effects, including death. Therefore, the aim of drug therapy is to achieve a level of medication in the blood or tissues that lies somewhere between the minimum effective dose and the maximum safe concentration of a drug.

This dosage level is referred to as a drug's *therapeutic range.* For instance, digitalis drugs and the sedative-hypnotic chloral hydrate have a very narrow therapeutic range, so the margin of effectiveness and safety is quite small. By contrast, other drugs such as penicillin and THC (the major psychoactive component of marijuana), have a much wider therapeutic range, and are considered relatively safe.

An index for rating the relative safety of drugs for use in large populations of humans has been identified as the therapeutic ratio, or **therapeutic index**.[13] Sometimes referred to as a drug's standard safety margin, the laboratory therapeutic index is usually defined as the ratio between the median lethal dose (LD_{50}) and the median effective dose (ED_{50}), and is represented by the following: $T.I. = LD_{50}/ED_{50}$.

Nevertheless, a more realistic method of calculating the T.I. in a therapeutic setting with human beings involves the use of the *effective dose in nearly all patients* (ED_{99}) and the *lethal dose in practically no patients* (LD_1). A ratio calculated on the basis of LD_1/ED_{99} yields a more meaningful interpretation of the therapeutic index. Of course, the greater this ratio, the safer the medication.

Age

In comparison with so-called average 18- to 65-year-old adults, both infants and the elderly generally display more sensitivity to the effects of drugs. Infants tend to have underdeveloped abilities to metabolize and excrete drugs. As a consequence, drug actions within their bodies tend to be prolonged. The elderly, too, are likely to have impaired ability to metabolize and eliminate drugs from their bodies, part of the phenomenon of aging. Poor absorption in some older people is also a factor in reducing the effects of certain drugs. In another instance, one drug has a special reputation for reacting differently in children than in adults. Ritalin, a powerful stimulant for adults, acts as a depressant in hyperactive children.

Body Weight

Giving the same amount of a drug to a 90-pound person and a 200-pound person is likely to produce significantly different results because of the greater concentration of the drug in the blood of the lighter-weight individual. Lightweight people usually experience a greater drug effect than heavier people when all other factors, including dosage, are similar. By contrast, the heavier individual with more blood and body fluids to dilute an absorbed drug thus reduces the concentration of the dissolved drug—the amount of the drug contained per unit volume of body fluid.

Gender

Although males and females respond similarly to drugs, females generally tend to be more sensitive to the effects of some drugs than males. This gender difference is often associated with the variable concentrations of proteins, lipids (fats), and water in the human body. For instance, a female who weighs exactly the same as a male and drinks exactly the same amount of an alcoholic beverage as the male will almost always have a higher blood-alcohol level. Such a condition is related to the higher proportion of fat and lower proportion of water typically found in the bodies of females in comparison with the bodies of males. While alcohol is readily soluble in fat, it is even more soluble in water.

Males, on the other hand, tend to have more body fluids, or a higher water content in which to dilute the alcohol consumed. As a consequence, females tend to become more intoxicated than males after drinking approximately the same amount of alcohol.

Other gender factors influencing drug effects include the fluctuating levels of female sex hormones during the menstrual cycle. In general, females absorb ethyl alcohol more rapidly during the premenstrual phase of the menstrual cycle. If these females happen to be taking oral contraceptives, however, they are still at considerable risk of intoxication if they drink alcoholic beverages. Simply stated, taking birth control pills tends to slow down the body's ability to metabolize ethyl alcohol. Thus, the drug effects of alcohol would be prolonged beyond the normal, expected period of influence.

Women also lack a recently identified stomach enzyme that functions to partially oxidize ethyl alcohol before it enters the bloodstream. Men, who tend to have such a stomach enzyme, are thus able to metabolize equal amounts of alcohol more rapidly than women. Again, females tend to have higher blood alcohol levels than men when they drink the same amount of an alcoholic beverage.

Of course, females should be extremely cautious about taking any drug during pregnancy, because many prescribed and recreational drugs cross the placenta and can then damage the embryo and fetus. At one time the placenta was considered a barrier that prevented toxic substances and harmful organisms from being transferred from the mother to the developing new life form. Today it is known that the "placental barrier" is crossed preferentially by fat-soluble compounds and by those substances having a molecular weight of less than 1,000. Most commonly used drugs, including psychoactive chemicals, have such characteristics and pass readily through the placenta. Rapid transfer of anesthetics, alcohol, barbiturates, cocaine, marijuana, morphine, and heroin occurs from the mother to the embryo or fetus.

Time

The length of time between taking a drug and observing the anticipated effect is referred to as the "onset of action." Some drugs act shortly after entering the body; others may require several hours or even days before their effects become apparent. After the onset of action, drugs will vary in terms of the time required to achieve their maximum effects, as well as the duration of time during which drugs continue to have an effect.

Disease

The presence or absence of a disease condition will often alter a person's response to a drug. For instance, aspirin reduces fever but has no effect in lowering normal temperature. People with impaired liver and kidney function often have difficulty metabolizing and excreting drugs and thus experience prolonged drug effects. Such people are unable to eliminate drugs from their bodies in a normal period of time. On the other hand, when a condition of diarrhea exists, some drugs are transported through the gastrointestinal tract so rapidly that drug absorption is significantly reduced.

Mind-Set

Often referred to as the *mind-set,* one's emotional state or climate is now recognized as having a potentially significant impact on drug responses. Temperament marked by anger, fear, sadness, joy, or any other emotion can bring about changes in various bodily processes, namely, secretion of gastric juices and hormones, and alteration of blood pressure, heart rate, pulse, and respiration. These bodily processes, in turn, influence drug absorption, distribution, metabolism, and excretion—all of which can modify the response to a drug.

However, taking a drug and having a particular expectation of that drug's effects also refers to the condition of mind-set. If an individual uses a drug, especially a psychoactive one, in anticipation of "getting high," feeling more powerful or secure, or experiencing a new altered state of consciousness, such a mind-set can and often does result in an exaggerated behavioral response, as expected. This mental predisposition is as important as pharmacology in determining whether the effect of a drug is ultimately perceived as desirable or undesirable, pleasant or unpleasant. For instance, experienced users are often able to get intoxicated on lower-potency marijuana than most first-time users are, presumably because experienced pot-puffers expect to do so, while the novice users may be terrified of losing their minds. Such beginners often have a negative response to the psychoactive drug. Similarly, the use of a fake or inert substance that produces a drug response (the so-called placebo effect discussed later in this chapter) is also based upon a mind-set of trust, belief in a physician's judgment, and expectation of relief.

Environmental Setting

Closely related to mind-set in changing a drug response are the various factors of the *environmental setting.*[14] The environment

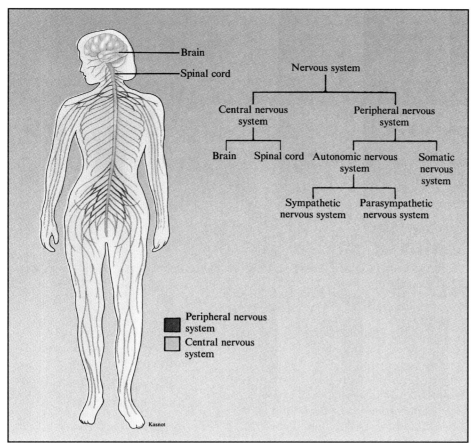

 3.2

The nervous system consists of the brain, spinal cord, and numerous peripheral nerves.

From Lester M. Sdorow, Psychology, *3d edition. Copyright © 1995 Wm. C. Brown Communications, Inc. Reprinted by permission of Times Mirror Higher Education Group, Inc., Dubuque, Iowa. All Rights Reserved.*

includes not only the physical place in which a drug is taken but also the psychosocial circumstances surrounding the drug use.

The impact of the environment on drug action can be very significant with mood- and behavior-modifying chemicals. For example, using a psychedelic drug in a controlled laboratory situation or among caring, protective friends will likely result in fewer "bad trips" than would be experienced in "street use" of the same drug or among uncaring drug takers. Also, the effect of drinking alcoholic beverages in celebration of New Year's Eve or an athletic victory may be quite different from the effect of using the same amount of beverage alcohol in the presence of one's parents, the college dean, or a disapproving loved one.

The influence of environmental setting on drug use was also apparent during the Vietnam War of the 1960s and 1970s. Many American soldiers smoked high-grade heroin, primarily to escape boredom and to help make time pass more quickly. Medical authorities had predicted that most of the soldiers would eventually become addicted. Few actually did when they returned to the United States. Apparently, the unique environmental setting of Army life in Vietnam shaped this pattern of drug use.[15] When the soldiers left the conflict in southeast Asia, most of them stopped using heroin.

The Nervous System

Although all drugs are capable of producing more than a single response, the so-called psychoactive substances—the major concern of this text—have their primary effect on the human nervous system. Therefore, this descriptive analysis will focus on the structure and function of the nervous system. It will provide a basic understanding of how drugs alter nerve function, mental processes, mood, feelings, consciousness, perceptions, and behavior. Subsequently, a brief consideration will be given to the effects of drugs on other body systems and to the role of chemotherapy in modern medical practice.

Organization of the Nervous System

The nervous system consists of specialized structures that control and coordinate the body's activities. Such functions are conducted in three basic ways: (1) *sensory reception*—the detection of stimuli from within and outside the body; (2) *interconnection*—the transmission of electrochemical messages from one part of the nervous system to another; and (3) *motor response*—the initiation of an appropriate response, such as a muscular contraction or glandular secretion, due to a message sent out to such parts by a nerve center.

As shown in figure 3.2, the nervous system has three major structures: the *brain,* the *spinal cord,* and the *peripheral nerves.* Each of these consists mainly of **neurons,** the functional and structural units of this body system. Neurons are specialized cells that can send electrochemical messages (impulses) to one another and to other cells outside the nervous system itself.

The nervous system is subdivided into two major parts:

1. The **central nervous system** (CNS) is composed of the brain and the spinal cord. Drugs of abuse and many of the commonly misused drugs have their primary effect on the central nervous system.

2. The **peripheral nervous system** consists of all the nerves that branch out from the central nervous system and connect it to other parts of the body, including the extremities. Anatomists and physiologists have subdivided the peripheral nervous system into two additional subdivisions:

a. The *somatic system*—the cranial and spinal nerves connecting the central nervous system to the skin and the skeletal muscles.

b. The *autonomic system*—the nerves that connect the central nervous system to the organs of the body cavity (the viscera), including the heart, stomach, intestines, and various glands. This subdivision's nerves function involuntarily and automatically without conscious control or effort.

The **autonomic nervous system** is sub-divided yet again into two more parts:[16] (1) the *sympathetic division,* which pre-pares the body for energy-expending activities; and (2) the *parasympathetic division,* which aids in restoring the body to a resting state after an emergency. The parasympathetic division tends to counterbalance the actions of the sympathetic division. Since these two subdivisions act in opposition to each other—the parasympathetic counterbalancing or opposing the action of the sympathetic—their function is described as *antagonistic.*

The Nerve Cell

As the basic unit of the nervous system, a nerve cell, or *neuron,* is capable of receiving stimuli and transmitting electrical messages or impulses. Depicted in figure 3.3, a neuron consists of a *cell body,* or *soma,* containing a nucleus, granular cytoplasm, and other structures common to all body cells.

Extending from the neuron are two types of *nerve fibers.* **Dendrites** are fibers that send nerve impulses toward the cell body; **axons** carry impulses away from the cell body. In general, each neuron has several dendrites but only one axon.

Originating in the dendrite, an electrical impulse is integrated in the cell body and then transmitted down the axon. Transmission of the impulse itself, known as the *action potential,* is accomplished through the loss of an electrical charge on the nerve fiber's membrane. Although psychoactive drugs do not act primarily on the axon, local anesthetics do, and thus block the transmission of pain impulses to the brain.

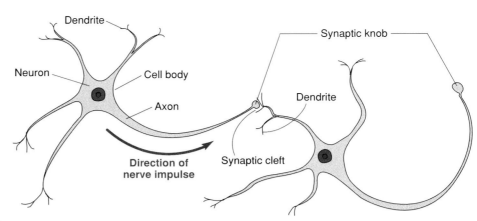

 3.3

For an impulse to continue from one neuron to another, it must cross the synaptic cleft at a synapse or junction between two neurons.

The junction between two nerve cells—the meeting place between the axon of one neuron and the dendrites of another neuron—is known as the **synapse.** Before an electrical impulse can be continued from one neuron to the next, it must cross a narrow space or gap named the *synaptic cleft,* illustrated in figure 3.4. The crossing-over process from axon to dendrite is accomplished not by any electrical discharge but by chemical transmission. It is at the synapse that other chemicals, specifically the psychoactive drugs, have their major effect.

Neurotransmitters

Rounded *synaptic knobs* at the ends of axons contain chemical factories called *synaptic vesicles.* These tiny, saclike structures manufacture chemical substances, the **neurotransmitters.** When an electrical impulse reaches the end of an axon, the following sequence of events occurs rapidly.

1. A nerve impulse reaches the synaptic knob.

2. The neurotransmitter substance ruptures from the synaptic vesicles into the synaptic cleft.

3. The neurotransmitter substance diffuses across the synaptic cleft.

4. The neurotransmitter substance reacts with the membrane of the dendrite on the other side of the cleft.

5. Electrical charge is lost on the dendrite membrane.

6. The nerve impulse is reestablished in the dendrite fiber and the transmission of the action potential continues.

7. The neurotransmitter substance rapidly decomposes to prevent continued stimulation of the dendrite.

It is through the repetition of these processes that a nerve impulse is conducted from one neuron to another.

Several neurotransmitter substances have been identified within the nervous system.[17] These include the following:

Acetycholine—an excitatory neurotransmitter (one that triggers a nerve impulse) released by axons both within and outside the central nervous system. It influences heart rate, learning, and memory.

Norepinephrine—one of the catecholamine neurotransmitters in the brain, associated with arousal reactions and moods. It influences sleep, appetite, blood pressure, heart rate, learning, memory, and affective disorders.

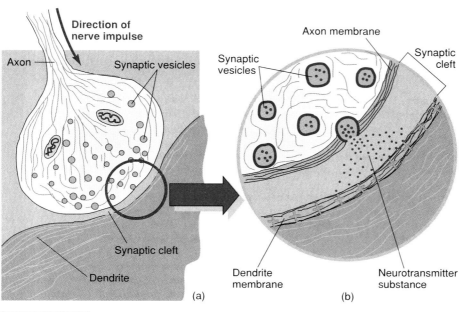

figure 3.4

(a) When a nerve impulse reaches the synaptic knob at the end of an axon, (b) synaptic vesicles release a neurotransmitter substance that diffuses across the synaptic cleft.

Dopamine—another catecholamine neurotransmitter in the brain, associated with body movement. It influences vision, motor control, appetite, euphoria, and schizophrenia.

Serotonin—a brain neurotransmitter associated with regulation of sensory perception, sleep, and body temperature. Alterations in the proper functioning of serotonin have been related to mental illnesses and certain drug-induced hallucinations.

Gamma-aminobutyric acid or GABA—an inhibitory neurotransmitter substance (one that blocks the transfer of a nerve impulse to an adjoining neuron) in the brain. When the normal functioning of GABA is disrupted at the synapses, convulsions may occur. GABA restrains brain activity with a reduction of arousal, aggression, and anxiety.

Glycine—an inhibitory neurotransmitter substance in the spinal cord.

Other presumed neurotransmitter substances include histamine, glutamate, adenosine triphosphate, prostaglandins, enkephalins, and endorphins. The latter two chemical substances will be discussed further in the chapter on narcotics (chapter 5).

The actions of two neurotransmitter substances are revealed in the antagonistic effect of the sympathetic and parasympathetic divisions of the autonomic nervous system. These opposing or counterbalancing effects are specified in table 3.1.

Drugs and Synaptic Transmission

Some drugs increase the excitability of neurons, whereas others reduce or inhibit such activity. For instance, caffeine, theophylline, and theobromine, found in coffee, tea, and cocoa, respectively, all increase nerve excitability, while hypnotics and anesthetics increase the threshold for excitation and thereby reduce nerve activity.

Nicotine mimics or intensifies the effect of acetylcholine, while atropine (a drug that decreases gastrointestinal movements) blocks the action of acetylcholine. The effect of atropine is thus described as

anticholinergic, that is, acting against acetylcholine that the cholinergic nerve fibers release.

By contrast, certain drugs prescribed to control hypertension (high blood pressure) are described as *adrenergic* blockers because they prevent the release of norepinephrine neurotransmitters from adrenergic nerve fibers or compete with adrenergic, neurotransmitter receptor sites in the heart.

The Brain

The brain is the most complex structure in the nervous system. This aggregate of 13 billion neurons contained within the skull controls and integrates all human behavior. Identified in figure 3.5 are several of the major structural and functional units within the brain.

Modification of mood and behavior resulting from the use of psychoactive drugs can be more easily understood when one is aware of the neuronal activities of the central nervous system.

Medulla Oblongata

The **medulla oblongata** is the direct upward continuation of the spinal cord within the skull. It is composed of both ascending and descending nerve fibers connecting the brain and spinal cord. Located herein are the *vital centers* responsible for controlling breathing (respiration center), blood pressure (vasomotor center), heart rate (cardiac center), contraction of heart musculature, functioning of the gastrointestinal tract, sleeping and waking, behavioral alerting, attention and arousal, coughing, sneezing, swallowing, and vomiting.

Opiates and barbiturates can so severely depress these centers that death may occur, often from respiratory failure. Antihypertensive drugs appear to exert their effect here too, depressing the center controlling the tone of blood vessels.

A complex network of nerve fibers within the core of the medulla has been identified as the *reticular formation.* Part of this formation is known as the *ascending reticular activating system* or, more simply, *ARAS.* The ARAS is involved in

table **3.1** Effects of Neurotransmitter Substances Upon Various Body Parts or Functions

Body Part or Function	Specific Response to Sympathetic Division Adrenergic Nerve Fibers Releasing Norepinephrine	Specific Response to Parasympathetic Division Cholinergic Nerve Fibers Releasing Acetylcholine
Pupil of the eye	Dilation	Constriction
Heart rate	Increases	Decreases
Bronchioles of the lungs	Dilation	Constriction
Muscles of the intestine wall	Slows peristaltic action	Speeds peristaltic action
Intestinal glands	Secretion decreases	Secretion increases
Coronary arteries	Dilation	Constriction
Blood distribution	More blood to skeletal muscles; less blood to digestive organs	More blood to digestive organs; less blood to skeletal muscles
Blood glucose concentration	Increases	Decreases
Salivary glands	Secretion decreases	Secretion increases
Tear glands	No action	Secretion
Muscles of gallbladder	Relaxation	Contraction
Muscles of urinary bladder	Relaxation	Contraction

controlling sleeping, waking, and behavioral alerting. Moreover, it serves as a filter of incoming sensory impulses. Ethyl alcohol, ether, and barbiturates tend to prevent or block normal activity in the ARAS, while amphetamines increase ARAS activity. However, if nerve stimulation into the ARAS is increased so rapidly as to intensify alertness beyond normal limits, hallucinations often occur. This is the case in the use of psychedelic drugs.

Pons

The pons is a rounded bulge on the underside of the brain stem that connects the medulla with the midbrain. It contains ascending and descending nerve fibers that relay impulses among the cerebrum, cerebellum, and spinal cord.

Midbrain

Also referred to as the mesencephalon, the midbrain is a short segment of the brain stem situated just above the pons. The midbrain contains bundles of nerve fibers that serve as motor pathways, or neuronal relays, between the cerebrum and lower parts of the nervous system. It also contains visual and auditory reflex centers that control

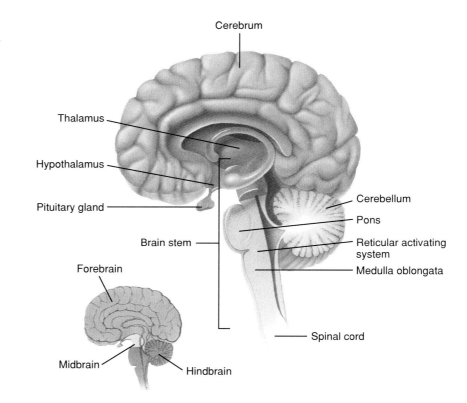

 3.5

The human brain with some of the major parts identified.

From Lester M. Sdorow, Psychology, *3d edition. Copyright © 1995 Wm. C. Brown Communications, Inc. Reprinted by permission of Times Mirror Higher Education Group, Inc., Dubuque, Iowa. All Rights Reserved.*

table 3.2 Functions of the Cerebral Lobes

Lobe	Functions
Frontal lobes	Motor areas control movements of voluntary skeletal muscles.
	Association areas carry on higher intellectual processes such as those required for concentrating, planning, complex problem solving, and judging the consequences of behavior.
Parietal lobes	Sensory areas are responsible for the sensations of temperature, touch, pressure, and pain involving the skin.
	Association areas function in the understanding of speech and in using words to express thoughts and feelings.
Temporal lobes	Sensory areas are responsible for hearing.
	Association areas are used in the interpretation of sensory experiences and in the memory of visual scenes, music, and other complex sensory patterns.
Occipital lobes	Sensory areas are responsible for vision.
	Association areas function in combining visual images with other sensory experiences.

From John W. Hole, Jr., *Human Anatomy and Physiology*, 6th ed. Copyright © 1993 Wm. C. Brown Communications, Inc. Reprinted by permission of Times Mirror Higher Education Group, Inc., Dubuque, Iowa. All Rights Reserved.

eye and head movements. Psychedelic drugs may induce auditory or visual hallucinations by acting on these reflex centers.

Cerebellum

This structure is a large, convoluted mass of nerve tissue situated below the cerebrum and behind the pons and medulla. The **cerebellum** communicates with other parts of the brain by various nerve tracts.

From a functional viewpoint, the cerebellum serves as a reflex center in coordinating and integrating skeletal muscle movements. Depression of the cerebellum, achieved by ethyl alcohol intoxication, results in loss of muscle coordination, staggering, and loss of balance.

Thalamus

The thalamus is part of the brain known as the diencephalon, and it is located between the cerebrum and the midbrain. In conjunction with the cerebral cortex, the thalamus functions as a central relay station of the brain, where all incoming sensory impulses, except for smell, synapse before being channeled to appropriate regions of the cerebrum. Additionally, it interprets sensations as painful or pleasurable and is associated with temperature and pressure.

Subthalamus

The small area situated beneath the thalamus and above the midbrain is called the subthalamus. It functions together with the cerebellum in controlling and coordinating motor activity.

Hypothalamus

Another portion of the diencephalon near the junction of the thalamus and midbrain is identified as the **hypothalamus.** It functions to maintain homeostasis by regulating various visceral (body cavity) activities and by linking the nervous system with the endocrine system by ductless glands.

The hypothalamus has several important functions. It controls heart rate, arterial blood pressure, water and electrolyte (chemical) balance, hunger (eating), body weight, movements and glandular secretions of the gastrointestinal tract, sexual behavior, and the synthesis of neurosecretory substances that stimulate hormonal production by the pituitary gland. Also functioning in the regulation of emotions and behavior, the hypothalamus is a prime site of action of many psychoactive drugs.

Limbic System

Components of the cerebrum interconnected with the thalamus and hypothalamus form a complex area of the diencephalon known as the limbic system. This system functions in the regulation of emotions, including fear, anger, pleasure, and sorrow. As such, it has a significant effect on human behavior, especially those aspects likely to promote survival.

Certain tranquilizing drugs, such as Valium and Librium apparently depress limbic system functions at dose levels below those that depress other brain functions. Rather than behavioral depression, these drugs result in tranquilization with its calming effect and relief of anxiety.

Cerebrum

The largest and most complex part of the brain, the **cerebrum** contains billions of neurons and nerve centers that have sensory, association, and motor functions. The cerebrum coordinates and interprets internal and external stimuli, and it is the site of higher mental functions such as memory and reasoning.

Composed of two large masses or hemispheres, the cerebrum is divided into various lobes. The *cerebral cortex* is the thin layer of gray matter that makes up the outermost part of the cerebrum. Beneath the cortex are masses of white matter containing many nerve fibers, and then more gray matter with neurons that relay impulses passing between the cortex and spinal cord.

Specific regions of the cerebrum perform various functions, as noted in table 3.2.

There is a consensus of opinion that many psychoactive drugs affect cerebral function either directly or indirectly. Stimulants, including amphetamines, increase neuronal activity, sometimes to the point of hallucinations. Depressant-type drugs, such as ethyl alcohol and barbiturates, decrease nerve cell function, thus affecting concentration and perception of stimuli.

Drugs and Other Body Systems

Although mind-changing psychoactive drugs are the major focus of this textbook, thousands of medications have been discovered and formulated to treat other body structures and functions. Some of these have their primary effects on the heart, blood vessels, kidneys, endocrine glands, stomach, intestinal tract, and various organs of the respiratory system, and are described in the following sections. A special box also details the various drug effects on human sexual functioning.

Cardiovascular-Renal System

This body system consists of the heart (cardio), blood vessels (vascular), and kidneys (renal). The heart is a four-chambered muscular pump that propels nutrient- and oxygen-rich blood throughout a closed system of tubes to the body's cells. Returning from the cells, the blood with its waste products is filtered through the kidneys. In addition to waste removal from the blood, the kidneys maintain the proper chemical balance of body fluids.

Four basic groups of drugs affecting the cardiovascular-renal system are described as follows.

Digitalis glycosides are used to enhance the force of heart contraction and to slow heartbeat in a failing heart. Employed in the treatment of congestive heart failure (inadequate and inefficient heart-pumping action) and arterial fibrillation (contraction of the heart's atrial chambers more often than the ventricles), digitalis is derived from the leaves of the purple foxglove plant.

Antiarrhythmic drugs such as quinidine correct abnormal heart rhythms. Most cardiac arrhythmias arise from disorders in the formation and normal conduction of nerve impulses in the heart musculature. Quinidine is compounded from the bark of the cinchona tree and is similar to quinine, a drug used in treating malaria. The therapeutic uses of the drug are based on quinidine's ability to decrease the excitability of heart musculature and slow the conduction of nerve impulses in the walls of the heart.

Nitroglycerin, a representative coronary blood-vessel dilator (vasodilator), increases the flow of blood supplying the heart muscle. Because of this action, nitroglycerin is called an antianginal drug—one that counters angina pectoris, the pain in the chest or arm experienced when there is a reduction of blood flowing to the heart muscle. The vasodilation effect relaxes the smooth muscles of the coronary blood vessels and thus increases blood flow to the oxygen-starved muscles of the heart. Administered under the tongue in nonexplosive tablet form, nitroglycerin is thought to lighten the work load of the heart. Such an action lowers the heart's oxygen requirements and contributes to the antianginal effect.

Antihypertensive drugs are used to control hypertension, the consistent elevation of blood pressure. Widely experienced in the general population, high blood pressure is often referred to as the "silent killer" because it has no outstanding signs or symptoms. Representative antihypertensive agents include Inderal, Catapres, and Aldomet. The treatment goal is to maintain blood pressure within normal limits without adversely affecting heart function or circulation of the blood. Such a goal is achieved through a variety of drug actions. These include depression of the vasomotor nerve center in the brain stem or higher brain centers (which results in a calming effect and a reduction in anxiety), and the depletion, blocked release, or altered synthesis of norepinephrine neurotransmitter substances at sympathetic nerve endings.

Diuretics, drugs that increase the production of urine, are also used in treating mild cases of hypertension. Diuretic agents such as Diuril increase the excretion of salts and water, resulting in a reduction of the blood-plasma volume (plasma is the liquid part of the blood) and a decrease in the work load of the heart. Other than their antihypertensive effect, diuretics are used mainly to treat edema, the swelling of body tissues caused by the accumulation of excess fluids. Edema is often associated with kidney disorders, cirrhosis of the liver, and congestive heart failure.

Endocrine System

The endocrine system is a network of various glandular organs that secrete chemical products or hormones directly into the blood. Major endocrine glands are identified in figure 3.6. Together with the nervous system, these "chemical messengers" from ductless glands maintain a constant internal body environment (homeostasis), regulate functions of metabolism, growth, and development, and modify certain types of behavior. Only a few of the many endocrine functions will be mentioned here.

When the pituitary gland's growth hormone (GH) is insufficiently secreted in childhood, body growth is limited—resulting in dwarfism. This form of hormone deficiency can be corrected by replacement therapy—the administration of a natural or synthetic hormone substance that will have the desired effect of the original.

Sometimes a drug introduced into the body can upset hormone function. Normally, another pituitary hormone, the antidiuretic hormone (ADH), functions to reduce excessive urine formation by the kidneys. However, the presence of ethyl alcohol in the central nervous system blocks the formation of ADH, and the kidneys work "overtime" in their output of urine.

The pituitary also secretes follicle-stimulating hormone (FSH) and luteinizing hormone (LH) in the female, and their hormonal counterparts in the male: FSH and ICSH (interstitial cell-stimulating hormone). These specific hormones are known as gonadotropins because they act on the gonads, or reproductive organs. The ovaries are directed chemically to initiate maturation of an ovum, production of estrogen (one of the female sex hormones), and ovulation. The testes respond to FSH by producing sperm, and they secrete androgen (the male sex hormones, the major one being testosterone) under the influence of ICSH.

The sex hormones themselves originate in the ovaries and testes, which also act as endocrine glands. In addition to their many functions related to the female

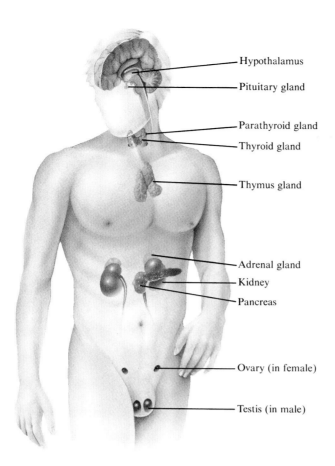

- Hypothalamus
- Pituitary gland
- Parathyroid gland
- Thyroid gland
- Thymus gland
- Adrenal gland
- Kidney
- Pancreas
- Ovary (in female)
- Testis (in male)

 3.6

Locations of major endocrine glands.

From Lester M. Sdorow, Psychology, *3d edition. Copyright © 1995 Wm. C. Brown Communications, Inc. Reprinted by permission of Times Mirror Higher Education Group, Inc., Dubuque, Iowa. All Rights Reserved.*

menstrual cycle and to the secondary sex characteristics of both sexes, sex hormones are the bases for various drug compounds, as noted below.

1. *Estrogen replacement therapy,* not without some risk to the patient, is used to provide relief from the distressing symptoms of menopause.

2. Commonly available oral contraceptive pills containing ethinyl estradiol (an estrogenic compound) and norgestrel (a progestogenic compound) can be used for *postcoital treatment when a contraceptive emergency arises.*[18] The treatment, known as the Yuzpe regimen, tends to be most effective if begun within the first twelve to twenty-four hours after unprotected intercourse. A synthetic androgen has also been used for emergency treatment in a regimen referred to as the Danazol treatment. No longer recommended for emergency postcoital contraception is a high-dose estrogen compound known as diethylstilbestrol (DES). Although effective, DES often resulted in severe side effects, particularly cancer and other health risks, in mothers and their female and male offspring.

3. The combination of estrogen and progesterone (another female sex hormone) is the chemical basis for *oral contraceptives,* pills that prevent pregnancy. The oral contraceptives act by blocking the pituitary gland's release of FSH and LH, by preventing the implantation of a fertilized egg in an unhospitable uterine lining, and/or by thickening the mucous plug in the cervix, thereby preventing sperm from entering the uterus.

4. A synthetic form of testosterone, the *anabolic-androgenic steroids* are drugs used by some athletes and bodybuilders to increase their muscle mass and weight. See also box 3.1.

Atop each kidney is another endocrine gland, the *adrenal.* One of the adrenal hormones is *cortisol,* which has been used in treating inflammatory conditions and reducing arthritic debilitation of the joints. Synthetic cortisonelike drugs are employed more effectively today and tend to reduce the undesirable side effects associated with cortisol.

Insulin, a hormone produced by specialized cells of the *pancreas,* enhances the entry of glucose (blood sugar) molecules into various body cells where the sugar is burned for energy or stored as a future source of fuel. If there is an impairment of insulin activity, the blood-sugar level increases until some of the surplus sugar spills over into the urine. This condition is the disease of *diabetes mellitus.*

Injection of insulin preparations replaces the deficient supply in the body and makes possible the utilization of sugars and starches. For some diabetics, *orally administered antidiabetic drugs* have been successful in lowering blood-sugar levels by stimulating the pancreas to secrete insulin. Drug therapy controls but does not cure diabetes.

Gastrointestinal System

Among the common disorders of the digestive system (mouth, pharynx and esophagus, stomach, the small and large intestines, plus associated organs) are *acid-related conditions, constipation,* and *diarrhea.*

Due to a variety of factors, gastric juices normally secreted by the stomach to assist in digestion begin to irritate the stomach, which undergoes a localized breakdown of its tissues. Sometimes the small intestine and esophagus are irritated too. The inner lining of these organs sustains a

Drugs and Sex: Selected Drugs and Their Possible Effects on Human Sexual Function

box 3.1

Drugs of abuse as well as frequently prescribed medications, identified here, can have undesirable effects on normal sexual functioning. Such drugs may impair an individual's sexual arousal, disrupt the sexual desire process, interfere with one's sexual performance, and therefore block sexual satisfaction.

Commonly Used Social or Recreational Drugs

Alcohol or ethyl alcohol in small doses tends to lessen sexual inhibitions, but in larger amounts it often reduces the male's ability to achieve erection and delays or reduces the female's experience of orgasm. Serum testosterone levels tend to decrease as blood alcohol levels increase, resulting in decreased sexual desire among males. At higher levels of intoxication, women tend to experience lowered levels of vaginal vasocongestion, which will inhibit sexual desire and possibly performance. Chronic use often leads to impotence, and among long-term alcoholics, sexual desire simply disappears. Eventually, the long-term female alcoholic may also experience menstrual disturbances, infertility, and a possible loss of secondary sex characteristics.

Amyl and *butyl nitrite* are inhalants that produce a brief "high" and also tend to enhance the sensation of orgasm. Due to its relaxation of the ringlike muscles around the anus, amyl nitrite has been used frequently by homosexual drug users.

Depressants, such as the sedative-hypnotics, tend to lessen inhibitions, may increase sexual desire, but may also produce inability to achieve erection, ejaculation, and orgasm in moderate to large doses.

Marijuana users experience varied effects, including relaxed sexual inhibitions, increased sexual pleasure, no impact whatsoever on sexual drive or performance, and also very negative feelings about sexual function. Erectile problems, lowered testosterone levels, disruption of normal sperm production, and—in the female—vaginal dryness, have all been reported. Enhanced sexual awareness is experienced more often when both parties are under the influence of marijuana.

Opioids, the narcotic analgesics, tend to impair sexual desire, performance, and satisfaction, and may even temporarily decrease female fertility, delay ejaculation, and reduce erections and orgasms during high-dose use. However, pain experienced by females during intercourse may be reduced.

Psychedelics, such as LSD, have been reported as both greatly increasing sexual desire and performance as well as producing totally asexual and nonerotic experiences. MDA, the so-called "love drug," may stimulate feelings of warmth and desire for communication, prerequisites for sexual interaction. Some MDA users remain motionless, however, during their drug experience.

Stimulants, specifically cocaine and amphetamines, are often considered aphrodisiacs, because they force the release of dopamine and norepinephrine neurotransmitters that are linked with natural sexual excitement. Cocaine may heighten sexual arousal and delay orgasm in fairly low doses. High-dose use, however, seems to correlate with high-risk sexual practices, while prolonged use often results in decreased sexual desire, erectile and ejaculation difficulties in the male, and anorgasmia (inhibited orgasm) in the female. Amphetamines typically increase sexual desire and delay orgasm in low doses, but high-dose use or prolonged use tends to have a negative impact on both sexual performance and satisfaction.

Stimulants, such as amphetamines, may either increase or decrease sexual desire and tend to reduce potency. Cocaine may heighten sexual arousal in fairly low doses, and delay orgasm, but regular use often results in decreased sexual desire.

Prescription Drugs

Antabuse, or disulfiram, an aversive drug used to deter abusive drinkers from alcoholic beverages, may cause reduced potency.

Cimetidine (Tagamet), a frequently prescribed antiulcer drug, may cause impotence and enlarged breasts in males and decreased sexual desire in females.

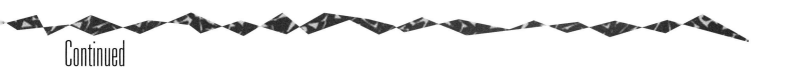

Continued

Conjugated estrogens (Premarin) can produce feminization, including loss of sexual desire, impotence, enlarged breasts, and shrinkage of the testes.

Guanethidine (Ismelin), used in treating hypertension (high blood pressure), prevents ejaculation. Other antihypertensives, such as clonidine (Catapres), may cause impotence or loss of sexual desire in females and males.

Levodopa (Larodopa), a drug used in treating Parkinson's disease, may be responsible for increased sexual desire in some men and women.

MAO inhibitors, including phenelzine (Nardil), used in treating psychological depression, may cause impotence.

Major tranquilizers, specifically thioridazine (Mellaril), sometimes cause ejaculatory problems.

Minor tranquilizers, the anti-anxiety drugs such as Valium and Librium, may reduce sexual desire and impair ejaculation.

Oral contraceptives may cause a reduction in sexual desire among some women.

Tolbutamide (Orinase), an oral antidiabetic medication, may cause prolonged, painful erections in some males.

Over-the-Counter Drugs

Aspirin can induce impaired spermatogenesis (formation of sperm), leading to reduced fertility in males.

Vitamin A in excessive dosages can result in menstrual disorders.

Vitamin C in doses of 1 gram or more can also impair spermatogenesis.

Ibuprofen may delay the onset of menstruation by as much as fourteen days.

The romantic link between alcohol and sex is greatly exaggerated. While small amounts may provoke sexual desire, larger amounts may spoil the capacity to perform or respond.

© *Bob Daemmrich/The Image Works*

Sources: Harold Doweiko, *Concepts of Chemical Dependency,* 2d. edition, pages 401–410, Brooks/Cole, Pacific Grove, Calif., 1993; and James Long and James Rybacki, *The Essential Guide to Prescription Drugs,* pages 1120–1126, Harper Perennial, New York, 1994.

long-term inflammation that can develop into an erosion of the lining, a form of self-digestion. The resulting lesion, or open sore, is referred to as an *ulcer.*

Immediate effects of heartburn, acid indigestion, and upset stomach, as well as the pain and discomfort of *gastric* (peptic) *ulcer disease,* are treated by drugs that hasten the healing of the ulcer and prevent its recurrence. Various antacids, both prescription and over-the-counter preparations, as well as antibiotics are now used in therapy. Gels, tablets, powders, suspensions, and gums relieve pain and tend to promote healing of the ulcer. Sodium bicarbonate, calcium carbonate, and aluminum and magnesium compounds—all types of antacids—neutralize gastric acid and reduce the digestive action of pepsin, a stomach enzyme (chemical) that breaks down protein substances. Frequently used drugs, including aspirin, ethyl alcohol, caffeine, and nicotine, should be avoided by people with ulcers. Such chemicals stimulate the secretion of gastric acid.

Laxatives are drugs that induce defecation. Among the most widely misused over-the-counter drugs, laxatives are taken to remedy constipation, the difficult passing of stools, and the decreasing frequency of bowel movements. Laxatives are usually classified as stimulants or initiators of peristaltic movements (alternate contraction and relaxation of the muscular walls), bulk formers, lubricants, and fecal softeners.

When fecal material moves more rapidly than normal through the large intestine, it is often expelled in a semisolid or fluid state. This condition is known as *diarrhea. Antidiarrheal* agents commonly used are those containing opiates or opiatelike synthetic compounds (Paregoric and Lomotil) and anticholinergic drugs, both of which reduce peristaltic movements of the large intestine. Drugs that *adsorb,* or gather in on their surfaces the poisons and bacteria responsible for diarrhea, are frequently sold without prescription to control diarrhea. Examples of *adsorbents* are Pepto-Bismol, Kaolin, Pectin, and Kaopectate.

Respiratory System

Included in the respiratory system are the nose, nasal cavity, sinuses, throat, larynx, trachea, bronchial tree, and the lungs. These organs filter incoming air and transport it to the lungs where gaseous exchanges occur.

Perhaps the most frequent disorder of this body system is the *common cold,* a viral infection of the upper portion of the respiratory tract. Cold symptoms include nasal discharge and congestion, cough, fever, aches, and pain. Although there is no cure for this viral-caused disease, various medications can provide some relief of symptoms. *Nasal decongestants* are vasoconstrictor drugs that reduce the flow of blood in the nasal membranes and thus shrink swollen nasal tissues. This action promotes nasal drainage and unobstructed air passage. *Antitussive agents,* such as codeine and Romilar hydrobromide, inhibit or suppress coughing; *antihistamines* are used widely to decrease mucus secretion and relieve a "runny nose." Aspirin and acetaminophen (Tylenol) act both as *analgesics* (pain relievers) and *antipyretics* (substances that reduce fever).

An allergy is a special sensitivity to some ordinarily harmless substance, such as, dust, dog dander, pollens, grasses, and mold spores. Collectively, these invading substances are called allergens because they can trigger the body's secretion of a powerful defensive chemical, *histamine.* The action of histamine in the area of the nose causes dilation of the blood vessels there, increased secretion of mucus and other nasal fluids, tissue swelling, sneezing, itching, and other discomforting symptoms. *Antihistamines* are used to block the histamine receptor sites on cells and thereby prevent histamine from having its undesirable effects. Pyrilamine (Neo-Antergan) and Chlorpheniramine (Chlor-Trimeton) Maleate are frequently used antihistamines. Because antihistamines tend to promote drowsiness—a secondary effect of these drugs related to central nervous system depression—they are often included in nonprescription sleep aids like Compoz and Sominex.

Asthma is a chronic, reversible obstruction of the airways, manifest by shortness of breath. Asthma attacks of breathing difficulty are due to the generalized narrowing or constriction of the bronchi, small air tubes within the lungs. Drugs employed in treating bronchial asthma are *ephedrine, epinephrine* (adrenaline), and *isoproterenol,* all of which cause the bronchi to dilate, thus restoring ease of breathing. Corticosteroid treatment has also proved effective in treating some cases of asthma.

Chemotherapy

As defined earlier in this chapter, **chemotherapy** is a special type of therapeutics in which drugs are used to kill or weaken organisms that invade the body or abnormal cells within the body. Such drugs are relatively more toxic to the "invaders" and "strangers" than to the patients being treated.

Chemotherapeutic agents act selectively against bacteria, fungi, viruses, multicellular organisms, and cancerous cells. Drugs that kill bacteria are described as *bactericidal,* while those that inhibit growth of bacteria are referred to as *bacteriostatic.* The effectiveness of such drugs depends upon their ability to interfere with various normal functions of the invading organisms, specifically, nutritional processes, synthesis of cell walls, nucleic acid, protein, and cell-membrane permeability.

Among the first chemotherapeutic agents were the *antiseptics* or *disinfectants,* substances capable of destroying microorganisms on the skin's surface. However, these were too toxic (poisonous) for internal use. After considerable research and accidental discovery, antimicrobial agents for internal use were developed. Such drugs are represented by

1. *sulfonamides* or *sulfa drugs*—synthetic antimicrobials and their derivatives used to combat certain bacterial microorganisms; and

2. *antibiotics*—drugs derived originally from other living cells such as molds.

Common antibiotics, used against a variety of bacteria and certain rickettsias and fungi, include the penicillins, tetracyclines, chloramphenicol, and streptomycin.

Drugs used in *cancer chemotherapy* to kill malignant cells are identified as *alkylating agents* that apparently interfere with cancer cell division, *antimetabolites* that interrupt the chemical processes of cancer cells, and *steroid hormones* that are selectively toxic against certain cancers originating in tissues under the influence of hormones.

One recent addition to the chemotherapeutic arsenal is *interferon* (IF). This is a natural substance produced by the body itself in minute amounts. Interferon's antitumor activity appears to be related to its antiviral properties of preventing viral replication in uninfected cells. Since some tumors appear to be related to viruses, interferon holds considerable promise in the protection of normal cells from cancer viruses.

Drug Dependence

Most people who use psychoactive drugs do so only as long as the problems and dangers associated with such use do not outweigh the perceived benefits. And most individuals are capable of using mind-changing drugs only occasionally and in moderate amounts. However, some find it extremely difficult or even impossible to control their use. This condition of uncontrolled drug use is generally referred to as drug dependence or drug addiction, the very heart of the modern drug problem.[19]

Often described as a psychological or physical condition (or both) in which a drug user needs regular doses of a chemical in order to function normally, **drug dependence** can occur in an individual who uses a drug periodically or on a continuous basis. Even though drug dependence is not exclusively associated with psychoactive drugs, the term is often used with reference to chemical mood and behavior modifiers.

Addiction

For many years, the word **addiction** was used to define compulsive use of drug substances, especially the narcotics and alcohol. Even today, the vast majority of people and many drug treatment and rehabilitation specialists use this term to describe drug taking in which the user's behavior is largely controlled by a substance that has a psychoactive effect and whose use is reinforcing. Addiction also involves compulsive use of a drug despite damage to the individual or to society. Furthermore, the drug-seeking behavior can take precedence over other life priorities.[20] Once the addictive state has developed, the drug becomes so important to the addict that he or she is completely uninterested in other people and activities.

During the recent past, considerable difficulty arose in distinguishing among the several interpretations of *addiction* and its companion term *habituation,* used to describe a drug that was merely habit forming. As compulsive drug use assumed even more varied dimensions with the newer recreational psychoactives, the World Health Organization eventually proposed substituting the more neutral term *drug dependence* for addiction.[21] More recent variations in drug-abuse terminology include *chemical dependency* and *substance abuse* (or *alcohol and other drug abuse*), more inclusive perhaps than the older terms.

Today, some authorities use the terms *drug addiction* and *drug dependence* as scientifically equivalent because both refer to the behavior of repeated intake of mood-altering and mind-changing substances. While *addiction* is the word used by the National Institute on Drug Abuse and other organizations when information is provided at a general level, the term *drug dependence* is preferred in the scientific and medical literature.

The Continuum of Drug Use and Drug Dependence (Addiction)

Although many people, including addiction therapists, believe that drug dependence is an either/or condition—it is either present or not—chemical dependence or addiction may be seen more accurately as a continuum or succession from moderate excess to severe, compulsive use. In one sense, drug dependence appears to evolve over a period of time, which varies from one person to another. As a consequence, an individual might be described as abstaining from drugs, using one or more drugs on a social basis, abusing a drug occasionally, abusing one or more drugs on a continuing basis, or being addicted to a drug.[22]

This concept of the evolving or developing nature of addiction views drug usage as a continuum ranging from nonuse to long-term addiction to one or more drugs. The following are the stages of the drug-use continuum:[23]

Total abstinence, or complete nonuse of all recreational psychoactive drugs, including alcoholic beverages.

Rare social use, or infrequent recreational use of a psychoactive drug, but without any drug-related problems.

Heavy social use/early problem use of psychoactive drugs in which frequent excessive use is accompanied by the onset of various drug-related problems, including legal, financial, social, occupational, and personal—a condition that might be considered drug abuse.

Heavy problem use/early addiction marked by frequent excessive use in association with drug-related problems, beginning medical complications, and the traditional withdrawal syndrome when unable to continue use of the drug.

Clear-cut drug addiction in which long-term compulsive use is characterized by the classic withdrawal syndrome following abstinence, multiple drug-related problems, various medical complications linked with drug abuse, use of psychological defense mechanisms (rationalization and projection) to explain abnormal drug use, and the possibility of death resulting from alcohol and/or other drug dependence.

As these stages or levels demonstrate, drug use can be classified according to various intensities and patterns, of which drug dependence or addiction is viewed as one extreme on the drug-use continuum.

Criteria for Psychoactive Drug Dependence

It is quite apparent that no single pattern of drug dependence fits all drugs or drug takers. While all psychoactive chemicals can produce a psychological dependence with repeated use, this particular condition is markedly present in the narcotic opioids, but only mildly present in caffeine and marijuana. With heroin, there is considerably more tolerance than in alcohol abuse, but there are more severe withdrawal symptoms associated with alcohol than are usually present with the narcotic drug. To account for such variations, a single multifactorial

category of substance dependence disorders has been proposed by the American Psychiatric Association. This category includes all major drugs of abuse, including caffeine.

According to the American Psychiatric Association's official diagnostic handbook, the *Diagnostic and Statistical Manual of Mental Disorders* (DSM-IV), substance dependence is a maladaptive (faulty or non-problem-resolving) pattern of drug use leading to clinically significant impairment or distress characterized by three (or more) of the following criteria, occurring at any time in a twelve-month period:[24,25]

Tolerance, distinguished by either of the following:

- There is a need for markedly increased amounts of the drug substance to achieve intoxication or the desired effect.

- There is a markedly diminished effect with continued use of the same amount of the drug.

Withdrawal, specified by either of the following:

- Characteristic withdrawal syndrome (combination of symptoms) develops when use of the drug has been stopped.

- The drug substance is often taken to relieve or avoid withdrawal symptoms.

(These criteria might not apply to marijuana, other cannabis preparations, hallucinogens, and phencyclidine.)

Impaired control

- The chemical substance is often taken in larger amounts or over a longer period of time than the drug taker intended.

Desire to quit or unsuccessful attempts to control

- There is a persistent desire or unsuccessful efforts to cut down or control substance use.

Time spent using drugs

- A great deal of time is spent in various activities needed to acquire the drug substance (including theft), to take the substance (as in chain-smoking), and recover from the drug's effects.

Neglect of activities

- Important social, occupational, or recreational activities are given up or reduced in order to seek or take a drug.

Drug use despite knowledge of problems

- Use of a drug continues despite knowledge of having a persistent or recurring physical or psychological problem that is caused or made worse by substance use. For instance, cocaine use continues despite an individual's awareness of cocaine-induced depression, or drinking of alcoholic beverages persists despite recognition that an ulcer has been made worse by repeated alcohol consumption.

While preoccupation with drug use, the evolving "love affair" between drug taker and drug substance, and the occurrence of drug-related problems can be observed by others, and therefore documented, only the drug abuser experiences several other aspects. These aspects deserve a more thorough analysis, especially psychological dependence, tolerance, physical dependence, and the withdrawal syndrome.

Psychological Dependence

A rather nonspecific term, *psychological* or *psychic dependence* refers to drug dependence without any physical complications. An individual who develops **psychological dependence** on a particular drug has a strong desire to repeat the use of that drug either occasionally or continuously for emotional reasons. Presumably, the persistent drug taking is related to the reinforcing or rewarding effects of the drug.

Although the body does not require the drug in a physical sense, the person has an intense craving or compulsion for it to maintain drug-induced pleasure and a feeling of well-being, to achieve a maximum level of functioning, to reduce tensions, or to dull reality. When drug seeking becomes compulsive and a regular behavioral pattern, psychological dependence has reached its peak intensity. Deprived of the drug, the user will typically experience a period of readjustment, accompanied by some degree of anxiety, irritability, and restlessness. No physical complications follow the discontinuance of drug usage.

It should be noted that an individual may be psychologically dependent on any given drug without being physically dependent on that drug. The opposite is also true: It is possible to be physically dependent on a drug without being psychologically dependent, although such occurrences are relatively rare and almost always involve the administration of a physician-prescribed narcotic analgesic in a medical facility. However, such a distinction between psychological and physical dependence might not be very relevant, since long-term users of drugs producing only psychological dependence act and function in much the same way as addicts of drugs that produce physical dependence.[26]

While psychological dependence is a characteristic of all drugs of abuse, the condition is often considered insignificant in comparison with physical dependence. Such is not the case! In chronic drug use, psychological dependence is increasingly viewed as more serious and more difficult to deal with than physical dependence.[27] Chemically dependent people involved only at the psychological level believe that they can control their drugs, that they are not using them to excess, and that they are not harming themselves or others. Such perceptions place them in a position where they risk their lives time and time again with both the quantity and the quality of their chemical usage.[28] Such individuals have no concept of what they are doing to themselves or to others.

Tolerance

An altered physiological state, **tolerance** develops with the repeated use of almost all drugs.[29] This condition is usually defined as a decreased response to the effects of a drug. As a consequence of this reduced sensitivity, the dosage must be increased to achieve the desired effects.

The onset of tolerance may be rapid or gradual, depending upon the drug used. However, this condition is not an all-or-none phenomenon, since a person may develop a tolerance to one aspect of a particular drug's action but not to another. It should also be noted that tolerance can accompany psychological dependence upon a drug without the occurrence of physical dependence. Nevertheless, the need to increase the dosage is more often seen in conjunction with the latter condition.

Usually the degree of tolerance varies with the drug and with other circumstances. Psychedelic drugs produce an extremely high tolerance very rapidly, while a high tolerance to the opioids and amphetamines also develops but at a much slower pace. A somewhat lower and more variable degree of tolerance develops with the repeated use of alcohol, nicotine, and marijuana.

Theories that explain the mechanisms of physiological or tissue tolerance may appear both contradictory or complementary. One major theory holds that tolerance is the result of alterations in how a drug is processed in the body after repeated doses are taken. Changes occur in the normal processes of drug absorption, distribution, metabolism, or elimination. For instance, the liver and other body organs destroy or break apart the drug substance more quickly due to a process called *enzyme induction* or excrete it more efficiently. As a result, less of the drug reaches the site of its action. Another contrasting theory is based on the reduced sensitivity of nerve-cell receptor sites that takes place over a long period of drug taking. This represents a form of cellular or tissue adaptation in which reaction to the drug is diminished. It is also possible that

the nerve cells (neurons) create additional receptor sites to accommodate the increased dosage of a drug.

In some instances, there is a condition known as *tachyphylaxis* or *acute tolerance,* which is an extremely rapid development of tolerance after just one or a few doses of the drug. LSD, amphetamines, and cocaine tend to show rapid development of tolerance, especially when large doses are used for short periods of time. This phenomenon may be due to the rapid exhaustion of a neurotransmitter or an accelerated loss of receptor sensitivity.

According to Sidney Cohen, the condition of *kindling* may be thought of as the exact opposite of tolerance.[30] In this form of "reverse tolerance," drug takers can become more sensitive to the effects of a given drug, rather than less sensitive. Analogous to igniting a wood fire, the so-called *kindling effect* spreads slowly at first, then suddenly erupts in a symptom compared to a briskly burning blaze. For instance, in cocaine use, the brain may become sensitive to the drug after repeated average doses, so that even low amounts of the stimulant may bring on seizures.

After long-term heavy use of alcohol, another example of "reverse tolerance" may also be evident. A liver damaged by the buildup of fat and the assaults of hepatitis and/or cirrhosis may no longer be able to metabolize effectively any alcohol consumed. Consequently, even small amounts of beverage alcohol result in elevated blood alcohol levels and the rapid experience of intoxication.

One additional concern with tolerance is the development of *cross-tolerance,* a condition in which the reduced pharmacological response to one drug results in a lessened response to another drug. Cross-tolerance, however, typically occurs among drugs belonging to the same class or related classes of chemical substances. For example, an individual tolerant to morphine is also tolerant to all other narcotic drugs, including heroin and methadone. However, such a person will not have a tolerance to alcohol and barbiturates, which belong to another class of psychoactive drugs.

Physical Dependence

An altered physiological state, physical or physiological dependence is induced by the frequent use of a drug and results in unwanted and adverse physical symptoms—the withdrawal syndrome—when drug use has stopped. Often described as a condition of physical need, **physical dependence** is presumed to have existed only when withdrawal symptoms occur.

The actual causes of this physical need are the temporary and compensatory changes in the cells of the nervous system. These changes in cellular functioning permit the nerve cells to work in their accustomed fashion in the presence of a particular chemical substance and take place over a period of several weeks or months. Thus physical dependence is a state of functional adaptation to a drug in which the presence of a foreign chemical becomes "normal" and necessary. In other words, the absence of a drug would constitute an abnormality, and the presence of a drug is required for normal function.

Often considered as the most hazardous aspect of drug abuse, physical dependence is likely to develop with continuing use of narcotics, barbiturates, minor tranquilizers, ethyl alcohol, and cocaine, and to a lesser degree with nicotine, caffeine, marijuana, and the amphetamines. Only use of the psychedelics and volatile inhalants does not result in physical dependence.

Cross-dependence is a condition in which a person who is physically dependent on one drug can prevent withdrawal symptoms by using other drugs in the same pharmacological class or a closely related drug class. For example, methadone can be substituted for heroin and prevents the occurrence of withdrawal when heroin use is discontinued. In general, those drugs that exhibit cross-tolerance will likely demonstrate cross-dependence to one another.

Withdrawal Syndrome

As mentioned above, the condition of physical dependence is revealed only when drug use is discontinued. If the drug is removed abruptly, "normal" cell function is disturbed, resulting in hyperexcitability (overactivity) or hypo-excitability (underactivity) of the nervous system.

Typically, when a person who is physically dependent on a central nervous system depressant (alcohol, barbiturates, or narcotics) stops using the drug, the *withdrawal symptoms* in evidence are restlessness, overactivity of the nervous system, and agitation—an uneven or disturbed form of stimulation. Withdrawal symptoms that occur after long-term use of cocaine, a central nervous system stimulant, are marked by psychic depression and uncontrolled drowsiness and excessive sleep. These drastic alterations in physical function and behavior, experienced after drug use is terminated, are known collectively as the classic **withdrawal syndrome,** *withdrawal sickness,* or the *abstinence syndrome.* Generally, the syndrome consists of symptoms broadly opposite to the drug's usual effects and produces a kind of "rebound" effect.[31]

Common signs and symptoms of the withdrawal syndrome may include watery eyes, runny nose, yawning, perspiration, restless sleep, irritability, loss of appetite, insomnia, tremors, nausea, vomiting, stomach cramps, diarrhea, elevation of heart rate and blood pressure, pain in muscles and bones, muscle spasms, convulsions, anxiety, depression, suicidal tendencies, and occasional psychotic episodes. Fortunately, not all of these functional changes are experienced by everyone who sustains the abstinence syndrome.

While the process of withdrawal can be painful and in some instances results in death, it nevertheless permits the nerve cells to return to their predrugged state and reduces the level of tolerance that has developed. In some instances, especially with heroin and other narcotics, a type of "prolonged" abstinence or withdrawal may be experienced in which elevated blood pressure, heart rate, and intense cravings suddenly recur many months and even years after the original withdrawal process. Similar to post-traumatic stress, the prolonged withdrawal phenomenon is possibly activated by exposure to particular sights, sounds, or odors. These stimuli cause the former addict to reexperience memories of the original withdrawal syndrome and the severe cravings for the drug. This rather strange condition may be the basis for relapse—the return of a person who has undergone withdrawal to the addictive or drug-dependent state once again.

With increasing frequency, multiple-drug dependence—evidence of polydrug abuse—is being reported by physicians and hospitals. In such cases, the individual goes through a series of withdrawal syndromes from each drug so abused.

Another potential hazard of polydrug abuse is drug interaction (see box 3.2).

The Placebo Effect

One of the more unusual aspects of pharmacology is the **placebo effect.** Derived from the Latin word meaning "I will please," a *placebo* is a preparation or treatment that has no specific effect on a patient's illness. Many view a placebo as a fake medicine, an inert substance that has no pharmacologic effect, such as a sugar pill or an injection of sterile water. Such nonmedicated items are administered for their psychological effect.

Although some physicians allegedly use placebos to fool or deceive patients, their rather suspect reputation is also due to their use in testing the effectiveness of new medicines. In clinical trial experiments, one group of patients receiving a new drug is compared with another group that is given an identical-looking placebo. This type of drug effectiveness testing is known as a *single-blind study.* When the identity of the medicine—placebo or active form—is withheld from both the test subjects and the evaluators, the drug testing design is called a *double-blind study.* If the active test drug fails to achieve better results than those obtained through the use of a placebo, the test drug is abandoned as useless and worthless.

Surprisingly, placebos can have a positive and even beneficial effect on many patients in certain circumstances. Placebos have been recorded not only as reducing pain, but also as healing ulcers, relieving hay fever, coughing, and elevated blood

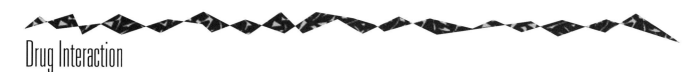

Drug Interaction

box 3.2

Double Trouble

Drug interaction is the phenomenon that occurs when one or more drugs present in the body alter the actions or effects of another drug present in the body at the same time. When drugs are taken in combination, the effects usually fall into one of the following categories.

Independent

Drugs taken together may work independently of each other, that is, neither one affects the drug actions of the other.

Antagonistic

Drugs taken together may interact so that the effect of either or both agents is blocked or reduced. The interaction "equation" is represented as 2 + 2 = 3.

An antagonistic interaction is likely to occur when the antibiotic tetracycline is taken at the same time with penicillin, another common antibiotic medication. Tetracycline reduces the effectiveness of the penicillin and may actually prolong an infection.

Another antagonistic drug interaction involves the combination of barbiturates and oral contraceptives. The headache remedy tends to reduce the effectiveness of the oral contraceptives.

The narcotic antagonist naloxone counteracts the effects of heroin or morphine overdose.

Additive

Drugs taken together may interact so that the net effect of the combination is the sum of the effects of the individual substances. The interaction "equation" may be represented as 2 + 2 = 4.

An additive effect is produced by the simultaneous consumption of two barbiturates, such as phenobarbital and secobarbital.

The interaction of narcotic analgesics with the phenothiazines (major antipsychotic drugs) may

result in either an additive effect or a potentiated drug interaction.

Potentiating or Synergistic

Drugs taken together may interact so that the effect of the two substances in combination is greater than merely additive. This phenomenon often occurs when one drug increases or potentiates the effect of the second drug by altering its distribution, its conversion into other chemicals, or its excretion from the body. In synergistic drug interactions, the effect of the second drug may be intensified or the duration of its action may be prolonged. The interaction "equation" is represented as 2 + 2 = 5.

An example of a potentiating drug interaction involves the use of a prescribed ulcer medication, Tagamet, together with alcoholic beverages. The antiulcer drug tends to increase blood-alcohol levels and may make drinkers more drunk if they do consume alcoholic beverages.

Listed below are some of the more dangerous combinations that can result when psychoactive drugs are taken together with other types of drugs or medication. These drugs

should never be combined without the consent and supervision of a physician:

Barbiturates in combination with tranquilizers, alcohol, drugs for high blood pressure, stimulants, cortisone, painkillers, diuretics, anticonvulsants, or birth-control pills

Tranquilizers in combination with barbiturates, antihistamines, alcohol, drugs for high blood pressure, stimulants, antidepressants, or painkillers

Stimulants in combination with barbiturates, tranquilizers, beer, drugs for high blood pressure, antidepressants, anticonvulsants, drugs for diabetes or digitalis

Antidepressants in combination with tranquilizers, alcohol, drugs for high blood pressure, stimulants, diuretics, anticoagulants, or asthma spray

Note: For a detailed listing of potentially harmful food and drug interaction, see box 12.5.
Source: National Clearing House for Alcohol Information, as modified, National Institute on Alcohol Abuse and Alcoholism, Department of Health and Human Services.

pressure, and enhancing physical performance. On the average, about one-third of individuals receiving placebos are helped.

The precise mechanisms of a positive placebo effect are not well understood, especially since no specific drug response is anticipated. Most believe that the placebo response arises from the person's own unique mental set and predisposition or from the entire environmental situation in which the inactive substance is taken.[32-33] It is now apparent that the patient's faith, beliefs, and expectations regarding the placebo, the physician's enthusiasm, and the context in which the substance is taken are all powerful elements in placebo-induced as well as in drug-induced responses.

Other factors that may explain how nonmedicines sometimes work have been proposed, including these:

* Increased production of endorphin neurotransmitters, morphinelike chemicals within the human body, that act on neuron receptors in the central nervous system to deaden pain.

* Activation of the body's immune system, a complex of biochemical processes that provide resistance to specific diseases.

* The patient's anxiety level, rather than gullibility or suggestibility. As the level of anxiety or free-floating fear increases, one's chance of responding favorably to a placebo increases.

As research into the positive placebo effect continues, some scientists believe that it can be used ethically as a powerful tool to enhance the benefits of modern medical practice.

Chapter Summary

1. Pharmacology is the study of the interaction of chemical agents with living organisms.

2. Since the introduction of chemical agents that have no relation to treating diseases, a drug is now defined as any chemical that affects living processes.

3. Drugs are most frequently administered orally, parenterally, and by inhalation.

4. After absorption, drugs are distributed in various patterns, metabolized by the liver, and excreted chiefly by the kidneys.

5. Structurally specific drugs interact with localized portions of cells, the receptors, in order to change cell functions.

6. Drugs can change cell function by stimulation, depression, blocking, replacement, killing or inactivating organisms, and by irritation.

7. Dosage, age, body weight, gender, time, disease, mind-set, and the environmental setting can affect drug actions within the human body.

8. The nervous system consists of the central nervous system (brain and spinal cord) and the peripheral nervous system, which is subdivided into the somatic and autonomic nervous system.

9. The sympathetic and parasympathetic subdivisions of the autonomic nervous system act in an antagonistic manner.

10. As the basic unit of the nervous system, the neuron consists of a cell body, one axon, and several dendrites.

11. An electrical impulse is transmitted from the axon of one neuron to the dendrite of another neuron by chemical substances, the neurotransmitters.

12. Psychoactive drugs have their major effect on the synapse, the junction between nerve cells, especially those in the specialized structures of the brain.

13. Specific drugs have a variety of actions on human sexual function and on the following body systems: cardiovascular-renal, endocrine, gastrointestinal, and respiratory.

14. Chemotherapy is the use of drugs to kill or weaken organisms that invade the body or abnormal cells within the body.

15. Major characteristics of drug dependence include various undesirable behaviors related with persistent drug use or abuse, such as increasing preoccupation with a drug, inability to fulfill common roles due to drug abuse, and not being able to stop drug use, as well as psychological and physical dependence, the development of tolerance, and the experience of withdrawal symptoms.

16. Drug interactions are categorized as independent, antagonistic, additive, and potentiating or synergistic.

17. A placebo is a nonmedicated preparation that has no specific pharmacologic effect on a patient's illness.

Review Questions and Activities

1. State the definition of pharmacology and distinguish among its three major subdivisions.

2. Explain the following terms as related to drug administration: *oral, rectal, parenteral,* and *inhalation.*

3. What are the basic patterns of drug distribution in the human body?

4. Describe the processes involved in the elimination of drugs from the body.

5. What is a drug receptor?

6. Distinguish among the following drug actions: stimulation, depression, blocking, replacement, killing or inactivation, and irritation.

7. Define threshold dose, median effective dose, maximum effect, and lethal dose.

8. How do factors such as age, body weight, disease, gender, and emotional states affect drug actions?

9. Identify the major parts and functions of the nervous system.

10. Define the following terms: *neuron, cell body, axon, dendrite, synapse, synaptic cleft.*

11. How is a nerve impulse transmitted from one neuron to another?

12. What is the significance of the following: acetylcholine, norepinephrine, dopamine, serotonin, GABA, and glycine?

13. What possible effects could psychoactive substances have on the functions of the medulla oblongata, ARAS, midbrain, cerebellum, hypothalamus, limbic system, and cerebrum?

14. Describe briefly the major actions of the following drugs: digitalis, nitroglycerin, antihypertensive agents, diuretics, insulin, antacids, laxatives, antihistamine.

15. What are some possible effects of using psychoactive drugs on human sexual function?

16. Differentiate between the following actions of antimicrobial agents: bactericidal and bacteriostatic.

17. What is the difference between an antiseptic and an antibiotic?

18. How do the following characteristics of drug dependence differ from one another: psychological dependence, physical dependence, tolerance?

19. In what way can addiction or drug dependence be viewed as a continuum?

20. What criteria have been established by the American Psychiatric Association to describe a drug-dependent individual?

21. Distinguish between an additive drug interaction and a potentiating drug interaction.

22. Explain how a placebo could possibly have a positive effect on a patient.

References

1. Bertram Katzung, ed., *Basic and Clinical Pharmacology,* 4th ed. (Norwalk, Conn.: Appleton & Lange, 1989), 1.
2. Andrew Weil and Winifred Rosen, *From Chocolate to Morphine,* rev. ed. (Boston: Houghton Mifflin, 1993), 9.
3. Charles Clayman, ed., *The American Medical Association Guide to Prescription and Over-the-Counter Drugs* (New York: Random House, 1988), 17–18.
4. Robert Julien, *A Primer of Drug Action,* 6th ed. (New York: W. H. Freeman, 1992), 2–8.
5. Christina Dye, *Drugs and the Body: A New Way to Understand Psychoactive Chemicals and Ourselves* (Tempe, Ariz.: Do It Now, 1989), 11–13.
6. Ibid., 13.
7. William Creasey, *Drug Disposition in Humans: The Basis of Clinical Pharmacology* (New York: Oxford University Press, 1979), 33–34.
8. John Hole, *Human Anatomy and Physiology,* 6th ed. (Dubuque, Iowa: Brown & Benchmark, 1993), 674.
9. Leslie Benet, Jerry Mitchell, and Lewis Sheiner, "Pharmacokinetics: The Dynamics of Drug Absorption, Distribution, and Elimination," in *Goodman and Gilman's The Pharmacological Basis of Therapeutics,* 8th ed. (New York: McGraw-Hill, 1990), 11.
10. Clayman, *AMA Guide,* 14.
11. Michael C. Gerald, *Pharmacology: An Introduction to Drugs* (Englewood Cliffs, N.J.: Prentice-Hall, 1981), 30–32.
12. Roberta Morgan, *The Emotional Pharmacy* (Los Angeles: Body Press, 1988), 32–37.
13. Katzung, *Basic and Clinical Pharmacology,* 24.
14. Tibor Palfai and Henry Jankiewicz, *Drugs and Human Behavior* (Dubuque, Iowa: Brown & Benchmark, 1991), 94.
15. Weil and Rosen, *From Chocolate to Morphine,* 25.
16. Hole, *Human Anatomy and Physiology,* 401.
17. Floyd Bloom, "Neurohumoral Transmission and the Central Nervous System," in *Goodman and Gilman's The Pharmacological Basis of Therapeutics,* 8th ed. (New York: McGraw-Hill, 1990), 244–68.

18. Robert Hatcher and others, *Contraceptive Technology,* 16th rev. ed. (New York: Irvington, 1994), 416–17.

19. Lester Grinspoon and James Bakalar, *Drug Abuse and Addiction: The Harvard Medical School Mental Health Review* (Boston: Harvard Mental Health Letter, 1993), 2.

20. C. Everett Koop, *The Health Consequences of Smoking: Nicotine Addiction: A Report of the Surgeon General* (Washington, D.C.: U.S. Government Printing Office, 1988), iv, 7.

21. N. B. Eddy, H. Halbach, H. Isbell, and M. H. Seevers, "Drug Dependence: Its Significance and Characteristics," *Bulletin of the World Health Organization* 32 (May 1965): 721–33.

22. Harold Doweiko, *Concepts of Chemical Dependency,* 2d ed. (Pacific Grove, Calif.: Brooks/Cole, 1993), 12–13.

23. Ibid.

24. American Psychiatric Association, *Diagnostic and Statistical Manual of Mental Disorders,* 4th ed. (Washington, D.C.: American Psychiatric Association, 1994), 181.

25. "DSM-IV Makes Changes in Substance-Related Disorders," *Substance Abuse Reports* 25, no. 15 (1 August 1994): 4–5.

26. Erich Goode, "Addiction and Dependence," in *Drugs in American Society,* 4th ed. (New York: McGraw-Hill, 1993), 28–34.

27. Robert O'Brien, Sidney Cohen, Glen Evans, and James Fine, *The Encyclopedia of Drug Abuse,* 2d ed. (New York: Facts on File, 1992), 257–58.

28. Hazelden Foundation, *Chemical Dependence: Psychological vs. Physiological* (Center City, Minn.: Hazelden Foundation, 1974), 2.

29. Grinspoon and Bakalar, *Drug Abuse and Addiction,* 4.

30. Sidney Cohen, *The Chemical Brain: The Neurochemistry of Addictive Disorders* (Irvine, Calif.: CareInstitute, 1988), 60.

31. O'Brien et al., *Encyclopedia of Drug Abuse,* 308.

32. Julien, *A Primer of Drug Action,* 41–42.

33. Palfai and Jankeiwicz, *Drugs and Human Behavior,* 91–94.

p a r t
t w o

The Depressants

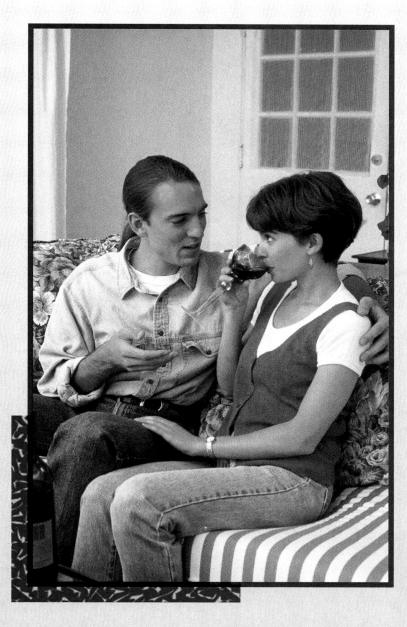

Questions of concern

1. When will the costs of alcohol abuse and alcoholism outweigh the perceived benefits of alcoholic beverage consumption?

2. Why are narcotics so frequently thought of as "devil drugs," the very worst of all abused psychoactive substances?

3. Wouldn't a tranquilized society be more peaceful and stable than our current tension-filled and stressful society?

drinki

alcoho

abuse,

and

chapter

4

alcohol: drinking, alcohol abuse, and alcoholism

Absorption
Abstinence
Alcoholics Anonymous (AA)
Alcoholism
Alcohol States of Consciousness (ASC)
Ambivalence
Antabuse
Beer
Blackout
Blood-Alcohol Concentration
Bootlegging
Breathalyzer
Co-alcoholism
Co-dependence
Congeners
Delirium Tremens
Detoxification
Distilled Spirits
Distribution
Dry-Drunk Phenomenon
Fetal Alcohol Syndrome (FAS)
Hangover
Intoxication
Loss of Control
Moonshining
Oxidation
Potentiation Effect
Problem Drinking
Prohibition
Pseudostimulation
Rapid Eye Movement (REM)
Social Drinking
Temperance
Tolerance
Wine
Withdrawal Symptoms

chapter objectives

After you have studied this chapter, you should be able to do the following:

1. Define the key terms for this chapter.

2. Estimate the number and percentage of American drinkers.

3. Describe the changes in tactics and goals of the American temperance movement that occurred before 1840.

4. Explain the significance of the Eighteenth and Twenty-First Amendments to the U.S. Constitution, and the Volstead Act, to the historical period known as the Prohibition Era.

5. Discuss how faulty attitudes about alcohol, drinking, and drinkers contribute to alcohol problems in modern society.

6. Describe several aspects of social drinking.

7. Discuss the use of alcoholic beverages as a mood modifier.

8. Distinguish between the concepts of awareness and unawareness in relation to alcohol use.

9. Compare the three major classes of beverage alcohol in terms of production, relative alcohol content, and the amount of alcohol per typical serving.

10. Identify at least five factors that can influence the absorption of ethyl alcohol.

11. Describe the process of alcohol oxidation.

12. Explain the phenomenon of intoxication in relation to blood-alcohol concentration, central nervous system depression, and gender differences in oxidizing alcohol.

13. Distinguish between the four alcohol states of consciousness.

14. Discuss the impact of mind-set and emotional setting on intoxication.

15. Identify short-term effects of alcohol on sensation and perception, emotions, sleep, motor skills, sexuality, and the function of the kidneys, heart, blood vessels, and liver.

16. Identify long-term effects of heavy alcohol consumption on the gastrointestinal system, the liver, nutritional status, the nervous system, the endocrine system, mental functions, the cardiovascular system, skeletal muscles, and the development of certain cancers and specific infectious diseases.

17. Explain the potentiation effect in terms of alcohol-drug interactions.

18. Describe the three principal features of fetal alcohol syndrome.

19. Discuss problem drinking in relation to auto accidents, disrupted family life, marital relationship, and criminal behavior.

20. Discuss the possible causes of alcoholism in terms of the agent (ethyl alcohol), the host (the drinker), and the environment (the psychosocial/cultural setting in which drinking occurs).

21. Describe several of the anticipated signs and symptoms that commonly occur in each of the four developmental phases of alcoholism.

22. Name the three general stages of alcoholism treatment and rehabilitation.

23. Distinguish among each of the following therapies for alcoholism: psychotherapy, family therapy, rational-emotive therapy, behavioral therapy, and transactional analysis.

24. Explain the basic nature and operational processes of Alcoholics Anonymous.

25. Describe several ways by which an individual can reduce problem drinking behavior.

Alcohol in Society

For centuries people have used beers, wines, and distilled spirits. Having originated spontaneously in nearly every culture, the phenomenon of drinking persists because individuals apparently like the effects it produces. Unlike tobacco and marijuana cigarette smoking, the use of alcoholic beverages has been an established custom in America for more than three hundred years. Most people consider alcohol a social beverage; too few recognize it as a "drink drug" with great potential for serious abuse.

Now a declining yet still significant part of our social fabric, drinking has long been viewed as a source of desirable, temporary mood modification and conviviality, on the one hand, and as a significant factor in personal and social disorganization, disease, and immorality, on the other. These contradictory effects have given rise to a somewhat ambivalent attitude toward alcohol use. Thus, while most Americans are "wet" (drinkers), many of these same individuals think "dry"—they feel guilty to some degree about using alcoholic beverages, view alcohol as one of the "forbidden fruits" or "demon rum," and are quite apprehensive about the pleasure derived from alcohol.

Americans spend more than $92 billion each year on beverage alcohol. In purchasing a variety of perceived benefits and pleasures, they pay over $13 billion in alcohol revenues or taxes, which amounts to only a small fraction of the federal budget—considerably less than 1 percent. Through alcohol abuse and alcohol dependence, they also generate a yearly expenditure of at least $99 billion.[1] Some analysts claim that the true cost is closer to $150 billion! This total estimated annual cost of national alcohol-related problems reflects expenditures for death expenses, reduced productivity in the workforce, lost employment, motor-vehicle crashes, crime, welfare programs, incarceration, and treatment and rehabilitation services.

At present, all states provide for the legal sale and consumption of beverage alcohol. However, specific restrictions controlling its manufacture, availability, and the time, place, occasion, and qualifications for drinking persist. For example, over 200 counties in 17 states allow "package" or container sales only, and another 400 counties in 15 states prohibit all sales of alcoholic beverages. Also, all states have a 21-year-old minimum drinking age, unless Congress allows future variance.

Despite the widespread availability and legal use of beverage alcohol, two illegal activities continue—**moonshining** (illicit production of distilled spirits) and **bootlegging** (secret and unlawful transportation and sale of beverage alcohol). The former practice is usually undertaken to avoid paying high federal and state taxes on distilled liquors. The latter is an attempt to make money by selling alcoholic beverages without having a state liquor license.

While drinking may still be considered a social norm, for the vast majority of Americans—nondrinkers and light, infrequent drinkers—alcohol use is not a very important part of their lives. In fact, just one-third of the total drinking-age population consumes more than 90 percent of all alcoholic beverages sold in the United States.[2]

Historical and Cultural Aspects

Whether by accident or by intent, beverage alcohol has played more than an inconsequential part in our national history. The earliest immigrants brought their own drinking attitudes and practices to their new homeland. According to legend, the Puritans landed at Plymouth Rock because their beers and victuals were running low. Contrary to popular belief, these early settlers considered alcohol as the "good creature of God," and beers and wines became normal parts of family life and festive occasions. It was also during the colonial period that many a Yankee fortune was amassed by manufacturing rum from supplies of West Indies molasses. The rum was then traded for slaves in Africa, giving rise to the infamous "trading triangle" of molasses, rum, and African slaves. New England traders and shippers had discovered a flourishing business.

From Temperance to Prohibition to Repeal

Early attempts to promote **temperance** were part of a moral crusade by several Protestant churches. Initially their aim was not abstinence but *moderation* in the use of beer and wine. People were actively discouraged from drinking whiskey and rum—popular distilled spirits. However, by the late 1830s this movement had evolved into a campaign for *total* **abstinence** from all alcoholic beverages. The temperance movement gradually switched from education and moral persuasion to political organization and the power of the ballot box to realize its goal. Leaders of this social and moral reform movement sought to legally repress the liquor trade and prohibit the sale of all alcoholic beverages.

Eventually the Prohibition Party, the Anti-Saloon League, and the Women's Christian Temperance Union were successful in their campaign to establish nationwide prohibition by amendment to the federal Constitution. This effort was truly extraordinary, inasmuch as the major force supporting prohibition, the women of America, had not yet been granted the right to vote.

Passing Congress with the necessary two-thirds majority, the Eighteenth Amendment to the U.S. Constitution was submitted to the states for ratification. By 1918, the needed thirty-six states had ratified the amendment that prohibited the manufacture, sale, or transportation of intoxicating liquors used for beverage purposes. The Volstead Act, passed in 1919, provided the amendment's enforcement. The constitutional amendment went into effect in January 1920 and ushered in the so-called Prohibition Era, America's "noble experiment." What was considered only immoral before was now also illegal.

The nearly fourteen-year period of national Prohibition (1920–33) was not particularly successful in eliminating the evil and harmful effects of "demon rum" and other alcoholic beverages from America. The Volstead Act was inadequately enforced, and organized crime grew into a vast network engaged in smuggling "bootleg booze." Ethnic minorities representing millions of drinkers felt that their natural folkways had been unjustly suppressed. And many who would never dream of violating other laws casually visited "speakeasies" or contracted with bootleggers for an ample supply of refreshing liquid.

After both drinkers and nondrinkers began to question the government's right to make moral judgments, and at the height of the Great Depression, America decided to end the noble experiment. Introduced by Congress, the Twenty-First Amendment to the U.S. Constitution repealed the Eighteenth Amendment and ended national Prohibition in December 1933. Thirty-six states had ratified the amendment in less than ten months. Other than federal taxation and production standards, the control of manufacture, distribution, and sale of alcoholic beverages reverted to the states.

Attitudes Toward Drinking

Many alcohol specialists believe that attitudes about alcohol and drinking are at the very core of our present alcohol problems. In effect, our "stupid thinking" about beverage alcohol contributes to our national "stupid drinking." Myths about alcohol still prevail—that everyone drinks; that drinking is sophisticated; that drinking is an essential part of a happy and successful life; that alcohol use improves thought, physical coordination, and social performance; and that "boozing" is a necessary ingredient of masculinity. Until such faulty perceptions are modified, efforts at promoting less-destructive drinking practices are not likely to be successful.

Although most Americans are identified as drinkers, the vast majority of our population of light, infrequent drinkers and abstainers consumes just 10 percent of all alcoholic beverages sold in the United States (see fig. 4.1). Nevertheless, there remains a strong disagreement about the significance of alcohol in terms of use and nonuse. Such conflict between the closely coexisting value structures of permissiveness and abstinence generates a considerable degree of confusion and mixed feelings regarding alcoholic beverages and their effects upon human behavior, health, and society.

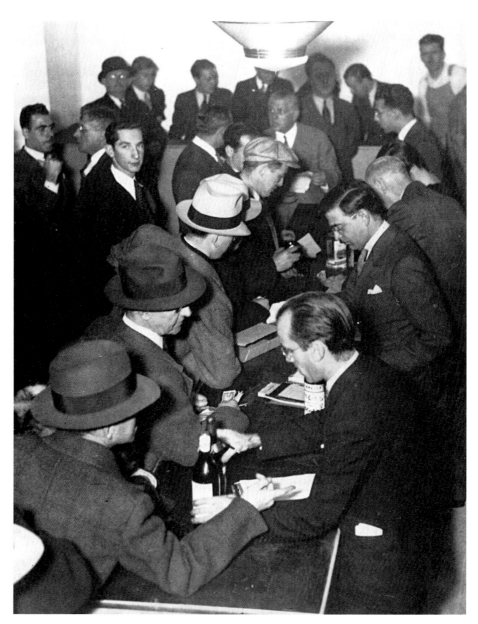

A "speakeasy" during the Prohibition Era. Although the 18th Amendment forbade the manufacture, sale and transportation of intoxicating liquors, some people could buy various alcoholic beverages at secret clubs and meeting places, if they spoke the proper password easily at the entrance door.
The Bettmann Archive

There is no consensus of opinion on the goodness or badness of drinking. There is no standard of moderation or agreement as to what constitutes responsible drinking. There are no strict controls for social use of alcohol or against abuse of alcohol. We often laugh at drunks who overdose on alcohol, but we rarely think that the person who has overdosed on sleeping pills or who has had a psychotic reaction to LSD is funny. (Does our reaction to intoxicated people subtly encourage drunkenness?)

Although heavy use of alcohol in combination with escape drinking—the use of alcohol to escape reality—often sets the stage for problem drinking, many Americans tend to associate heavy consumption with manliness, admire the individual who can hold his or her liquor, and largely approve of escape drinking when confronted with personal problems. Out of one side of our mouths we warn our children not to drink; out of the other side, we sip a cocktail. And when junior gets "bombed" on booze, we thank God that he was not involved with dope or one of those hard drugs.

Although national prohibition ended nearly 65 years ago, the temperance movement, Prohibition, and repeal may have been responsible for a number of beliefs and attitudes that contribute to our present alcohol problems.[3] The following are examples.

Drinking is immoral. It is disapproved by many churches and often linked with gambling and illicit sex.

Nice women do not drink. The alcoholic female, therefore, is to be condemned more so than the alcoholic male.

At one time, the sale of alcoholic beverages was illegal, but many people broke the law. Perhaps this is a factor in the continuing disrespect for drinking laws today.

The federal government once said that buying beverage alcohol was illegal. Now the government permits such purchases. Does the government really know what is best for its citizens?

All drinking is the same. Therefore, little or no distinction is made between alcohol use and alcohol abuse. Many people do not recognize any differences among various drinking patterns, such as social drinking, occasional excessive drinking, progressive excessive drinking, and chronic alcoholic drinking.

The alcoholic will eventually lose his or her job, his or her family, and self-respect, and will end up as a skid-row bum. The stereotype of the alcoholic as a "down-and-outer" was born, and now we fail to detect the

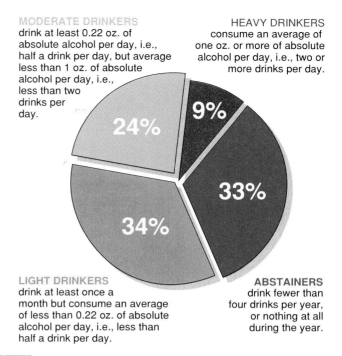

MODERATE DRINKERS drink at least 0.22 oz. of absolute alcohol per day, i.e., half a drink per day, but average less than 1 oz. of absolute alcohol per day, i.e., less than two drinks per day.

HEAVY DRINKERS consume an average of one oz. or more of absolute alcohol per day, i.e., two or more drinks per day.

LIGHT DRINKERS drink at least once a month but consume an average of less than 0.22 oz. of absolute alcohol per day, i.e., less than half a drink per day.

ABSTAINERS drink fewer than four drinks per year, or nothing at all during the year.

figure 4.1

American Drinking Practices. Most of the drinking-age population in the United States either abstains from alcohol use or drinks very little. It is also apparent that significant numbers of individuals move from one drinking category to another over a period of years. Some former drinkers become abstainers, and some nonusers eventually become drinkers.

Source: National Institute on Alcohol Abuse and Alcoholism.

alcoholic in the early stages of problem drinking because the individual still has a job and a family.

Such moralistic and contradictory attitudes create a good deal of confusion about what is acceptable drinking behavior. Some people feel uncomfortable about drinking or not drinking.

In a society with such mixed feelings and cultural **ambivalence**—the perception of both positive and negative aspects occurring in the same thing at the same time—many alcohol-related problems, including alcohol abuse and alcohol dependence, are likely to exist. The contrasting and often contradictory nature of our attitudes and practices regarding alcohol become apparent in several areas of concern:

1. The different moralities of alcohol use, as reflected in different religious denominations. ("Drinking is evil." "Alcohol is a gift of God.")

2. The varying reactions of individuals to inebriation. These range from horror and contempt to admiration and hilarity.

3. The conflict over the major focus in alcohol education. Shall it be on abstinence, moderation, or alcoholism?

4. The crazy-quilt pattern of government laws and college regulations—many of them unenforceable—regarding the purchase and consumption of alcohol. After the repeal of national Prohibition, individual states set their own legal drinking ages, usually from 18 to 21 years of age. In response to a sudden increase in the number of drunken teenagers and young adults involved in fatal auto accidents, several states enacted higher drinking ages. Then, in 1984, the U.S. Congress, in effect, adopted a

national drinking age of 21 by pressuring states to increase their minimum drinking ages or risk the loss of federal highway funds. Each state still determines the hours during which beverages can be sold, and sets standards for granting permits to distributors, sellers, and even bartenders. And most states (as well as the federal government) increase the "vice tax" on booze when expenditures require additional revenues. Prohibition sentiment lives on in our age of affluence and permissiveness.

5. The confusion as to the nature of alcoholism. It is variously described as alcohol dependence, a disease, a basic personality defect, a form of self-indulgence, a lack of will power, a personal health problem, and a sociolegal problem.

6. The difficulty in reducing public intoxication. The standard procedure of arrest, jailing, and release, followed soon by the rearrest, jailing, and release of the same person (the "revolving-door routine") does not appear to reduce the incidence of public intoxication or alcoholism. Such punitive measures will not give way to medical treatment and rehabilitation until society perceives chronic alcohol abuse and alcohol dependence (alcoholism) as both a health problem and a drug problem.

In this ambivalent, drinking society, with its mixed feelings about alcohol use and nonuse and the many contradictions regarding drinking behavior, everyone appears to "do his or her own thing" with relation to beverage alcohol. Could such highly prized diversities in attitudes and practices actually promote the self-destructive and antisocial use of alcohol so prevalent in America today?

Personal and Social Uses of Alcohol

For many people, there will probably always be the need for an adaptive mechanism—a means of altering an individual's

inner being of feelings and perceptions in relation to his or her surroundings.[4] Alcohol serves that function well.

Social Drinking

By definition, drinking is the consumption of beverages containing ethyl alcohol. From a sociological viewpoint, drinking is described as a particular group's customary way of using beverage alcohol. Such a custom is learned by other members of that group and is continued by the group because drinking serves to promote interpersonal relations and to enhance feelings of camaraderie and solidarity (see box 4.1). The pleasure derived from drinking is primarily reciprocal; that is, drinking by one of the group brings satisfaction to the other drinkers. Alcohol is seen as the "social lubricant" in which the conscience is dissolved

and rigid inhibitions are lowered. For Americans, this form of learned drinking behavior—**social drinking**—is the common way of using alcoholic beverages.[5]

Ritualistic Drinking

Ritualistic use of alcohol is seen in religious ceremonies wherein wine is sacred and drinking is an act of communion. Other cultural ceremonies—celebrating birth, birthdays, engagements, marriages, anniversaries, good fortune, sometimes even death—are also traditionally celebrated with alcoholic beverages.

Dietary Drinking

For some, alcohol is an essential part of one's dietary intake, a complement to certain foods or, like cooking wine, a basic

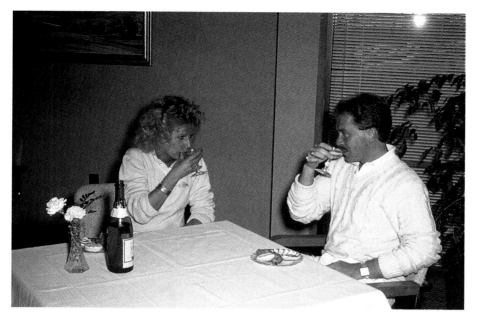

Drinking that tends to promote interpersonal relationships and feelings of camaraderie is often referred to as social drinking, while dietary drinking describes the use of alcoholic beverages as compliments to certain foods or as basic ingredients in special food dishes. The couple above seem to combine the two types of drinking.

© James L. Shaffer

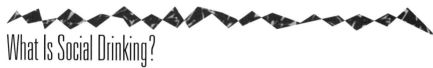

What Is Social Drinking?

Social Drinking Is

A glass of wine to enhance a meal

A drink or two while you are having fun

Sipping and eating

Using alcohol as a beverage

Drinking and talking with friends

Never having to say you are sorry for what you did while drinking

Knowing when to say when

Social Drinking Is Not

Three fast martinis before lunch

Having a drink to have fun

Gulping drinks on an empty stomach

Forgetting what you did while drinking

Drinking and worrying alone

Showing off how much you can hold

Using alcohol as a problem solver

Where does social drinking end and problem drinking begin? There is no simple answer. However, here is one good description: *If you need a drink to be social, that's not social drinking!*

Source: *Social Drinking*, Operation Threshold, United States Jaycees, 1975. Funded by the National Institute on Alcohol Abuse and Alcoholism.

ingredient in special food dishes. When alcohol is served along with meals and integrated with routines of family living, the risks of excessive use and intoxication are considerably diminished.

Mood Modification Drinking

There is little doubt that the major reason so many people use alcoholic beverages is to change their conscious experience.[6] This alcohol-induced state of awareness is usually perceived as a sensation of feeling better, feeling less bad, or just feeling different. Alcohol can produce a tranquilizing effect that reduces tension and anxiety. Stressful situations are often more easily tolerated, irritations of daily living seem to diminish, and relaxation is often promoted or enhanced. In some instances, drinking may provide a pleasant and relatively safe way to feel "high" or even powerful with one's peers or strangers.

Although thoughts of power, aggression, and even sexual conquest tend to increase regularly with increased drinking among men, female social drinking is sometimes related to enhancing or increasing traditional aspects of femininity, such as personal warmth, lovingness, expressiveness, and affectionateness. However, heavy use among females has been associated with attempts to escape temporarily from gender-role conflict.[7]

According to Sigmund Freud, an early twentieth-century researcher in the emerging field of psychology, drinking was one way of satisfying hidden dependency needs that adults are forbidden to express. As such, alcohol abuse could express a secret desire for support and care from others, while maintaining an appearance of adult sophistication and independence—qualities often linked with alcohol use.

A more contemporary explanation of using and abusing alcohol focuses on the basic motivation of satiation or excessive satisfaction.[8] Drinking becomes an antidote or countermeasure for psychic pain. Psychologically, binging on alcohol is an attempt to cut off negative feelings by reducing stimulation from both the internal and the external environment.

Recent research also suggests that the desire for altered states of consciousness or intoxication (i.e., being influenced by a drug's effects) is an acquired motivation similar to the basic drives of hunger, thirst, and even sex.[9] Accordingly, humans have a natural need to change their awareness from time to time, in response to environmental stressors or just plain boredom, or in an effort to decrease feelings of fatigue, tension, and anxiety. This concept values intoxication for its alleged ability to enliven daily experiences, vitalize one's perceptions, and serve as a unifying symbol that encourages solidarity or unity among fellow drinkers.

Thus, although alcohol relaxes individuals, temporarily frees them from their inner selves and conflicts, brightens the world, and heightens pleasures, it is possible that even more practical (though not easily understandable) reasons are responsible for the widespread and continuous use of beverage alcohol:[10] alcohol's ability to increase *awareness* and psychic stimulation, resulting in variations in thought processes, ideas, and activities. Allowing for liquor's power to induce *unawareness*, also, the temporary relaxation provided by alcohol may promote an enlarged "life scope" and create feelings of exhilaration and new enthusiasms. As such, beverage alcohol allegedly plays an integral role in the human struggle for survival and in the mental evolution of the human being.

Unfortunately, millions of drinkers use alcohol to produce *unawareness* (narcosis) exclusively. They do not wish to return to reality but seek a hiding place from the world in a bottle. Frequent drinking for narcosis only is the type that often leads to alcohol dependency and reduced life expectancy.

Thus, alcohol can serve a variety of personal and social uses. Some of these are less problem producing than others.

Alcoholic Beverages

The term *alcohol* generally denotes a specific chemical compound, ethyl alcohol. One of several chemicals in the "alcohol

 table 4.1 Selected Nonprescription Medications That Contain Ethyl Alcohol

Type of Medication	Alcohol Content (%)
Antidiarrhea medication	
Imodium A-D	5.25
Pepto Diarrhea Control	5.25
Astringent	
Witch hazel	14.00
Internal analgesic	
Excedrin PM liquid	10.00
Tylenol Adult Extra Strength liquid	7.00
Vitamin preparation	
Centrum	6.60
Mouthwash preparation/dental rinse	
Cepacol	14.00
Listerine	26.90
Plax	8.50
Scope	16.60
Toothache/cold sore/canker sore remedy	
Anbesol	70.00
Orajel Mouth-Aid	70.00
Zilactin Medicated Gel	80.00
Cough/cold/allergy medication	
Benadryl cold liquid	10.00
Cheracol Plus cough syrup	8.00
Comtrex	20.00
Contac Severe Cold	18.50
MediFlu	19.00
NiteTime Relief (Plus)	25.00
Nyquil	25.00
Tylenol Max Strength Cough	10.00

Source: Author's recent analysis of nonprescription medications available for sale in drug stores, department stores, and groceries.

family," ethyl alcohol is a thin, clear, colorless fluid with a mild, aromatic odor and pungent taste. It is capable of being mixed with water in all proportions, is diffusible through body membranes, and is the essential and characteristic ingredient of beverage alcohol. Ethyl alcohol is also present in many nonprescription medications (see table 4.1) and often is used in the preparation of chemical detergents, flavorings, and fragrances. When added to gasoline, ethyl alcohol improves the octane rating; mixing 10 percent ethanol with 90 percent gasoline produces the motor fuel gasohol.[11]

The ethyl alcohol contained in beverages is derived from certain grains and fruits by *fermentation*. In this natural chemical process, yeast cells act on the sugar content of the grain or fruit juice and convert the sugar to carbon dioxide

and alcohol. Rarely does one consume pure alcohol. Intake is accomplished in the form of alcoholic beverages classified as either wines, beers, or distilled spirits.

Wine

Made from the fermented juice of grapes or other fruits, **wine** typically has an alcohol content of 10 to 14 percent by volume. There are five basic types of wines: red, white, and rosé, and sparkling wines or champagne, which contain carbon dioxide (all referred to as table wines); and dessert or cocktail wines (with alcohol contents ranging from 15 to 24 percent). The higher alcohol content of the dessert wines, such as sherry, port, Madeira, and the vermouths, is the result of adding *neutral high-proof spirits* (ethyl alcohol) or brandy to a table wine.

Although the original "light" wines with reduced caloric value did not prove to be very popular, the more recent wine variants, the "wine coolers," became an overnight success. Syrupy sweet, fruity beverages with little or no alcohol taste, wine coolers are blends of red or white wine, fruit juice, carbonated water, and sugar. They typically contain from 1.5 percent to 6.0 percent alcohol by volume. Such concoctions are extremely popular among junior and senior high school students, who consume about 35 percent of all wine coolers sold in the United States.[12]

Beer

Including both the regular and the newer low-calorie "light" varieties with less alcohol, **beers** are derived from cereal grains—barley, rye, corn, and wheat. The process of beer making is referred to as brewing and includes the conversion of cereal broth starch to a fermentable sugar, fermentation, and storage. The resulting product contains from 3.6 percent to 6 percent alcohol by volume, though the typical alcohol content of popular beers is about 4 percent to 4.5 percent—characteristic of the traditional "regular beers."

Light beers, by contrast, contain fewer calories per serving. The alcohol content is usually about 3.2 percent by volume, but may be as high as 4.7 percent. Reflecting perhaps the increased health consciousness of Americans and the growing awareness of alcohol abuse, the newer "low-alcohol beers" contain about 1.8 percent of ethyl alcohol. Recently marketed so-called non-alcoholic beers are "near beers" that contain less than 0.5 percent alcohol by volume. These products are referred to as "brews"—not beers—because they would have to contain a higher alcohol content to be considered a beer, according to federal government regulations.[13] Nevertheless, the National Council on Alcoholism and Drug Dependence warns that the new brews may have sufficient alcoholic content to trigger a response among recovering alcoholics that could lead to a relapse into problem drinking.

After brewing, the resulting clarified fluid is carbonated and bottled or canned. Besides water and alcohol, beer contains minute substances called **congeners**, as do all alcoholic beverages. Common congeners are dextrins, maltose, certain soluble minerals and vitamins, organic acids, acacia or gum arabic, salts, and carbon dioxide. Some of these are added to preserve, stabilize, enhance flavor, and produce or promote foaming.

Most American beers are lager beers and have a light color and a relatively low alcohol content of 4.0 percent to 4.5 percent by volume. Malt liquor has a delicate, aromatic flavor and between 5 percent and 6.9 percent alcohol content, though recent versions have been brewed with an alcohol content of 9.5 percent. Malt beverage "coolers" have a much lower alcohol content, ranging from 3.2 percent to 4.8 percent. More bitter than malt liquor are ale, stout, and porter—high-powered beers with "full-bodied" taste and an alcohol content of 6 to 7 percent by volume.

One of the latest variants in the ever-expanding beer family is a concoction named "ice beer." This particular kind of beer is brewed at an extremely cold temperature. This innovative marketing gimmick of brewers has an alcohol content equal to that of many malt liquors—between 5 and 6 percent.

Distilled Spirits

Whiskey, vodka, gin, and brandy are **distilled spirits** and are made from fermented mixtures of cereal grains or fruits that are heated in a still. Rum, another distilled spirit, is derived from molasses, and tequila is made from the fermented juice of the cactuslike century plant, the mescal.

Because alcohol has a lower boiling point than other substances in the fermented mixture, ethyl alcohol boils off first when the mixture is heated. The invisible vapors or spirits are cooled and condensed. These distilled fluids have a relatively high alcohol content, along with some water and flavoring ingredients. The alcohol content of such distilled beverages, ranging from 40 to 50 percent by volume, is indicated by the term *proof*. Proof is twice the percentage of alcohol by volume. Thus, a whiskey labeled 90 proof contains 45 percent alcohol by volume.

Another type of distilled spirits is liqueur, a sweet alcoholic drink made by mixing or redistilling spirits with or over fruits, flowers, plants, nuts, beans, seeds, or cream. These flavoring agents impart their essence to the particular liqueur, such as Creme de Cacao (cacao is a vanilla bean), Kahlua (coffee), and Cointreau (orange).

In an attempt to increase market share, distillers also market a "mixed-drink cooler," or "breezer," a fruit-flavored beverage containing about 4 percent alcohol by volume. This product resembles a wine cooler, but the added alcohol is a distilled spirit. Such a mixture amounts to a diluted mixed drink.

Equivalent Servings

The major types of alcoholic beverage—beer, wine, and distilled spirit—differ as to alcohol content. Nevertheless, a typical serving of any one beverage contains approximately the same amount of ethyl alcohol as does a typical serving of any other alcoholic beverage, though specific servings vary in terms of volume (see box 4.2).

Referred to as the "equivalent amount," this quantity of ethyl alcohol is about one-half ounce. Thus, people who drink one glass of table wine, one 12-ounce wine cooler, one 12-ounce can of beer, or one "shot glass" of "hard liquor" with 1.25 ounces of whiskey are all consuming approximately the same amount of alcohol. In terms of typical servings, then, distilled spirits are not "stronger" or "harder" than beer or wine. And beer and wine coolers are not insignificant or harmless beverages.

There are, however, limitations to the concept of "equivalence" in servings of alcoholic beverages. The typical serving of beer is predetermined at the brewery at the time of canning or bottling, but the typical servings of wines and distilled spirits tend to vary according to the person who pours them. Sometimes mixed drinks—combinations of hard liquor and soda or fruit juice—contain two or more shots of "hard liquor." And martinis and Manhattans, two commonly served cocktails, are prepared by adding distilled spirits to wine. In these instances, the equivalency rule does not apply.

box 4.2

Alcohol Equivalencies and Drinking

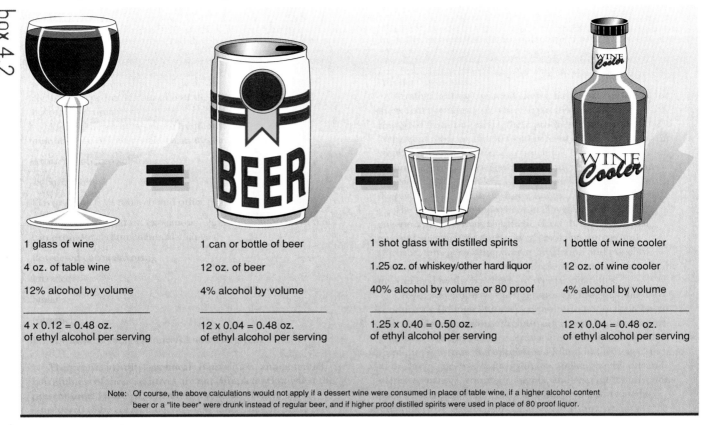

1 glass of wine	1 can or bottle of beer	1 shot glass with distilled spirits	1 bottle of wine cooler
4 oz. of table wine	12 oz. of beer	1.25 oz. of whiskey/other hard liquor	12 oz. of wine cooler
12% alcohol by volume	4% alcohol by volume	40% alcohol by volume or 80 proof	4% alcohol by volume
4 x 0.12 = 0.48 oz. of ethyl alcohol per serving	12 x 0.04 = 0.48 oz. of ethyl alcohol per serving	1.25 x 0.40 = 0.50 oz. of ethyl alcohol per serving	12 x 0.04 = 0.48 oz. of ethyl alcohol per serving

Note: Of course, the above calculations would not apply if a dessert wine were consumed in place of table wine, if a higher alcohol content beer or a "lite beer" were drunk instead of regular beer, and if higher proof distilled spirits were used in place of 80 proof liquor.

Alcohol within the Body

As it enters the body, alcohol is subjected to three basic body processes—absorption, distribution, and oxidation. These processes are described in this section. The relatively small amount of ethyl alcohol that is not oxidized is eventually eliminated unchanged in the urine, sweat, and breath. However, there is no scientific basis for the belief that intoxicated people can urinate, sweat, or breathe themselves sober!

Absorption

Once the beverage is swallowed and conveyed to the stomach, the process of **absorption** begins. Unlike other foods, alcohol requires no digestion and passes readily through the walls of the gastrointestinal tract, where tiny blood vessels pick up the alcohol. About one-fifth of the total alcohol consumed is absorbed in the stomach. The major site of absorption, however, is in the small intestine. A number of factors can influence absorption.

1. *Concentration of alcohol.* The greater the concentration of alcohol in a beverage, the more rapid will be the rate of absorption. Given the same quantity of alcoholic beverages, two ounces of whiskey will produce a higher blood-alcohol level or **blood-alcohol concentration** than two ounces of beer. (Blood-alcohol level or concentration is the ratio of alcohol present in the blood to the total volume of blood, expressed as a percentage.)

2. *Amount of alcohol.* The more alcohol consumed at any one time, the longer the absorption period will be.

3. *Rate of drinking.* Rapid consumption through gulping a drink will likely result in an elevated blood-alcohol level. Drinking in small, divided amounts prevents high concentrations of alcohol because less is available for absorption.

4. *Amount of food in the stomach.* The presence of food in the stomach delays the absorption of alcohol, especially when milk products and foods high in protein are consumed before drinking. Diluted by the food contents, alcohol is retained for a longer period in that body organ where absorption occurs more slowly than in the small intestine.

5. *Body weight.* The more a person weighs, the lower will be the blood-alcohol level. Heavier people have more body fluids in which the alcohol is diluted.

6. *Body chemistry and emotions.* During the premenstrual phase of the menstrual cycle, females tend to absorb alcohol more readily. If

box 4.3

Why Women Can't Hold Their Liquor Like Men

It has been known for many years that females tend to be more vulnerable than males to the effects of alcohol. Such a gender difference traditionally has been related to the overall smaller body size of most females and the lower proportion of water in the bodies of women in comparison with men's bodies. As a consequence, females have less body fluid and a lower water content in which to dilute any alcohol consumed. Women, therefore, become more intoxicated than men after drinking the same amount of beverage alcohol.

Recent studies suggest yet another factor that tends to make alcohol even more risky for women than for men.[a] According to both American and Italian scientists, women are also more susceptible to alcohol's effects because they have less of a protective stomach enzyme that breaks down (oxidizes) a portion of the alcohol consumed before it enters the bloodstream. Men tend to produce higher amounts of gastric alcohol dehydrogenase than do women, and as a result, men do not get as tipsy as women on the same number of drinks.

Because women have less of the gastric (stomach) enzyme than men, females will absorb up to nearly 30 percent more alcohol into the bloodstream than males of the same weight who have drunk an equal amount of beverage. Therefore, when women of average size drink one serving of beverage alcohol, it will have nearly the same effects as two drinks for average-size men.[b]

Other findings of the studies indicate the following:

Women who drink small amounts of alcohol may be more adversely affected than men in their ability to drive and perform other similar tasks requiring close attention and coordination.

Drinking on a full stomach is more desirable than consuming alcohol on an empty one. Because food in the stomach delays the absorption of alcohol, the gastric enzyme has more time to oxidize some of the alcohol before it enters the bloodstream or passes into the small intestine where absorption occurs more rapidly.

The lower amount or total absence of the stomach enzyme may also explain why women alcoholics tend to experience more liver damage than do alcoholic men. The livers of females work harder to break down alcohol and thus become subject to more wear and tear on that particular body organ.

[a]Mario Frezza et al., "High Blood Levels in Women: The Role of Decreased Gastric Alcohol Dehydrogenase Activity and First-Pass Metabolism," *The New England Journal of Medicine* 322, no. 2 (11 January 1990): 95–99.

[b]Anastasia Toufexis, "Why Men Can Outdrink Women," *Time,* 22 January 1990, 61.

women are taking oral contraceptives (birth control pills), they also will absorb alcohol more rapidly. Unique patterns of body functioning may determine individual reactions to alcohol. Anger, fear, stress, nausea, the condition of the stomach tissues, and even fatigue have been identified as factors affecting the emptying time of the stomach.

Distribution

Having passed through the capillary walls of the small blood vessels in the intestines, the alcohol is now circulated to all parts of the body. Eventually it is distributed evenly in the body's fluids and cells, achieving a concentration proportionate to the water content and blood supply of the organ or tissues in question. The **distribution** of alcohol continues a general dilution process begun when the beverage was consumed. Regardless of the original alcohol concentration, the blood-alcohol level (or concentration) rarely exceeds 0.60 percent. At this level, nearly all drinkers would likely be dead. The moderate drinker's blood-alcohol level approximates only a few hundredths of 1 percent by comparison.

Oxidation

Most of the alcohol consumed, absorbed, and distributed—more than 90 percent— is combined eventually with oxygen. This process of **oxidation** results in the formation of water and carbon dioxide and the production of heat and energy.

First, a special gastric enzyme (alcohol dehydrogenase) breaks down about 20 percent of the alcohol in the stomach itself before the alcohol enters the bloodstream.[14] This "first-pass" metabolism of ethyl alcohol appears to be more effective in males than in females, but less effective in alcoholics than in nonalcoholics (see box 4.3).

After the remaining alcohol passes into the bloodstream, the process of oxidation continues in the liver. There, alcohol dehydrogenase enzyme also acts as a catalyst in changing more of the alcohol into acetaldehyde, a toxic substance. Very rapidly this by-product is further oxidized to acetic acid in a chemical process occurring within both the liver and other organs. Authorities disagree as to the site of the third phase of oxidation, in which acetic acid is changed to water and carbon dioxide, the process yielding about seven calories of energy per gram of alcohol.

While the rate of alcohol oxidation varies from person to person due to size of liver, enzyme activity, diseases of the liver, and certain drug reactions, the average rate of disposition is estimated to be one-third of an ounce of pure ethyl alcohol or two-thirds to three-fourths of an ounce of whiskey per hour, or the equivalent in beer or wine. This is fairly constant for each person. Because of the liver's limited oxidation capacity, individuals are advised to consume no more than one serving of beverage alcohol per hour.

Activities to increase the oxidation rate of alcohol have not been successful, except in experiments with intravenous administration of fructose and dialysis of the blood. These are rarely available to the vast majority of drinkers. The use of black coffee, cold showers, stimulant drugs, and exposure to fresh air have no significant effect on increasing alcohol oxidation. The intoxicated person may be more alert but is still drunk and still impaired! Time is the only practical thing that will sober up an individual who has consumed alcohol.

At extremely high blood-alcohol levels, another liver enzyme system, the so-called microsomal ethanol oxidizing system (MEOS), becomes activated.[15] After long periods of heavy alcohol consumption, the MEOS appears to increase its activity significantly, allowing for greater oxidation of ethyl alcohol. Such a function allows some alcohol-dependent individuals to drink extremely large amounts of alcohol without apparent effect.

Intoxication

The most noticeable consequences of alcohol use pertain to *mood and behavior modification*. Such alterations of feelings and conduct are due to the action of alcohol on the central nervous system, specifically the brain, and are in direct proportion to the *blood-alcohol level (BAL)* or *blood-alcohol concentration (BAC)*.

Most drinkers who have a relatively low BAC from taking one drink in an hour will experience only mild effects, such as slight changes in feeling, heightening of existing moods, and very little impairment of mental function, if any. However, definite impairment begins in a BAC zone ranging from 0.03 percent to just below 0.10 percent. As the BAC increases, the degree of mental inefficiency increases. Feelings of relaxation and sedation are experienced, and the control of voluntary muscles declines in the performance of fine motor skills. These changes are manifestations of alcohol's *progressive, depressant action* on the brain, as represented in table 4.2.

 4.2 Alcohol Intoxication: Progressive States of Impairment with Increasing Blood-Alcohol Concentrations (BAC)

BAC	Possible Effects of Alcohol
0.01%	Usually mild effects, if any; slight changes in feeling; heightening of moods.
0.03%	Feelings of relaxation and slight exhilaration; minimal impairment of mental function.
0.06%	Mild sedation; exaggeration of emotion; slight impairment of fine motor skills; increase in reaction time; poor muscle control; slurred speech.
0.09%	Visual and hearing acuity reduced; inhibitions and self-restraint lessened; increased difficulty in performing motor skills; judgment is now clouded.
0.10%	Legal evidence of driving under the influence of alcohol in most states.
0.12%	Difficulty in performing gross motor skills; blurred vision; unclear speech; definite impairment of mental function.
0.15%	Major impairment of physical and mental functions; irresponsible behavior; general feeling of euphoria; difficulty in standing, walking, talking; distorted perception and judgment.
0.20%	Mental confusion; decreased inhibitions; gross body movements can be made only with assistance; inability to maintain upright position; difficulty in staying awake.
0.30%	Severe mental confusion; minimum of perception and comprehension; difficulty in responding to stimuli; general suspension of sensibility.
0.40%	Almost complete anesthesia; depressed reflexes; state of unconsciousness or coma likely.
0.50%	Complete unconsciousness or deep coma, if not death.
0.60%	Death is most likely now, if it has not already occurred at somewhat lower BACs following depression of nerve centers that control heartbeat and breathing. Such a person is "dead drunk."

Source: Charles Carroll and Dean Miller, *Health: The Science of Human Adaptation*, 5th ed. Copyright © 1991 Wm. C. Brown Communications, Inc., Dubuque, Iowa.

Functional impairment increases rapidly and more noticeably after the BAC reaches 0.10 percent and takes several forms: decreased inhibitions, less efficient vision and hearing, unclear speech, difficulty in performing gross motor skills, deterioration of judgment, and a general feeling of euphoria. Studies reveal that with a BAC between 0.10 percent and 0.15 percent, about 65 percent of drinkers display definite signs of physical and mental impairment. At a BAC of 0.20 percent, nearly all drinkers display profound and obvious signs of intoxication—difficulty in walking and speaking, and irresponsible and often antisocial behavior.

Intoxication is a temporary state of mental chaos and behavioral dysfunction resulting from the presence of ethyl alcohol in the central nervous system. Alcohol is being consumed faster than it can be oxidized. Like other sedatives, it has a depressant action on the various control centers in the brain, and it interferes with the transmission of nerve impulses at the synapse. As the brain becomes more anesthetized, the drinker has difficulty maintaining an upright position, experiences dulled perception and minimal comprehension, and finally loses consciousness. If the BAC exceeds 0.60 percent, the drinker's brain becomes so depressed that breathing and heartbeat cease, and death results.

Mechanism of Impairment

Traditionally, it has been thought that the higher brain centers of the cerebral cortex that control judgment and inhibit or restrain behavior are depressed first. Then, as the presence of alcohol in the central nervous system increases, paralysis of the lower brain centers, including the medulla, occurs and results in poor coordination, confusion, disorientation, stupor, coma, or death.

However, more-recent investigations indicate that the nerve cells (neurons) within the brain's "arousal centers," the ascending reticular activating system (ARAS), are extremely sensitive to depression by alcohol.[16] Such depression tends to induce a state of disinhibition (unrestrained behavior) and mild euphoria, accompanied by talkativeness, animated feelings, noisy behavior, increased levels of activity, and expansiveness of the personality. These changes in behavior and mood are generally referred to as **pseudostimulation**—apparent, yet false or deceptive, stimulation. However, as the level of alcohol in the neurons increases, the cerebral cortex also becomes depressed and the state of disinhibition and euphoria ceases.

The precise mechanism of brain impairment is not completely known or understood. It is likely that alcohol temporarily alters the cell membranes of neurons and thus changes specific membrane functions, including neurotransmitter activity. Several possibilities may be considered relevant:[17]

1. Alcohol produces its effects by dissolving the cell's membrane and then disturbing and disordering either the lipids (fats) or proteins (nitrogen organic compounds) in the neuron's thin outer layer of tissue. This process of disordering neuronal membranes is now referred to as membrane fluidization and indirectly inhibits both neurotransmitter production and the transmission of nerve impulses over the synapse.

2. Alcohol's presence in the neurons appears to potentiate or intensify the receptor function of GABA (gamma aminobutyric acid), a neurotransmitter that blocks the transfer of an electrical or chemical signal across the synapse of a nerve cell. Alcohol's effects on this particular neurotransmitter receptor might contribute to ethanol's anxiety-reducing, sedation, and motor impairment actions.

3. Glutamate is a major excitatory neurotransmitter in the central nervous system. Alcohol tends to block glutamate receptor function. Significant decreases in the function of these specific receptors may result in loss of consciousness, severe sensory and movement impairment, and even respiratory failure— particular hazards of excessive drinking, referred to as overdose poisoning or acute intoxication.

4. During an individual's use of alcohol, both dopamine- and serotonin-dependent neurotransmitters are changed. For instance, alcohol intake produces an increase in dopamine levels, which in turn contributes to the reinforcement or rewards associated with long-term alcohol abuse. However, the primary roles these neurotransmitters and their respective receptors play in alcohol intoxication, as well as the sites responsible for controlling neurotransmitter levels in the brain, are not completely known and remain the focus of ongoing research.

Alcohol States of Consciousness

Although scientists do not agree on the initial site of impairment, there is no doubt that intoxication produces an altered state of consciousness in individuals. Behavioral and biological differences suggest, however, that the period of mood and behavior modification is not a unitary or single state. Rather, the duration of alcohol effects is a time composed of several different states of consciousness, depending on whether the blood-alcohol concentration is increasing (the ascending limb of the blood-alcohol curve) or decreasing (the descending limb of the blood-alcohol curve).[18]

Four **alcohol states of consciousness (ASC)** during intoxication have been identified.[19]

ASC-1: the time of alcohol absorption and increasing blood-alcohol concentrations, characterized by talkativeness, laughter, motor incoordination, impaired performance on various cognitive, motor, and sensory tasks, and poor memory

ASC-2: the time beginning after the peak blood-alcohol concentration has been obtained and the blood-alcohol level is declining, during which the drinker becomes quiet and tired, but impaired performance is beginning to improve

ACS-3: the time beginning about halfway between peak blood-alcohol concentration and zero blood-alcohol level, in which the individual feels confident that he or she is perfectly sober, yet a detectable blood-alcohol concentration is still present

ASC-4: the time during which all traces of alcohol have disappeared from the body, but for up to 32 hours after drinking, positional alcohol nystagmus (PAN) eye movements can be detected in which the eyeballs involuntarily oscillate laterally, vertically, or in a rotary manner

Psychological Aspects of Intoxication

While the presence of alcohol in the central nervous system is the basis for intoxication, the psychological makeup of the drinker and the psychological atmosphere of drinking are important factors influencing intoxicated behavior.

The drinker's emotional makeup or temperament has been labeled as the *mind-set*. This factor is important in producing behavioral reactions accompanying alcohol use as well as any drug use. A person who drinks with the expectation of getting "high" will often display a form of "psychological intoxication" before "physiological intoxication" is possible. The author recalls an incident in which a nonalcoholic fruit drink was served to several people at a party. Before the beverage was consumed, the adult guests, most of whom were infrequent or light drinkers, were told that vodka had been added to the drink, but no taste would be detected. The results were amazing! After just a few sips, some of the guests claimed they felt warmer; a few mentioned the feeling of dizziness; the conversation became more animated; and the activity level of several guests increased markedly. This situation is a good example of the psyche's influence on the body.

Not only the individual's mind-set but the *emotional climate* or *setting of drinking* also sets the stage for certain behaviors. Imagine the excitement that surrounds a victory celebration of an athletic contest or the completion of an academic semester. The psychological atmosphere of these events predisposes drinkers to somewhat boisterous, excessive, and even bizarre behavior. The same individuals consuming the same amount of beverage in a more controlled, restrained setting would likely behave in a more mature way. Since a controlled atmosphere does not permit the peculiar actions of manifest intoxication, few if any are evidenced. Could it be that drinking serves as a convenient and socially approved excuse for some to act in a carefree, careless, and irresponsible manner?

For many years, law enforcement officials have determined whether individuals were intoxicated by using field sobriety tests, such as the nystagmus gaze test for variations in the visual tracking of objects, the walk-and-turn test, and the one-leg stand. However, because the mood or mind-set of the consumer, along with the psychological atmosphere of drinking, will likely influence the drinker's responses to alcohol, estimating the degree of impairment by observation has proved very unreliable.

Therefore, chemical tests for an objective evaluation of intoxication have been developed and involve the determination of alcohol levels in the blood and the breath. The tests are based on the constant proportion between alcohol concentrations in blood and in the breath. Several breath analysis instruments are available, namely, the *alcosensor, alcometer, drunkometer, intoximeter,* and *Breathalyzer*. The **Breathalyzer,** along with newer high-technology modifications of this device, is being used increasingly by law enforcement officials to identify alcohol-impaired drivers.

Short-Term Effects of Alcohol

Specific body parts and functions can be influenced directly or indirectly by alcohol. Short-term effects include the following:

Sensation and Perception

Decreases in both visual and hearing acuity.

Altered sensitivity to odors and taste.

Reduced sensitivity to pain due to the masking of fatigue.

An appearance that time passes more rapidly.

Underestimation of the speed of moving objects.

Increased sensation of thirst, possibly due to shifting of water from within the body's cells to the spaces between the cells.

Emotions

Feelings of elation.

Decreased fear.

Increases in risk-taking behaviors.

Emphasis on aggressive humor more than nonsense humor.

Reduced inhibitions.

Sleep

Induced sleep because of alcohol's depressant effect on the brain. But regular use over a period of time deprives an individual of **rapid eye movements (REM)** or dreaming sleep, resulting in anxiety, tiredness, and impaired concentration.

Kidneys

Increased urinary output due to the *diuretic effect* of alcohol on the pituitary gland. Alcohol blocks this gland's production of a special chemical substance, the antidiuretic hormone. Without this hormone, which regulates the reabsorption of water before it is voided, the urine volume is increased, but not to the point of dehydration.

Heart and Blood Vessels

Temporary increases in both heartbeat and blood pressure.

Dilated peripheral blood vessels in arms and legs. This blood vessel expander effect leads to a loss of body heat while producing a feeling of added warmth.

Constriction of the arteries supplying the heart.

Liver

An accumulation of fat cells that are considered the forerunners of other liver diseases is often associated with prolonged use of alcohol.

Motor Skills

Impairment of most types of performance, although individual susceptibility varies at BAC of 0.10 percent or below.

Increased swaying.

Interference with sensorimotor coordination, as in tracking a moving object.

Hangover

Temporary, acute physical and psychological distress following excessive consumption of alcoholic beverages. The experience known as a **hangover** has been related to the amount of *congeners* (nonalcohol components) in beverage alcohol; the type of food eaten and liquor consumed; various emotional influences and expectations; the impact of physical factors, including loud and dark drinking environments; and physical factors, especially fatigue. Nausea, gastritis, headache, and anxiety experienced during a hangover are painful reminders of disrupted body functions that could not be felt while one was intoxicated. A hangover is the body's reaction to excessive drinking and represents a pronounced withdrawal syndrome from relatively large amounts of alcohol. Despite some innovative hangover cures, the only effective cures have been the use of analgesics for headaches and the healing powers of time.

Sexuality

Small doses of alcohol may facilitate sexual activity by helping one to overcome a lack of confidence or feelings of guilt. But while alcohol may provoke desire, larger amounts may spoil the capacity to perform or respond (see box 3.1).

Long-Term Effects of Alcohol

Prolonged, heavy consumption of alcoholic beverages can result in one or more tragic, often life-threatening consequences:

Gastrointestinal system disorders and diseases—These include irritation and inflammation of the esophagus, stomach, small intestine, and pancreas.

Liver disorders and diseases—These involve altered functions in the largest and most chemically complex body organ. Alcohol is now recognized as having a direct, toxic effect on liver tissue, the *hepatotoxic effect*. The trauma consists, first of all, of a fatty liver, which is reversible if drinking ceases. If heavy consumption persists, the fatty liver condition may develop into a chronic inflammation of liver tissue known as *alcoholic hepatitis*, which can be fatal. In some cases, this condition may evolve into *alcoholic cirrhosis*, characterized by the shriveling and hardening of the liver, in which functioning liver cells are replaced by scar tissue. Such disease can develop in spite of adequate dietary intake. The incidence of alcoholic cirrhosis is one indicator of

the extent of alcohol abuse and alcoholism. Presently, alcoholic cirrhosis ranks among the twelve leading causes of death in America.

Hypoglycemia—This is a serious condition in which blood-sugar levels are lowered beyond the normal range. Chronic drinking usually places considerable stress on the liver, thus interfering with the body's ability to produce glucose (blood sugar) and to store it as glycogen. Because of the poor nutritional status of many alcoholics, the glycogen reserves are often depleted, predisposing such individuals to the development of hypoglycemia when food is not eaten for 24 hours or more. Since the brain and spinal cord, which govern basic life processes, depend upon glucose for proper functioning, hypoglycemia brings about a physiological crisis that can be damaging to the body and result in death.

Nutritional deficiency—This is one of the most common yet most undetected problems associated with long-term alcohol use. Alcohol basically interferes with the nutritional process by adversely affecting digestion, storage, utilization, and excretion of nutrients.[20] Because alcohol itself is highly caloric, some alcoholics take in as much as 50 percent of their

total daily calories from alcohol. While taking in the "empty" calories deficient in vitamins, minerals, essential amino acids, and essential fatty acids, heavy drinkers often decrease their intake of nutrients from other food sources. Diminished appetite, vomiting, and diarrhea also contribute to nutritional imbalance. Heavy consumption also disrupts normal processes of digestion by causing gastritis (inflammation of the stomach lining), stomach ulcers, and intestinal lesions or sores, which interfere with proper transport, absorption, and activation of vitamins and minerals. The end result is *malnutrition* that contributes to certain brain diseases, liver disease, pancreatitis, abnormal fetal development, suboptimal health, anemia, convulsions, and malfunction of the small bowel. Though severe malnutrition may be relatively rare, the effects of the subtle nutritional disturbances become more significant as intake of alcohol increases.[21]

Nervous system diseases—Often combined with malnutrition, these surface as impairments of normal nerve cell functioning and cognitive deficits, especially those of problem solving, abstract thinking, concept shifting, psychomotor performance, and difficult memory tasks.[22] For the most severe alcoholics, serious organic impairments of brain function are common complications. Two such mental disorders are *dementia* associated with alcoholism and *alcohol memory disorder*. These disorders are not mutually exclusive, and aspects of each often coexist in the same patient. When linked with alcoholism, dementia surfaces as a general deterioration of intellectual abilities and a disintegration of behavior and personality, but without a clouding of consciousness. By contrast, alcohol memory loss disorder, often called Korsakoff's psychosis or Wernicke-Korsakoff syndrome, is described as short-term memory impairments and behavioral changes that occur without clouding of consciousness or general loss of intellectual abilities.

Wernicke's syndrome—Related to thiamine (part of the vitamin B complex) deficiency, this syndrome is characterized by total bewilderment and disorientation, paralysis of the motor nerves of the eye, rhythmical oscillation of the eyeballs, loss of muscular coordination, and diseases of the peripheral nerves. *Korsakoff's psychosis*, often seen in conjunction with Wernicke's disease, includes severe amnesia, the recitation of imaginary experiences, and remarkable personality alterations. Chronic alcohol consumption has also been associated with numerous impairments of the central nervous system and the peripheral nervous system. In addition to these manifestations of alcohol's *neurotoxic effect* (poisonous to nervous tissue) are the occurrence of tolerance and physical dependence, as described in chapter 3.

Endocrine system disorders—These especially affect the hypothalamus, pituitary, and gonads. The production and release of certain chemical regulators (hormones) are altered significantly. In males this results in reduced testosterone levels, causing sexual impotence, loss of

libido, breast enlargement, loss of facial hair, and wasting away of the testes, common to male alcoholics. In females, heavy use of alcohol sometimes contributes to menstrual disturbances, premature cessation of menstruation, or even ovarian failure and atrophy, leading to infertility.

Mental disorders—Usually occurring as part of the alcohol withdrawal syndrome, these are identified as alcohol psychoses, alcoholic hallucinosis, and affective disorders, including disturbances of mood, accompanied by a full or partial manic or depressive syndrome. Alcoholics often have high levels of depression, and alcohol can increase depression.

Cardiovascular diseases—These affect the heart and blood vessels and are common in patients who have been chronic alcoholics for more than ten years. Long-standing use of substantial amounts of alcohol contributes to cardiomyopathy (disease of the heart muscle) and premature heartbeats or total loss of rhythmic beating in the heart's upper chambers.

Heavy drinking, often defined as consuming more than two cocktails or three glasses of beer or wine daily, is now related to a 40 percent increased risk of high blood pressure. Middle-aged women and men who drink even more are likely to experience a 90 percent greater risk. Alcohol is also associated with phlebitis (inflammation of the veins) and varicose (unnatural and permanently distended) veins. In addition, research now indicates that heavy drinkers are more than three times as likely as nondrinkers to have a stroke or cerebral vascular accident (CVA).[23] This increased risk pertains only to hemorrhagic stroke, in which small blood vessels in the brain rupture or burst. Moreover, this risk is independent of hypertension or high blood pressure. Light and moderate drinkers, by comparison, are more than twice as likely to have such strokes.

In contrast with long-term, heavy consumption, drinking just one or two servings of beer, wine, or distilled spirits

daily has appeared to confer a protective effect against heart attack among some drinkers. Early claims of such a cardio- (heart) protective effect due to drinking alcohol, particularly red wine, were sensationalized by attention given to the "French paradox"—the low rate of heart disease among French citizens who regularly consume foods very rich in saturated fats and cholesterol. Nutrition scientists and medical specialists typically associate such a diet with an increased, not a decreased, incidence of coronary heart disease. This seemingly contradictory situation persists because the same French people also consume moderate amounts of red wine almost on a daily basis. Apparently the daily intake of moderate amounts of red wine somehow results in a protective effect against coronary heart disease.

Researchers have now concluded that a moderate intake of any alcoholic beverage, not just red wine, reduces the risk of coronary heart disease.[24] Moreover, extensive data suggest that alcohol's beneficial effect is due in large part to an increase in blood levels of total high-density lipoprotein (HDL) as well as both subfractions, HDL_2 and HDL_3. (Lipoprotein is a combination of a blood lipid, or fat, and a protein substance that transports or carries fats in the blood, including cholesterol and triglycerides.)

In this major study, one alcoholic drink was defined as a twelve-ounce glass of beer, or its equivalent in wine or distilled spirits. Individuals who consumed more than one, but fewer than three, drinks per day reduced their heart attack risk by half.

Despite this favorable aspect of moderate alcohol use, drinking any amount of alcohol can have risks for some people, as noted earlier in this section. In terms of ethyl alcohol, the difference between daily small to moderate amounts and large quantities may be the difference between preventing and causing disease.[25] There are other, safer ways of raising HDL levels, including regular exercise and the replacement of saturated fat with monounsaturated fats in one's diet. Encouragement of alcohol use to reduce the likelihood of the occurrence or recurrence of heart disease seems unwise. Even moderate drinking poses serious risks—hypertension (elevated blood pressure), alcohol-related auto accidents, and fetal damage in pregnant women.

Myopathy—This is an abnormal condition or disease of muscular tissues, characterized by muscle weakness, cramps, and wasting away of skeletal musculature.

Cancer—Cancer, or uncontrolled cell growth, is frequently observed in patients who are alcohol dependent or who have alcohol-related cirrhosis. Heavy drinking increases the risk of developing cancer of the tongue, mouth, throat, esophagus, and liver, and is often associated with cancer of the pancreas, large intestine, and rectum. Though still controversial, relatively new research suggests that alcohol may also increase the risk of breast cancer in women as much as 2 times in comparison with women who do not drink.

There is now little doubt that heavy drinking is related significantly to many kinds of malignant cancer. But the precise mechanism of alcohol's involvement remains somewhat a mystery. Studies of laboratory animals have failed to show that pure ethyl alcohol is carcinogenic (cancer-causing) in and of itself.

Consequently, it is now believed that some of the congeners or other contaminants in alcoholic beverages may be the culprit in drinking-related cancers. Alcohol itself may prove to be more of a cocarcinogen: a promoter, or a vehicle bearing a causal agent. For instance, alcohol appears to interact with tobacco to increase the risk of certain cancers and with the condition of cirrhosis to increase the development of liver cancer.

Infectious diseases—These, particularly pneumonia and tuberculosis, are common to alcohol abusers. The neglect of nutrition, impairment of lung clearance and phagocytosis (a process whereby white blood cells ingest and digest specific bacteria), and decreased immune response mechanisms make alcohol abusers prone to respiratory infections.

Alcohol-drug interactions—Mixing alcoholic beverages with other drugs can have unpleasant and even fatal effects. The effects of alcohol-drug interactions can range from the relatively minor drowsiness that comes with mixing a cocktail with an antihistamine all the way to loss of consciousness and death. How much a person is affected by the combination of alcohol and certain prescription drugs, as well as over-the-counter drugs, depends on several factors: body size, weight, age, sex, health status, genetic makeup, and the person's ability to process or change consumed substances before their elimination from the body. One fact seems fairly certain: People who drink a lot or who take a lot of medicines run a greater risk of encountering alcohol-drug reactions.

Perhaps the most dangerous alcohol-drug interaction is related to the **potentiation effect**. In *potentiation*, or *synergism*, the joint effect of two drugs taken together is greater than the sum of the effects of the two drugs taken individually. Mix alcohol, a central nervous system (CNS) depressant, with another CNS depressant, and the pharmacologic effect on the body is multiplied or exaggerated. Sometimes the result is drowsiness and difficulty in walking, talking, driving, and thinking. Performance skills, judgment, and alertness can be slowed down dangerously. Some combinations of alcohol with barbiturates, tranquilizers, and prescription painkillers can be fatal.

Alcohol and drugs can also interact so as to reduce the effectiveness of certain drugs (anticonvulsants and anticoagulants). Long-term alcohol abuse can even produce the opposite effect, so that some drugs will remain in the body longer than they should, thus increasing the likelihood of serious side effects. A detailed listing of various alcohol-drug interactions appears in table 4.3.

Prenatal Alcohol Abuse

Ethyl alcohol is now widely recognized as a powerful teratogen, a drug capable of interfering with the development of an embryo and fetus and responsible for one or more birth defects. Moreover, alcohol is now associated with a wide range of adverse effects in children of women who drink during pregnancy. And an estimated 5 to 10 percent of pregnant women in America drink at levels high enough to place their children at risk for the harmful effects of fetal alcohol exposure.[26]

Fetal Alcohol Syndrome

For many years it has been observed that children of alcoholic mothers have been born alcohol dependent or physically addicted to alcohol; that is, they experience withdrawal signs and symptoms at birth. Although physicians and laypeople alike have long suspected that drinking could affect the unborn in even more insidious and permanent ways, it was not until 1973 that pediatrician David W. Smith discovered a direct association between drinking alcohol and birth defects.

The evidence of medical research now suggests the existence of a common pattern of birth defects and mental retardation among some children born of alcoholic women or those who drank excessively during pregnancy. These structural and functional abnormalities have been identified as **fetal alcohol syndrome (FAS)**. While all of the defects related to prenatal exposure to alcohol have not yet been established, we now know the following:

- Alcohol can be very toxic to the fetus, independently of the effects of malnutrition.

- Adverse effects of prenatal exposure to alcohol exist along a continuum, with the complete FAS syndrome at one end of the spectrum and

table 4.3 Alcohol-Drug Interactions

Drug	Possible Effects of Combining This Drug with Alcohol
Analgesics	
Narcotics	Increased central nervous system (CNS) and respiratory depression.
Nonnarcotics	Increased gastrointestinal blood loss and damage to the stomach lining.
Aspirin	
Darvon	Increased CNS depression.
Acetaminophen	Development of liver disorders in long-term drinkers.
Antidepressants	
Tricyclics	Enhanced CNS depressant effects and impairment of motor skills.
Monoamine oxidase inhibitors	Increased sedative effects; nausea, vomiting, and headache.
	Increased blood pressure.
	Hypertensive crisis with Chianti wine and beer.
Antidiabetic agents	
Insulin	Increased chance of hypoglycemia resulting in increased drug effect in the body.
Diabinese and Orinase	Possible disulfiram-like reaction in the body.
Antihistamines	CNS depression ranging from minimal to prominent effects of these drugs synergized by alcohol.
Antihypertensive agents	May increase sedation with initial treatment.
Anti-infective agents	Possible disulfiram-like reaction.
Central nervous system stimulants	
Cocaine	No interactions have been reported.
Amphetamines	Antagonized CNS depression.
	No motor coordination improvement.
Nicotine	Clinically important drug interaction not established, but cocarcinogenic effect is possible.
Hallucinogens	
Cannabis	Additive effect.
	Mental and motor impairment.
LSD	Reported but questionable precipitation of LSD flashbacks.
Oral contraceptives	Prolonged elevated blood-alcohol levels.
	Slowed rate of elimination of alcohol from the body.

Source: National Center for Alcohol Education, National Institute on Alcohol Abuse and Alcoholism, modified.

incomplete features of FAS, including more subtle mental and behavioral deficits, on the other.

- Harmful effects of prenatal alcohol exposure on child development can vary from child to child and depend primarily on the pattern and extent of alcohol exposure prior to birth.

- FAS may vary with the race, income, and drinking history of the mother, as well as her medical status and other socioeconomic factors.

- After a woman gives birth to a child with FAS, the probability that her subsequent children will also have FAS is about 70 percent.

Principal Features of FAS

The main features associated with fetal alcohol syndrome are grouped into three major categories:[27, 28]

Growth deficiency—Alcohol-exposed infants tend to be smaller in weight, length, and head circumference. Some studies indicate that such growth deficits persist well into childhood. Such children are often only about 65 percent of normal birth length and 38 percent of normal birth weight.

Central nervous system damage—The most commonly observed problem is mental retardation. Difficulty with

learning, attention, memory, and problem solving are common, along with incoordination, impulsive behavior, and speech and hearing impairments. Sometimes these problems in learning skills persist well into adolescence and even adulthood. According to the Office for Substance Abuse Prevention, children who suffer mental retardation due to alcohol abuse by their mothers typically display alarming amounts of disturbed physiological functioning and maladaptive behavior, in contrast with Down syndrome children, who are usually complacent, happy, and compliant.[29]

Drug	Possible Effects of Combining This Drug with Alcohol
Sedative-hypnotics	
Barbiturates	Enhanced CNS and respiratory depression.
	Cross-tolerance to sedative effect among sedative-hypnotics and with alcohol.
	Potentially lethal combination in large doses.
	Nausea.
Nonbarbiturates	Vomiting.
Tranquilizers	
Minor (anti-anxiety agents)	Caution should be used when driving or operating machinery.
	At social drinking levels, there is considerable synergism or CNS depression.
	At more than social drinking, increased sedation and CNS depressant effects occur.
	Cross-tolerance to sedative effect.
	Additive or synergistic increase of CNS depressant effect.
	Combination can lead to death by accidental overdose or by suicide.
Major	Additive CNS depression.
	Impairment of muscle coordination and judgment; caution should be used when driving or operating machinery.
Miscellaneous	
Disulfiram	Disulfiram plus alcohol, even in small amounts, produces flushing,
(Antabuse)	throbbing in head and neck, nausea, vomiting, breathing difficulties, sweating.
	In severe reactions, there may be serious cardiovascular and respiratory problems, convulsions, and death.
Methotrexate	Increased risk of liver disorders.
Phenytoin	Drowsiness, reduces effectiveness of drug in preventing seizures.
(Dilantin)	
Prednisone	Irritation of the stomach.
(Deltasone)	
Warfarin	Increased anti-blood-clotting effect.
(Coumadin)	Easy bruising.

Head and facial abnormalities—The most frequently observed characteristics are shortness of the palpebral fissures (the slits between the opposed lids of the closed eyes); a short, upturned nose with an underdeveloped ridge between the base of the nose and the upper lip; a sunken nasal bridge; folds on the inner aspect of the eyelids; a thin upper lip; an underdeveloped midface; and growth retardation of the jaw. While these abnormalities are individually subtle, jointly they characterize a distinctive face, as noted in figure 4.2.

Other major and minor malformations of the human body may also be present among the FAS patient population.

There is likely to be an increase in abnormal structures of various organ systems, including cardiac (heart), urinary, genital, and skeletal systems (e.g., peculiar palmar creases), and limited joint movements of the fingers and elbows.

Fetal Alcohol Effects or Alcohol-Related Birth Defects

Developmental effects of prenatal alcohol exposure that are less severe than FAS are classified as fetal alcohol effects (FAE) or alcohol-related birth defects (ARBD). Children of alcohol-abusing or alcoholic mothers may display signs in just two of the three defining categories of FAS. Less severe clinical findings include low birth weight, subtle behavioral

problems, abnormalities of the mouth or heart, and evidence of mild neurological difficulties. This category of alcohol-exposed individuals is undoubtedly much larger, less easily identified, and often more problematic in terms of social behavior than children with full FAS.

Mechanism of Impairment

Nearly 5,000 infants—one in every 750—are born with FAS every year. An estimated 36,000 newborns are affected by FAE in any one year. Yet the precise manner by which alcohol consumption contributes to harmful fetal and neonatal growth and development has not been fully established. It is likely that much of the trauma occurs early in the first trimester of pregnancy, when harmful

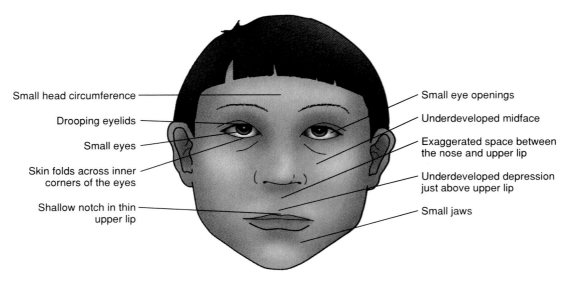

Small head circumference

Drooping eyelids

Small eyes

Skin folds across inner corners of the eyes

Shallow notch in thin upper lip

Small eye openings

Underdeveloped midface

Exaggerated space between the nose and upper lip

Underdeveloped depression just above upper lip

Small jaws

 4.2

Frequently occurring facial and head characteristics as seen in children with the Fetal Alcohol Syndrome typically present a "pushed-in-face" effect.

From Harry Avis, Drugs and Life. *Copyright © 1990 Wm. C. Brown Communications, Inc. Reprinted by permission of Times Mirror Higher Education Group, Inc., Dubuque, Iowa. All Rights Reserved.*

exposure to alcohol affects fetal organ development and results in related, major birth defects. At this time, when signs of pregnancy are few and many women are not yet aware that they are pregnant, binge drinking is especially perilous.[30]

Since alcohol in the mother's body crosses the placenta and enters the fetal bloodstream, the direct embryotoxic effect of alcohol has been implicated in producing abnormalities, along with alcohol's primary oxidation by-product, acetaldehyde. Distributed by the fetal blood to all parts of the fetal body, the alcohol can bathe the cells of the brain and exert a damaging effect. The fetal liver cannot oxidize alcohol as readily as the mother's can, so the alcohol circulates in the fetus for a longer time before elimination.

There are other possible mechanisms of trauma: Alcohol might interfere with the delivery of maternal nutrients to the fetus, impair the supply of fetal oxygen, derange protein synthesis and metabolism, or stimulate excess production of certain prostaglandins, chemicals that regulate cellular functions of the body

and possibly cause fetal malformations.[31] Alcohol's possible effect on the father's sperm cells prior to fertilization has also been investigated for its possible contribution to FAS or FAE. Although ethyl alcohol might interfere with male reproductive function, there is no firm evidence that paternal alcoholism accounts for the specific congenital defects seen in FAS or FAE.

Although no one knows how much alcohol is too much and therefore damaging to the developing embryo and fetus, the FAS risk for human infants seems to increase markedly when the mother's daily consumption is three ounces (six drinks) or more. Between 30 and 40 percent of infants born to women who consume this amount have some FAS defects. However, the severity of the syndrome might be related more closely to how much is drunk at one time during pregnancy than to frequency of drinking. Binge drinking of more than five drinks on any occasion and drinking during the first two months of pregnancy are two of the strongest maternal predictors of later neurobehavioral deficits among their children.[32]

Prevention of FAS and FAE

In 1981, the U.S. Food and Drug Administration issued its first official, written warning on alcohol and pregnancy. This new advisory declared that even women who drank as little as one ounce of alcohol (the amount contained in about two glasses of table wine) twice a week during pregnancy experience significant increases in spontaneous abortion and giving birth to smaller babies or infants with birth defects. Alcoholics and heavy drinkers are more likely to give birth to babies with severe FAS.

In advising expectant mothers and those considering pregnancy that they may be harming their unborn children by drinking even small amounts of alcohol, the Food and Drug Administration and many physicians now reject the concept of safe or moderate drinking during pregnancy. Until the exact amount of alcohol that might be safe is known, most medical authorities now recommend abstinence from alcohol during pregnancy and breast-feeding, pending confirmation of alcohol's role in relation to fetal development.[33]

The Short Michigan Alcoholism Screening Test (SMAST)   *Adapted from the SMAST (Selzer, 1975)*

Screening tests have been formulated to identify individuals who may have a particular health problem but whose symptoms have not yet become highly visible. One of the more frequently used screening tests for alcoholism is the Michigan Alcoholism Screening Test (MAST). Originally developed by Melvin Selzer, the first MAST had 24 items. A revised list of just 13 questions, which are typically self-administered, is now used with a high degree of effectiveness by clinicians.

1. Do you feel you are a normal drinker? (By normal we mean you drink *less than* or *as much as* most other people.)
2. Does your wife, husband, a parent, or other near relative ever worry or complain about your drinking?
3. Do you ever feel guilty about your drinking?
4. Do friends or relatives think you are a normal drinker?
5. Are you able to stop drinking when you want to?
6. Have you ever attended a meeting of Alcoholics Anonymous?
7. Has drinking ever created problems between you and your wife, husband, a parent, or other near relative?
8. Have you ever gotten into trouble at work because of drinking?
9. Have you ever neglected your obligations, your family, or your work for two or more days in a row because you were drinking?

10. Have you ever gone to anyone for help about your drinking?
11. Have you ever been in a hospital because of drinking?
12. Have you ever been arrested for drunken driving, driving while intoxicated, or driving under the influence of alcoholic beverages?
13. Have you ever been arrested, even for a few hours, because of other drunken behavior?

Scoring and evaluation of the SMAST: An answer to any of the questions that corresponds to the following responses is assigned a value of one point:

1. No, 2. Yes, 3. Yes, 4. No, 5. No, 6. Yes, 7. Yes, 8. Yes, 9. Yes, 10. Yes, 11. Yes, 12. Yes, 13. Yes.

In individuals who score two points, alcoholism is suggested; in those who score three or more points, alcoholism is assessed.

Based on current yet somewhat contradictory estimates, the overall occurrence of FAS in the United States is estimated to be approximately 1 to 3 for every 1,000 live births. However, the risk of FAS for African Americans is nearly seven times higher than for whites, and among southwest plains Native Americans, the prevalence of FAS is alarmingly high—at 1 case for every 102 live births. The National Institute on Alcohol Abuse and Alcoholism suggests that several factors may play a role in such differences, including cultural influences, alcohol consumption patterns, nutrition, metabolic differences, and even some type of genetic susceptibility.[34] Such statistics indicate that fetal alcohol syndrome is now a leading known cause of mental retardation and birth defects, along with Down syndrome and spina bifida. Of these three major causes of birth defects, FAS is the only one that is potentially preventable.

Problem Drinking: Personal and Social Aspects

Problem drinking refers to alcohol consumption that results in damage to the drinker, the drinker's family, or the drinker's community. Problem drinkers include not only alcohol-dependent individuals and long-time alcohol abusers, but also moderate and light drinkers who drive after excessive drinking and cause accidents, those who engage in drinking to become intoxicated, and those who drink when such imbibing is contraindicated by some medical condition. Some problem drinkers even engage in the "sport" of competitive consumption to determine who can hold more.

In other words, problem drinking is a form of substance abuse as well as a consequence of substance abuse. Use of alcohol continues despite a persistent social, occupational, psychological, or physical problem related to such consumption. Problem drinking is also a form of substance abuse because alcohol intake recurs when such use is dangerous to oneself or to others or both (see box 4.4).

Problem Drinking and the Individual

For the person involved, alcohol abuse can result in intoxication, death or injury by accident, loss of a job, disruption of family life, quarreling and fighting, and certain deficiency and metabolic diseases often associated with excessive drinking.

Dependence on alcohol as a psychological crutch to hide or mask problems of everyday living is particularly hazardous, especially for young people. Youths who are dependent on alcohol may never develop and practice decision-making skills for coping with the perplexities and disappointments of reality. Furthermore, it is probable that alcohol, not marijuana, is the first mood modifier used by many people who later become dependent on other drugs.

Alcohol-Impaired Driving and Auto Crashes

With the arrest of nearly 1.7 million drivers each year for driving while intoxicated—an arrest rate of 1 for every 90 licensed drivers—*alcohol-impaired driving* has become this nation's most socially accepted violent crime. In the United States, traffic crashes continue to be the greatest single cause of death for every age group between 6 and 33 years old—greater than deaths from other drugs, wars, or disease.[35] Of those crashes, about 45 percent are caused by someone's excessive consumption of alcohol combined with driving a car, motorcycle, truck, or bus.

According to the National Highway Traffic Safety Administration, alcohol-related motor-vehicle crashes claim about 17,700 lives each year. Nearly 38 percent of all traffic fatalities involve a driver or pedestrian with a blood-alcohol concentration (BAC) greater than or equal to 0.10 percent—the current legal definition of intoxication in most states. Another 7 to 8 percent of fatalities involve a driver or pedestrian with some blood-alcohol level, that is, a BAC of 0.01 to 0.09 percent.

Every hour, almost two Americans are killed by an alcohol-impaired driver. Most victims of these fatal crashes (about 66 percent) are drinking drivers, drinking pedestrians, and drinking bicyclists. The other 33 percent are nondrinking drivers, nonoccupants (primarily pedestrians and bicyclists), and passengers. In addition to alcohol-related traffic deaths, another half-million people—one person every minute—sustain injuries as a result of alcohol-related crashes. After the vehicular wreckage is hauled away, the human wreckage is left behind, including permanent brain damage, spinal cord injuries, lost or permanently deformed limbs, blindness, and impotence—lifetimes crippled with disability, lifetimes haunted by nightmares of how it all happened.[36]

An analysis of statistics from the National Highway Traffic Safety Administration and the Behavioral Risk Factor Surveillance System further describes the dimensions of alcohol-impaired driving in the United States.

- Nearly 2 out of 5 Americans will be involved in an alcohol-related crash in their lifetime.

- Most people who drink and drive are not heavy drinkers, but moderate and light drinkers.

- The prevalence of drinking and driving is highest among men, young adults, and divorced or separated people.

- Drinkers who prefer beer are more likely to drive after drinking and to believe that driving while intoxicated is less serious than do drinkers who prefer wine or liquor.

- Nearly 9 out of 10 teenage automobile accidents involve alcohol.

- More than three-fourths of all fatal crashes that occur between 8 P.M. and 4 A.M. on any night of the week involve alcohol.

- A much higher percentage of fatal crashes on weekends (62 percent) than on weekdays (39 percent) involve a driver with a detectable blood-alcohol level.

- A much higher percentage of fatal crashes at night (70 percent) than during the daytime (23 percent) involve a driver with a detectable blood-alcohol level.

- Even though the minimum legal drinking age is now set at 21 years in all states, more than one-third of fatally injured drivers under 21 had known blood-alcohol concentrations of 0.01 percent or above.

- The amount of alcohol consumed by people arrested for driving under the influence is usually very high. On the average, their BACs register the pure-alcohol bloodstream equivalent of ten to twelve drinks in a four-hour period, or BACs greater than 0.15 percent.

In light of these revealing facts, it should not be surprising that more than 340 Americans—the number of passengers on a large, fully occupied jetliner—die each week due to alcohol-impaired driving.

Studies of traffic accidents consistently show that the relative probability of being involved in a crash and the probability of a driver's causing an accident both increase as the blood-alcohol concentration or level increases (see figure 4.3). At a blood-alcohol concentration (BAC) of 0.06 percent, a drinking driver is twice as likely as a sober driver to cause an accident. But when a BAC of 0.10 percent is reached, a drinking driver's chances of having an accident are 6 to 7 times higher than if his or her BAC were zero. If the BAC rises to 0.15 percent, the driver's chances of crashing are 25 times greater. These BACs are not characteristic of the social drinker, however. To reach a concentration of 0.15 percent within two hours after eating, a 160-pound man would have to consume ten one-ounce drinks of 86 proof whiskey, all within one hour. The same drinker would reach the same state of intoxication with one-third less quantity if the alcohol were taken on an empty stomach. Even six or seven drinks within one hour is a lot of drinking.

Alcohol also has a potentiating effect on injury once a crash happens.[37] In a crash of a given severity, those vehicle occupants who have been drinking alcohol are likely to sustain greater injury than those who have not been consuming alcohol. When alcohol is present, the general difference in probability of serious injury or death from a crash is about twofold. However, in certain types of crashes, the differences between those with and without alcohol are more than fourfold.

The connection between drinking and alcohol-impaired driving is more complex than a mere depressant effect on the brain. It is commonly recognized that many of those who drink and drive do not display the obvious signs of intoxication: reporting double vision, giving evidence of slurred speech and/or bloodshot eyes, and inability to walk a straight line. Yet they are under the influence of alcohol. Slightly impaired judgment, reduced tolerance to glare, underestimation of speed and distance, drowsiness, a false sense of security,

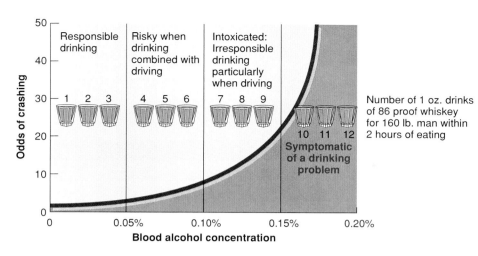

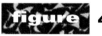 **4.3**

Drinking and highway safety: Odds of a crash after drinking.

Source: National Highway Traffic Safety Administration.

slower reaction time, narrowed peripheral vision, a lessening of depth perception, a reduction of cue-taking, an inflated ego, and undue expansion of aggression all take their toll on the driver's ability.

Also affected at BACs as low as 0.01 to 0.02 percent are three essential driving skills: tracking, information processing, and attention sharing.[38] A relatively difficult psychomotor task, tracking or steering is a driver's ability to maintain a vehicle within lane limits and in the correct direction, while monitoring the driving environment for other important information. Information processing, on the other hand, involves a person's ability to interpret and integrate complex sensory information. Alcohol-impaired drivers require more time to read street signs or recognize and respond to traffic signals than the nonimpaired do. Such drivers look at fewer sources of information, acquire less total sensory input from the driving environment, and tend to restrict their vision to the center of the roadway.

The third essential driving skill adversely affected by even small amounts of alcohol is attention sharing, the ability to divide one's awareness between two or more sources of visual and/or sound information. In driving, two major tasks must be performed at the same time—maintaining a vehicle in the proper lane and direction, and monitoring the driving environment for vital information, including vehicles, traffic signals, pedestrians, and various road hazards. But the alcohol-impaired driver, confronted with the need to divide his or her attention between the tasks, tends to favor one task over the other. Typically, alcohol-impaired drivers restrict their vision to the center of the visual field and fail to observe important events in the driving environment. Divided attention deficits often begin in the 0.02 to 0.10 percent BAC range, the very lowest blood-alcohol levels that can be reliably measured.

In order to reduce the alcohol-related carnage on American highways, the National Highway Traffic Safety Administration set a BAC of 0.10 percent as indicative of intoxication while operating a motor vehicle. This level of blood alcohol was eventually adopted by most states as *prima facie* (sufficient) evidence of driving under the influence of alcohol. However, thirty-seven states and the District of Columbia have also enacted "per se" laws that specify that it is unlawful to drive with a blood-alcohol level of 0.10 percent or higher. An additional nine states have now adopted lower "per se" limits of 0.08 percent or less. Only four

states and the Commonwealth of Puerto Rico have no "per se" law at the present time. In recognition that in most people driving skills are adversely affected beginning at a BAC of just 0.05 percent, several states are now discussing the desirability of setting even lower "per se" limits. You might benefit by determining your consumption limits now, as illustrated in table 4.4.

Under provisions of the Commercial Motor Vehicles Safety Act of 1986, Congress authorized the U.S. Department of Transportation (DOT) to set new limits for alcohol use by truck and bus operators.[39] In 1989, the DOT adopted a BAC limit of 0.04 percent for commercial drivers, commercial shippers, and aviators, while other authorities have proposed for the same groups a zero-tolerance or zero alcohol standard level; that is, any amount of alcohol in the blood would be disallowed. Until individual states also adopt such limits, their application will not be effective. However, some states have already adopted the zero-tolerance standard for teenage drivers; these states suspend the driver's licenses of teenagers found operating a motor vehicle with any detectable blood-alcohol level. Several states have also enacted laws that revoke the driver's licenses of those under 21 years of age who commit any drug offense or drop out of school.

The safest policy is not to drive after drinking. If you do drink and then drive, know and stay within your own personal limits as well as the legal limits. Of course, you can help promote the health and welfare of all those who drive on the highways by keeping an intoxicated person from driving. Car keys should be calmly yet firmly taken away from such a person if he or she insists on operating a motor vehicle. If possible, arrange for someone else to drive the drunk person's car, and take the person home yourself, call a taxi, or have the individual stay overnight. Remember, friends do not let friends drive drunk!

Until recently there has been a general public indifference about, or a lack of commitment to, solving the drunk-driving problem. Many people still believe that drinking-and-driving behavior is acceptable until the drunk driver causes an accident that harms another person. Because such occurrences are relatively infrequent, the public has empathy for the typical convicted drinking driver. He or she is perceived as an otherwise law-abiding citizen who just got caught doing two legal and widely practiced activities in an illegal combination. Such an attitude has caused juries to be swayed by sympathy, has undermined support for campaigns such as "If you drink, don't drive," and remains the biggest obstacle to solving the drinking-driver problem.

Recently, outraged parents and friends of young victims of alcohol-impaired drivers have formed action groups that lobby and influence legislators, police, prosecutors, and judges to "crack down" on drunk drivers. Despite tremendous indifference and sometimes vocal opposition, several organizations, such as Remove Intoxicated Drivers (RID), but especially Mothers Against Drunk Drivers (MADD), have been quite successful in enacting tougher laws dealing with sentencing violators. Now in its second decade, MADD has also been a major force in raising the drinking age in all fifty states, promoting "designated driver" programs, and advocating the rights of those victimized by drunk drivers.[40] Without question, MADD has been responsible for developing a new social and moral code in America concerning drinking and driving.

An ever-increasing number of driving-while-intoxicated (DWI) countermeasures is now available to help end the national epidemic of alcohol-impaired driving. Following are specific countermeasures various federal and state commissions have proposed. Has your state or local community adopted any of them?

- Reduction of the blood-alcohol concentration indicative of driving while intoxicated from 0.10 percent to 0.04 percent by the year 2000. Establishment of a limit of 0.00 percent (zero tolerance) for drivers under the age of 21.

- Enforcement of "dram shop acts"—either by formal statute or by judicial decision or precedent—that impose liability for damages on social hosts, including fraternities and sororities, who furnish alcoholic beverages to their guests.

 4.4 Know Your Drinking Limits

Chart for Responsible People Who May Sometimes Drive after Drinking!									
Approximate Blood-Alcohol Percentage									
Drinks in One Hour	Body Weight in Pounds								Adversely Affected
	100	120	140	160	180	200	220	240	
1	.04	.03	.03	.02	.02	.02	.02	.02	Rarely
2	.08	.06	.05	.05	.04	.04	.03	.03	
3	.11	.09	.08	.07	.06	.06	.05	.05	
4	.15	.12	.11	.09	.08	.08	.07	.06	
5	.19	.16	.13	.12	.11	.09	.09	.08	Possibly
6	.23	.19	.16	.14	.13	.11	.10	.09	
7	.26	.22	.19	.16	.15	.13	.12	.11	
8	.30	.25	.21	.19	.17	.15	.14	.13	Definitely
9	.34	.28	.24	.21	.19	.17	.15	.14	
10	.38	.31	.27	.23	.21	.19	.17	.16	

Subtract .01 percent for each 40 minutes of drinking.

One drink is 1 oz. of 100 proof liquor, 12 oz. of beer, or 4 oz. of table wine.

Surest Policy Is . . . Don't Drive After Drinking! Know Your Limits

The safest policy is not to drive after drinking. If you do drink and then drive, then know and stay safely within your own personal limits. Even this chart is only a guide, not a guarantee.
Driving after excessive drinking is dangerous and punishable by law. The operator of a motor vehicle is presumed by law to be impaired when the percent of alcohol in his/her blood is above the .10 level. The above table indicates the relationship between number of drinks (taken by normal adults) and the legal limits. If your weight is between two of those shown, use the lower weight.
The legal limit is **not** the same as your own personal, safe limit.

Source: Courtesy of Distilled Spirits Council of the United States, Inc.

- A ban on open containers of alcoholic beverages in motor vehicles.

- Institution of a "sobriety checkpoint" program—now determined to be constitutional by the U.S. Supreme Court—in which all motorists in a specific area are stopped without selection or discrimination and observed for obvious signs of intoxication. If such signs are apparent, the motorists are asked to take a breath test, usually at the site of the checkpoint.

- Enactment of a 0.08 percent or lower blood-alcohol level "per se" law that makes driving with such a blood-alcohol level illegal in itself, without need for establishing probable cause in order to stop an obviously drunken driver.

- Adoption of a "presumptive level" of 0.08 percent or lower BAC that establishes *prima facie* evidence of driving under the influence of alcohol.

- Confiscation of a driver's license on the spot (administrative license revocation) for those who are found to have equaled or exceeded the legal BAC limit. License suspension or permanent revocation might follow such action.

- An automatic charge of vehicular homicide imposed for death or serious injury occurring while driving under the influence of alcohol.

- A ban on "plea bargaining" in cases of driving under the influence. In effect, the plea-bargaining process drops charges against a defendant for one serious criminal offense in exchange for an admission of guilt to another, lesser offense. This common legal practice would be forbidden in DUI cases.

- Mandatory jail sentences for driving on a suspended or revoked driver's license.

- Use of preliminary roadside breath tests (or newer saliva tests) to screen potential drunk drivers at the site of apprehension, prior to administering more sophisticated breath analysis tests to confirm the original findings.

- Provision of a system in each state to fund comprehensive alcohol-impaired-driving programs, and drinking-and-driving education in worksites, communities, health care agencies, and schools.

- Reduction of the availability of beverage alcohol by eliminating "happy hours" and other reduced-price promotions, limiting hours and density of sales outlets, and requiring impaired-driver prevention training of sellers and servers.

- A matching of alcoholic beverage ads with an equal number of pro-health and pro-safety messages.

- Restrictions on certain advertising and marketing practices, especially those that appeal to "underage" young people. This action would ban the use of sports figures and other youth role models from promoting beer and forbid breweries from sponsoring rock concerts and sporting events.

- Increased excise taxes on alcoholic beverages, and equal taxation of beer, wine, and distilled spirits, based on alcohol content.

The Family and Problem Drinking

Alcohol abuse and alcohol dependence within the family setting often result in a serious psychological and social disorder that many now consider a family disease. Truly, the family is not at ease, and family relationships are not only disrupted but also disrupting. Undeniably, each member of the family can be victimized by the disturbing effects of problem drinking on the stability, unity, values, attitudes, and goals of the family unit. Countless millions of American adults have been exposed to problem-producing family drinking through endangered physical, mental, social, economic, and even spiritual welfare; unhappy and unfulfilling marriages; broken homes resulting from desertion and divorce; impoverishment; and sometimes violence involving both spouse abuse and child abuse.

The family and marital interactions of alcohol-abusing people have become a growing area of research recently. We now know that evidence linking alcohol abuse and family violence is not simply one of cause and effect. Indeed, the husband who beats his wife is sometimes a battering father, but alcohol consumption may be coincidental to the circumstances that end with the abuse. Sometimes the drunken father is the target of violence from the wife and even the children. To complicate the family situation, violence is often interspersed with periods of calm that mistakenly encourage the victim to believe that the personal abuse will not be repeated. And in some instances, alcohol abusers can hold all other family members psychologically hostage to their threats of misbehavior or embarrassment, so that problem drinkers "get their way" and nonproblem drinkers allow the alcohol abuse to continue through their own silence and inaction.

The role of alcohol in violence is not well understood, although personal violence is frequently associated with alcohol consumption by the offending perpetrators. In fact, alcohol is present in more than one-half of all incidents of domestic violence.[41] And the most common pattern of such violence includes drinking by both husband and wife. It should be noted, however, that the majority of drinkers, even heavy drinkers, never engage in violent behavior. It should also be emphasized that drinking by victims is neither an excuse for nor a direct cause of spousal abuse, but such alcohol use may contribute to their own increased risk of victimization.[42]

In reality, heavy-drinking females are often married to heavy-drinking males, which places such wives in an environment in which their potential exposure to violence is higher. Also, heavy drinking is still more socially stigmatizing for females than for males, and drunken females are more likely than drunken males to be viewed as obnoxious (drunken females are also likely to be viewed as unfeminine). Therefore, such wives might be seen as more socially acceptable targets of violence, even by their intoxicated husbands. In addition, alcohol abuse by the husband, wife, or both could indirectly contribute to family violence by complicating already existing economic and child-care difficulties.

Nevertheless, police records and victimization survey responses recorded by the National Institute on Alcohol Abuse and Alcoholism typically indicate somewhat higher rates of alcohol involvement among offending assailants than among their victims.[43] Moreover, the rate of physical violence significantly increases when male partners increase their alcohol consumption.[44] When such involvement occurs within the family, husbands might use their excessive drinking as an excuse for beating their wives. They believe that if they are drunk, they cannot be held responsible for their actions. For others, alcohol abuse may be an attempt to lessen rage, but as drinking increases, assault and aggression become more likely due to loss of inhibitions and loss of the ability to control rage.

Even when spouse abuse is absent from the marital relationship, problem drinking typically afflicts the couple with some type of sexual problem that often threatens the marriage. Such problems include loss of libido or sexual interest among both males and females, inhibited sexual excitement, impotence in males, and anorgasmia (lack of orgasmic response) in females. Of course, chronic, excessive use of alcohol diminishes both sexual performance and sexual desire.

Parents with alcohol problems also have a high potential for neglecting and abusing their own children. Alcohol abuse is a contributing factor in about one-third of all child-abuse cases, including sexual abuse. There appears to be an alarming similarity between child abusers and alcohol abusers. Among these shared characteristics are low self-esteem, low tolerance

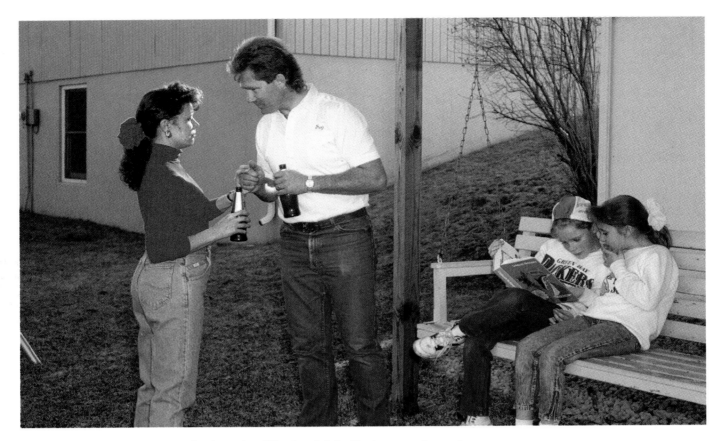

Children of alcoholic parents appear to develop coping skills when their families become endangered by a problem drinker. However, the children are at increased risk for experiencing various psychological problems as well as for alcoholism.

© James L. Shaffer

for frustration, impulsive behavior, difficulty in experiencing pleasure, and a lack of understanding of the needs and abilities of infants and children. And child-abusing families, like alcohol-abusing families, often share social isolation from friends and neighbors, and tend to have parents who themselves were abused as children.

Children of Alcoholics

Currently, it is estimated that there are 29 million Americans who may be designated as *children of alcoholics* (COAs). Nearly 7 million of them are under 18 years of age, and almost 3 million of this group will likely develop alcoholism, other drug problems, and/or other serious coping problems.[45] Moreover, about half of all COAs will likely marry alcoholics and are thus at risk of re-creating the same kinds of stressful and unhealthy families in which they themselves grew up.

There is no doubt that all children are affected adversely by family alcohol abuse and suffer negative consequences. However, the larger proportion of COAs seem to function fairly well and do not develop serious problems during childhood or adulthood. Apparently many COAs make positive adjustments to their family's alcoholism and other alcohol-related problems.

Many children of alcoholics, however, are at an extremely high risk for developing alcohol and other drug problems, and often live with overwhelming tension, stress, and, especially, fears.[46] Some have high levels of anxiety and depression, others do poorly in school, and still others experience problems with coping. Among the most frequently observed differences in COAs are deficits in mental functioning: in perception, reasoning, intuition, and the process of gaining knowledge. While these children tend to achieve lower scores, they nevertheless test within normal ranges for intelligence and knowledge of specific academic subjects.[47] However, they often experience school problems, repeat grades, fail to graduate from high school, and require referrals to school counselors and psychologists.

Nearly fifteen years ago, when COAs were first identified as a special population with unique needs and problems, a standard group of symptoms—the *COA syndrome*—was formulated to describe children of alcoholics:[48, 49]

- Toleration of bizarre behavior displayed by parents as normal and acceptable

- Inability to trust others

- Difficulty in expressing inner feelings

- Experience of depression, and increased risk for mental illness

- Development of guilt feelings for supposedly causing a parent's alcoholism

- Loss of self-esteem and perception of self and family as oddities

- Feeling of helplessness in controlling oneself and life's events

- Belief in a magical person who will eventually save the child from harm

- Development of an inward life focus to escape from the turmoil of the home

In addition, COAs were commonly observed assuming one of the following distinctive coping roles within the family system.[50]

The family hero or "junior mom" caretaker, who is also quite successful both at home and at school.

The scapegoat, who is something of an angry rebel and is often involved in unapproved social behavior.

The lost child or "angel," who withdraws to the background, never causes trouble, has no opinions, feels unimportant, and isolates himself or herself from others.

The mascot, who manages to defuse explosive and tense situations, often through humor, by focusing attention on himself or herself.

Recently, critics of the theory of the COA syndrome have contended that many children of nonalcoholic though strongly dysfunctional families—those marked by sexual or physical abuse and incest—also share some of the same characteristics as COAs. Although the uniqueness of the COA syndrome may be abandoned, the pain created within a child who grows up in an alcoholic home is still acknowledged as significant and serious. The revised COA syndrome appears to include the following characteristics:[51]

- A greater likelihood of becoming an alcohol or other drug abuser

- A strong predisposition toward having psychiatric symptoms as an adult

- A moderately significant increased risk for marital difficulties

- More impulsive behavior as a child

- Delayed language development, fine motor coordination, and sociability

- A higher incidence of cognitive (mental) disorders as a child

Although most COAs have few common psychological factors that distinguish them from other children who experienced a disadvantaged childhood, one researcher has found that a disproportionate number of children born to alcoholic or drug-addicted parents have abnormal brain-wave patterns. Such differences appear to correlate strongly with certain behavioral characteristics, including impulsivity, social deviance, and lower IQ.[52]

Co-dependence

For the past several years, the terms **co-dependence** and **co-alcoholism** have been used to describe the unusual coping mechanisms, attitudes, and behaviors that family members sometimes develop in response to a problem-drinking parent, spouse, child, or sibling. Co-dependence is the foundation of the COA syndrome and also serves as the basis for the diseased behavior of adult children of alcoholics.

The so-called co-dependent or co-alcoholic supposedly denies the existence of problem drinking in a family member and appears to overlook or minimizes the seriousness of family dysfunction. The nonproblem drinker or nondrinker frequently begins to view the strange drinking behaviors of a loved one as normal, and sometimes cooperates in the elaborate cover-up of making excuses and rationalizing to explain alcohol-abuse situations and their consequences. Unwittingly, the co-alcoholism of family members tends to promote problem drinking by delaying any attempts at intervention that are needed to get the alcohol abuser into treatment and rehabilitation. Though this is somewhat controversial, co-alcoholism or co-dependency is increasingly viewed as a disease or "subdisease," characterized by a preoccupation and extreme dependency (emotionally, socially, sometimes physically) on another person or on a substance (such as alcohol, drugs, nicotine, or sugar) or on a behavior (such as working, gambling, or sexual acting out).[53] Co-alcoholics display a number of common behavioral traits:[54]

- They are often so-called "good" persons who make themselves indispensable to others.

- They tend to be sufferers, servers, and selfless to the point of hurting themselves in service to one or more family members or friends.

- Co-alcoholics who are children—sometimes referred to as "para-alcoholics" who do not have the choice to stay in or leave a particular situation or relationship—tend to develop allergies, skin problems, asthma, bed wetting, and learning disabilities and often are accident-prone or suicidal.

However, the most important characteristic of co-alcoholism is commonly identified as "*external referenting*." This is a condition in which a person perceives herself or himself as having meaning or significance only in relation to what is outside of the self, or external sources.[55] Lacking intrinsic meaning or self-worth, the external-referenting co-alcoholic will do almost anything to maintain a relationship, including total psychological self-abandonment.

External referenting also involves a number of other important tendencies, including the formation of "cling-clung" relationships that offer security but are usually nongrowing and static in nature. In addition, because of a lack of personal psychological boundaries, such an individual often takes on another's sadness, happiness, fears, and confusion, and persistently attempts to please others in order to gain acceptance and security. The external-referenting individual also displays an unusual inability to trust his or her own perceptions unless they are approved or confirmed by others.[56]

Because alcohol abuse is so pervasive today, the chances of interacting with a relative or friend who drinks too much are not remote. At least four other people are affected by the disturbing behavior of each of America's problem drinkers and alcoholics. From yet another perspective,

What to Do When Someone Close Drinks Too Much

box 4.5

With knowledge, compassion, and patience, the person with "someone close who drinks too much" can play a key role in his or her turnabout, treatment, and recovery from problem drinking.

Such help is usually given in three stages:

1. Learn about the illness of alcoholism and various sources of treatment.
2. Guide the "someone close" to treatment.
3. Support the person during and after treatment.

While waiting for the "right time" for medical and psychological intervention and treatment, the following do's and do not's are recommended for the person who knows someone close who drinks too much.

Do:

Try to remain calm, unemotional, and factually honest in speaking with the problem drinker about his or her behavior and its day-to-day consequences.

Let the problem drinker know that you are reading and learning about alcoholism, attending Al-Anon or Alateen, and the like.

Discuss the situation with someone you trust—a clergyperson, social worker, friend, or some individual who has experienced alcoholism either personally or as a family member.

Establish and maintain a healthy atmosphere in the home, and try to include the alcoholic member in family life.

Explain the nature of alcoholism as an illness to the children of the family.

Encourage new interests and participate in leisure-time activities that the problem drinker enjoys. Encourage him or her to see old friends in nondrinking situations.

Be patient and live one day at a time. Alcoholism generally takes a long time to develop, and recovery does not occur overnight. Try to accept setbacks and relapses with calm and understanding.

Refuse to ride with the alcoholic person if he or she insists on drinking and driving.

Do Not:

Attempt to punish, threaten, bribe, preach, or try to be a martyr. Avoid emotional appeals that may only increase feelings of guilt and the compulsion to drink.

Allow yourself to cover up or make excuses for the alcoholic person or shield the person from the realistic consequences of his or her behavior.

Take over his or her responsibilities, leaving the person with no sense of importance or dignity.

Hide or dump bottles, or shelter the problem drinker from situations where alcohol is present.

Argue with the alcoholic person when he or she is drunk.

Try to drink along with the problem drinker.

Accept, above all, guilt for another's behavior.

Source: National Institute on Alcohol Abuse and Alcoholism.

---

then, there are nearly 50 million people who are sharing alcohol problems and who are potential helpers in assisting those who are close and who drink to excess. Some ideas for coping with these relatives and friends are listed in box 4.5.

Alcoholism

In this section, alcoholism will be described in terms of various definitions, prevalence, possible causes, signs and symptoms, and treatment and evaluation.

Overview

The most prominent and extreme form of problem drinking is **alcoholism**. Now

considered a complex illness or disability, alcoholism is more than just alcohol abuse, though it almost always involves the recurrent use of beverage alcohol that contributes to a variety of personal and social problems. Alcoholism is more appropriately considered as the *disease of alcohol dependence*. The alcohol-dependent person cannot consistently exert control over his or her intake of alcohol.[57]

Society in general and even the medical profession have had considerable difficulty in understanding and defining alcoholism. Over the past two centuries, many differing and even conflicting concepts of alcoholism have emerged. Some of these remain to the present day—alcoholism is a sin, a vice, a personality weakness, a bad habit, willful misconduct—and add to confusion

and controversy about the precise nature of this psychoactive substance dependence disorder.

It was not until 1946 that E. M. Jellinek proposed the modern disease concept of alcoholism and described the condition as *any use of beverage alcohol that causes any damage to the individual drinker, to society, or both*. Known as the "father" (originator) of the disease concept of alcoholism, Jellinek later identified several *species* or types of alcoholism, as noted below:[58]

> *Alpha alcoholism*—an entirely psychological reliance on alcohol to relieve physical and psychic pain. There is no loss of control or inability to abstain.

Is alcoholism really a disease?

Point:

Most surveyed Americans and the following prestigious health organizations consider alcoholism a disease that requires medical treatment: the American Medical Association, American Psychiatric Association, American Psychological Association, World Health Association, and National Council on Alcoholism and Drug Dependence. Those who live with alcoholics, as well as experienced alcohol treatment specialists and recovering alcoholics, also tend to view alcoholism as a disease. The "disease concept" more appropriately explains than does the "behavior disorder concept" why alcoholics so frequently mistreat and abuse the people they love the most. Moreover, the disease model is very helpful in convincing alcoholics to admit their alcohol problems and in getting them treated effectively. Despite the fact that alcoholism's cause or causes remain largely unknown, and that signs and symptoms of pathological alcohol consumption vary considerably from one alcoholic to another, alcoholics are typically "dis-eased," or not at ease. They are usually not at ease with themselves, their families, or with society.

Counterpoint:

Considering alcoholism as a disease has no scientific basis whatsoever. Alcoholism is better described as a "behavior disorder" or habit that is under considerable voluntary control of the drinker. In fact, there is no typical pattern of drinking behavior, which actually ranges widely from one problem drinker to another. If alcoholism were a disease, signs and symptoms would be similar among those affected, there would be no ability to control alcohol consumption on a temporary basis, and there would be no environmental or social factors considered as precipitating the condition. Additionally, there is no precisely identified cause of alcoholism that applies to all alcoholics, and labeling people as diseased only serves to excuse the continuance of the condition and remove any element of self-respect from problem drinking. Thus, alcoholism may be considered a symptom of some underlying personality or mental depression. It certainly isn't a disease!

on Alcoholism and Drug Dependence adopted a new, revised definition of alcoholism that gives greater consideration to basic behavioral changes symptomatic of the disease.[60] Earlier, the two organizations emphasized biological tolerance and physical dependence, which appear when the disease has already adversely affected behavior.

According to the revised definition, alcoholism is a *primary, chronic disease* with genetic, psychosocial, and environmental factors influencing its development and manifestations. The disease is *often progressive* and *fatal*. It is characterized by continuous or periodic *impaired control over drinking, preoccupation with the drug, alcohol, use of alcohol despite adverse consequences*, and *distortion in thinking*, most notably *denial*.

Following are brief explanations of the major terms in this lengthy definition:

> *Primary* means that alcoholism as an addiction is not a symptom of some underlying disease state, but is a distinct disease condition separate from other physical or emotional disorders often associated with the alcoholismic state.

> *Chronic* refers to the long-term duration of the alcoholismic state. Once this condition has developed, an individual remains an alcoholic and is not likely able to resume controlled drinking.

> *Disease*—a condition of distress, uneasiness, or any departure from health—suggests that alcoholism is an involuntary disability that places those affected at a disadvantage in relation to those who are not alcoholismic.

> *Progressive* indicates that alcoholism moves through various stages of development the longer it persists, and tends to worsen over time.

> *Fatal* describes the ultimate outcome of alcoholism, death, unless intervention and/or treatment stops the progressive nature of the disease. Premature death may come from overdose and physical complications of the brain, liver, and heart, as well

Beta alcoholism—a type of alcoholism in which severe medical complications occur, such as nerve irritations, gastric disturbances, and cirrhosis of the liver. There is neither physical nor psychological dependence. No withdrawal symptoms are manifest.

Gamma alcoholism—the most prevalent form of alcoholism seen in America. It is characterized by psychological dependence, physical dependence, tolerance, loss of control, and withdrawal symptoms.

Delta alcoholism—the predominant form of alcoholism in France. It is

similar to the gamma type except that instead of loss of control, there is inability to abstain.

Lesser types of alcoholism are identified as periodic, explosive, weekend, and fiesta drinking.

More recently, the American Medical Association defined alcoholism as "an illness characterized by significant impairment that is directly associated with persistent and excessive use of alcohol."[59] Manifested as drug dependence, alcoholism involves a progressive preoccupation with drinking, leading to physical, mental, or social dysfunction.

In 1990, the American Society of Addiction Medicine and the National Council

as by alcoholism-related suicide, homicide, and motor-vehicle accidents.

Impaired control identifies the alcoholic's inability to limit alcohol use on any drinking occasion or the inability to limit with any consistency the duration of the drinking episode, the amount consumed, and/or the behavioral consequences of drinking.

Preoccupation highlights the exaggerated attention and all-consuming expenditure of energy given to acquiring alcohol, using alcohol, and experiencing the effects of alcohol.

Adverse consequences are those alcohol-related impairments in physical health, psychological functioning, interpersonal relationships, occupational roles, as well as legal, financial, or spiritual problems.

Denial, an integral part of the disease and an obstacle to recovery, includes not only a refusal to acknowledge the seriousness of drinking-related problems, but also a full range of psychological maneuvers or processes aimed at reducing awareness of the fact that alcohol use is the cause of, rather than the solution to, an individual's problem.

Yet another definition is offered by the American Psychiatric Association (APA). This professional organization views alcoholism as a *disease* marked by a *pathological* (diseased) *pattern of alcohol use or impairment in* one's *social or occupational functioning due to alcohol,* and in which *either tolerance or withdrawal symptoms* are present. The APA considers alcoholism a psychiatric substance dependence disorder that is defined in terms of undesirable behavior associated with regular use of alcohol. Specific diagnostic criteria that can be applied for determining alcohol dependence have already been identified in chapters 1 and 3 in descriptions of drug dependence.

Alcoholism appears to be one of those "equal opportunity" illnesses affecting millions of individuals without respect to race, color, creed, sex, ethnic group, marital status, geographical location, or socioeconomic standing. Nevertheless, over the past several years, studies have revealed some unusual variations in the prevalence of this disabling condition.

1. Approximately 5 to 7 percent of all adults—about 10 percent of all adult drinkers—are likely to be alcohol-dependent at some point in their lives. Several million additional adults and perhaps as many as 3 million teenagers have serious drinking problems or experience adverse personal or social problems due to alcohol abuse.

2. In the past, alcoholics have tended to be 35 to 55 years old. However, an alarming increase in adolescent-onset alcoholism has been noted recently. Factors frequently cited for this increase in teenage alcohol dependency include the easy availability of beverage alcohol, the toleration of drunkenness by parents, the growing use of alcohol to cope with the pressures and conflicts of adolescence, exposure to parental problem drinking patterns, and the recent emphasis in alcohol advertisements on youth drinks, such as "pop wines," or wine-coolers. Furthermore, current statistics indicate that males in their late teens and early twenties have the highest incidence of alcohol-related problems and problem drinking behaviors.

3. Alcoholism is involved in at least one-fourth of all admissions to general hospitals. The medical and social costs run to tens of billions of dollars per year—more than the cost of cancer and respiratory diseases combined. Among males aged 25 to 44 years, alcohol abuse is a major factor in four of the leading causes of death—accidents, homicide, suicide, and alcoholic cirrhosis of the liver.

4. Contrary to popular belief, alcoholics are not always drinking uncontrollably and are not even always drinking. Many alcohol-dependent individuals seem to be either abstinent or drinking without symptoms in any given month of alcohol use.

5. Less than 5 percent of all alcoholics are found on skid row. Most manage to hold jobs and maintain homes where they are sheltered or tolerated by a spouse and children. The stereotyped image of the alcoholic as the skid-row inebriated bum often deceives the "respectable" alcoholic and his or her family into minimizing the seriousness of problem drinking. Alcoholism is an illness that can occur in people in all walks of life.

Possible Causes of Alcoholism

Without alcohol, there would be no alcoholics. However, most people who use beverage alcohol do not develop into problem drinkers. Therefore, while alcohol is a necessary factor in alcoholism, it is not the sole causative agent. Additionally, alcoholism does not result from drinking a particular alcoholic beverage. Furthermore, though many alcoholics share common personality disorders as noted below, no well-defined "alcoholic personality" has been identified. It is probable that such behavioral difficulties are the result, rather than the basic cause, of alcohol abuse.

Alcoholics display such varying backgrounds and characteristics, and so many possible causative factors have been proposed, that some authorities believe many alcoholisms or forms of alcoholism exist rather than a single disorder. While disturbed psychological functioning may be visibly dominant in the development of alcoholism, there is no good evidence that most alcoholics began abusing alcohol because they were "anxious, depressed, insecure, poorly reared, dependent on their mothers, subjected to child abuse, raised in unhappy families, or emotionally unstable in childhood or adolescence."[61]

Indeed, recent research has questioned some long-held ideas about the causes of alcoholism. Nevertheless, physical or biological factors, family origin, ethnic differences, and susceptible personality types are all recognized as powerful factors in the development of alcoholics. Though

The typical alcoholic American

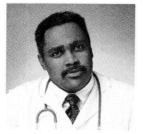

Doctor, age 54

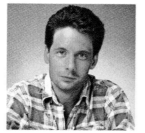

Farmer, age 35

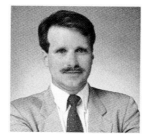

Unemployed, age 40

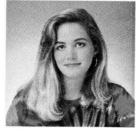

College student, age 19

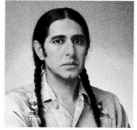

Counselor, age 38

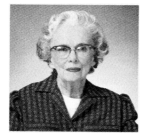

Retired editor, age 86

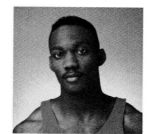

Dancer, age 22

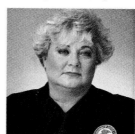

Police officer, age 46

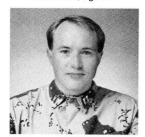

Military officer, age 31

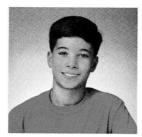

Student, age 14

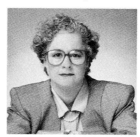

Executive, age 50

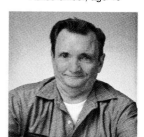

Taxi driver, age 61

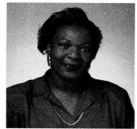

Homemaker, age 43

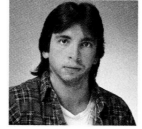

Bricklayer, age 29

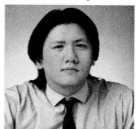

Computer programmer, age 25

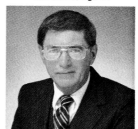

Lawyer, age 52

There's no such thing as typical. We have all kinds.
10 million Americans are alcoholic.
It's our number one drug problem.

For information or help, contact:
CSAP's National Clearinghouse for Alcohol and Drug Information, P.O. Box 2345, Rockville, MD 20847-2345
1-800-729-6686

U.S. DEPARTMENT OF HEALTH AND HUMAN SERVICES • Public Health Service • Substance Abuse and Mental Health Services Administration
Prepared and published by the Center for Substance Abuse Prevention

DHHS Publication No. (ADM) 92-1801

 4.4

U.S. Department of Health & Human Services.

research may yet reveal a single cause, many authorities argue for a multicausal or multifaceted origin of alcoholism, and focus on both "nature" (hereditary, biological, physical) factors as well as "nurture" (psychosocial, cultural, environmental) factors.[62] Several of these factors are described in the following sections dealing with

- the agent (ethyl alcohol),

- the host (the person in whom alcoholism develops), and

- the environment (the psychosocial and cultural setting in which alcohol dependence occurs).

The terms *agent, host,* and *environment* are often used to categorize factors or possible causes in the development of any disease or disorder.

Agent-Related Causative Factors

In this category are those properties or characteristics of ethyl alcohol that might contribute to alcohol dependency.

1. Alcohol is a central nervous system *depressant-type drug.* As such, it is capable of altering consciousness and producing a calming and tranquilizing effect.

2. As a *relatively fast-acting drug* in inducing an altered state of consciousness, alcohol carries an increased potential for abuse.

3. In addition to being a central nervous system depressant, ethyl alcohol is also a *psychomotor agitant.* This latter drug effect is usually unrecognized until the calming effect of alcohol has worn off. Then the shaking, tremors, and nervousness that accompany withdrawal are considered evidence of the effect of the "uneven stimulant" and sufficient to cause the drinker to resume his or her alcohol intake.

4. Related to the foregoing factor, alcohol is a psychoactive *drug capable of producing physical dependence* that is *manifested by withdrawal symptoms.* One of the factors maintaining alcohol dependence is the discomfort of withdrawal.

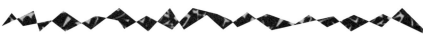

Selected Gender and Ethnic Differences in Drinking, Alcohol Abuse, and Alcoholism in the United States

Men are somewhat more likely than women to drink at all, and are particularly more likely to drink frequently and heavily.

Alcohol abuse is much more prevalent among males of northern European descent than among males of Mediterranean descent, regardless of other psychological, social, and family conditions.

Nearly one-third of the estimated 15 million alcohol-abusing or alcohol-dependent Americans are women.

Adult females' role deprivation—loss of one's role as wife, mother, or worker—seems to increase women's risk for abusing alcohol.

The time period between onset of drinking-related problems and entry into treatment appears to be shorter for women than for men. This more-rapid progression of problem-related drinking and its consequences is referred to as "telescoping."

Overall, African American and white men have similar drinking patterns, although black men have higher abstention rates than do whites. The same pattern tends to exist for women, with more black women than white abstaining.

Among African Americans, individuals with higher "racial consciousness" are less likely to be involved in alcohol abuse or tolerant of such behavior.

Hispanic American males generally tend to drink heavily and to have a disproportionate number of alcohol-related problems, including alcohol dependence, compared to African American and white males.

Hispanic American females are at considerably lower risk for developing alcohol-related problems than are white American females.

Among Native Americans, alcohol use varies tremendously from tribe to tribe, although most young Native American males report experimentation with alcohol, which can be very serious. Native American women drink much less than Native American men do.

An estimated 75 percent of all traumatic deaths and suicides among Native Americans are alcohol-related.

When considered together, Asian Americans and Pacific Islanders display lower prevalences of alcohol abuse, alcoholism, and adverse consequences of drinking than other racial and ethnic minorities do.

A relatively high proportion of heavy drinkers exists among Japanese American and Filipino American males. By contrast, Chinese American men and women tend to have significantly lower prevalences of alcohol use and abuse.

Alcohol-dependent individuals, as noted above, tend to abuse alcohol in order to avoid withdrawal and to feel normal again.

Host-Related Causative Factors

This category includes those factors associated with the individual drinker, the so-called host. The drinker presents a unique combination of genetic, biochemical, and psychological forces that somehow predispose that host to alcoholism.

1. *Heredity* is now considered a major predisposing causal factor in many cases of alcoholism. There is no doubt that alcoholism runs in families, even when children are

separated from their alcoholic parents and reared by nonalcoholismic adoptive parents.[63] The evidence for such genetic influences is now compelling, although the precise mechanism of inheritance has not yet been identified. Two types of genetic predisposition have been described.[64, 65]

- *Male-limited susceptibility* occurs only in males, is highly heritable, gives rise to severe early-onset alcoholism requiring extensive treatment, and is associated with serious lawbreaking activity.

- *Milieu-limited susceptibility*, that is, environmentally dependent susceptibility, occurs in both sexes, accounts for most male and female alcoholism, gives rise to late onset of the illness, is not as severe as male-limited alcoholism, is not usually associated with the legal system, and requires some environmental stimulus or cofactor to be expressed as alcoholism.

Quite possibly, rather than a specific "alcoholism gene," a genetic predisposition might involve multiple genetic factors that combine with a heavy-drinking environment to produce an increased risk of consuming large quantities of alcohol.[66] Some drinkers might be disabled from adequately judging the effects of alcohol. Consequently, such individuals might become drunk before they know what is happening to them.[67] However, the abnormal response of the alcoholic to the intake of alcohol may also be influenced by other physical factors that interfere with alcohol's metabolism or chemical processing in the human body.

2. Alcoholism, especially the early-onset type beginning before age 20, may indicate a *deficit in or lack of serotonin*, a neurotransmitter that regulates mood, aggression, and impulses. Atypical levels of certain other neurotransmitters may also play a role in predisposing an individual to alcohol dependence.

3. Another theory proposes that alcoholics have a *shortage of endorphins*, the body's own pain-relieving and euphoria-producing chemicals manufactured by the brain. Abnormal alcohol consumption might make up for this endorphin deficiency.

4. *Unusual brain electrical activity*, revealed by analysis of electroencephalographic (EEG) patterns, has been found among alcoholics and children of alcoholics. Abnormalities discovered include fast EEG activity, increases in slow alpha energy, and reduced amplitude of P3 brain waves. Such findings do not tend to occur in nonalcoholics, and they suggest that the brains of alcoholics and those at risk of becoming alcoholic process information differently from the nonalcoholismic population. These variations in brain electrical activity might serve as "markers" or indicators of a predisposition to alcohol dependence before such a condition develops.

5. Certain *biochemical differences* might also play a role in the development of alcoholism. Faulty enzyme systems that function in the metabolism of ethyl alcohol and acetaldehyde may account for considerable differences in how people process and eliminate alcohol. For instance, many Japanese and Chinese exhibit an intolerance to alcohol, sometimes referred to as the "Oriental flushing phenomenon," based on an absence or low amount of aldehyde dehydrogenase. After small amounts of alcohol are consumed, such individuals often display a cutaneous (skin) flush (reddening) on the face and upper body, and experience unpleasant feelings of warmth and queasiness. Frequently there is also an increase in heart rate and a decrease in blood pressure. These signs and symptoms of the flushing phenomenon constitute a powerful deterrent to heavy drinking among Orientals.

There is also the possibility that a defect in the metabolism of acetaldehyde produces addictive substances, known as *tetrahydroisoquinolines* (THIQs or TIQs), that may be the precursors or forerunners of opiate alkaloids. Such products of oxidation could serve as the common physiological basis for all types of chemical dependencies.

6. While the so-called alcoholic personality has been largely discounted as a factor in alcoholism, two personality types appear to be somewhat susceptible to alcohol abuse—the mostly male "antisocial personality" and the "borderline personality," found usually in females. Though most alcoholics display neither personality type, an underlying common problem of controlling impulses may be the basis for each. The male antisocial personality type is characterized by an extremely high rate of alcohol problems, whereas the female borderline personality type is described as lacking in self-esteem, manifest in chronic boredom or anger, and marked by difficult interpersonal relations and psychotic episodes.

7. Another quite popular theory often used to explain the basis of alcoholism has been related to an individual's *unique reaction to stress*. Alcohol is used as an escape or relief from various forms of psychological distress, especially loneliness, anxiety, depression, frustration, insecurity, unhappiness, and sometimes even guilt. Some individuals might also drink to self-medicate their panic attacks.

Despite scientific investigations proving that chronic use of alcohol actually makes people more depressed, anxious, and withdrawn and less self-confident, many noninsightful alcohol abusers persist in "relief drinking." Perhaps these individuals drink in anticipation of relief from distress or the perceived euphoria experienced during earlier drinking episodes. Regardless of the original motive or precipitating intention, it is likely that many alcohol-dependents eventually drink to feel normal again or to avoid the pain of withdrawal.

Environment-Related Causative Factors

Psychosocial and cultural forces have a significant influence on the development of alcoholism. Frequently identified factors in this category include the following:

1. The *availability and accessibility of alcoholic beverages* determine if ethyl alcohol is the "drug of choice." Widespread promotion of this legal psychoactive substance, its relatively low cost, and its general social acceptability all combine to make alcohol the most abused drug in the United States.

2. The *absence of clear guidelines for nonabusive alcohol use* in certain populations, the existence of ambivalent attitudes, and conflicting values regarding alcohol often lead to general confusion as to what constitutes acceptable drinking behavior. Unwittingly, our *culture may be encouraging alcoholism* by accepting "relief drinking," by promoting drinking unrelated to family activities and mealtime, by enshrining alcohol use as a status symbol, and by tolerating and perceiving intoxication as funny or manly.

3. *Learning theory* also suggests that children who see parents using alcohol to solve or escape from daily problems will themselves adopt such drinking habits. In addition, children who are served "kiddie cocktails" may be subtly encouraged to drink to gain adult approval and learn that alcohol is only a social beverage rather than a dangerous thing.

4. According to some behavioral scientists, when society permits a large gap to develop between expectations or goals and the means for achieving them, many people express their *alienation* through retreatism and rebellion, as represented in alcoholism. And if society labels alcoholism as *deviant behavior*, those so labeled become forced by society into playing a deviant role.

5. One of the more intriguing theories offered to explain the occurrence of alcoholism is based on the cultural importance a particular ethnic group places on *individualism*. In French, Irish, and American societies, children are encouraged to be "on their own" psychologically. Unable to achieve emotional release through associations with other people, these individualists tend to find emotional release by drinking alcohol. By contrast, Japanese and Jews tend to have relatively low rates of alcohol dependency, because in these ethnic groups children are not expected to be independent. Indeed, children are reared to become emotionally dependent upon other family members, who often indulge infants and tolerate dependent behavior in adulthood.[68]

Signs and Symptoms of Alcoholism

Better known than the causes of alcoholism are the signs and symptoms, often described in a series of developmental phases or stages. E. M. Jellinek first established the following four-phase description based on his analysis of recovering alcoholics: (1) the so-called prealcoholic phase; (2) the prodromal or early-warning phase; (3) the crucial phase; and (4) the chronic phase. This initial description was later refined and expanded by other alcoholism and drug dependence specialists, including Great Britain's Max M. Glatt, who depicted the development of and recovery from alcoholism in chart form (see fig. 4.5).

The general phases of alcoholism are identified and explained as follows:

Phase 1: During this initial contact-with-alcohol phase, the evolving alcoholic drinks first for social reasons, but eventually changes the motivations for consumption to include those of anticipated stress reduction and relief from psychological tension or pain. Soon the developing alcoholic seeks out drinking occasions, begins to increase consumption (dose), becomes defensive about his or her intake, and typically associates with new drinking partners who accept the heavier drinking behavior and more frequent intoxication. It is during this phase that alcohol and drinking become significant parts of daily living. In essence, the drinker's all-consuming "love affair" with drink begins to grow and flourish.

Phase 2: In this phase, the alcoholic tends to drink in secret in order to hide the consumption level, and develops several of the early warning signals, such as feelings of guilt about drinking; lying about drinking behavior when confronted by others; an extremely pleasant response to alcohol; drinking before joining others in drinking situations; drinking due to worry, tiredness, or depression; the need for increased intake to produce desired effects (**tolerance**); and the experience of alcohol-induced amnesia, the **blackout** or memory blank-out. Soon there is no social motivation for drinking. What began as a trend earlier is now the exclusive motivation for intake of alcohol—the expectation of euphoric relief.

Eventually, the alcoholic is preoccupied with procuring a source of alcohol and begins to drink alone, inventing occasions for imbibing if none exist. Intake increases rapidly as guzzling becomes the norm. Sometimes the drinker is unable to abstain. More often, the alcohol abuser cannot control drinking once it has begun, evidence of the **loss of control**

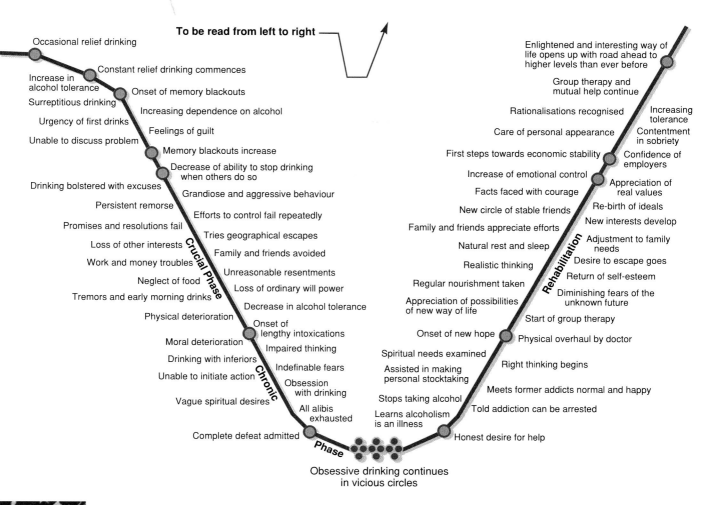

To be read from left to right

Occasional relief drinking

Constant relief drinking commences

Increase in alcohol tolerance

Onset of memory blackouts

Surreptitious drinking

Increasing dependence on alcohol

Urgency of first drinks

Feelings of guilt

Unable to discuss problem

Memory blackouts increase

Decrease of ability to stop drinking when others do so

Drinking bolstered with excuses

Grandiose and aggressive behaviour

Persistent remorse

Efforts to control fail repeatedly

Promises and resolutions fail

Tries geographical escapes

Loss of other interests

Family and friends avoided

Work and money troubles

Unreasonable resentments

Neglect of food

Loss of ordinary will power

Tremors and early morning drinks

Decrease in alcohol tolerance

Physical deterioration

Onset of lengthy intoxications

Moral deterioration

Impaired thinking

Drinking with inferiors

Indefinable fears

Unable to initiate action

Obsession with drinking

Vague spiritual desires

All alibis exhausted

Complete defeat admitted

Crucial Phase

Chronic Phase

Obsessive drinking continues in vicious circles

Enlightened and interesting way of life opens up with road ahead to higher levels than ever before

Group therapy and mutual help continue

Rationalisations recognised

Increasing tolerance

Care of personal appearance

Contentment in sobriety

First steps towards economic stability

Confidence of employers

Increase of emotional control

Appreciation of real values

Facts faced with courage

Re-birth of ideals

New circle of stable friends

New interests develop

Family and friends appreciate efforts

Adjustment to family needs

Natural rest and sleep

Desire to escape goes

Realistic thinking

Return of self-esteem

Regular nourishment taken

Diminishing fears of the unknown future

Appreciation of possibilities of new way of life

Start of group therapy

Onset of new hope

Physical overhaul by doctor

Spiritual needs examined

Right thinking begins

Assisted in making personal stocktaking

Stops taking alcohol

Meets former addicts normal and happy

Learns alcoholism is an illness

Told addiction can be arrested

Honest desire for help

Rehabilitation

---

figure 4.5

A chart of alcohol addiction and recovery.

From Max Glatt, *"Group Therapy in Alcohol"* in The British Journal of Addiction, *vol. 54, no. 2. Copyright © Max Glatt. Reprinted by permission of Dr. Glatt and the National Council on Alcoholism and Drug Dependence.*

phenomenon—inability to determine with any consistency the duration of drinking or the amount consumed.

A physiological dependency is now established, and if denied a regular dose, the alcoholic will experience **withdrawal symptoms** or the withdrawal syndrome—restlessness, tremulousness or involuntary shaking of the body, insomnia, feelings of depression and anxiety, loss of appetite, mental confusion, and hallucinations and seizures (convulsions), typically occurring within 6 to 48 hours after the last drink.[69] The term **delirium tremens** denotes the intensification and most severe form of the

withdrawal symptoms, which usually follow heavy drinking that has lasted over an extended time period. Characterized by vivid and terrifying hallucinations, complete disorientation and confusion, and severe agitation with almost continuous motor activity, this medical emergency usually develops between 48 to 96 hours after the last drink. Fortunately, only a small minority of individuals undergoing withdrawal experience delirium tremens.

Phase 3: Now there is an intensification of all forms of alcohol abuse experienced earlier—more

solitary drinking, avoidance of family and friends, and an increase in memory blackouts and passouts. When sober, the alcoholic may regret what was said or done while drinking. To prove that he or she still has everything under control, the drinker will often attempt to restrict personal consumption by going "on the wagon" (an abrupt cessation of drinking). Usually such action is only temporary, excessive intake is resumed, and morning drinking becomes the norm in an attempt to stabilize one's rather chaotic life. Sometimes a form of reverse tolerance develops as a result of liver damage. In such an instance, the alcoholic appears to be easily intoxicated on a small dose that would rarely have affected behavior earlier in the disease. A series of physical, mental, and social changes now occurs in the alcohol-dependent individual. These may include nervous and gastrointestinal disorders, cirrhosis of the liver, malnutrition, the overuse of defense mechanisms to justify drinking, and a general deterioration in interpersonal relationships. Chain-drinking and extended "benders" are characteristic of this phase of the illness. Hospitalization for alcoholism or an alcohol-related problem is frequently required during this phase.

Phase 4: Progression to this stage usually develops after a number of years of excessive intake. Drinking bouts often last for several days at a time. When the alcoholic gets the "shakes" in the morning upon awakening, more alcohol is consumed to quiet the "nervous" condition. The person is drunk on important occasions and has increasing numbers of blackouts and passouts. Completely oriented around alcohol, the alcohol abuser displays a complete ethical breakdown, unreasonable fears, increased reverse tolerance, and loss of motor coordination. Now, the drinker's "love affair" with the alcoholic beverage is complete, and that relationship takes priority over all other people and all other life activities. At this point, alcoholics drink to live and live to drink. The medical complications may be so severe that either institutionalization or death occurs unless there is some form of intervention.

Not every alcoholic experiences all of the foregoing signs and symptoms. Moreover, there is great variation in the order in which the abnormal behaviors occur. It should also be noted that while alcoholism is a devastating disablement, it tends to display a somewhat inconsistent symptomatology; that is, the alcoholic does not always behave the same way with regard to alcohol. Especially in phase 2 or 3, the alcoholic may enter a stage of remission—a temporary, periodic absence of symptoms—during which time he or she does not get drunk after starting to drink. This phenomenon should not be viewed as a complete cure, because another characteristic of alcoholism is the tendency to have a *relapse*, a return to problem-causing alcohol use again. Consequently, the prevention of relapse is an important part of the alcoholic's recovery.

Treatment and Rehabilitation

Modern therapies for alcoholism are considered usually in three general stages: (1) **detoxification**; (2) provision of *medical care* for health problems related to heavy alcohol consumption; and (3) *changing the long-term behavior* of the alcohol abuser so that destructive drinking patterns are discontinued.

Detoxification is the process of "drying out," or ridding the body of alcohol, in which the alcoholic experiences the withdrawal syndrome. Sometimes medications are administered to prevent convulsions and produce a healthy appetite and sound sleep. Nutrient-rich diets and high-strength vitamins are often prescribed, along with the provision of encouragement and emotional support. This stage can require several days. Special therapies are also begun for various health problems. In some cases, body organs that have been damaged begin to heal themselves, as long as the recovering alcoholic stops using alcohol and starts eating properly.

However, unless the destructive behavior pattern of the alcoholic is altered significantly, the individual runs a high risk of repeated, uncontrolled drinking episodes. Relapses are common and are often fueled by the **"dry-drunk" phenomenon**. This term denotes the alcoholic's state of mind when he or she is not drinking. Poisonous to the alcoholic's well-being, the dry-drunk syndrome is characterized by a lack of insight, pomposity in personal behavior, an exaggeration of self-importance, an overestimation of one's abilities and intelligence, insensitivity to the needs and feelings of others, a rigid judgmental outlook, tense impatience, and a constant dissatisfaction with life.[70] This grandiose, unrealistic, and even childlike behavior must be altered if recovery from alcoholism is to be accomplished to any appreciable degree.

Common treatment approaches, applied in a variety of therapeutic settings, include the following.

Drug therapy or pharmacotherapy—the use of drugs in the treatment of a disease. In treating alcoholics, the drug most commonly used is a deterrent drug that tends to discourage people from resuming drinking once they have stopped. One such drug is disulfiram (**Antabuse**), which interferes with alcohol oxidation and prolongs the presence of toxic acetaldehyde in the body. If alcohol is consumed, the patient experiences a series of severe physical effects—flushing of the skin, throbbing head and neck, pulsating headache, breathing difficulty, nausea, copious vomiting, sweating, thirst, chest pain, very rapid heartbeat, fainting, marked uneasiness, weakness, inability to remain upright, blurred vision, and confusion.[71] Forewarned of the consequences of drinking, the alcoholic usually responds with abstinence and a willingness to continue therapy. Use of this drug provides the alcoholic with the motivation to avoid drinking. Thus, the taking of Antabuse is a form of *aversion therapy*, treatment that helps a patient stay away from some potentially harmful substance or practice.

Another drug, lithium, has been employed to a limited degree in alcoholism therapy because of its effectiveness in treating affective (emotional) disorders commonly found in alcoholics. Sometimes the tricyclic antidepressants are given to treat the initial symptoms of withdrawal, including anxiety, depression, and bodily discomfort.

Naltrexone, a drug sometimes used in the treatment of opiate addiction, has been approved recently by the Food and Drug Administration as a treatment for alcoholism. Marketed under the brand name of Revia, Naltrexone tends to reduce the craving for alcohol and helps prevent relapse. The first new drug used to fight alcoholism in nearly half a century, Naltrexone acts on the brain to block the pleasure sensations associated with drinking alcoholic beverages.

Psychotherapy—purposeful conversation between two or more people through which trained therapists help clients achieve greater self-understanding and objectivity in viewing others, and more maturity in the resolution of personal problems. Such a process involves intense self-analysis for the purpose of modifying attitudes, emotional states, and behavior. In addition to individual psychotherapy, there are the self-expressive psychodrama and group therapy, with its feature of mutual support.

Family therapy—a form of psychotherapy based on the proposition that disturbed relationships among various family members may have contributed to or resulted from the destructive drinking of one family member. This form of treatment emphasizes family interactional factors, in addition to individual problems of the alcohol abuser, and proposes changes in the communication patterns of family members. As such, all family members are treated as a unit, rather than isolating the alcoholic and treating that person apart from his or her family.

Behavioral therapy—a general form of psychotherapy that is based on the application of human learning theories in a clinical setting. Behavioral therapists emphasize changing the coping patterns of

alcohol-dependent individuals rather than changing the underlying causes of self-destructive alcohol abuse.

Some behavioral therapies focus on assertiveness training and improving communication skills and problem-solving methods. For example, rational-emotive therapy—the basis for Rational Recovery and Secular Organizations for Sobriety self-help groups—helps alcoholics cope with psychic discomfort, express feelings, identify drinking pressures, and change personal habits. Such treatment emphasizes that drug-dependent people can gain control over their own actions, reaffirm the value of sobriety, and eventually overpower alcohol. This basic belief stands in sharp contrast with the philosophy of Alcoholics Anonymous, which emphasizes personal powerlessness over alcohol.

A therapeutic approach referred to as behavior modification seeks to describe both undesirable and desirable patient behavior. Early therapy featured aversion techniques based on punishing the alcoholic if he or she drank. Today, newer behavior modification techniques consist of a variety of behavior-rewarding modeling, and guiding experiences in an attempt to change drinking patterns and other dysfunctional responses to life situations.

Transactional analysis—a form of group therapy that examines in depth the various verbal exchanges between people. This therapy denies the disease concept of alcoholism. The transactional analyst simply refuses to participate in the "games" alcoholics play, thus leaving them without an incentive to play them. Furthermore, the therapist assigns responsibility for alcoholic behavior to the patient, and tries to instill positive expectancy and hope in the individual problem drinker.

Alcoholics Anonymous—one of the most successful approaches in recovery from alcoholism. **Alcoholics Anonymous (AA)** is a fellowship of

problem drinkers who want help in maintaining sobriety. Voluntary membership involves an emotional commitment that the alcoholic is powerless over the control of alcohol and that only a power greater than the self can restore soundness of mind. The famous "Twelve Steps" of AA express the philosophy and recovery process of this international association.[72] Offering hope of recovery from alcoholism is an essential feature of Alcoholics Anonymous. Such hope is provided by both example and supportive interrelationships with other members of this self-help fellowship. Each person is expected to become involved with the Twelve Steps of AA, an ongoing process referred to as "working the program" (see box 4.7).

The Twelve Traditions of AA are the operational principles of the fellowship and express the importance and significance of the group in relationship to its membership, nonmembers, and society in general (see box 4.8).

At present, Alcoholics Anonymous has an estimated membership in excess of 1.5 million people in 114 countries around the world. Despite its evident spiritual orientation, AA continues to thrive, based on singleness of purpose, group autonomy, self-supporting financial operation, maintenance of nonprofessional status, noninvolvement in public controversy, and personal anonymity. Patterned closely after AA are the Al-Anon family groups for spouses and friends of recovered and recovering alcoholics and Alateen groups for children of alcoholics.

The therapies just described are offered through many individuals and groups in numerous types of facilities. There are enlightened physicians; community mental health centers; pastoral counseling programs in churches; and general hospitals offering emergency medical services, inpatient care, and outpatient care through clinics. There are also specialized

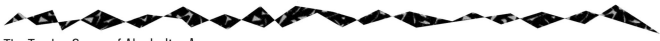

The Twelve Steps of Alcoholics Anonymous

box 4.7

1. We admitted we were powerless over alcohol—that our lives had become unmanageable.
2. Came to believe that a Power greater than ourselves could restore us to sanity.
3. Made a decision to turn our will and our lives over to the care of God as we understood Him.
4. Made a searching and fearless moral inventory of ourselves.
5. Admitted to God, to ourselves, and to another human being the exact nature of our wrongs.
6. Were entirely ready to have God remove all these defects of character.
7. Humbly asked Him to remove our shortcomings.
8. Made a list of all persons we had harmed, and became willing to make amends to them all.
9. Made direct amends to such people wherever possible, except when to do so would injure them or others.
10. Continued to take personal inventory and when we were wrong promptly admitted it.
11. Sought through prayer and meditation to improve our conscious contact with God as we understood Him, praying only for knowledge of His will for us and the power to carry that out.
12. Having had a spiritual awakening as the result of these steps, we tried to carry this message to alcoholics and to practice these principles in all our affairs.

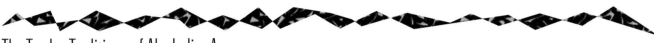

The Twelve Traditions of Alcoholics Anonymous

box 4.8

1. Our common welfare should come first; personal recovery depends upon AA unity.
2. For our group purposes there is but one ultimate authority—a loving God as He may express Himself in our group conscience. Our leaders are but trusted servants; they do not govern.
3. The only requirement for AA membership is a desire to stop drinking.
4. Each group should be autonomous except in matters affecting other groups or AA as a whole.
5. Each group has but one primary purpose—to carry its message to the alcoholic who still suffers.
6. An AA group ought never endorse, finance, or lend the AA name to any related facility or outside enterprise, lest problems of money, property, and prestige divert us from our primary purpose.
7. Every AA group ought to be fully self-supporting, declining outside contributions.
8. Alcoholics Anonymous should remain forever nonprofessional, but our service centers may employ special workers.
9. AA, as such, ought never be organized; but we may create service boards or committees directly responsible to those they serve.
10. Alcoholics Anonymous has no opinion on outside issues; hence the AA name ought never be drawn into public controversy.
11. Our public relations policy is based on attraction rather than promotion; we need always maintain personal anonymity at the level of press, radio, and films.
12. Anonymity is the spiritual foundation of all our traditions, ever reminding us to place principles before personalities.

hospitals that treat only alcoholism and drug abuse and their associated health problems; mental hospitals that provide residential care; Veterans Administration hospitals; and "halfway houses" where recovering alcoholics receive semicustodial care while adjusting to independent living after institutionalization. Experience has indicated that when treatment and rehabilitation services are coordinated within a job-related or employer-sponsored alcoholism program, recovery rates are considerably higher than ordinarily achieved in other settings.

Reduction of Problem Drinking: Personal Actions

Whether or not there is healthy or responsible drinking is still debatable. Many have chosen an alcohol-free lifestyle and thereby avoid personal involvement with alcohol abuse. And yet millions more have decided to interact with this potentially dangerous drug in order to derive various perceived benefits. Since the United States has given up any attempt at prohibition, those who wish to drink must be concerned with reducing the many problems related to alcohol abuse. This strategy will certainly demand responsible decisions regarding alcohol use. Parents who want to minimize the risk of their children becoming victims of alcohol abuse would be wise to begin early to teach their children about making responsible decisions.

Parents Who Drink and Their Children

Research indicates that Italians, Orthodox Jews, Greeks, Spaniards, Chinese, and Lebanese all use alcohol regularly and in quantity, yet tend to have few alcohol-related problems. These cultures have long histories of relatively safe drinking and share certain common practices in their use of alcohol. Perhaps Americans should consider and adopt these "immunizing" practices.

> The children are exposed to alcohol early in life, within a strong family or religious group.
>
> Parents present a consistent example of moderate drinking.
>
> The beverage is viewed mainly as an accompaniment to food and is usually taken with meals.
>
> The beverages commonly used are wine and beer.
>
> Drinking has no moral connotation. It is considered neither a virtue nor a sin.
>
> Drinking is not viewed as proof of adulthood or virility.
>
> Abstinence is socially acceptable.
>
> Excessive drinking or drunkenness is not condoned.
>
> Alcohol use is not the prime focus for an activity.
>
> Most importantly, there is wide agreement among members of the group on these "ground rules" of drinking.

Host and Hostess Responsibilities

The American house party is another setting in which responsible decisions about alcohol use can help reduce problem drinking. The host and hostess can decide what drinking atmosphere will prevail. Will drinking be the major focus, or will alcohol be used merely as an adjunct to a rewarding social occasion? If true hospitality involves more than plying guests with alcohol, there are some procedures that responsible party givers can follow to promote party togetherness and still keep things under control. These party responsibilities, formulated by the National Institute on Alcohol Abuse and Alcoholism, appear in box 4.9.

For Those Who Drink

Alcohol abuse is everyone's problem. Whether nonuser, moderate or social drinker, or alcoholic, everyone is directly or indirectly affected by alcohol abuse. Whether alcoholism is perceived as a personal threat or not, and whether drinking is viewed as good or bad, the most important thing to remember is that ethyl alcohol is a drug with the potential for adverse drug effects, even when used in social settings.

Social drinking is usually "moderate," but the limits of appropriateness are likely to vary from one drinker or drinking group to another. Consequently, promoting so-called responsible drinking behavior may be less than adequate as a method of reducing alcohol problems and alcohol abuse. In a similar manner, urging drinkers to "party sensibly," "know their limits," and "know when to say when" may sound like good advice. But these recommendations have been criticized as lacking in specificity and dealing with glittering generalities that cannot be applied easily.

By contrast the "Zero-One-Three" strategy offers straightforward, unambiguous guidelines for "moderate drinking." Included are specific, short, and easy-to-apply principles for conducting moderate drinking behavior. Notice that both nondrinkers and drinkers are considered and that the message "It's always OK not to drink" is reinforced in the "Zero = zero alcohol" portion of the safety promotion concept (see fig. 4.6).

In addition, the following suggestions are also offered for those who wish to preserve alcohol use as a nondestructive part of social functions, to avoid the mental chaos of intoxication, and to minimize the risks of alcoholism.

1. Integrate alcohol use with leisure activities, eating, and social functions.

2. Conduct drinking among friends or within the family setting, where social controls are more likely to function.

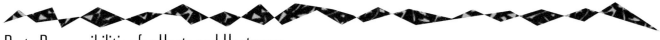

Party Responsibilities for Hosts and Hostesses

box 4.9

The home setting	Provide seats for all, plan for people movement and keep the lights on.
The bartender	Choose a bartender of known discretion. The eager volunteer may turn out to be a pusher who uses the role to give every glass an extra "shot."
Pace the drinks	Serve drinks at regular, reasonable intervals. The length of the interval will depend on whether the guests are enjoying the company or the drinks more. A drink-an-hour schedule means good company prevails.
Don't double up	Many people count and pace their drinks. If you serve doubles, they'll be drinking twice as much as they planned. Doubling up isn't hospitality; it's rude.
Don't push drinks	Let the glass be empty before you offer a refill. And then don't rush, especially if someone comes up empty too fast. When a guest says "no, thanks" to an alcohol drink—don't insist.
Push the snacks	Do this while your guests are drinking, not after. This is important because food slows down the rate at which alcohol is absorbed into the bloodstream. It also slows down the rate at which people drink.
Serve nonalcoholic drinks, too	One out of three adults chooses not to drink at all. Occasional drinkers sometimes prefer not to. Offer a choice of drinks besides alcohol—fruit and vegetable juices, tea, coffee, and soft drinks.
Offer more than drinks	When guests focus on the drinks, the party is slipping. Stir up conversation. Share a laugh. Draw out a guest talent. A good host or hostess has more to give than just food and drinks.
Serving dinner	If it's a dinner party, serve before it's too late. A cocktail hour is supposed to enhance a fine dinner, not compete with it. After too many drinks, guests may not know what they ate or how it tasted.
Set drinking limits	When a guest has had too much to drink, you can politely express your concern by offering a substitute drink—coffee, perhaps. This is a gentle way of telling a guest that he or she has reached the limits you have set for your home.
Closing the bar	Decide in advance when you want your party to end. Then give appropriate cues by word and action that it's time to leave. A considerate way to close the drinking phase is to serve a substantial snack. It also provides some nondrinking time before your guests start to drive home.

Source: National Institute on Alcohol Abuse and Alcoholism.

3. Pace your consumption of alcohol by sipping drinks and becoming involved in conversation. Take your second drink no sooner than one hour after the first. Do not drink fast!

4. Avoid drinking on an empty stomach. Eat ice cream, meat, eggs, or cheese, or drink milk or cream before ingesting alcohol, and also eat while you drink.

5. Dilute distilled spirits with water so as to retard alcohol absorption; always use plenty of ice cubes; and beware of unfamiliar drinks with unknown alcohol content.

6. Drink in well-lighted, quiet places. Dark and noisy places produce tenseness, which in turn may give rise to overdrinking.

7. Deliberately avoid beverage alcohol when confronted with problems or the need to relax.

8. Watch carefully your personal drinking pattern for early signs and symptoms of problem drinking. Remember, if you need a drink to be social, that is *not* social drinking!

For Safer Fall Activities Follow These Lower Risk Guidelines For

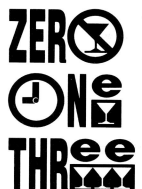

Zero = Zero Alcohol. Especially if you're under 21, driving, chemically dependent or pregnant.

One = One drink per hour sets the pace for moderate drinking. **AND**
Three = No more than three drinks per day, and never daily.

WEEKENDS

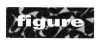 **4.6**

The "Zero-One-Three" strategy for lower-risk drinking.
From the Enjoy Michigan Safely Coalition, Michigan Substance Abuse and Traffic Safety Information Center, Lansing, Mich. Reprinted by permission.

Chapter Summary

1. Continuing a long-term custom, a majority of Americans use alcoholic beverages as a legal and socially approved form of drug taking.

2. The "temperance movement" began as a promotion of moderate use of beverage alcohol and evolved into a moral crusade aimed at mandating total abstinence by law.

3. Enforcement of national Prohibition began in 1920 after passage of the Eighteenth Amendment to the U.S. Constitution. After nearly fourteen years, the "noble experiment" ended when the Twenty-First Amendment was approved in 1933, repealing the provisions of the Prohibition amendment.

4. The emotional legacy of Prohibition and the conflict between permissive use and abstinence have generated a cultural ambivalence toward alcohol. This condition, in which both positive and negative aspects of alcohol are perceived jointly, has contributed to numerous alcohol problems.

5. Patterns of alcohol use range from nondrinking to chronic (long-term) alcoholic drinking. General uses of beverage alcohol include social, ritualistic, dietary, and mood modification drinking. Alteration of mood may result in tranquilization, feelings of powerfulness, enhancement of femininity, satisfaction of dependency needs, increased awareness, and increased unawareness.

6. Alcoholic beverages are classified as beers, wines, and distilled spirits, each having varying amounts of ethyl alcohol. However, a typical serving of any one beverage contains approximately the same amount of alcohol, 0.5 ounce.

7. Once an alcoholic beverage is consumed, it undergoes processes of absorption, distribution, and oxidation. If intake of alcohol exceeds the body's ability to eliminate it, the blood-alcohol concentration will increase. As BACs increase, the depressant effect of alcohol is manifested as intoxication, a temporary state of mental chaos and behavioral dysfunction.

8. The duration of alcohol effects is a time composed of several different states of consciousness, depending on whether the blood-alcohol concentration is increasing or decreasing. Behavioral reactions accompanying intoxication are influenced by the drinker's mind-set and the emotional climate of drinking.

9. Short-term effects of alcohol are evidenced in alteration of sensation, perception, emotions, sleep, and motor skills, and in changes in kidney, heart, blood vessel, liver, and sexual functions. Of course, a hangover is always a possibility following excessive consumption.

10. Long-term effects of alcohol consumption, often heavy and prolonged intake, can develop into gastrointestinal disorders, liver diseases and dysfunction, nutritional deficiency, diseases of the nervous system, endocrine system disorders, mental disorders, cardiovascular diseases, certain cancers, undesirable alcohol-drug interactions, fetal alcohol syndrome, and alcoholism.

11. With regard to problem drinking, alcohol abuse is related to nearly half of all highway deaths, serious family dysfunction including marital violence and child abuse, numerous sexual problems, and many crimes, such as public intoxication, sex offenses, assault, and murder.

12. Alcoholism is the disease of alcohol dependence in which a drinker cannot consistently exert control over the intake of alcohol; a primary, chronic disease that is often progressive in nature and fatal, involving preoccupation with alcohol use despite adverse consequences,

and distortions in thinking, especially denial. Among the possible causes of this complex illness are factors relating to alcohol itself; the drinker with unique genetic, biochemical, and psychological forces; and the psychosocial and cultural setting in which drinking occurs.

13. Treatment for alcoholismic individuals begins with detoxification, includes medical care for specific health problems, and progresses to changing long-term behaviors that have contributed to destructive drinking patterns. Specific treatments include drug therapy, (e.g., Antabuse, Naltrexone), psychotherapy, family therapy, behavioral therapy, transactional analysis, and the self-help techniques of groups like Alcoholics Anonymous.

14. Reduction of problem drinking begins with "immunizing" strategies employed by parents with their own children, relies upon responsible actions taken by hosts and hostesses at drinking parties, and ultimately depends upon the prudent actions of drinkers who wish to preserve alcohol use as a nondestructive part of social functions.

Review Questions and Activities

1. What percentage of Americans are estimated to be drinkers? Survey class members to determine if they approximate national percentages of users and nonusers.

2. What is the difference between moonshining and bootlegging activities?

3. Explain what is meant by the infamous "trading triangle" in colonial times.

4. Identify the historical factors that led to the adoption of national Prohibition in the United States.

5. State the provisions of the Eighteenth Amendment to the U.S. Constitution.

6. Describe how the emotional legacy of the Prohibition Era has contributed to modern alcohol problems.

7. Name four manifestations of cultural ambivalence as related to alcohol use in America.

8. How would you describe social drinking? Do you believe there is such a thing as social use of alcohol?

9. What is meant by ritualistic, dietary, and mood modification drinking?

10. How does drinking for increased awareness differ from drinking for increased unawareness?

11. Describe the similarities and differences among beers, wines, and distilled spirits.

12. Name several factors that influence the absorption of alcohol.

13. What is meant by the term *blood-alcohol concentration*?

14. What are the various intermediate and end by-products of alcohol oxidation?

15. Why can't women hold their liquor like men?

16. Explain the various changes that are likely to occur as an intoxicated person's blood-alcohol concentration increases from 0.03 percent to 0.30 percent.

17. What is the relation of pseudostimulation to alcohol intoxication?

18. How does alcohol state of consciousness #1 differ from ASC-2?

19. Name several short-term and potential long-term effects of alcohol consumption on physical and mental health status.

20. Why does nutritional deficiency often develop in a heavy drinker?

21. What is meant by the neurotoxic effect of alcohol? How does this differ from alcohol's hepatotoxic effect?

22. Give an example of an alcohol-drug interaction that will likely produce a potentiation or synergistic effect.

23. What are the possible consequences of alcohol's embryotoxic effect?

24. Why is an intoxicated person a menace to society when he or she attempts to drive an automobile under the influence of alcohol? What can you do to prevent such an individual from driving?

25. Explain why alcohol abuse or alcoholism is often referred to as a "family disease."

26. State three definitions of alcoholism that reveal various characteristics of this complex illness.

27. Identify at least three agent-related, three host-related, and three environment-related factors that might cause or contribute to alcoholism.

28. Describe the progressive nature of alcoholism by citing specific signs and symptoms typical of the four phases of this disease.

29. What therapies are used in treating alcoholics? You may want to attend an open meeting of Alcoholics Anonymous and report on your findings.

30. To what extent do you agree or disagree with the recommendations in the text to reduce problem drinking?

References

1. Institute for Health Policy, Brandeis University, *Substance Abuse: The Nation's Number One Health Problem* (Princeton, N.J.: Robert Wood Johnson Foundation, 1993), 16.
2. "Let's Have a Drink: Changing Patterns of Beverage Consumption in the U.S. 1990," *Bottom Line on Alcohol in Society* 10 (1990): p. 17.
3. National Institute on Alcohol Abuse and Alcoholism, "Influences of American History and Popular Media on Drinking Practices in America," in *Planning a Prevention Program* (Washington, D.C.: U.S. Government Printing Office, 1978), 95–96.

4. Ronald K. Siegel, *Intoxication: Life in Pursuit of Artificial Paradise* (New York: Dutton, 1989), 10.

5. David Pittman and Helene Raskin White, *Society, Culture, and Drinking Patterns Reexamined* (New Brunswick, N.J.: Rutgers Center of Alcohol Studies, 1991), 175.

6. Andrew Weil and Winifred Rosen, *From Chocolate to Morphine*, rev. ed. (Boston: Houghton Mifflin, 1993), 14.

7. Marian Sandmaier, *The Invisible Alcoholics: Women and Alcohol Abuse in America* (New York: McGraw-Hill, 1980), 91.

8. Harvey B. Milkman and Stanley G. Sunderwirth, *Craving for Ecstasy: The Consciousness and Chemistry of Escape* (Lexington, Mass.: Lexington Books/D.C. Heath, 1987), 18.

9. Siegel, *Intoxication*, pp. 10, 207–27, 313.

10. Morris Chafetz, *Liquor: The Servant of Man* (Boston: Little, Brown, 1965), 150–74.

11. *World Book Encyclopedia* (Chicago: World Book, 1992), 335.

12. Department of Health and Human Services, Office of the Inspector General, *Youth and Alcohol: A National Survey—Drinking Habits, Access, Attitudes, and Knowledge* (Washington, D.C.: National Clearinghouse for Alcohol and Drug Information, 1991), 6.

13. "Looks, Smells, Tastes Like Beer," *Bottom Line on Alcohol in Society* 10 (1990): 26–28.

14. Mario Frezza and others, "High Blood Alcohol Levels in Women: The Role of Decreased Gastric Alcohol Dehydrogenase Activity and First-Pass Metabolism," *New England Journal of Medicine* 322, no. 2 (11 January 1990): 95–99.

15. Nancy M. Lee and Charles E. Becker, "The Alcohols," chapter 22 in *Basic and Clinical Pharmacology*, 4th ed., ed. Bertram Katzung (Norwalk, Conn.: Appleton & Lange, 1989), 278–79.

16. Robert Julien, *A Primer of Drug Action* (New York: W. H. Freeman, 1992), 75.

17. National Institute on Alcohol Abuse and Alcoholism, *Alcohol and Health: The Eighth Special Report to the U.S. Congress* (Rockville, Md.: National Institutes of Health, 1993), 88–94.

18. Theodore Rall, "Hypnotics and Sedatives: Ethanol," chapter 17 in *Goodman and Gilman's The Pharmacological Basis of Therapeutics*, 8th ed., ed. A. G. Gilman, T. W. Rall, A. S. Nies, and P. Taylor (New York: McGraw-Hill, 1990), 371.

19. Ben Morgan Jones and Marilyn K. Jones, "States of Consciousness and Alcohol: Relationship to the Blood Alcohol Curve, Time of Day, and the Menstrual Cycle," *Alcohol Health and Research World* 1, no. 1 (fall, 1976): 10–15.

20. National Institute on Alcohol Abuse and Alcoholism, "Alcohol and Nutrition," *Alcohol Alert* no. 22, PH 346 (October 1993): 1–3.

21. Charles Lieber, "Alcohol and Nutrition: An Overview," *Alcohol Health and Research World* 13: 197–205.

22. National Institute on Alcohol Abuse and Alcoholism, "Alcohol and Cognition," *Alcohol Alert* no. 4 (May 1989): 1–2.

23. Richard Donahue, Robert Abbott, Dwayne Reed, and Katsuhiko Yano, "Alcohol and Hemorrhagic Stroke: The Honolulu Heart Program," *Journal of the American Medical Association* 255, no. 17 (2 May 1986): 2311–14.

24. J. Michael Gaziano and others, "Moderate Alcohol Intake, Increased Levels of High-Density Lipoprotein and Its Subfractions, and Decreased Risk of Myocardial Infarction," *New England Journal of Medicine* 329, no. 25 (16 December 1993): 1829–34.

25. Ibid.

26. Claire Coles and Kathleen Platzman, "Fetal Alcohol Effects in Pre-school Children: Research, Prevention, and Intervention," chapter 4 in *Identifying the Needs of Drug-Affected Children: Public Policy Issues*, Office for Substance Abuse Prevention (OSAP) Prevention Monograph No. 11, USDHHS Publication No. ADM-92-1814 (Washington, D.C.: U.S. Government Printing Office, 1992), 59.

27. Nancy Day, "The Effects of Prenatal Exposure to Alcohol," *Alcohol Health and Research World* 16, no. 3 (1992): 238–44.

28. National Institute on Alcohol Abuse and Alcoholism, *Alcohol and Health*, 203.

29. Office for Substance Abuse Prevention, "Introduction," in *Identifying the Needs of Drug-Affected Children*, 2.

30. George Steinmetz, "The Preventable Tragedy: Fetal Alcohol Syndrome," *National Geographic*, February 1992, p. 36.

31. Paddy Cook, Robert Peterson, and Dorothy Moore, *Alcohol, Tobacco, and Other Drugs May Harm the Unborn*, USDHHS Publication No. ADM-90-1711 (Washington, D.C.: U.S. Government Printing Office, 1990), 15.

32. Ibid., p. 18.

33. Enoch Gordis, "Fetal Alcohol Syndrome: A Commentary," *Alcohol Alert* no. 13, PH 297 (July 1991): 3.

34. National Institute on Alcohol Abuse and Alcoholism, "Fetal Alcohol Syndrome," *Alcohol Alert* no. 13, PH 297 (July 1991), 2.

35. National 3D Prevention Month Coalition, *National Drunk and Drugged Driving (3D) Prevention Month Background and Resource Guide* (Washington, D.C.: U.S. Department of Transportation, 1993), 3.

36. C. Everett Koop, *Surgeon General's Workshop on Drunk Driving: Proceedings* (Washington, D.C.: U.S. Government Printing Office, 1989), 6.

37. David A. Sleet, Alexander C. Wagenaar, and Patricia F. Waller, "Introduction: Drinking, Driving, and Health Promotion," *Health Education Quarterly* 16, no. 3 (fall 1989): 319–33.

38. Herbert Moskowitz and Marcelline Burns, "Effects of Alcohol on Driving Performance," *Alcohol Health and Research World* 14, no. 1 (1990): 12–14.

39. "How Much Is Too Much?" *Bottom Line on Alcohol in Society*, 10 (1990): 18–23.

40. Robert J. King, "From the Executive Office," *MADD in Action* 9, no. 2 (May–August 1990): 2.

41. James J. Collins, "Epidemiology of Alcohol-Related Violence," *Alcohol Health and Research World* 17, no. 2 (1993): 93–100.

42. National Institute on Alcohol Abuse and Alcoholism, *Alcohol and Health*, 247.

43. Ibid.

44. Robert N. Parker, "The Effects of Context on Alcohol and Violence," *Alcohol Health and Research World* 17, no. 2 (1993): 117–32.

45. Office for Substance Abuse Prevention, *Some Questions and Answers about Children of Alcoholics*, USDHHS Publication No. ADM-92-1914 (Rockville, Md.: National Clearinghouse for Alcohol and Drug Information, 1992).

46. Donald Jorgensen and June Jorgensen, *Secrets Told by Children of Alcoholics* (Blue Ridge Summit, Pa.: Tab Books, 1990), 21–44.

47. National Institute on Alcohol Abuse and Alcoholism, *Alcohol Alert: Children of Alcoholics: Are They Different?* (Rockville, Md.: Public Health Service, Alcohol, Drug Abuse, and Mental Health Administration, 1990), 1–2.

48. Judith Seixas and Geraldine Youcha, *Children of Alcoholism: A Survivor's Manual* (New York: Perennial Library/Harper & Row, 1985).

49. Sharon Wegscheider, *Another Chance: Hope and Health for the Alcoholic Family* (Palo Alto, Calif.: Science and Behavior Books, 1981).

50. William H. Crisman, *The Opposite of Everything Is True: Reflections on Denial in Alcoholic Families* (New York: William Morrow, 1991), 72–78.

51. Tom Dunkel, "Dealing with Demons of a New Generation," in *Annual Editions: Drugs, Society, and Human Behavior 94/95* (Guilford, Conn.: Dushkin, 1994), 128–30. (Originally published in *Insight*, 1993.)

52. "Children of Alcoholics: Are They Different from the Rest of the Population?" *Bottom Line on Alcohol in Society* 13, no. 1 (spring 1992): 64–67.

53. Sharon Wegscheider-Cruse, *The Miracle of Recovery* (Deerfield Beach, Fla.: Health Communications, 1989), 35.

54. Anne Wilson Schaef, *When Society Becomes an Addict* (San Francisco: Harper & Row, 1988), 30.

55. Ibid.

56. Anne Wilson Schaef, *Co-dependence: Misunderstood—Mistreated* (San Francisco: Perennial Library/Harper & Row, 1986), 45–52.

57. George E. Vaillant, "The Alcohol-Dependent and Drug-Dependent Person," chapter 31 in *The New Harvard Guide to Psychiatry*, ed. Armand M. Nicholi, Jr. (Cambridge: Belknap Press/Harvard University Press, 1988), 702.

58. E. M. Jellinek, *The Disease Concept of Alcoholism* (New Brunswick, N.J.: Hillhouse Press, 1960), 35–38.

59. American Medical Association, *Manual on Alcoholism*, 3d ed. (Chicago: American Medical Association, 1977), 4.

60. Robert Morse and Daniel Flavin, "Report for the Joint Committee of the National Council on Alcoholism and Drug Dependence and the American Society of Addiction Medicine to Study the Definition and Criteria for the Diagnosis of Alcoholism," *Journal of the American Medical Association* 268, no. 8 (26 August 1992): 1012–14.

61. Lester Grinspoon, James Bakalar, and others, "Alcohol Abuse and Dependence," *Harvard Medical School Mental Health Review* (1990): 5.

62. Donald Goodwin, *Is Alcoholism Hereditary?* 2d ed. (New York: Ballantine, 1988), 83–156.

63. National Institute on Alcohol Abuse and Alcoholism, "The Genetics of Alcoholism," *Alcohol Alert* no. 18, PH 328 (October 1992): 1–3.

64. George E. Vaillant, *The Natural History of Alcoholism* (Cambridge: Harvard University Press, 1983), 64–74.

65. National Institute on Alcohol Abuse and Alcoholism, *Alcoholism: An Inherited Disease* (Washington, D.C.: U.S. Government Printing Office, 1985), 18–27.

66. Mark Schuckit, "A Clinical Model of Genetic Influences in Alcohol Dependence," *Journal of Studies on Alcohol* 55 (1994): 5–17.

67. Grinspoon, Bakalar, and others, "Alcohol Abuse and Dependence," 5.

68. Goodwin, *Is Alcoholism Hereditary?* 149.

69. National Institute on Alcohol Abuse and Alcoholism, "Alcohol Withdrawal Syndrome," *Alcohol Alert* 5 (August 1989): 1.

70. R. J. Solberg, *The Dry-Drunk Syndrome* (Center City, Minn.: Hazelden Educational Services, 1980), 3–4.

71. Rall, "Hypnotics and Sedatives: Ethanol," 378.

72. Alcoholics Anonymous World Services, *Alcoholics Anonymous*, 3d ed. (New York: Alcoholics Anonymous World Services, 1976), 59–60.

chapter

5

narcotics

Opioid Analgesics

chapter objectives

After you have studied this chapter, you should be able to do the following:

1. Define the term *narcotic*, revealing its major effects and general characteristics.

2. Classify common opioids as natural, semisynthetic, synthetic, or endogenous.

3. Identify several common side effects and adverse drug reactions associated with using narcotics.

4. Explain how the following narcotics are related in their derivation or origin: opium, morphine, China White heroin, and codeine.

5. Distinguish the unique status of an "exempt narcotic" from opioids such as morphine and methadone.

6. Explain how lifestyle could influence the health of a person abusing heroin.

7. Compare the effects of methadone and LAAM with those of morphine-based drugs.

8. Define the following terms: *narcotic antagonist, opioid receptor, enkephalins, endorphins,* and *"designer heroin."*

9. Describe drug dependence as an endorphin deficiency.

10. Discuss the historical influences in the early part of the twentieth century that led to the enactment of the first Federal Food and Drug Act of 1906 and the Harrison Narcotics Act of 1914.

11. Identify the major provisions of the Comprehensive Drug Abuse Prevention and Control Act of 1970 that affected the availability, distribution, and possession of narcotics.

12. Distinguish from one another each of the following, pertaining to the treatment of narcotic-dependent individuals: psychotherapy, detoxification, therapeutic communities, methadone maintenance, Narcotics Anonymous, and narcotic antagonists.

13. Explain the meaning of the term *cold turkey* as it relates to the condition of narcotic drug dependency.

14. Discuss the pros and cons of methadone or LAAM maintenance as a technique for reducing problems of heroin dependency.

15. Describe the major elements of the "multimodality approach" to the treatment of narcotics dependency.

General Characteristics of Narcotics

Although the term **narcotic** has several meanings—one of which refers to all illegal drugs of abuse—it will be used exclusively in this text to describe a family of drugs having both a stupor- or sleep-inducing action and an analgesic (pain-relieving) action. Sometimes the narcotic drugs are called **opioids** or *opiates* because they are derived from the opium poppy plant or made synthetically to have the same drug actions of morphine, a major ingredient of opium.

As shown in figure 5.1, the opioids may be classified as

1. *natural substances*, such as opium, morphine, codeine, and thebaine;

2. *semisynthetic narcotics*, such as heroin, hydromorphone

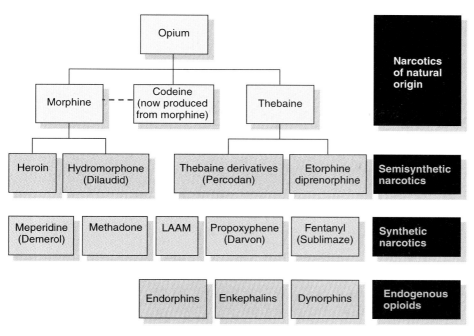

 5.1

The narcotics: Opioid analgesics.

(dihydromorphinone), thebaine derivatives, and etorphine, all produced by modifying the chemicals contained in opium;

3. *synthetic products* made entirely in the laboratory, such as meperidine (Demerol), methadone, and propoxyphene (Darvon); or

4. *endogenous opioids*, recently discovered natural, internal bodily substances, now identified as enkephalins, endorphins, and dynorphins, that originate within the body and have opioid-like effects within the body.

Although the opioids have been used medically for **analgesia** (pain relief), treatment of diarrhea, and the relief of coughing, they are also addictive. Their heavy use or even occasional use over a long period of time will likely result in opioid abuse and dependence, characterized by daily use, inability to stop usage, constant or repeated intoxication with a narcotic drug, overdoses, tolerance, and withdrawal reaction or abstinence syndrome.[1]

Once again, it should be noted that words such as *addictive, addiction*, and *addict* have been replaced by the more modern, precise, and accurately descriptive terms *dependency producing, drug dependence*, and *drug* or *chemically dependent person*, respectively. However, the **"addiction"** terminology still appears frequently in current professional literature and mass-media reports dealing with narcotics and compulsive drug use. Such persistent popularity of addiction terms is often related to the influence of tradition and the ease of speaking and spelling these words. Nevertheless, when used in this and following chapters, "addiction" words should be interpreted in their more appropriate meanings.

Many artificial morphine-like drugs have been produced in the laboratory to duplicate the medical usefulness of, yet avoid the chemical dependence often associated with, the opioids. Some of these newer nonnarcotic drugs are presently used for the relief of coughing. However, morphine, codeine, and the synthetic narcotics still play vital roles in the medical relief of pain.[2] In fact, morphine remains the stan-

dard against which new analgesics are measured, because no other drug has been proven to be clinically superior in relieving severe pain and the pain of terminal illness.[3]

Because of the euphoria-producing effects of the narcotics and the likelihood of their misuse and abuse, they are rarely used alone to induce sleep. In addition to pain relief and a general feeling of well-being, opioids also produce drowsiness that leads to sleep. With high doses, these drugs cause a clouding of mental function due to central nervous system (CNS) depression. Unlike other CNS depressants, there is usually no loss of motor coordination or consciousness, and no slurring of speech, unless a very large dose is administered or the person is already ill or fatigued.

Behavioral effects of the narcotics usually depend upon whether the individual is experiencing pain or is pain-free. When given a therapeutic dose of morphine, for instance, a patient in pain and suffering from anxiety tends to experience relief from the pain as well as from overwhelming fear. However, when pain is not present, a person taking the same dose may develop mental distress, such as fear and nervousness as well as nausea.

Common side effects include constipation, constriction of the eye's pupil, and respiratory depression that leads to irregular breathing. Less commonly experienced are nausea, vomiting, dizziness, and shortness of breath. There is little doubt, however, that the most attractive nonmedical effect of the opioids is the experience of well-being, ranging from a mild euphoria to a tingling sensation often interpreted as a sexual orgasm. In such a state, the user becomes detached from the worries and concerns of daily existence.

When used medically, narcotics are given orally or by intramuscular injection. When abused, they may be smoked, sniffed (**"snorting"**), or self-administered by either subcutaneous (**"skin-popping"**) or intravenous (**"mainlining"**) injection.

And unlike ethyl alcohol and the barbiturates, the opioids, even when they are abused, generally do not cause physical damage to the brain, liver, or heart. And unlike the stimulant drugs—cocaine and amphetamine—the opioids do not induce psychotic experiences or increase susceptibility to seizures.[4] The health problems so often associated with the abuse of narcotics are typically related to the neglect of personal health and safety, as detailed later in this chapter.

Narcotics of Natural Origin

Included in this section are those opioids that are present in or produced by nature, that is, not artificial or synthetic in their origin.[5]

Opium

Known as the "mother drug" because it is the main source of nonsynthetic narcotics, **opium** is produced from the opium poppy, *Papaver somniferum.* Cultivated in many countries around the world, the poppy flower is grown in large quantities in Turkey, India, Burma, China, Thailand, Laos, and Mexico. Opium is derived from the unripe poppy pod, which is slit with a knife. Milky fluid oozes from the seedpod, which is allowed to "bleed" overnight. Early the next day, the dried exudate is scraped off the leaves and air-dried to yield a brownish gum known as "crude" or "raw" opium. An alternate method of harvesting opium is the industrial poppy straw process, in which chemical substances known as alkaloids are extracted from the mature dried plant. This extract may be either a liquid, a solid, or a fine brown powder.

The dried raw opium or extract generally is smoked, with inhalation of its vapors. Sometimes, though, the crude opium is swallowed. Widely used throughout the world until the beginning of the twentieth century, opium is not often abused in America because of its strength of action and massive bulk, which interferes with trafficking. With current drugs of abuse that produce an even greater euphoria, opium seems to have lost its cultural popularity, except among recently arrived Asian refugees on the West Coast of the United States.

Only a small amount of opium is imported for making antidiarrheal preparations. Most of the legally imported opium

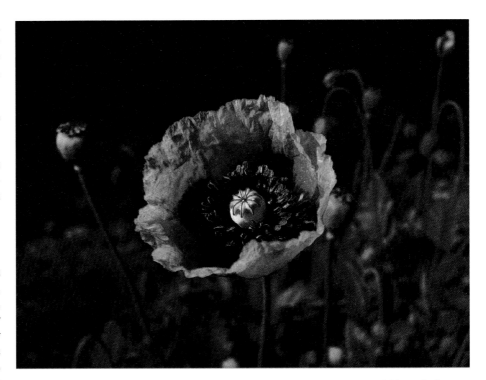

A close-up view of the poppy, Papaver somniferum, from which opium is produced. This particular poppy is the main source of nonsynthetic narcotics.

© *Karl Weidmann/Photo Researchers, Inc.*

gum and almost all of the illegal substances destined to enter America are chemically treated for the constituent alkaloids (basic nitrogenous compounds) of the "mother drug." Legal derivatives of opium include morphine, codeine, Dilaudid, and metopon, all of which have valid medical uses. The major illegal narcotic derived from opium is heroin.

Morphine

The chief alkaloid ingredient of opium, ranging from 4 percent to 21 percent concentration, is **morphine**. It is used medically as a sedative and an analgesic, being one of the most effective drugs known for relief of pain. Large doses have been used to provide anesthesia during heart surgery because morphine, unlike most anesthetics, has no depressant effect on the cardiovascular system. Sometimes morphine is also used to control postoperative pain and pain associated with cancerous conditions.

Manufactured in several different forms, morphine is usually available in tablets and injectable preparations. The white crystal form is illegal. When taken orally, morphine has a bitter taste. It is more frequently administered by subcutaneous, intramuscular, or intravenous injection; the latter method is most frequently used by morphine-dependent individuals. Known on the street by names like "Big M," "Miss Emma," "white stuff," "M," "encel," "hocus," "unkie," "hard stuff," and "morpho," morphine is often obtained for illegal use through theft, diverted shipments, and counterfeit prescriptions. Used nonmedically, morphine produces a typical "high," a feeling of extreme well-being, and then drowsiness. Tolerance and physical dependence develop rapidly among users, depending, of course, upon the frequency of use and potency or dosage of the drug consumed.

A very small portion of the morphine obtained from opium is used for medical purposes. Most of this opioid is converted to several other medically useful drugs, particularly codeine and hydromorphone (Dilaudid), both of which are described in this chapter.

Codeine

Occurring naturally as a minor alkaloid ingredient in raw opium, **codeine** is more often produced from morphine. In terms of chemical structure, codeine is closely related to morphine, although it is less potent and thus produces less pain relief, sedation, and respiratory depression. Codeine is marketed in tablets for oral administration, in combination with aspirin or acetaminophen (Tylenol), in liquid preparations for relief of coughs (**antitussives**), and in injectable forms. Potentially addictive, codeine infrequently causes physical dependence when taken under medical supervision for only a short time. As such, it is the most widely used naturally occurring narcotic in medical practice.

Particularly effective as an antitussive, codeine is also sold in over-the-counter, nonprescription cough products in some states.[6, 7] Such availability without a prescription demonstrates the **exempt narcotic** status of codeine. An exempt narcotic is a drug preparation that contains a narcotic substance but can be purchased without a physician's written prescription. Most states require that the purchaser be an adult, have personal identification, and sign a special record book at the pharmacy when buying such a drug. An exempt narcotic preparation usually contains less than one grain of narcotic per fluid ounce of the liquid product.

As an exempt narcotic, codeine has been somewhat appealing to certain drug abusers. The syrup form of codeine, as found in cough syrup and Tylenol #4 medicine, is frequently used in combination with gluthethimide (Doriden), a nonbarbiturate sedative-hypnotic. Known as "hits," this mixture is used by those who want the effects of heroin but are reluctant to use drugs intravenously. Still others

who are dependent on "harder" drugs make the rounds of drugstores to purchase large quantities of codeine-containing cough suppressants when other opioids are temporarily not available on the street. The liquid is then boiled down until only a white, powdery residue remains that is eventually prepared for injection into a vein. Some people drink the codeine cough syrup to experience a "drunken glow," the result of a slight narcotic experience in combination with alcohol—nearly 40 percent of the total mixture. Such drug abuse has declined somewhat in recent years, due largely to codeine's removal from its exempt status in several states.

Thebaine

One of the minor components of opium, *thebaine* is chemically similar to both morphine and codeine. However, thebaine has stimulant effects rather than depressant ones, and it is not used in this country for medical purposes. It is converted into various other medically important compounds, including codeine, naloxone, and etorphine. Thebaine itself is controlled in Schedule II of the Controlled Substances Act.

Semisynthetic Narcotics

This section describes some of the more significant semisynthetic or half-synthetic opioids, substances that have been derived indirectly from a natural narcotic by modifying the chemicals contained in opium.

Hydromorphone

Commonly known as Dilaudid, *hydromorphone* is a semisynthetic narcotic analgesic derived from morphine. Marketed in both tablet and injectable form, it is shorter-acting and more sedative than morphine. Its potency is two to eight times as great as that of morphine. Therefore, it is a highly abusable drug, often illegally procured through fraudulent prescription or theft.

Oxycodone

Synthesized from thebaine, *oxycodone* is similar to codeine but more potent. It also has a higher dependence potential. Taken orally, it is marketed in combination with other drugs, especially Percodan, for the relief of pain. Drug abusers often take Percodan by mouth or dissolve Percodan tablets in water, filter out insoluble material, and then "mainline" the active drug.

Etorphine

Derived from thebaine, *etorphine* is more than a thousand times as potent as morphine in its analgesic, sedative, and respiratory depressant effects. As such, its potential for human use is distinctly limited by the danger of overdose. One form of this semisynthetic narcotic is used by veterinarians to immobilize large, wild animals. Another thebaine derivative, diprenorphine, counteracts the effects of etorphine. The production and distribution of both drugs are strictly regulated by the Controlled Substances Act.

Heroin

Of all the narcotics, heroin accounts for nearly 90 percent of the opioid abuse in the United States. One of the more powerful dependency-producing drugs, **heroin** is a semisynthetic drug made by treating morphine with acetic anhydride to yield diacetylmorphine. In 1898 it was introduced into medical practice as a cough suppressant under the name *heroin*. This name is derived from a German word meaning long or powerful. Heroin's impact on both individuals and society is described appropriately by this original meaning!

Characteristics of Heroin

Initially, the use of heroin in medical practice met with worldwide acceptance. There were fewer undesirable side effects than with morphine, and most people and physicians were unaware of heroin's potential for causing drug dependency. However, within twenty years, heroin had gained a bad reputation in the United

States—a reputation evident in the slang words describing the drug: *junk, smack, scag, H,* and *hard stuff.*

Pure heroin is a white powder with a bitter taste. It may vary in color from white to dark brown due to impurities remaining from the manufacturing process or the presence of additives. Since 1924, its production and importation have been outlawed in the United States, where heroin is no longer used medically. Recent experiments with cancer patients to determine its possible use as a pain-relieving drug, however, may rehabilitate heroin's therapeutic value in the future.

The very possession of heroin is illegal. Bought "on the street" from a "pusher" or dealer, heroin is invariably mixed or "cut" with other substances, including powdered milk, sugar, starch, quinine, and even strychnine and arsenic. Consequently, users seldom know precisely what they are buying.

More Potent Forms of Heroin

During the 1980s, a cheaper and more powerful form of heroin, known as "black tar" or "tootsie roll," became widely available throughout the United States. Resembling roofing tar, black tar is a crudely processed heroin that originates in Mexico. It is still sold on the street in extremely small pieces that can be "cut down" to a powder form. This new form of heroin ranges between 40 to 80 percent pure at the dealer level, a figure that is nearly forty times higher than regular heroin of an earlier time.

Then, in the 1990s, a potentially even more dangerous form of heroin, known as "China White," was introduced into this country by secret Chinese "triads," or criminal societies.[8,9] With a purity of nearly 90 percent, China White is now widely smoked or snorted. No longer confined to the inner city, use of China White has appeared in trendy metropolitan clubs where middle-class teenagers often snort heroin to counteract the effects of cocaine. Increasing numbers of college students reportedly snort heroin in order to relax when they are anxious about exams.[10]

Smokers and snorters do not need a syringe to get a fix, and thus they avoid the fear of HIV infection and AIDS often associated with a "dirty" needle.

Presently, intranasal use, or snorting, accounts for over 45 percent of heroin use in the United States. Nevertheless, many heroin users eventually move up from smoking and snorting to injecting themselves with China White, especially when tolerance begins to progress. Because of this drug's extremely high potency, overdoses are likely to be fatal. There is little doubt that the increased purity and low cost of both black tar and China White have led to a general increase in heroin use in the United States, and to a sudden rise in heroin-related emergencies at the nation's hospitals.

The Heroin "Rush"

In preparation for "skin-popping" or "mainlining," illegally procured heroin is typically mixed into a liquid solution.

Because of its chemical nature, heroin that is injected directly into a vein can reach the central nervous system much more rapidly than morphine. Shortly after mainlining, the user experiences a tingling sensation, the so-called **"rush"** of intense well-being or euphoria. This short-lived jolt is caused by the introduction of a foreign substance into the bloodstream, where sudden changes in blood pressure occur. The faster the drug reaches the nervous system, the better the rush seems to the user.

In addition to the euphoria of the rush, common reactions may include reddening of the face and constriction of the pupils of the eyes. Emotionally, there is a feeling that everything is fine. Some people also report a reduction of aggressive tendencies, depressed appetite and sex

Opioid Overdose and First-Aid Treatment

box 5.1

Overdose of an opioid is usually the result of an addict's accidental injection of impure "street heroin," for instance, rather than any inherent properties of the drug itself. Accustomed to specific doses of impure "street heroin," opioid-dependent individuals sometimes unknowingly buy drug packets that have not been "cut" as much as usual. Injection of the so-called right dose becomes an overdose. Such accidental overdosing with high-potency heroin occasionally leads to death.

Symptoms of Opioid Overdose

Stuporous condition, or deep sleep, cannot be aroused easily

Low respiration (slow or shallow breathing)

Blueness of lips and skin

Pinpoint pupils of the eyes

Needle marks on the body

First-Aid Treatment of Opioid Overdose

Try to keep the overdose victim awake by talking

Maintain an open airway

Give mouth-to-mouth resuscitation if needed

Place the unconscious person on his or her side

Monitor the unconscious person's vital signs—breathing, pulse, temperature

Call paramedic/ambulance service for transportation to a medical facility

---

drive, and a generalized decline in the level of physical activity. Tensions are reduced; worries disappear; the sharp edges of reality are dulled. Eventually, a period of stuporous inactivity follows in which splendorous daydreams occur. This calm, tranquil, carefree, forgetful state of mind, the so-called "high," lasts from three to six hours. It is both the allure of heroin and the undoing of the heroin user who takes the drug with any regularity.

Heroin Dependency

Within several weeks of continued use, the drug taker often needs to increase the dose in order to achieve the desired "high." Tolerance to heroin develops rapidly. Quite often the individual no longer experiences euphoria but is compelled to continue taking the drug in order to prevent withdrawal. Now the user has become physically dependent on the drug.

Eight to twelve hours after the last dose is taken, withdrawal symptoms appear if another "fix," or injection of heroin, is not procured. Perspiration,

tearing, tremors, chills, diarrhea, nausea, and sharp abdominal and leg cramps occur and become progressively worse for two or three days. After a week, the heroin abuser is free of withdrawal symptoms, but minor depression and insomnia may last for several months. Although the withdrawal process is painful, death from withdrawal occurs only in extreme cases. Of course, if a fetus has been drugged sufficiently while still in its heroin-using mother's uterus, the newborn infant will likely experience the heroin withdrawal process. Such withdrawal symptoms may last several weeks or months. Many babies so afflicted eventually die.

Potential hazards associated with abusing narcotics are related to the specific opioid used, its source, potency, dose, and the way it is used. The physical dangers so often reported with heroin and other opioid abuse are more closely related to the unhealthy lifestyle many addicts lead. Diseases, injuries, and deaths commonly observed are caused by uncertain dosage levels, use of unsterile needles and other paraphernalia, contaminants in

the drug itself, or the combination use of heroin with other drugs, especially barbiturates and/or alcohol (box 5.1).

There is no doubt that heroin in particular and opioids in general are drugs capable of inducing a powerful drug dependency. Most people find the struggle to free themselves from such drugs to be long and difficult, and practically impossible. Therefore, the assumption is widely held that anyone who uses heroin with any frequency will inevitably develop tolerance to and physical dependence on the drug.

This assumption is now being challenged by the discovery of people who have used heroin with some regularity and have avoided drug dependency. Apparently these occasional users (referred to as "chippers") space out their drug intake and limit their doses to extremely small amounts of low-potency heroin. Studies of Vietnam War veterans indicate that nearly three-quarters of those who used heroin at least five times while in Vietnam became addicted, but among veterans who used heroin in the United States after their return from Vietnam, only 28 percent became drug dependent. Some analysts believe the difference in the percentage of addiction was due to the high purity of heroin in Vietnam (nearly 90 percent). At the time of these studies, heroin in the United States had a purity of only about 5 percent. However, others contend that the "peacetime drug setting" of America versus the "wartime setting" of Vietnam was the important factor.

It is now apparent that the development of narcotics dependency is related to a number of factors: frequency of drug use, potency of the drug itself, dosage consumed, and the setting of use as well as the mind-set of the user. In some cases, physical dependency to heroin develops several months, or as long as a year and a half, after "experimental" use begins.

Unlike the physical trauma frequently associated with the abuse of alcohol and barbiturates, continuing use of heroin and the other opioids does not damage the brain, liver, or heart.[11] However, heroin abusers are subject to numerous life-endangering conditions, because they tend to neglect their health, fail to detect common signs of illness, and frequently resort to intravenous injecting of opioids with shared needles. Commonly observed problems include the transmission of HIV, AIDS, viral hepatitis (hepatitis B virus), inflammation of the heart's lining, blood poisoning, tetanus, malaria, syphilis, blood vessel inflammation, heart valve infection, malnutrition, festering sores on the arms and legs, the toxic effects of overdose, withdrawal syndrome, and even the rare possibility of degenerative nerve damage.

In spite of all these problems, the heroin-dependent individual soon has but two concerns: fear of running out of the drug and fear of running out of accessible veins for injection.

Synthetic Narcotics

In contrast with opioids derived directly or indirectly from sources of natural origin, synthetic narcotics are produced entirely within the laboratory. Some of these are described below. Research has been accelerated to find a drug that retains the analgesic properties of morphine but avoids the dangers of tolerance and physical dependence. To date, no such drug has been synthesized that is not susceptible to abuse.

Meperidine

The very first synthetic narcotic ever produced was *meperidine*. Chemically unlike morphine, it does resemble the opium extract in its analgesic potency. It is used widely today under the brand name Demerol for the relief of moderate to severe pain. Available in pure form and in products containing other medications, it is administered orally or by injection. Tolerance and dependence occur with long-term use, and large doses can result in convulsions.

A designer analogue of meperidine, known for several years as MPPP, was formulated again in 1982 by an "underground" chemist. However, during its production, the derivative of Demerol was accidentally contaminated with a toxic by-product,

named **MPTP** (1-methyl-4-phenyl-4-propionoxypiperidine). This Demoral look-alike, sold in the "street market" as China White, new heroin, or synthetic Demoral, is not easily distinguished from authentic heroin or cocaine.

MPTP is extremely neurotoxic (nerve damaging) and attacks the part of the brain that regulates movement, resulting in permanent symptoms like those of Parkinson's disease. Use of this "designer heroin" causes arthritis-like symptoms at first, such as stiffness, tremors, body seizures, and difficulty in speaking, and eventually results in a stiffening body paralysis.

MPTP and other meperidine derivatives have been sold not only as designer heroin, but also as methamphetamine, PCP, and cocaine (see box 5.2).

Methadone

Synthesized during World War II, **methadone** produces many of the same effects as heroin and morphine. Chemically, it is unlike either of those narcotics. Originally introduced in the United States as an analgesic, methadone was first promoted during the 1960s as a treatment for narcotic-dependent individuals.

The effects of methadone differ considerably from those of morphine-based drugs, in that methadone tends to suppress opioid withdrawal symptoms, shows persistent effects with repeated use, and has a longer duration of action, lasting up to twenty-four hours.[12] Consequently, methadone needs to be given only once a day in heroin detoxification and maintenance programs. Such therapeutic use relieves the physical craving for heroin and prevents both the "high" as well as the onset of **withdrawal symptoms**. The use of methadone in a maintenance therapy program for heroin addicts is described in more detail later in this chapter.

Methadone is nearly as effective when given by mouth as it is by injection. However, tolerance and dependence may occur, and withdrawal symptoms are more prolonged, though they develop more slowly and are less severe, than for most other opioids.

LAAM

Chemically related to methadone, levo-alpha-acetyl-methadol (**LAAM**) is another synthetic narcotic. Recently approved by the Food and Drug Administration for clinical use as a treatment for heroin and other opioid addictions, LAAM has a much longer duration of action—from 48 to 72 hours—than does methadone.[13] This important characteristic permits a reduction in clinic visits and the elimination of take-home medicine in heroin detoxification and methadone maintenance programs.

Propoxyphene

Another close relative of methadone, *propoxyphene* was first marketed in 1959 under the trade name **Darvon**. It has been used for the relief of mild to moderate pain, with millions of prescriptions written each year. Darvon is somewhat less dependence-producing than other opioids and also less effective as an analgesic. This prescription drug is available today in propoxyphene-only preparations as well as in combination with aspirin (Darvon with ASA), with acetaminophen (Darvocet, Wygesic), and with both aspirin and caffeine (Darvon Compound and Darvon Compound-65).

An early controversy has continued up to the present time about Darvon's effectiveness as an analgesic. When it was first manufactured in 1957, Darvon was widely promoted as a safe, nonaddicting substitute for codeine.[14] Since then, the drug has been limited by the U.S. Food and Drug Administration in terms of how, when, and for how long physicians could prescribe the drug. In addition, the FDA has also warned the public about the dangers associated with overdose and combination use of Darvon with other central nervous system depressants, especially alcoholic beverages.

There is no doubt that Darvon is less potent than codeine. In fact, some medical authorities claim that a dose of propoxyphene is less effective than a normal dose of aspirin tablets. Because

box 5.2

Designer Drugs

Narcotics

For many years, illegal drugs have been defined in terms of their chemical formulas. To avoid such legal restrictions and outwit officials of the Drug Enforcement Administration, so-called underground chemists have modified slightly the molecular structure of certain illegal drugs to produce chemical variants or analogues known as "designer drugs." (An analogue is a substance derived from a chemically similar compound.) These chemically engineered analogues can be several hundred times stronger than the drugs they are designed to imitate.

The narcotic analogues—now outlawed—can cause symptoms such as those seen in Parkinson's disease: uncontrollable tremors, drooling, impaired speech, paralysis, and irreversible brain damage.

Type	Street Name	Appearance	Methods of Use
Analogues of fentanyl (narcotic)	Synthetic heroin "China White"	White powder resembling heroin	Inhaled through nasal passages Injected
Analogues of meperidine (narcotic)	Synthetic heroin MPTP (new heroin) MPPP PEPAP	White powder	Inhaled through nasal passages Injected

propoxyphene can be misused and abused, and due to its dependency-producing qualities and potential for accidents and overdoses, Darvon has been placed in Schedule IV of the Controlled Substances Act.

Fentanyl

In 1968 another synthetic narcotic, **fentanyl**, was introduced as an intravenous analgesic-anesthetic. Because of its almost immediate and very short duration of action—about one to two hours—it is used today in surgical procedures for the control of pain.[15]

Marketed under the trade name Sublimaze, fentanyl is an extremely potent drug. A dose of just 0.1 milligram is approximately equivalent in pain-killing activity to 10 milligrams of morphine.[16] In a medical setting, fentanyl is used only by injection. Although there are no legally produced oral forms of this drug, there is evidence that some individuals now abuse fentanyl by smoking or snorting special preparations of this substance.

Due to fentanyl's extreme potency, there is considerable risk of respiratory depression and a significant decrease in blood pressure and heart rate resulting in death. It has been reported that some addicts have died so rapidly after using this drug that when they are found, the needle was still in their arms.[17]

By manipulating the chemical structure of fentanyl, so-called street chemists have created numerous designer heroins or fentanyl analogues, including alpha-methyl fentanyl and 3-methyl fentanyl. Each new "designer" analogue differs in potency, toxicity, and length of action. While each fentanyl derivative mimics heroin's rush and tends to delay or forestall withdrawal symptoms, certain potent analogues have caused sporadic outbreaks of death from overdosage.[18]

Fentanyl derivatives have been sold to unsuspecting drug users under the names "China White," "synthetic heroin," "Mexican Brown," and "Persian White." Available in powder form, these designer drugs are often diluted with lactose, powdered sugar, or mannitol. Sometimes the fentanyl analogues are mixed with heroin to improve somewhat poor quality or with cocaine. The analgesic potency of designer heroin ranges from 200 to 3,000 times stronger than morphine in the human body (see box 5.2).

Endogenous Opioids

Recent investigations into the chemistry of brain function revealed that many natural body chemicals—identified as neurotransmitters in chapter 3—serve as communicators by which certain nerve cells send and receive messages. Some of these endogenous ("made-within the body") chemicals were found to act in much the same way as opioid drugs.

During the 1970s, researchers discovered that morphine appeared to bind or attach to natural receptors (specific sites) in the brain.[19] If such receptors exist, it was reasoned, the body itself must be producing some type of morphine-like chemicals. After intense investigation, scientists discovered natural bodily substances resembling morphine that produce morphine-like effects—euphoria and pain reduction—and also use the same brain receptors as morphine.[20] This linkage of naturally occurring neurochemicals with opioid-like effects provided a new, physical basis for understanding how psychoactive drugs can cause addiction or dependence.

Pertinent research findings related to the **endogenous opioids** (the "morphine within") are summarized below.

1. The specific and rapid effect of narcotic antagonists, or "blockers," such as naloxone (Narcan), suggested that the antagonists and the narcotics (morphine or heroin) were in competition for common attachment sites in the brain.

2. The human brain and gastrointestinal tract were then found to contain specific **receptors** or sites where opioid molecules attach in order to produce the characteristic effects of narcotics. These receptors appear to be concentrated in the limbic system and the thalamus with its associated

box 5.3

New-Wave Narcotics

Heroin appears to be making a big comeback among Americans. Today some young people are scared by the devastating effects of crack cocaine and choose heroin instead. Others prefer the mellower high and cheaper cost of heroin in comparison with crack. With high-purity heroin available now at "bargain basement" prices, snorting or sniffing is "in," while injecting heroin is on the decline. The needle is "out," due to the threat of contracting HIV and AIDS.

But an alarming number of drug abusers also dabble in "new-wave" narcotics—esoteric combinations of two or more psychoactive drugs, one of which is an opioid. Some of these new-wave narcotics are identified below.

Narcotic	Used in Combination With	Anticipated Effects	Common or Street Name
Codeine (from Empirin #4 and Tylenol #4)	Doriden (a CNS depressant)	• Euphoria • Sedation	Loads, Four Doors, Hits
Talwin (partial narcotic antagonist with analgesic effect)	Pyribenzamine (an antihistamine)	• Heroin-like rush with prolonged euphoria	T's and Blues
Heroin	Cocaine (a CNS stimulant)	• Smoother stimulating effect • Reduced excitability after crashing	Speedball, Goofball, Dynamite, Hot Rocks
Heroin	Marijuana (a sedative/psychedelic)	• Euphoria • Relaxation • Pain reduction	Atom Bomb, Dusting
Morphine	Cocaine (a CNS stimulant)	• Smoother stimulating effect • Reduced excitability after crashing	C & M
Heroin	Morphine (a narcotic) and cocaine (a CNS stimulant)	• Smoother stimulating effect • Reduced excitability after crashing	Cottonbrothers

structures—areas of the brain involved with pain perception, emotions, and behavior control.

3. Opioid receptors were originally thought to be attachment sites for some naturally occurring, internal bodily substance resembling a narcotic. Eventually, such substances were extracted from the brain and the pituitary gland and were named **enkephalins** (from the Greek word meaning "in the head").

4. Shortly after enkephalins were identified, another pituitary extract was also found to have opioid activity. This latest chemical was named **endorphin** (the "morphine within"). It was found to be 40 times more powerful than the enkephalins and 100 times more potent than

morphine. The term *endorphin* is now used to describe any natural, internal bodily substance that has opioid-like activity, including the enkephalins and the more recently identified dynorphins, another form of endogenous opioids. These particular endorphins are compounds consisting of amino acids, the building blocks of proteins.[21]

5. These opioid neurotransmitters are thought to be used by the brain to control and moderate emotions.

6. The endorphins (endogenous opioid peptides) can be displaced from the brain by opioid drugs (heroin and morphine) that use the same receptor sites in the brain to reduce an individual's awareness of pain.

With the identification of many endorphins, scientific inquiry has been accelerated in an attempt to explore the likely relationship between these internal morphinelike substances and several scientifically puzzling conditions, as indicated below:

Drug dependence might be an endorphin deficiency. Within a theoretical framework, endorphins act somewhat like hormones (body-regulating chemicals in the blood) in a negative feedback relationship with the pituitary gland. When the concentration of a particular circulating hormone is high, the pituitary gland that triggers the release of the hormone stops production. On the other hand, when the concentration of that same hormone falls below necessary levels, the pituitary speeds up production once again to supply the need.

Applied to drug dependence, this theory suggests that the use of morphine or heroin effectively ties up the receptor sites and fools the natural feedback system. Natural endorphin production is halted. When the external narcotic is also withdrawn, the system experiences an acute shortage of endorphins that cannot be quickly supplied by the manufacturing centers. Thus narcotic withdrawal symptoms appear. It seems likely, then, that long-term use of any narcotic would produce an endorphin shortage. If so, this deficiency could explain the craving for a particular narcotic that exists even after a drug-dependent person goes through withdrawal.

Pain is typically relieved; that is, an individual is enabled to tolerate pain better by the use of some narcotic drug. Endorphins also have potent analgesic effects. Perhaps the endorphins are one's private, internal supply of morphine that is released to alleviate severe pain associated with shock or trauma, including emotional stress.

Placebo relief of pain may be produced by the release of endorphins that act as neurotransmitters on nerve cells to deaden pain. This effect occurs when a pharmacologically inert substance is given to a person instead of an active drug.

Acupuncture, an ancient Chinese procedure for reducing pain and treating various diseases by the insertion of extremely fine needles into the body, might produce its analgesic effect when the inserted needles trigger the brain's production of endorphins.

Schizophrenia, other mental illnesses, and even specific behavioral roles, may be the result of altered endorphin production and function. Though this view is still controversial, some researchers believe that certain symptoms of schizophrenia may be due to either an excess or a deficiency of endorphin activity. Some endorphins have caused hallucinations and are possibly an important factor contributing to a variety of mental illnesses and abnormal mental functioning.

Sexual activity might be related to endorphins that function as regulators of sexual behaviors. People who possess high levels of endogenous (internal) opioids will probably be sexually inactive, but those with low levels should, according to this view, be highly sexual.

The **natural "high"** of exercise is likely the result of increased production of endorphins. People who exercise vigorously often experience a feeling of elation similar to a druglike high. This perceived condition of euphoria is known among joggers as "runner's high" and occurs with regular, sustained exercise.

Researchers now relate physical conditioning with increased blood levels of endorphins. Although still somewhat controversial, these findings suggest that daily exercise (e.g., jogging and running) can be addictive. Joggers frequently complain of unsettled feelings and being out-of-sorts when they miss their daily "fix" of exercise. Without their sustaining endorphins, they experience withdrawal symptoms from the "morphine within." Upon resuming their regular exercise, the joggers' moods and emotions seem to improve with elevation of their endorphin levels.

Continuing scientific investigations suggest that endorphins are fundamental to normal physiological functioning. Endorphins are now thought to influence our "appetite clocks," reproductive hormone cycles, the onset of puberty, pregnancy and labor, and even esthetic and emotional experiences of thrills, laughter, and tears.[22]

Historical and Legal Perspectives

The pursuit of the poppy for recreational purposes as well as medical ones is not of recent origin. Opium use dates back to at least 3000 B.C., when ancient Egyptians derived significant benefits from their "joy plant." It is likely that early Greeks, Romans, and Arabians were aware of both the healing power and the addicting quality of opium.

Over the centuries, the smoking of opium became widespread in much of the Middle East and Far East. By the seventeenth century, opium was firmly established in Europe. A profitable trade between the Orient and Great Britain developed around the exportation and importation of opium. This international arrangement was jeopardized temporarily by the Chinese emperors who attempted to prohibit the cultivation and use of opium through strict antiopium laws, and eventually by the Opium Wars of the nineteenth century.

Until the beginning of the nineteenth century, opium was the sole narcotic. Then in 1806 a German pharmacist, Friedrich Serturner, isolated the principal active ingredient of opium. After using this opium extract, he and his associates named the new drug morphine, after Morpheus, the Greek god of sleep. Although the dangers of opium dependence were well known, the hazards of morphine abuse were not recognized for many years. The new opium extract was hailed as a "wonder drug" in the treatment of pain and relief of diarrhea. Less than fifty years after its initial introduction, the abuse of morphine—and many other drugs—was enhanced by the perfection of the hypodermic syringe.

By the dawn of the twentieth century, the addictiveness of morphine was finally acknowledged. The "cure" had become worse than the diseases for which morphine had been taken. Then in 1898 the Bayer Company of Germany introduced a new "wonder drug." It was derived from morphine, supposedly nonaddicting, and yet more powerful than morphine as an analgesic. Heroin, as the new drug was named, was promoted as a treatment for morphine dependency and withdrawal. The medical profession was slow in recognizing the addictive nature of heroin, while opium and morphine addicts were switching rapidly to heroin as the "drug of choice." Heroin soon reigned supreme and unrestricted.

The first nationwide response to the growing epidemic of narcotic abuse in America was the passage of the original **Pure Food and Drug Act** of 1906. This law prohibited interstate commerce in misbranded and adulterated drugs. A particular target of the law was the secretly formulated "cure-all" patent medicines. Many of these nonprescription drugs contained either opium or morphine in combination with alcohol. Now the drug makers would have to reveal the narcotic contents on the labels of their products and assure the purity of their medicines.

In 1914, the federal government officially entered the area of narcotics control with the enactment of the **Harrison Narcotics Act.**[23] This law established a mechanism of recordkeeping for the importation, manufacture, distribution, sale, and prescription of narcotic drugs. While this effectively outlawed the nonmedical use of heroin, physicians were still allowed to prescribe narcotics; and numerous over-the-counter medications containing small amounts of opium, morphine, heroin, and cocaine were permitted to be sold. Because cocaine was considered to be a "stepping-stone" to heroin abuse, it was mistakenly classified as a narcotic.

With the enactment of the Harrison Narcotics Act, dispensing narcotics to known addicts was forbidden. Clinics that had been established to provide opioid drugs to "registered addicts" on a maintenance or continuing dose level were closed within a few years. These policies effectively ended the medical profession's involvement in the treatment of drug dependency for nearly 40 years. Then, in 1924, the importation of heroin was outlawed. Deprived of medical sources for their supply of narcotics, addicts eventually turned to the black market and to crime to finance their drug dependency. Amazingly, the cultivation of the opium poppy in the United States was not banned by Congress until 1942.

During the decade of the national economic depression, the federal government constructed two narcotics "farms" for the compulsory treatment of criminals convicted of drug addiction. Both facilities also admitted patients on a voluntary basis. Under the direction of the Public Health Service, the hospital "farms" were established in Lexington, Kentucky (1935) and Fort Worth, Texas (1938). Treatment at these hospitals usually consisted of withdrawing the drug-dependent individual by giving progressively smaller doses of

The Narcotic Paradise

During much of the nineteenth century, the United States could properly be called the narcotic's paradise. Millions of people pursued the poppy and its natural and semisynthetic derivatives. The following examples demonstrate the prevalence of narcotic use and abuse during one phase of American history.

Opium was legal and a major ingredient in numerous patent medicines, such as "snake oil," teething syrups for infants, cough medicines, and painkillers.

Physicians legally prescribed opium, then morphine, and—by the end of the century—heroin.

Medications containing opium and morphine could be ordered by mail, if such preparations were not available at groceries and drugstores.

Children were routinely given opium-containing drugs to quiet them down and to treat colic (abdominal pain).

In an age when drinking alcohol was often considered unladylike or too embarrassing, women took narcotic medications in the form of elixirs for

"female troubles" (menstrual cramping and menopausal discomfort).

Alcoholics desiring to give up liquor often took opium or morphine for a quick cure. They were quickly converted from being alcoholics to being "opioidolics."

Opium was legally imported, and later morphine was legally manufactured from opium.

Despite its dependency-producing potential, opium's reputation was quite favorable, as reflected in its nickname—God's Own Medicine, or "G.O.M."

In the United States, morphine was first used extensively during the Civil War (1861–65) as an analgesic for battle wounds. Because tens of thousands of soldiers eventually became drug dependent, morphine addiction was soon known as the "soldier's disease."

When first introduced on the American drug scene, heroin was thought to be a cure for morphine dependence.

Historical Sources: Edward M. Brecher and the editors of *Consumer Reports, Licit and Illicit Drugs*, pages 3–7, Consumers Union, Mt. Vernon, N.Y., 1972; and Michael Burkett, *The History and Use of Opiates: Facts, Myths, Realities*, Do It Now Foundation, Phoenix, Ariz., 1975.

morphine. Such treatment was not generally successful, and many patients returned to addictive behavior soon after discharge.

Until new methods of treating drug dependency were developed in the 1960s, the federal government's policy toward drug abuse was to encourage public compliance with restrictive drug laws. This was to be accomplished by imposing high fines and severe prison sentences for first conviction. Increasingly, the United States relied on its criminal justice system to control and punish the narcotics user. Treatment and prevention concerns were largely ignored.

The present era of drug law enforcement was spearheaded by a federal

government "war on drug abuse" begun in the late 1960s. The **Comprehensive Drug Abuse Prevention and Control Act** of 1970 replaced the crazy-quilt pattern of criminal drug laws and became the legal foundation for reducing the consumption of illicit narcotic and nonnarcotic drugs. Under the provisions of the Controlled Substances Act portion of the legislation, all psychoactive drugs were categorized into five schedules according to their presumed potential for abuse and their current acceptability in medical practice.[24]

Additionally, this legislation established mechanisms for reducing the availability of controlled drugs, procedures for bringing substances under control, penalties for the

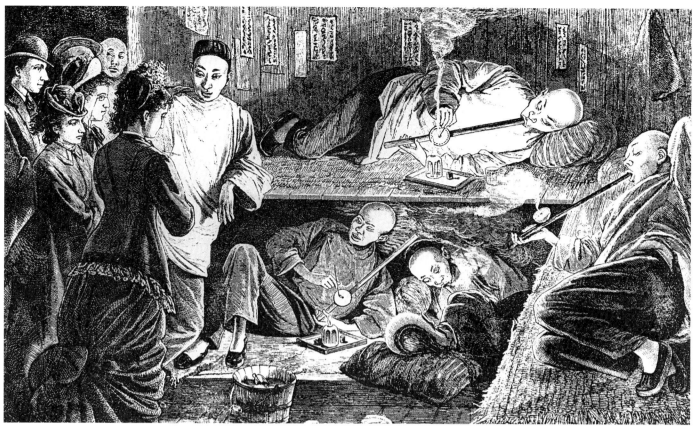

The pursuit of the poppy for recreational purposes is not of recent origin. Shown here are some citizens of San Francisco as they observe newly arrived Chinese immigrants in a popular opium den on Kearney Street in 1878.

The Bettmann Archive

manufacture, distribution, and possession of controlled drugs, criteria for determining control requirements and prescription status, and international obligations for the control of specific drugs. Under the provisions of the Controlled Substances Act, the federal drug bureaucracy was restructured and expanded. In recent years, the drug law-enforcement functions of the federal government have evolved through a series of bureaus, special offices, agencies, and administrations, and are now under the Department of Justice, as described in chapter 13.

Despite the persistent efforts of drug enforcement agencies at all levels of government, it appears practically impossible to forbid entirely the personal use and abuse of illicit drugs in American society. Perhaps there are limits to what laws and law enforcement can achieve in this area of human endeavor.

Treatment of Narcotic-Dependent Individuals

Before 1900, the treatment for opium and morphine dependence consisted of managing the withdrawal syndrome through *detoxification*. In this process, the blood level of the opioid was gradually lowered by decreasing dosages of some opium-based patent medicine in order to wean addicted patients from the more potent opioid drug. Eventually both drugs were completely withdrawn from the body. Occasionally, patients were simply deprived of their drugs and then observed and restrained during the withdrawal process. This sudden withdrawal of a narcotic without medical treatment is often called the "cold turkey" method. The gooseflesh

effect—one of the common withdrawal symptoms—resembles that of a plucked turkey.

Even during those "primitive days" of drug-abuse treatment, it was recognized by many that a permanent cure depended upon the reeducation of the patient's attitude after detoxification had been achieved. However, little attention was paid to the psychological and sociological aspects of the drug-dependence and drug-treatment processes. Until the full effects of the Harrison Narcotics Act were felt, many physicians and even some "walk-in" clinics supplied addicted patients with small "maintenance" doses of narcotics. Such treatment was eventually stopped as provisions of the new federal legislation were implemented.

When the federal government opened the two Public Health Service Hospitals for narcotic-dependent individuals in the 1930s, the major therapeutic effort was the "institutional-aftercare model of treatment." This therapy mandated inpatient hospitalization in a drug-free environment and detoxification. Emphasis was then placed on rebuilding physical health status and providing vocational rehabilitation services, counseling, and various social services. After completing a prescribed time of institutional care in the hospital, the patient returned to the nonmedical community but was closely supervised to ensure total abstinence from narcotics. This supervision was conducted through a parole system in which former patients reported at regular intervals to designated officials.

Currently, several therapies are available for the modern treatment of opioid dependence. These include detoxification; pharmacological treatments, involving maintenance therapy and the use of narcotic antagonists; therapeutic communities; psychotherapy; self-help groups; and acupuncture. Each of these major treatments is described below.[25–29]

Detoxification

Unless an addict is to be placed on a so-called maintenance program, the first and basic treatment is still **detoxification**, as noted earlier in this section. Defined as controlled withdrawal from an opioid under medical supervision, detoxification is only the first step in recovery from narcotics dependence.

Several drugs may be used in the detoxification process to help the addict become drug-free. Oral methadone, better known for its major role in maintenance therapy, is given in progressively smaller doses each day for one to two weeks. This procedure gradually lowers both the blood level of the opioid drug and the tolerance threshold to prevent withdrawal from occurring. Another medication, levo-alpha-acetyl-methadol (LAAM), recently approved, may also be employed for acute detoxification. Within a medical setting, clonidine is sometimes used for rapid detoxification, because this drug suppresses withdrawal symptoms. Although still controversial, buprenorphine shows promise as another drug that may be utilized in the detoxification of opioid-dependent individuals, as well as in maintenance therapy, described below.

Maintenance Therapy

A somewhat controversial form of treating opioid dependence, maintenance therapy involves the continuing use of a drug that is similar in action to the drug for which it substitutes. In this section, two synthetic narcotics—methadone and LAAM—as well as narcotic antagonists are described in relation to maintenance therapy for heroin addiction and other opioid dependencies.

Methadone

A synthetic opioid, **methadone** was developed by German scientists during World War II as a substitute for morphine. In America, methadone was used initially in the detoxification of opioid-dependent patients.

However, methadone was first used on a large-scale basis in the mid 1960s when two physicians, Vincent Dole and Marie Nyswander, pioneered their **methadone maintenance** (continuing use of methadone) program. They recommended that minimal dosages of methadone be used on a regular basis to stabilize heroin patients. This would enable narcotic-dependent individuals to live as functioning members of society, in contrast to the alternating euphoria and desperation associated with illegal heroin use.

Unlike heroin, whose effects last about 4 hours, methadone's effects last approximately 24 hours. Methadone can be administered orally, while heroin is injected intravenously. In effect, methadone use reduces the addict's craving for a drug; eliminates the "rush" of sensation following injection of heroin, as well as the dangers associated with needles; and permits the patient to move toward conventional patterns of living and improved social functioning. Agencies providing such maintenance services also offer extensive counseling and life reeducation programs for the recovering addict.

During the first several weeks of maintenance treatment, patients visit a licensed or registered practitioner six days each week and take liquid oral doses of methadone under supervision. Gradual reduction of the methadone dose is encouraged, although total abstinence from methadone is not always a primary goal.

Critics of maintenance programs view methadone as little more than a substitute of one addictive drug for another. Proponents of such therapy consider methadone maintenance as a lesser evil than heroin dependence. At the very least, methadone permits the heroin addict to abandon a criminal lifestyle, if only for a short time.

Methadone maintenance has certainly had a major impact on the treatment of narcotic addicts. However, it is not a "cure-all." Many people on methadone either continue or start using alcohol or some other dependency-producing drug, thus complicating the therapeutic and rehabilitative processes.

LAAM

Levo-alpha-acetyl-methadol (**LAAM**) is only the second synthetic narcotic drug approved by the Food and Drug Administration to treat heroin and other opioid addictions through outpatient clinic maintenance programs. Like methadone, LAAM blocks the "highs" of other opioids and suppresses the symptoms of withdrawal, such as increased blood pressure and temperature, rapid heartbeat, gooseflesh, runny nose, tremors, insomnia, vomiting, abdominal cramping, restlessness, headaches, and drug craving.

The major advantage of LAAM is that its effects last for 48 to 72 hours after a dose is taken, compared to just 24 hours for methadone. Methadone must be given daily; LAAM use allows patients to reduce their clinic visits to only three per week. Consequently, with fewer required visits to a clinic, patients can lead a more normal life, and clinics have the option to treat more patients than with methadone.

In addition to methadone or LAAM maintenance therapy, licensed clinics and hospitals must also provide comprehensive medical services, counseling, vocational rehabilitation, and general treatment plans for narcotics-dependent patients.

Narcotic Antagonists

Research for an effective analgesic that is not dependency-producing has led recently to the development of a class of chemical compounds known as **narcotic antagonists**. These drugs tend to block and even reverse the effects of narcotics and are therefore useful in treating opioid dependence. Some of these antagonists have analgesic activities, while others totally lack any narcotic action.

Naltrexone and *cyclazocine* chemically prevent heroin from having any effect on the opioid-dependent person, except the shortening of the withdrawal syndrome. Another antagonist, naloxone (Narcan) is used frequently for the treatment of narcotic poisoning, that is, as an antidote for opioid overdose. A "partial antagonist," *pentazocine* (Talwin) provides effective analgesia but also possesses narcotic antagonistic activity. When taken orally, pentazocine has little potential for abuse. Intravenous self-administration, however, has led to instances of drug dependence. Nevertheless, the narcotic antagonists seem to be ideally suited for individuals who wish to leave therapies such as methadone maintenance and therapeutic communities.

Therapeutic Communities

The concept of drug-free **therapeutic communities**, directed by ex-addicts, was first established in 1958 as a basic treatment for narcotic and other drug dependencies. This approach to therapy was based on the belief that only former addicts could break through the shell of projection, denial, and lying common to the narcotics addict. The ultimate goal of such residential communities is to enable an addicted individual to develop a socially productive, drug-free lifestyle.

Synanon, the original such community, was founded in Los Angeles, California, by Chuck Dederich in 1958. Somewhat controversial, hostile encounter sessions called "Synanon Games" became a central feature of this program. Former addicts were used as role models for patients, who were provided communal support for human error, human alienation, and mental and physical dysfunction through the process of group therapy.

In addition to encounter group therapy, these communities also used tutorial learning sessions, remedial and formal education classes, assignment of jobs within the residence, and eventually "living-out" situations within the local community. Those who entered the Synanon program became committed to a drug-free, highly disciplined lifestyle and to indefinite residence in the Synanon facility.

Before long, other residential therapeutic communities developed, such as Daytop Village, Phoenix House, and Gateway House. Some of the more recent communities have even added degreed professionals to their staffs to complement the nondegreed former addicts and alcohol abusers. However, all of these groups have maintained their hostility to the use of drugs for either "withdrawal" or "maintenance." Additionally, all have programs of varying lengths aimed at changing personal lifestyle patterns of self-destructive behavior. The basic goal of therapeutic communities is to bring about a change in living—specifically, abstinence from drugs, elimination of criminal behavior, and development of employable skills, self-reliance, and personal honesty.

In recent years, therapeutic communities have begun to serve criminal offenders and socially disadvantaged people, including the unemployed and newly arrived immigrants, in addition to drug abusers.

Psychotherapeutic Approaches

In general, **psychotherapy** is any form of treatment that uses psychological, rather than physical, means or medications in helping patients cope with various mental problems and mental disorders. Psychotherapeutic procedures feature verbal and nonverbal communication between a patient (or client) and a trained therapist. Goals of verbal therapy attempt to promote deeper self-understanding, provide insights into oneself and one's personal meaning, and bring disturbed and dysfunctional people into closer contact with the split elements of their mental lives. Such therapy tends to analyze and then resynthesize the self and also permits the individual to vent rage, frustration, and hate without fear of condemnation.

Psychotherapy has recently expanded beyond inner conflicts and unconscious drives and now deals with interpersonal relationships and events outside the self. Several forms of group therapy and family therapy have evolved from this new approach. For instance, an individual's problems are frequently viewed as being rooted in relationships with others, especially family members. Thus the entire family becomes involved in treatment. Role-playing, in which individuals assume different characters within the family for purposes of expression and interpretation of behavior, is one technique sometimes utilized in family therapy.

Because heroin addicts often display antisocial personality traits, have difficulty forming meaningful relationships, and are frequently aggressive and manipulative, psychotherapeutic procedures have severe limitations. Indeed, psychotherapy is not a panacea in treating opioid-dependent individuals. Yet some patients have benefited from such techniques as well as from less-structured counseling provided by recovering addicts or other trained therapists at drug-free outpatient clinics. In many instances, psychotherapeutic techniques have been combined successfully with other treatment approaches.

Narcotics Anonymous

Over the past forty years, many self-help groups have been formed in which recovering addicts offer help to others seeking recovery from opioid dependence. In Narcotics Anonymous (NA), members employ a twelve-step program similar to that of Alcoholics Anonymous. On a voluntary basis, NA members meet regularly to promote and stabilize their own recovery. Founded in 1953, Narcotics Anonymous now has close to four thousand groups in the United States and throughout the world. (See box 5.5.)

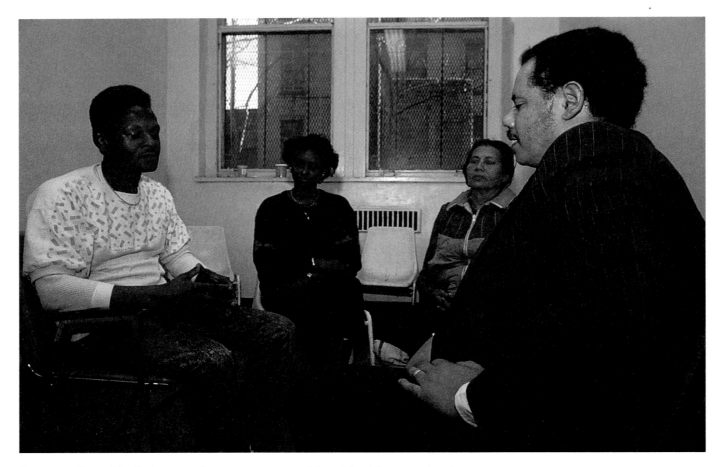

Group counseling and family therapy are important components of the multimodality approach to the treatment of narcotics dependency. Pictured here are former heroin addicts who are now alcoholics in a counseling session at a methadone clinic.

© J. Griffin/The Image Works

Acupuncture

Recently, a form of alternative medicine has emerged on the health care scene. The ancient art of acupuncture, as practiced in Asia for thousands of years, has generated considerable interest among physicians and dentists, and it might have some beneficial application in the treatment of heroin addiction.

According to the traditional Chinese definition, acupuncture is a procedure of treating certain diseases and alleviating pain by the insertion of extremely fine needles into the human body at specific points called loci. After initial insertion, which causes only a slight feeling of soreness and swelling, the stainless steel or copper needles are twisted for varying lengths of time by manual twirling or by electrical stimulation.

Since the introduction of acupuncture into the United States in the 1970s, scientific investigations have been undertaken to learn more about its therapeutic applications. Specifically, its use in reducing the pain of withdrawal from heroin has been researched, as has the procedure's seeming ability to relieve chronic pain and to produce surgical anesthesia. However, to date, the precise mechanism of acupuncture's effectiveness has not been established.

According to traditional Chinese medicine, stimulation of points, or loci, along a channel, or meridian, close to the skin surface supposedly affects the internal organs attached to that particular channel. Stimulation is provided by the insertion of needles in a patient's skin. Such action allegedly restores a balance in the flow of vital energy throughout the

channels and various bodily organs. Western medical researchers generally dismiss this unscientific explanation for the apparent functions of acupuncture. The efficacy of acupuncture, they contend, is likely based on the inserted needles' interference with the transmission of pain signals from the body to the brain or the brain's production of painkilling neurochemicals, the endorphins.

A Multimodality Approach to Treatment

It is apparent that at the present time there is no single therapy for all opioid dependents. It is also recognized that the most important predictor of therapeutic success is time spent in treatment. Consequently, the individual addict must be matched with an individualized comprehensive

box 5.5

Narcotics Anonymous

Narcotics Anonymous (NA) is a fellowship of men and women learning to live without drugs. The NA program is one of complete abstinence from all drugs and its primary purpose is to bring the message of recovery to other addicts. Although NA is not a religious organization, its programs consists of a set of spiritual principles through which members recover from an apparently hopeless state of mind and body.

There is just one requirement for membership—the desire to stop using drugs. However, the members are guided along their way to recovery by the Twelve Steps of Narcotics Anonymous and the fellowship meetings where interacting with, talking with, and helping other addicts become the very means of staying clean from drugs. Members believe that their addiction provides a common ground for understanding one another and for handling their painful past.

According to the Twelve Step program of NA, members admit their powerlessness over their addiction and come to believe that a power greater than themselves could restore them to sanity. Basic to recovery from addiction are two healing forces—forgiveness and gratitude—that are learned by practicing the Twelve Steps of Narcotics Anonymous. Forgiveness releases the grip others have on recovering addicts for real or imagined wrongs. Gratitude for being clean helps recovering addicts to break old habits that promoted the continuing use of drugs.

Source: Modified from *Treatment to N.A.* Hazelden Foundation, Center City, Minn., 1988.

therapeutic program to assure maximum effect. A **multimodality therapeutic approach**, one with several components or aspects, would properly identify a full range of treatment services to meet the physical, mental, social, and spiritual needs of each patient. Such a comprehensive program might include the following:

Rapid admission to a health care facility on a voluntary or compulsory basis for necessary medical care, including emergency procedures.

Detoxification under supervision, with or without the use of other drugs to ease the discomfort of withdrawal.

Medical services, including tuberculosis skin testing, HIV counseling, and random urine testing for drugs of abuse. In maintenance programs, individualized dosage will be determined to control withdrawal symptoms without causing sedation or other effects of intoxication.

Extensive vocational rehabilitation leading to the acquisition of job skills that, in turn, will improve the self-image of the individual and provide the basis for independent living.

Transitional care in a "halfway house" or a residential center until the patient is ready for complete, full-time reentry into the community.

Long-term outpatient care provided in a hospital, public clinic, or day center, offering counseling, casework, psychotherapy, spiritual renewal, and the optional use of methadone maintenance or narcotic antagonists.

Provision of emergency services through "crash pads," information and referral centers, free clinics, telephone hot lines, as well as in hospital emergency rooms.

The Intervention Process

A desirable element of any treatment program is the drug abuser's willingness to cooperate with those who can help. This willingness is not usually present at first and is often difficult to achieve. Indeed, for many years it was firmly believed that no treatment could be effective unless drug abusers wanted to change their lives and truly sought out help on their own. Only then were these people ready for treatment.

Before such a state of "psychological and spiritual readiness" was reached, drug-dependent individuals presumably had to "hit bottom;" they had to recognize the seriousness of their dependency, admit their need for help, and ask for help. Frequently, this recognition followed the breakdown of elaborate psychological defense mechanisms that allowed the addicts to deny their need for assistance, and it was often reached only after loss of health, family and friends, job, and self-respect. Between the proverbial "devil and the deep blue sea," the drug abuser was now ready for help.

One of the most significant developments in the substance abuse field during the past several years was the discovery that drug abusers, including alcoholics, do not always have to wait to "hit bottom" before they can be helped. A relatively new process, referred to as **intervention**, can now be implemented to help drug abusers identify their need for making lifestyle changes and for seeking help for their drug problems before "hitting bottom." Intervention helps a drug-dependent person become aware of and desire the path to recovery.

The process of intervention involves compassionate communication in which family members and friends of the drug-dependent person describe and explain the adverse consequences of continued drug abuse as they experience them. Through planned and rehearsed nonjudgmental confrontation, a directed self-evaluation of the drug abuser, identification of treatment options, and a statement of expectation on the part of family members, the intervention process can interrupt drug abuse and drug dependence before they progress to their most devastating phase. The intervention process is described more fully in chapter 13 as a secondary prevention technique.

Chapter Summary

1. Narcotics are psychoactive drugs that induce sleep and relieve pain. Derived from the opium poppy plant or made synthetically to have narcotic drug actions, these drugs are also known as opioids or opiates.

2. Opioids are classified as natural substances, semisynthetic narcotics, synthetic products, and, more recently, internal bodily substances (endogenous opioids) that have opioidlike effects within the human body.

3. Continuing use of opioids frequently leads to opioid dependence—inability to stop usage, constant or repeated intoxication, overdoses, tolerance, and withdrawal symptoms—often described as addiction.

4. Certain narcotics have legitimate medical uses. Morphine sedates and relieves pain; codeine acts as an antitussive; dihydromorphinone (Dilaudid) is a powerful analgesic; and methadone and LAAM are used in treating heroin-dependent individuals.

5. Heroin, a powerful, dependency-producing derivative of morphine, is considered the most frequently abused narcotic in America.

6. Many physical dangers associated with heroin abuse are related to uncertain dosage levels, use of unsterile needles for injection, contaminants in the heroin sample used, and the combination use of heroin with barbiturates and/or alcohol.

7. Heroin withdrawal, though not usually fatal, can be very painful and includes sweating, tearing, tremors, chills, diarrhea, nausea, sharp abdominal and leg cramps, mental depression, and insomnia.

8. Research has revealed the existence of natural, internal bodily chemicals (endogenous opioids) that have opioidlike effects. Known as endorphins, or "the morphine within" the head or body, these substances are thought to possibly be related to drug dependence (a deficiency of endorphins), toleration of pain, acupuncture, mental illness, and the natural "high" of vigorous exercise.

9. The widespread and indiscriminate therapeutic use of opium, morphine, and heroin (especially in "patent medicines"), in the nineteenth and early twentieth centuries in America, led to enactment of the Federal Pure Food and Drug Act of 1906 and the Harrison Narcotics Act of 1914.

10. Presently, the legal foundation for reducing the illicit use of narcotic and nonnarcotic drugs is the Comprehensive Drug Abuse Prevention and Control Act of 1970. This drug law categorizes most psychoactive drugs into five schedules of decreasing restrictiveness according to their presumed potential for abuse and current acceptability in medical practice.

11. Treatment of opioid dependency might involve detoxification and psychotherapy, participation in therapeutic communities, admission to methadone or LAAM maintenance programs, and use of narcotic antagonists. Sometimes the intervention process is used to help drug abusers discover their need for help before their drug dependency progresses to an advanced state.

12. A multimodality approach to treating opioid dependency meets various physical, mental, social, and spiritual needs of addicts through rapid admission for medical care, supervised detoxification, placement in a halfway house or long-term outpatient clinic program, extensive counseling and psychotherapy, and a spiritual reawakening often achieved through participation in Narcotics Anonymous. Sometimes methadone or LAAM maintenance or narcotic antagonists are also employed.

Review Questions and Activities

1. In what ways are the various narcotic drugs classified?

2. What are the major drug actions or effects of opioids?

3. Describe some of the legitimate therapeutic uses of the opioids—specifically, morphine, codeine, and methadone.

4. Distinguish between the heroin "rush" and the heroin "high."

5. Explain why there are so many physical dangers associated with heroin abuse, since heroin itself does not usually cause long-term physical damage or illness.

6. Interview a local police officer who specializes in narcotics investigations and related criminal offenses. Do narcotics violations involve illegal drugs other than the opioids? Are narcotics a significant part of the "drug scene" in your community or not? Explain.

7. Investigate the lives and works of poet Samuel Taylor Coleridge and author Thomas De Quincey and their involvement with laudanum (tincture of opium).

8. Report on one or more of the following literary works dealing with opioids: Dean Latimer and Jeff Goldberg's *Flowers in the Blood: The Story of Opium* (New York: Franklin Watts, 1981); Richard Ashley's *Heroin: The Myths and the Facts* (New York: St. Martin's Press, 1972); Arnold Trebach's *The Heroin Solution* (New Haven: Yale University Press, 1982); Jean Cocteau's *Opium: The Diary of a Cure* (New York: Grove Press, 1980); Nelson Algren's *The Man with the Golden Arm* (New York: Penguin, 1977); Peter Maas's *China White* (New York: Simon & Schuster, 1994).

9. Explain how opioids such as methadone and LAAM can be used in the treatment of heroin dependency.

10. Discuss the probable relationship between the endorphins and drug dependence as well as general physiological functioning.

11. Describe the use of opium, morphine, and heroin as therapeutic drugs during the part of American history before the enactment of the Harrison Narcotics Act and the Comprehensive Drug Abuse Prevention and Control Act.

12. What factors are thought to play a part in the development of opioid dependency?

13. What are the unique features of a "therapeutic community" as a treatment approach to drug dependency?

14. How does a methadone maintenance program work as a treatment for heroin dependency?

15. What would likely happen if an individual no longer dependent on an opioid were to take a narcotic antagonist?

16. How does an opioid detoxification program differ from the "cold turkey" treatment?

17. Do you believe that psychotherapy and Narcotics Anonymous are effective means of reducing opioid abuse? Explain.

18. What opioid-like drugs have been identified as "China White" on the illegal street market?

References

1. Lester Grinspoon and James Bakalar, *The Harvard Medical School Mental Health Review: Drug Abuse and Addiction* (Boston: Harvard Mental Health Letter, 1993), 25.
2. Robert Julien, *A Primer of Drug Action* (New York: W. H. Freeman, 1992), 194.
3. Jerome Jaffe and William Martin, "Opioid Analgesics and Antagonists," chapter 21 in *Goodman and Gilman's The Pharmacological Basis of Therapeutics*, 8th ed., ed. A. G. Gilman, T. W. Rall, A. S. Nies, and P. Taylor (New York: McGraw-Hill, 1990), 489.
4. Grinspoon and Bakalar, *The Harvard Medical School Mental Health Review*, 25.
5. Unless otherwise indicated, the basic description of the opioid drugs is derived from Drug Enforcement Administration, U.S. Department of Justice, *Drugs of Abuse* (Washington, D.C.: U.S. Government Printing Office, 1989), 12–23.
6. Editors of Consumer Reports Books, *The New Medicine Show* (Mount Vernon, N.Y.: Consumers Union, 1989), 27.
7. *Physicians' Desk Reference*, 48th ed. (Montvale, N.J.: Medical Economic Data Production Company, 1994), 1902, 2038, 2665.
8. Peter Maas, "The Menace of China White," *Parade*, 18 September 1994, 46.
9. Peter Maas, *China White* (New York: Simon & Schuster, 1994).
10. "Heroin's New Purity Creates New Customers: Snorters," *Substance Abuse Report* 24, no. 24 (15 December 1993), 1–3.
11. Grinspoon and Bakalar, *The Harvard Medical School Mental Health Review*, 25.
12. Joseph Ternes and Charles O'Brien, "The Opioids: Abuse Liability and Treatments for Dependence," *Addiction Potential of Abused Drugs and Drug Classes* (New York: Haworth Press, 1990), 27–45.
13. Deborah Goodman, "Heroin Addiction— From Research to Treatment: SAMHSA Leads the Way," *Substance Abuse and Mental Health Services Administration SAMHSA News* 2, no. 2 (spring 1994), 8, 15.
14. Jim Parker, *Darvon, Darvocet, and Other Prescription Narcotics* (Tempe, Ariz.: Do It Now, 1990), 2–3.
15. Harold Doweiko, *Concepts of Chemical Dependency*, 2d ed. (Pacific Grove, Calif.: Brooks/Cole, 1993), 118–19.
16. *Physicians' Desk Reference*, 1098.
17. Doweiko, *Concepts of Chemical Dependency*, 119.
18. Jerome Jaffe, "Drug Addiction and Drug Abuse," chapter 22 in *Goodman and Gilman's The Pharmacological Basis of Therapeutics*, 8th ed., ed. A. G. Gilman, T. W. Rall, A. S. Nies, and P. Taylor (New York: McGraw-Hill, 1990), 559.
19. Tibor Palfai and Henry Jankiewicz, *Drugs and Human Behavior* (Dubuque, Iowa: Brown & Benchmark, 1991), 153.
20. Andrew Weil and Winifred Rosen, *From Chocolate to Morphine*, rev. ed. (Boston: Houghton Mifflin, 1993), 28–29.
21. Grinspoon and Bakalar, *The Harvard Medical School Mental Health Review*, 24.
22. Janet Hopson, "A Pleasurable Chemistry," *Annual Editions: Drugs, Society, and Behavior 94/95* (Guilford, Conn.: Dushkin, 1994), 59–62. (Reprinted from *Psychology Today*, July–August 1988, 29–30, 32–33.)
23. Bureau of Justice Statistics, U.S. Department of Justice, *Drugs, Crime, and the Justice System: A National Report* (Washington, D.C.: U.S. Government Printing Office, 1992), 80.
24. Ibid., 82, 84.
25. Barry Stimmel and the Editors of Consumer Reports Books, *The Facts about Drug Use: Coping with Drugs and Alcohol in Your Family, at Work, in Your Community* (New York: Haworth Medical Press, 1993), 155–70.
26. "Pharmacological Treatments for Opiate Dependence: Methadone and More," *Substance Abuse Report* 25, no. 1 (1 January 1994): 1–2.
27. "Maintenance Pharmacotherapy: Turning Addicts into Taxpayers," *Substance Abuse Report* 25, no. 12 (15 June 1994): 3.
28. "How Pharmacotherapies Work: Agonists and Antagonists," *Substance Abuse Report* 25, no. 1 (15 June 1994): 4–5.
29. Dixie Farley, "New Drug Approval Approach Boosts Fight against Heroin Addiction," *FDA Consumer* 28, no. 9 (November 1994): 11–15.

chapter

6

sedative-hypnotics

The Other Depressants

Antianxiety Agent
Appetitive Drug Use
Automatism
Barbiturate
Benzodiazepine
Bromide
Cross-Dependence
Cross-Tolerance
Depressant
Escape-Avoidance Drug Use
Flurazepam
Hypnotic
Inhalant
Major Tranquilizer
Methaqualone
Minor Tranquilizer
Potentiating Drug Interaction
Rauwolfia serpentina
Reserpine
Sedative
Sedativism
Synergistic Drug Interaction
Triazolam
Valium
Xanax

chapter objectives

After you have studied this chapter, you should be able to do the following:

1. Describe the general pharmacological effects of the sedative-hypnotic drugs.

2. Identify the major types or families of psychoactive drugs that are central nervous system depressants and also produce a calming effect, induce euphoric intoxication, and promote sleep.

3. Explain why sedative-hypnotics are frequently misused and abused.

4. Differentiate between appetitive motivations and escape-avoidance motivations in relation to the use of sedative-hypnotics.

5. Describe the general characteristics shared by nearly all of the sedative-hypnotics.

6. Distinguish between potentiating and synergistic drug interactions.

7. Define the following terms: *cross-tolerance, cross-dependence,* Rauwolfia serpentina, *automatism,* and *maximum tolerance level.*

8. Explain how automatism and maximum tolerance level may be contributing factors to barbiturate overdose.

9. Describe the process of barbiturate withdrawal.

10. Identify three nonbarbiturate sedative-hypnotics.

11. Discuss the brief history of the popularity of methaqualone (Quaalude) as a recreational drug.

12. Distinguish major tranquilizers from minor tranquilizers in terms of their drug actions.

13. List five brand names of antianxiety drugs.

14. Discuss the alleged controversies surrounding the use of antianxiety drugs in the general population.

15. Explain why many young people may become involved in the abuse of inhalants.

16. Identify three inhalants that have become popular among some adults.

Introduction

This chapter examines those psychoactive drugs that have been used to restore sleep to the sleepless and to calm the anxious patient—persistent goals of medical practice. When chemical alternatives to the opioids were developed, there was international praise for the new drugs that would help people achieve what the narcotics could not bring—tranquilization by day and relaxing sleep by night. It was not long, however, before the new sleep inducers and antianxiety agents were found to have serious and sometimes health-threatening characteristics.

When taking less than sleep-inducing doses of these new drugs, many people experienced a pleasant, euphoric state of intoxication, known as a "high." This calm "high," achieved through the "downer" drugs, soon became the focal point for millions of recreational drug abusers. At last, one could get drunk without booze!

These depressant, nonalcoholic, nonopioid drugs—barbiturates and nonbarbiturate sedative-hypnotics, the antianxiety minor tranquilizers, and the inhalants—are the major focus of this chapter, along with the people who use them and abuse them.

6.1 Depressants: Sedative-Hypnotic Drugs and Inhalants

Barbiturates	Inhalants
Amobarbital (Amytal)*	Benzene
Butabarbital (Butisol)	Butane
Hexobarbital (Sombucaps)	Gasoline
Phenobarbital (Luminal)	Toluene
Secobarbital (Seconal)	Naphtha
Pentobarbital (Nembutal)	Carbon tetrachloride
Amobarbital/Secobarbital (Tuinal)	Acetone
	Methyl ethyl ketone
Minor Tranquilizers	Freons
	Propane
Meprobamate (Miltown, Equanil)	Nitrous oxide
Benzodiazepines	Amyl nitrite, butyl nitrite
Alprazolam (Xanax)	Organic nitrogen room odorizers
Chloridazepoxide (Librium)	
Clonazepam (Clonopin)	**Major Tranquilizers**
Clorazepate (Tranxene)	
Diazepam (Valium)	Reserpine (Serpasil)
Flurazepam (Dalmane)†	Phenothiazines
Lorazepam (Ativan)	Chlorpromazine (Thorazine)
Oxazepam (Serex)	Prochlorperazine (Compazine)
Prazepam (Centrax)	Mesoridazine (Serentil)
Temazepam (Restoril)†	Butaperazine (Repoise)
Triazolam (Halcion)†	Thioridazine (Mellaril)
	Haloperidol (Haldol)
Nonbarbiturate Sedative-Hypnotics	
Chloral hydrate (Noctec)	
Glutethimide (Doriden)	
Methaqualone	
Methyprylon (Noludar)	
Ethchlorvynol (Placidyl)	

*Common trade names occur within parentheses. Many of these drugs are sold under a variety of trade names.

† These drugs are used almost exclusively as a bedtime sedative to induce sleep.

Drugs That Calm and Promote Sleep

Drugs that slow down mental and physical functions of the body are known generally as central nervous system (CNS) **depressants**. Because these chemical agents tend to produce a calming effect, relax muscles, and relieve feelings of tension, anxiety, and irritability, they are also described as having a sedative or sedating effect. Such drugs are referred to as **sedatives**.

At higher dose levels, sedatives also produce drowsiness and eventually a state resembling natural sleep. Drugs that have such a sleep-inducing effect are called **hypnotics**. This hypnotic effect has nothing whatsoever to do with the artificially induced state of suggestibility often associated with the word *hypnosis*. Nevertheless, the combination term *sedative-hypnotic* appropriately identifies the major pharmacological effects of these drugs. In reality, almost any drug that calms, soothes, and reduces anxiety is also capable of relieving insomnia (sleeplessness).[1]

Ethyl alcohol and the narcotic analgesics, such as morphine and heroin, are also classified as CNS depressants but are discussed in separate chapters. Along with the sedative-hypnotics, they are considered "down" drugs, or "downers," as they too decrease activity and reduce excitement. Having limited therapeutic applications today, alcohol has achieved near-universal acceptance as a recreational drug. Thus it deserves special consideration in this text as America's number one psychoactive drug and number one drug problem. Although the narcotics and the sedative-hypnotics share many of the same actions, the latter drugs have no practical pain-relieving properties. Unlike the narcotics, intoxicating doses of the sedative-hypnotics almost always result in impaired judgment, slurred speech, and loss of motor coordination.

Due to chemical differences, the sedative-hypnotics include several related families of drugs having common characteristics but somewhat diverse effects and therapeutic uses. The family members of the sedative-hypnotic classification are (1) barbiturates, (2) nonbarbiturate sedative-hypnotics, (3) minor tranquilizers, and (4) abused inhalants that have mind-changing actions similar to those of alcohol, barbiturates, and benzodiazepines.[2] Because their abuse potential is so high, all but the inhalants are strictly regulated under the provisions of the Controlled Substances Act. The prescribed sedative-hypnotics and commonly abused volatile solvents and chemicals are listed in table 6.1, along with examples of common trade-name drugs.

A fifth family member, the **major tranquilizers** or antipsychotics, are also sedative-hypnotics. Unlike the minor tranquilizers, these major antipsychotics are not controlled drug substances. Moreover, these major tranquilizers produce their desired effect almost exclusively among psychotic patients, have virtually no addictive potential, and are not typically abused substances.

Sedative-hypnotics are among the most widely prescribed psychoactives in the United States. Taken under medical supervision, they have improved the quality of life for millions of people.

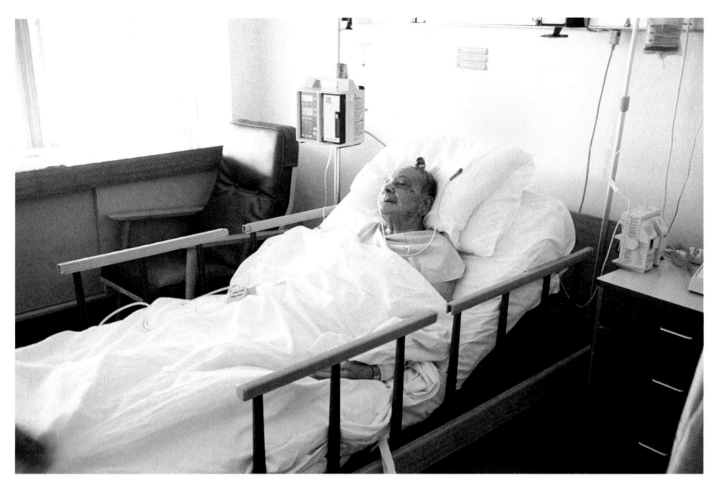

Many elderly people have used sedative-hypnotic drugs for years to relieve minor anxieties and to secure proper sleep—an unrelenting human desire. Such persistent dependence on these drugs is broken only upon hospitalization.

© Tony Freeman/PhotoEdit

Beneficially employed for the specific treatment of insomnia and the relief of anxiety and tension, the sedative-hypnotics have also become important additions to surgical anesthesia because of their sleep-inducing actions. One drug, phenobarbital, is often the drug of choice in controlling grand mal epileptic seizures.

Although their use in medical practice has declined steadily and rather significantly over the past twenty years, barbiturates are still used as surgical anesthetics but only occasionally as sleeping pills. Specific barbiturates designated as "short-acting" and "intermediate-acting" were once the favorites of drug abusers. However, with a reduction in their prescription and manufacture, barbiturates are not as likely to be diverted from approved medical use today.

Among the most frequently abused nonbarbiturates are glutethimide (Doriden), methyprylon (Noludar), ethchlorvynol (Placidyl), and, until its United States production ceased in 1983, methaqualone (Quaalude, Sopor)—all prescribed to induce sleep. Benzodiazepines (frequently used minor tranquilizers) are often prescribed as antianxiety medicines as well as sleep-promoting medications. These tranquilizers are commonly abused, typically by individuals who want to counteract the unpleasant, or enhance the pleasant, effects of another drug that is actually more highly valued, such as alcohol, an opioid, or a stimulant.[3]

Motivational Factors in Misuse and Abuse

The unrelenting human quest for sleep, along with physicians' over prescription of "sleeping pills," is the basis for much misuse and abuse of the sedative-hypnotics. People who have difficulty sleeping or who have trouble coping with stress, the pressures of modern living or anxiety, sometimes overuse or become dependent on sedatives. Patients on prescribed barbiturates soon discover that taking smaller doses produces a feeling of drowsy well-being while still awake. Similar to the pleasant feelings of alcohol intoxication, the response attracts those who do not really need these drugs and promotes overuse by those who do.

Misuse of the sedative-hypnotics is thought to be quite extensive. Many people, especially the elderly, have used these drugs for years—out of habit or by tradition—to relieve minor anxieties and to secure "proper" sleep. Such prolonged drug taking is often preferred by patients to eliminate the underlying causes of their fears and the ensuing insomnia.

Recreational drug use often includes a desire for some pleasure or an escape from worry. Certain individuals value the feelings of relaxation and tranquility, the sensation of decreased tension, and the tingling euphoria resulting from use of the sedative-hypnotics. The enjoyment of such effects describes **appetitive drug use**, or drug-taking behavior motivated by the hunger or desire for pleasurable responses and sensations. While others may also enjoy the various pleasures of intoxication, their primary concern in drug taking is, by contrast, to get relief from unpleasant sensations, tension, disturbed interpersonal relationships, fears, and anxieties. Such motivation for taking drugs is called **escape-avoidance drug use**. These two basic motivations—desire for pleasure (appetite use) and relief from tension (escape-avoidance use)—represent the extremes on a spectrum of psychological factors that give rise to drug-taking behavior.

As with alcohol, sedative-hypnotic intoxication can also bring about a temporary period of disinhibition. Desirable social behaviors may vanish, and internal feelings of anger, rage, and even depression may be released. Contrary to common belief, this emotional upheaval is sometimes enjoyed by drug takers.

On occasion, heroin abusers take sedative-hypnotics to potentiate the effects of narcotics. Stimulant users often take sedatives to moderate or offset the undesirable, jittery feelings that stimulants produce. Alcoholic beverages are also used together with various sedative-hypnotics, especially the minor tranquilizers.

Whether they are used for recreation, self-medication, or merely to prevent withdrawal symptoms, the depressant drugs are frequently taken with little consideration of possible adverse consequences. Moreover, they are often acquired not only within a legitimate and supervised patient-physician relationship, but also as a result of illicit prescribing, inadequate medical supervision of a patient's medical condition, and patient manipulation of the prescriber. Nonprescription channels of acquiring these drugs include thefts at the retail or wholesale levels, prescription forgeries, smuggling, illegal manufacture, and "street sales."

General Characteristics

Several effects of the sedative-hypnotics are shared by nearly all drugs in this classification because of their pharmacologic similarity.[4]

1. These sedative-hypnotics tend to produce a *widespread depression,* or slowing down of the brain and central nervous system, including a reduction in the state of wakefulness. Used primarily for their calming and sleep-inducing effects, they are prescribed variously as antiepileptic agents, muscle relaxants, and antianxiety drugs. Some of the sedative-hypnotics are used to produce general anesthesia, that is, drug-induced absence of all sensation.

2. With increasing dosage, nearly all of these drugs produce a variety of behavioral alterations in a continuum of sedation. Beginning with relief from anxiety at low doses, the behavior progresses to disinhibition (a state of euphoria), sedation, hypnosis, general anesthesia, coma, and then, at high doses, death, resulting from depression of the brain's respiratory center. It should be noted, however, that the benzodiazepines do not induce general anesthesia.

3. The combined effects of sedative-hypnotics can be described as both *additive* and *potentiating* or *synergistic* with respect to depressant characteristics, described in chapter 3. Both **potentiating** and **synergistic drug interactions** result in an exaggerated depressant effect on the central nervous system when sedative-hypnotics, narcotics, or ethyl alcohol are taken in combination. As such, these two descriptive terms are often used interchangeably. (More precisely, potentiation involves one drug's intensifying the action of another, while synergism describes the cooperative, facilitative, supraadditive effect of two or more drugs that have the same drug action.) The combination use of barbiturates and alcohol or two or more sedative-hypnotics—a common practice for those who want to increase the "high"—contributes frequently to the problem of drug overdose and even death.

4. With repeated use over a prolonged period of time, these drugs are capable of inducing *psychological dependence, tolerance,* and *physiological dependence.* Such dependency on sedative-type psychoactive drugs has become known as **sedativism**, an all-too-common American affliction.

5. To a remarkable degree, both **cross-tolerance** and **cross-dependence** are exhibited by the sedative-hypnotics. In cross-tolerance, the tolerance to one drug, *A,* results in a lessened or reduced pharmacological response to another, *B* of the same drug class, even though the person never used drug *B* before. By contrast, cross-dependence is a condition in which one drug can prevent withdrawal symptoms associated with physiological dependence on a different drug. Significantly, any sedative-hypnotic can be substituted for any other in the same drug class.

Historical Perspectives

The use of depressant drugs has its origin in antiquity. For legitimate as well as sinister purposes, secret potions of herbs, opium, alcohol, or cannabis were employed to induce both stupor and sleep. Although the legendary oracle of Delphi—an ancient Greek priestess—did not know the precise scientific reasons for carbon dioxide's effects, the inhaled gas permitted her to make her predictions in a trancelike state. During the nineteenth century, "ether frolics," "chloroform jags," and nitrous oxide ("laughing gas") demonstrations popularized the inhalation of vapors to produce an altered state of consciousness.

Rauwolfia serpentina, the Indian snakeroot shrub common to India and Southeast Asia, had been used for centuries to treat many diseases, including high blood pressure and even mental disorders. It was not until the 1950s that *Rauwolfia's* active ingredient, **reserpine**, was used clinically as an antipsychotic agent. Reserpine ushered in the age of the "major tranquilizers," which revolutionized treatment of the mentally ill. Because of reserpine's adverse side effects, the derivative of the Indian snakeroot was soon replaced by the phenothiazine family of antipsychotic agents.

The very first drug introduced as a sedative-hypnotic was **bromide**. In the 1860s, potassium bromide entered the practice of medicine as a treatment for epileptic convulsions. Due to its irritating effects on the gastrointestinal tract and its tendency to accumulate in the body, leading to chronic bromide intoxication (bromism), bromide was replaced by the barbiturates upon their introduction in the early 1900s.

Synthesized first in 1862, barbiturates were initially utilized in medical practice under the name *barbital*. Unlike the acid, from which it was derived, barbital not only sedated but also induced sleep. Since the introduction of barbital, more than 2,500 barbiturates have been synthesized. Only about 50 of these drugs have ever been distributed as prescribed medications.

Although *chloral hydrate* and *paraldehyde* were synthesized and marketed before 1900, the barbiturates proved so successful as sedative-hypnotics that they remained the number one depressant-type medication until 1960. Still prescribed today, barbiturates have been replaced in large measure by the newer minor tranquilizers—benzodiazepines. These relatively new antianxiety drugs, also referred to as anxiolytics (dispellers or dissolvers of anxiety), are generally less sedating, much safer, and slower to induce tolerance, and they demonstrate greater antianxiety effects with less sedation than the barbiturates.[5,6] However, they are dependency-producing drugs.

Barbiturates

Among those drugs employed as hypnotics, sedatives, anesthetics, and anticonvulsants are the **barbiturates**. Of the nearly fifty derivatives of barbituric acid ever marketed for medical use, fewer than fifteen are in common use today. Easy to use, barbiturates almost always come prepared in capsule or tablet form. A few of them are injectable.

Still prescribed for conditions requiring central nervous system depression, small doses of barbiturates tend to calm nervous individuals, while large doses cause drowsiness and sleep. Short-term effects are similar to those of alcohol intoxication, with a reduction of tension and anxiety, a calming relaxation, slower reaction time, and varying degrees of motor incoordination. However, these drugs are not effective as painkillers.

Since the early 1970s, safer, less toxic, and less sleep-producing benzodiazepines have been replacing the medical use of barbiturates. As physicians reduced their prescribing of the barbiturates, a corresponding decline in barbiturate-related suicides has also occurred.

Though not strongly supported by clinical studies, the several barbiturates are classified according to their onset and duration of action, as well as their therapeutic uses, as follows.[7,8]

1. *Ultrashort-acting barbiturates* with rapid onset of effects are used as surgical anesthetics. These drugs produce anesthesia within 1 minute after intravenous administration. Their rapid onset and brief duration of action (from 15 minutes to 3 hours) make them undesirable for purposes of abuse. Examples of ultrashort-acting barbiturates include thiopental (Pentothal), hexobarbital (Evipal), and thiamyl (Surital).

2. *Short-intermediate-acting barbiturates,* used mostly as sedative-hypnotics, have an onset time of action between 15 to 40 minutes after administration by mouth. The duration of action lasts up to 6 hours, a characteristic that makes these drugs the preferred barbiturates of most abusers. These drugs are sold in capsules and tablets, as well as in a liquid form or suppositories. Representing this classification are the following barbiturates: secobarbital (Seconal), amobarbital (Amytal), pentobarbital (Nembutal), butabarbital (Butisol), talbutal (Lotusate), and aprobarbital (Alurate). Two of these barbiturates, amobarbital and secobarbital, are combined and sold under the trade name Tuinal.

3. *Long-acting barbiturates* have onset times of up to 1 hour after use, but their durations of action approach 16 hours. Their relatively slow onsets of action discourage these barbiturates from being used for episodic intoxication. Consequently, they are not usually distributed on the illicit market. In medical practice, these barbiturates are used as sedatives, hypnotics, and anticonvulsants in the control of epilepsy. Frequently prescribed barbiturates include phenobarbital (Luminal), mephobarbital (Mebaral), and metharbital (Gemonil). Unlike other barbiturates, phenobarbital does not usually produce the "high" typical of depressants.

The many years of barbiturate use in medical practice and barbiturate abuse have revealed both the benefits and problems of these sedative-hypnotics. For instance, prescribed for only short periods of time, barbiturates are relatively safe when taken under medical supervision. However, the aftereffects of such legitimate use can include a residual depression of the central nervous system (a "hangover") on the day following use.[9] This hangover is characterized by motor incoordination, listlessness, nausea, and emotional disturbances—all related to barbiturates' disruption of normal REM, (rapid eye movement) or dream, sleep.

Nonmedically approved uses of the sedative-hypnotics include the simultaneous consumption of barbiturates and amphetamines, CNS stimulants. Such a

Overdose with Depressants and First-Aid Treatment

Among the frequently abused depressants are both the barbiturate and the nonbarbiturate sedative-hypnotics, the minor tranquilizers, and ethyl alcohol. Although all of these drugs tend to slow down body function, the actual physical symptoms of overdose may vary considerably, depending on the specific drug used, the method of administering the drug, and the particular stages of intoxication reached by the drug user.

Symptoms of Depressant Overdose

Confused behavior, often with slow and slurred speech.

Aggressive behavior is possible.

Slow, shallow, or irregular breathing.

Glazed eyes with slow reaction to light.

Person may be either semiconscious or unconscious. Coma is a possibility.

Individual is difficult to keep awake.

If individual falls asleep, he or she is difficult to awake.

Muscles may be either flaccid or rigid.

First-Aid Treatment of Depressant Overdose

Try to keep overdose victim awake by talking.

If individual falls asleep or becomes unconscious, watch for sudden cessation of breathing.

Give mouth-to-mouth resuscitation, if possible.

Maintain an open airway to promote unobstructed breathing.

Place unconscious person on his/her side.

If person is conscious, consider diluting the drug taken, inducing vomiting, and then transporting the individual to the nearest medical center as soon as possible.

Be watchful of possible emotional depression and suicidal tendencies.

---

combination is alleged to produce super-mood elevation. The same combination involves an alternating cycle of sedation and stimulation, that is, taking amphetamines during the day to overcome a drowsy hangover, and then ingesting barbiturates at night in order to overcome insomnia. "Speed freaks" also use barbiturates to produce sleep after several days of almost continuous amphetamine injection.

Illegally sold barbiturates pose special hazards for drug abusers. In addition to their high price, barbiturates manufactured and packaged as "street drugs" lack quality control. Street-obtained downers, for example, often contain toxic contaminants and very little of the hoped-for sedative-hypnotic. Illegally sold barbiturates, especially those in capsule form, are often cut with weaker drugs or with traces of tranquilizer, strychnine, arsenic, laxative, heart medication, or inactive substances, such as milk sugars. Homemade capsules may appear genuine, but any red capsule is sometimes offered as Seconal and any yellow capsule may masquerade as Nembutal.

The main reasons for the declining medical uses of barbiturates relate to the risks of fatal overdose, the rapid increase of tolerance, the disruption of normal rapid eye movement (REM), or dream, sleep, and the sheer addictiveness of these drugs.[10]

Barbiturate Overdose

The long-term use of barbiturates has the potential for serious, even lethal, effects, especially among those who increase their prescribed dosage without medical advice or abuse nonprescribed forms of these drugs (see box 6.1). Even occasional recreational use or self-medication may precipitate an overdose condition resulting in respiratory depression, collapse of the blood-circulatory system, kidney failure, and coma. Taking just 10 times the hypnotic dose is highly toxic and sometimes fatal, while 15 to 20 times the hypnotic dose in usually fatal.

Among those who develop a tolerance, a "maximum tolerance" level is eventually established for each kind of barbiturate. Unfortunately, this maximum tolerance, or uppermost dosage limit or cutoff point, is never precisely known to the barbiturate abuser until it is too late for preventive action. The usual dose becomes dangerously close to the lethal dose. For instance, if a person having a maximum tolerance of 25 barbiturate capsules per day were to take in 23 or 24 capsules just to achieve a desired "high," then consuming only a few extra capsules could easily result in an overdose condition. This is assumed to be what

happened to Judy Garland, the famous singer-actress who died allegedly of barbiturate overdose.

Of course, overdosing can occur well under the maximum-tolerance level if barbiturates are combined with alcohol or some other depressant drug. Alcohol enhances the toxic effect of the barbiturate.

For many years, physicians believed that a major factor in barbiturate overdose and death was a condition known as **automatism.** According to this automatism explanation, people using hypnotics would forget about having taken their sleeping pills and would thus continue to consume multiple doses during a particularly restless night. Blood levels of barbiturates would thereby become damagingly high, even lethal. Extensive research, however, found that overdose associated with genuine forgetfulness for taking pills was quite rare. In fact, nearly all cases of alleged automatism were related to suicidal intent or the denial of suicidal tendencies.

Barbiturate Dependence

As indicated earlier, tolerance, psychological dependence, and physiological dependence occur rather easily with the barbiturates. Tolerance to the euphoric effects builds quickly after a few weeks.

Many people find that taking just one barbiturate the first day produces a desired high. By the second or third day, the same dose only makes them sleepy. To get high, they must increase the daily dosage. This pattern is repeated over and over again until the dose required for the euphoric effect builds to a high of twenty-five or more capsules per day. But as tolerance increases, the overdose threshold remains relatively unchanged; it does not increase proportionately. Too often the outcome of barbiturate abuse is overdose and death.

While differing from person to person, physical dependence occurs when large quantities of barbiturates (four to six times the average hypnotic dose) are taken for a prolonged period of time, often within two to six months after the initial excessive dose.

Barbiturate Withdrawal

Most people do not understand how serious and extremely dangerous withdrawal from barbiturates can be. Unlike heroin-dependent individuals, those who experience barbiturate withdrawal symptoms cannot "kick" their drug alone. They must receive medical assistance in a hospital because the abstinence syndrome for barbiturates *is* a medical emergency.

Within just 12 hours after the last dose, the dependent person without medical care begins returning slowly to a nonintoxicated state. Several hours later, this individual usually begins to experience nervousness, weakness, insomnia, nausea, and tremors of the arms and legs. Then, 48 to 72 hours later, the withdrawal symptoms intensify. The person begins to vomit, has a drop in blood pressure, and develops extreme weakness, delirium, hyperexcitability, fever, and severe body convulsions or seizures. Death can occur from physical exhaustion and collapse of the cardiovascular (heart-blood vessel) system. There is little doubt that barbiturate withdrawal with convulsions is more dangerous than withdrawal from opioid drugs (narcotic analgesics).

Nonbarbiturate Sedative-Hypnotics

In this section, three nonbarbiturate sedative-hypnotics—chloral hydrate, glutethimide, and methaqualone—and other similar hypnotics are discussed.

Chloral Hydrate

One of the oldest sedative-hypnotics still in use today, chloral hydrate was first synthesized in 1862. Advantages originally associated with use of this drug included its lack of side effects in therapeutic doses, such as hangover and respiratory depression. However, the popularity of chloral hydrate declined substantially after barbiturates were introduced in 1903.

A liquid marketed in syrups and soft gelatin capsules, chloral hydrate induces sleep shortly after a normal therapeutic dose. The sleep typically lasts about five hours. At one time, the hypnotic drug was added to an alcoholic beverage to concoct the infamous "Mickey Finn" or "knockout drops"—a potent, quick-acting, and sometimes lethal sleep-inducing preparation.

In addition to its continued use as a daytime sedative and a short-term hypnotic, chloral hydrate keeps children calm during dental procedures and during CAT scans. Sometimes this drug is also prescribed for newborn infants who are on ventilators.

Easily capable of producing a drug dependency with symptoms of withdrawal resembling those of alcohol dependence, chloral hydrate is rarely used as a "recreational" drug today. The hypnotic is primarily misused by older adults who take the prescribed drug as a sedative despite its tendency to cause gastric disturbances. Recently, studies conducted by the Environmental Protection Agency suggest the possibility that chloral hydrate might cause cancer as well as genetic damage. If this drug proves to be a carcinogen, its limited use, especially among the elderly, will further decline.

Glutethimide

First introduced in 1954 as a substitute for the barbiturates, glutethimide was distributed under the trade names Doriden and Dormtabs. This drug treatment for sleeplessness was supposedly less toxic and less dependency-producing than barbiturates. Neither of these hoped-for characteristics was demonstrated in medical practice. Although considered as somewhat obsolete by many physicians, Doriden is prescribed only occasionally today.

Within 30 minutes of oral intake, glutethimide produces a sedative-hypnotic effect that lasts approximately 6 hours. At 10 times the hypnotic dose, the drug is likely to induce severe intoxication. The lethal dose is estimated at 20 to 40 times the usual hypnotic dose. Because of Doriden's relatively long duration of action, it is very difficult to reverse overdoses, which often result in death. In terms of lethality, glutethimide is considered several times more hazardous than barbiturates.

Methaqualone

A synthetic drug originally marketed under the trade name Quaalude, **methaqualone** was first introduced in the United States in 1965 as a safe, effective, and non-dependency-producing medicine to replace the dangerous barbiturates. By the late 1970s, it became one of the most frequently prescribed sedative-hypnotics. Additionally marketed under the brand names Sopor, Mequin, Somnafac, Parest, and others, methaqualone—like many other sedative-hypnotics—was not usually effective for more than two weeks when taken regularly for insomnia.

Because of its alleged safety and widespread availability, methaqualone soon became a popular recreational drug, known variously as "ludes," "sopors," "sopes," "lemmons," and "714s." The chief nonmedical attractions were that the drug produced a euphoric, alcohol-like high, a general feeling of relaxation, and the anticipated enhancement of sexual performance, since methaqualone was thought to have aphrodisiac properties.

In reality, Quaalude proved to be quite similar to barbiturates in its drug effects, and it reduced sexual performance. Nevertheless, methaqualone became one of the leading drugs of abuse in the 1970s and early 1980s, because drug takers' mind-sets, physical settings for drug use, and personal expectations about the drug's effects were more powerful than the drug's pharmacological effects.[11]

Relatively safe when used wisely under medical supervision, methaqualone could

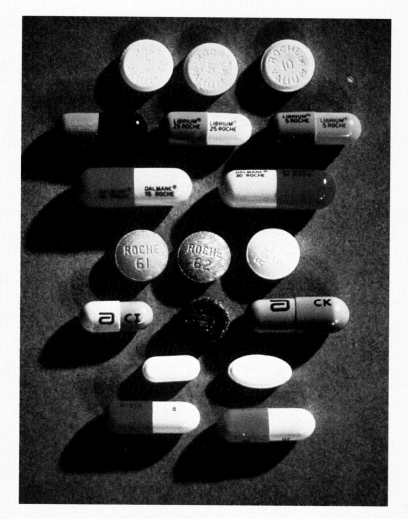

Benzodiazepines pictured here are often prescribed as antianxiety medications, but certain ones are promoted as hypnotics or as anticonvulsant drugs.

Courtesy of the Drug Enforcement Agency

their genuine American counterparts. Frequently, the former drugs contain methaqualone substitutes such as diazepam (Valium), phenobarbital, antihistamines, PCP (angel dust), or completely inactive substances. In many instances, not even experienced abusers are certain of what they have purchased.

Other Nonbarbiturate Hypnotics

Several other nonbarbiturates are also available for use as sleep-inducing medications. Two of these, *methyprylon* and *ethchlorvynol*, are still commonly prescribed, but much less now than in the past. Three others—*flurazepam, temazepam,* and *triazolam*—all belong to the **benzodiazepine** drug group of antianxiety medications but are promoted almost exclusively as hypnotics. These latter three benzodiazepines are now among the most frequently prescribed sleeping pills.

Although methyprylon (Noludar) and ethchlorvynol (Placidyl) may help people fall asleep and stay asleep, with regular use their effectiveness rarely lasts for more than one or two weeks. Methyprylon is very toxic and sometimes fatal in overdose situations. However, it does not have the extremely high mortality associated with glutethimide overdose.

Ethchlorvynol is marketed as a hypnotic agent with a rapid onset and short duration of action. Like methyprylon, ethchlorvynol can produce death at as low as fourteen times the hypnotic dose, although there is considerable individual variation. With overdose there may be low blood pressure, decreased breathing and heart rate, and coma.

Marketed under the brand name *Dalmane,* **flurazepam** is one of the most widely prescribed hypnotics in current medical practice. Due to its relatively long duration of sedative action, flurazepam is used primarily to treat insomnia characterized by difficulty in falling asleep and frequent nighttime and early awakenings.[12] Dalmane is not used for daytime sedation because its metabolites (breakdown by-products) have sedative effects and tend to accumulate in the body. When used on consecutive nights, the drug increases gradually in the patient's body and is thought to result in reduced alertness and impaired visual motor coordination

cause loss of inhibitions and motor coordination, dizziness, sleep, and hangover the next day. Prolonged use sometimes led to tolerance and both psychological and physical dependence. Overdose was common and occasionally fatal, especially when combined with an alcoholic beverage. Without medical supervision, withdrawal from methaqualone often proved deadly.

Such a reputation of toxicity and fatal consequences was responsible for the reclassification of methaqualone from its uncontrolled prescribed drug status first to a Schedule II drug and eventually to a Schedule I drug, under provisions of the

Controlled Substances Act. While this reclassification reduced the nonmedical abuse of methaqualone, such restrictions did not eliminate the problem. Continuing widespread abuse soon led to its demise in 1983, when the sole manufacturer stopped production of Quaalude.

Many varieties of "street" or "bootleg" methaqualone have surfaced up to the present time. Illegally manufactured "sopors" that are processed secretly, and then smuggled into the United States from Great Britain and Canada (under the brand name of Mandrax) and South America, have been prepared to resemble

during the waking hours of the day. Because there has been a high incidence of adverse effects, older adults have been cautioned to avoid using this drug.

Nevertheless, flurazepam possesses certain desirable properties not shared by other hypnotic agents. It is often effective as long as 28 nights; it promotes more sleep time on the first 3 nights of therapy; it avoids the problem of rebound insomnia when therapy is discontinued. Tolerance to the effects of flurazepam develops more slowly than to the barbiturates. Furthermore, medically supervised use of this drug does not typically result in physical dependence unless it is taken for more than three months. Even after massive doses, most people do not experience a toxic reaction unless flurazepam is taken along with alcohol or some other CNS depressant.

Since its introduction in the early 1980s, **triazolam** (*Halcion*) has become one of the most widely used sleeping medications in the United States. A benzodiazepine hypnotic, Halcion has a rapid onset and a short duration of action. Consequently, it is less likely than some of the other benzodiazepines to cause drowsiness the following day. Its primary use as a hypnotic is for the short-term treatment of insomnia.

In spite of Halcion's popularity and apparent effectiveness, special concerns have arisen about its widespread use, especially regarding its causing memory loss, increased wakefulness during the last third of the night, and increased signs of daytime anxiety or nervousness. In addition, numerous reports of serious adverse reactions to taking this medicine have been reported to the U.S. Food and Drug Administration. Harmful reactions have included amnesia to events occurring after taking the drug, anxiety, anorexia (loss of appetite for food), agitation, bizarre and aggressive behavior, confusion, delirium, depression, hallucinations, paranoia, seizures, suicidal thinking, and a feeling of detachment from reality.[13]

Because some patients have experienced serious psychiatric side effects when using Halcion, this medication was recently taken off the market in the United Kingdom and severely restricted in Canada.[14] In the United States, the Food

and Drug Administration has required the manufacturer of Halcion to provide consumers with more detailed information about the risks and benefits of this drug.

Temazepam (Restoril) is another benzodiazepine hypnotic that has a relatively long duration of sedative action. This characteristic makes the drug especially useful for people who tend to wake early. Although Restoril has had many fewer reported dangerous side effects (adverse reactions) than other benzodiazepines, the main disadvantage of this hypnotic is its tendency to cause a hangover—a drowsy, light-headed feeling—the following day. Like all the benzodiazepines, the continued use of Restoril can result in drug dependence. In addition, the sleep-inducing effects of this medication may decline with time.

Several drugs intended for other medical purposes also possess sleep-inducing characteristics. Some of these are prescribed as such by physicians. Examples include prescription-only sedating antihistamines (Atarax, Vistaril, and Benadryl); an antipsychotic drug, such as thioridazine (Mellaril) used in treating severe mental disorders; and an antidepressant, such as amitriptyline (Elavil). Over-the-counter hypnotics are discussed in chapter 11.

Self-Care for Inducing Sleep

While various drug and nondrug therapies have been developed for the condition of insomnia, many people have found relief from sleeplessness by engaging in one or more forms of self-care or self-medication.[15] Some of these acceptable alternatives are listed below:

1. Do not take naps during the day or go to bed earlier than usual.

2. Change the bedroom environment so that it is as quiet and dark as possible. Use special window shades that eliminate most external light and electronic devices that emit rest-promoting sounds that mask many noises from within and outside one's home. Maintain a comfortable room temperature for sleeping and keep it consistent from night-to-night.

3. Do not consume caffeine-containing beverages (coffee, tea, and cola drinks) or chocolate within eight hours of your anticipated bedtime.

4. Do not eat a heavy meal in the evening, especially just before retiring. Drink a mixture of warm milk and "instant breakfast" to which a spoonful of malt has been added. Milk and malt are high in the chemical tryptophan (an essential amino acid found in food), which can have a natural sedative effect.

5. Engage in exercise on a daily basis. Regular physical activity tends to promote a good night's sleep.

6. Take an unhurried warm bath about three hours before bedtime. This procedure tends to be relaxing. Other bedtime routines, such as reading a pleasant book, listening to music, or watching TV just before retiring, can also help promote sleep.

7. Do not use any drugs that might affect the central nervous system. Chief offenders tend to be alcohol, tobacco, nose drops, and nasal decongestants, in addition to caffeine. Under a physician's care, change the intake of any prescribed medicine that might also affect the central nervous system.

8. Each day, get up early at the same time, even when you have slept poorly and especially on nonworking days. This consistent behavior will help you avoid the "late-sleeping syndrome"—the feeling of being "out-of-sorts" after sleeping late in the morning.

9. If sleeplessness is the result of worry or grief, try to resolve your own basic problem by confiding in a friend, joining a support group, or consulting a counselor.

10. Resist the urge to be a clock watcher at night. Turn the clock to the wall or reposition your bed to avoid looking at the clock.

Another nondrug approach to insomnia is the use of a behavior therapy technique called "systematic desensitization."

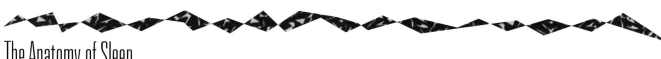

The Anatomy of Sleep

Sleep consists of two distinct phases or states: rapid eye movement sleep (referred to as REM sleep or dreaming sleep), and non-REM or NREM sleep (known as orthodox or slow-wave sleep).

REM sleep has been described as a very active brain in a paralyzed body. On the psychological level, REM sleep is characterized by dreaming, and on the physiological level by activation of the brain's nerve cells, increased blood flow in the brain, and bursts of extra ocular and middle-ear muscle activity. In the normal adult, REM sleep constitutes about 20 to 25 percent of the total night's sleep, or 90 to 120 minutes per night. REM sleep occurs in approximately three to five regularly spaced periods about 70 to 100 minutes after sleep onset and recurs at intervals of about 90 minutes from the onset of one period to the next.

NREM sleep, by comparison, is usually subdivided into four stages on the basis of relatively distinguishable electronencephalographic (EEG) brain-wave patterns.

Stage 1 is a brief transitional stage between wakefulness and sleep. This stage makes up about 5 percent of the total night's sleep.
Stage 2 constitutes from 40 to 60 percent of total sleep in young adults.
Stages 3 and 4 are characterized by a specific EEG pattern known as delta waves, and constitute nearly 10 to 20 percent of total sleep. Most stages 3 and 4 sleep occurs during the first 1 to 3 hours of night sleep in young adults.

Normal sleep almost always begins with NREM sleep. As a person falls asleep, he or she enters stage 1, then stage 2, which is followed by stages 3 and 4. After sleeping for nearly 1 1/2 hours, the individual enters the first period of REM sleep, which is usually brief (5 to 15 minutes). The NREM/REM cycle then begins again and is repeated throughout the night.

Most people do not understand that there are wide individual differences in the amount of sleep required each night. Older adults do not realize that sleep patterns typically and normally change with age. Indeed, many senior citizens firmly believe that the "Eleventh Commandment" dictates at least 8 hours of sleep per night. In reality, as adults enter middle and old age, stages 3 and 4 of NREM sleep decrease markedly, and sleep tends to become progressively more fragmented, shorter, and shallower, with brief arousals and longer periods of wakefulness. Experience suggests that most people suffer some degree of insomnia from time to time and have no lasting ill effects.

All of the currently prescribed hypnotics appear to alter one's sleep pattern in one way or another. While flurazepam has a relatively small effect on REM sleep, it has a highly potent suppresssant effect on stages 3 and 4. On the other hand, barbiturates, glutethimide, ethchlorvynol, and the antihistamines tend to suppress REM sleep. Although the overall effects of REM sleep deprivation or stage 4 deprivation may be slight or even subtle, one complaint about REM-suppressing drugs should be considered. When these drugs are discontinued, total amounts of REM sleep on subsequent nights may increase dramatically for several days or weeks. This "REM rebound" may be associated with vivid dreams or nightmares. On occasion, some depressant users also experience "daymares" — disturbing nightmarelike visualizations that occur while the persons are awake and cause panic reactions.

Source: Modified from Institute of Medicine, *Sleeping Pills, Insomnia, and Medical Practice*, pages 18–20, National Academy of Sciences, Washington, D.C., 1979.

In this process, an individual engages in various relaxation exercises—a modification of Herbert Benson's relaxation response or a similar procedure. Then the person visualizes scenes related to going to bed while in a relaxed state. The ultimate goal is to associate bedtime with a sense of relaxation that is incompatible with anxiety (see box 6.2).

Minor Tranquilizers

The term **minor tranquilizer** is somewhat misleading because it implies that such a drug acts like a "major tranquilizer," but to a lesser degree. Nothing could be more incorrect! The major tranquilizers, such as chlorpromazine (Thorazine) and reserpine (Serpasil), relieve symptoms of severe mental disorders, such as schizophrenia and paranoia; they are therefore more appropriately called "antipsychotics." The minor tranquilizers, on the other hand, function more like sedative-hypnotics. Because these minor tranquilizers are useful in treating anxiety and neurotic conditions, the preferred descriptive term for the minor tranquilizer is **antianxiety agent**. It should be noted that while the antianxiety drugs do in fact tranquilize a person, the antipsychotics seldom produce such a state in a non-psychotic individual. Consequently, the major antipsychotics are rarely abused drugs, and, unlike the minor tranquilizers, they are not even controlled substances.

Meprobamate

Ushering in the era of antianxiety drugs, meprobamate was first marketed in the mid 1950s under the trade names Miltown and Equanil. This drug not only possessed a muscle-relaxant effect but was

A Thumbnail Sketch of Valium, One of the Most Frequently Prescribed Psychoactive Drugs in America for Over 20 Years

box 6.3

Generic Name: Diazepam, a benzodiazepine derivative.

Brand Name: Valium; also available generically.

Controlled Drug Status: Prescription required, Schedule IV.

Pharmacology: Appears to act on the limbic system, thalamus, and hypothalamus to induce a calming effect by enhancing the action of GABA (gamma-aminobutyric acid), a neurotransmitter that blocks the arousal of higher brain centers.

Indications for Use: Management of anxiety disorders or for short-term relief of the symptoms of anxiety; also used at bedtime to produce a calming effect that promotes sleep; sometimes used in treating muscle spasms, symptoms of acute alcohol withdrawal, and certian convulsive disorders.

Dosage forms: Capsules, concentrate, injection, oral solution, and tablets.

Should Not Be Taken if Patient: Has glaucoma or myasthenia gravis, or is an infant under 6 months of age.

Possible Side Effects: Drowsiness, lethargy, unsteadiness in stance and gait, increase in level of blood sugar in some cases of diabetes.

Possible Mild Adverse Effects: Allergic reactions, especially skin rashes, dizziness, fainting, blurred vision, double vision, slurred speech, nausea, menstrual irregularity.

Possible Serious Adverse Effects: Allergic reactions (especially jaundice), impaired resistance to infection manifest by fever and/or sore throat, acute excitement, hallucinations, rage, eye pain, possibly glaucoma, emotional depression.

Precautions to Be Observed if: Used by infants and children, by those over 60 years of age, by women during pregnancy and while nursing infants, and combining use with consumption of alcoholic beverages. Avoid driving a vehicle, operating machinery, and engaging in hazardous activities while using Valium.

Drug-Dependency Potential: Psychological dependence, tolerance, physical dependence, and withdrawal syndrome similar in character to those seen with barbiturates and alcohol may occur following sudden discontinuance.

Effects of Overdose: Definite drowsiness, weakness, feeling of drunkenness, staggering gait, tremor, stupor that may progress to deep sleep or coma.

Effects of Extended Use: Reduction of white blood cells and impairment of liver function.

Possible Effects on Sexual Function: Changes in the pattern and timing of menstruation. While small doses may be used to relieve anxiety causing male impotence and inhibited female sexual responsiveness, larger doses can lower sexual desire, impair male potency, and inhibit female orgasm.

Sources: James Long and James Rybacki, *The Essential Guide to Prescription Drugs*, pages 419–423, Harper Perennial, New York, 1994; and *Physicians' Desk Reference*, PDR 48th edition, 1967–1969, Medical Economic Data Production Company, Montvale, N.J., 1994.

---

also found to be an antianxiety agent. It was soon prescribed widely for relief of anxiety, tension, and muscle spasms.

The success of this new "minor tranquilizer" was related to its calming effects without producing sleep when taken at low therapeutic doses. Meprobamate was able to provide relief from anxiety and free-floating fears without heavy sedation. After several years of clinical use, meprobamate was found to be somewhat less toxic than barbiturates. With excessive use, however, psychological and physical dependence developed. Whether or not the new "minor tranquilizer" provides more relief from anxiety than the barbiturates do is still debated.

Benzodiazepines

Meprobamate's initial success was soon followed by the discovery of a new family of antianxiety drugs, the benzodiazepines. In 1960, *chlordiazepoxide* (Librium) was marketed and widely prescribed as a wonder drug in the "age of coping." Just three years later, *diazepam* (Valium), another tranquilizing agent chemically similar to chlordiazepoxide, entered medical practice. Valium proved to be five to ten times more potent than Librium.

Since its introduction, **Valium** has become the most frequently prescribed psychoactive drug in American medical

history. For more than twenty years it has been one of the most widely prescribed drugs in the world (see box 6.3). Only in the past few years has Valium's "therapeutic popularity" been exceeded by **Xanax**, another member of the benzodiazepine family and a chemical relative of diazepam. Alprazolam (Xanax) is promoted as not having the "buzz" effect of Valium, and it is particularly useful in treating panic disorders, anxiety accompanied by agitated depression, and various phobias, including the fear of open spaces (agoraphobia). In addition, Xanax has a somewhat shorter duration of action than Valium.

Tranquilizers, Other Sedative-Hypnotics, and Driving *Why Take the Risk?*

Tranquilizers are central nervous system depressants (drugs that slow down the body) and help relieve tension and anxiety. Major and minor tranquilizers, such as chlorpromazine (Thorazine) and diazepam (Valium), can have pronounced effects on driving skills.

Studies show that prescribed doses of tranquilizers can affect driving skills by slowing reaction time and interfering with eye-hand coordination and judgment. Warnings that caution against taking these medications while driving are often ignored. Recent research suggests that driving skills are most impaired in the first hour after a tranquilizer is taken.

Flurazepam (Dalmane) is a widely prescribed sleeping pill. Studies show that this drug accumulates in the body, and the buildup can impair driving skills, even the morning after. Elderly people must be especially careful when driving the day after taking this drug, since the drug remains in their bodies longer than it does in younger persons.

Other sedative-hypnotic drugs, including barbiturates and Quaaludes, are chemical sedatives that calm people or help them sleep. Sleepy drivers are a hazard on the road. Mixing these drugs with alcohol can double the effects of both and is extremely dangerous.

If your doctor prescribes a tranquilizer or sedative, make a point to discuss how the drug will affect your ability to drive safely. Driving requires a combination of thought and motor skills, a great deal of common sense, and a concern for the safety of everyone on the road. Safe driving requires an observant eye, a steady hand, and a clear head. By mixing drugs with driving, you are only asking for trouble. Why take the risk?

Source: Modified from *Drugs & Driving: Why Take the Risk?* National Institute on Drug Abuse, 1985.

In general, the various benzodiazepines currently in use differ mainly in the duration of their effects, and are grouped as follows:[16]

Long-acting benzodiazepines— drugs that stay in the body longer and need to be taken only once or twice per day or every other day:

diazepam (Valium)
clonazepam (Clonopin)
chlordiazepoxide (Librium)
flurazepam (Dalmane)
prazepam (Centrax)
clorazepate (Tranxene)

Intermediate-acting benzodiazepines—shorter-acting drugs that are eliminated more quickly from the body; can be taken three or four times per day or at night:

temazepam (Restoril)
alprazolam (Xanax)

Short-acting benzodiazepines— shortest-acting in this drug group; are eliminated most rapidly from the body and can be taken three or four times per day or at night:

oxazepam (Serax)
lorazepam (Ativan)
triazolam (Halcion)

With the exception of Dalmane, Restoril, and the controversial Halcion (all promoted as hypnotics) and Clonopin (used as an anticonvulsant), the benzodiazepines have been widely prescribed as antianxiety drugs for nearly a quarter of all psychiatric patients, as well as for people with arthritis and chronic heart disease. The primary purpose of these "minor tranquilizers" is to reduce psychic tension and anxiety disorders (the intense fear of impending doom without obvious threat) or for the temporary relief of the symptoms of anxiety. However, most medical authorities do not believe that these drugs should be prescribed to relieve anxieties that are part of the ordinary stresses of everyday life.

Generally, the benzodiazepines are effective sedatives but are less sleep-inducing than other drugs in the sedative-hypnotic classification. In most patients, judgment and motor coordination are not seriously impaired and a lethal overdose is rare, because there is little depression of breathing. Nevertheless, there are many possible adverse effects, especially among the elderly. Some common undesirable side effects include mental confusion, drowsiness, shakiness, slurred speech, staggering, weakness, constipation, depression, headache, skin rash, insomnia, and even hallucinations.[17] All of these symptoms are usually reversed by adjusting or discontinuing the dose (see also box 6.4).

There is no doubt that extensive use of antianxiety drugs has led to their misuse and abuse. Because these drugs are available for quick comfort during a particular "life panic"—job pressures, family problems, marital difficulties, or stressful academic pressures—overdosing is common and is a frequent cause of visits to hospital emergency rooms. Since the benzodiazepines seldom induce respiratory depression, it is extremely difficult to commit suicide by overdosing with these drugs. However, these "minor tranquilizers" in combination with alcohol or other CNS depressants can be deadly. One of the less publicized potential dangers associated with the use of benzodiazepines is the occurrence of *impaired anterograde memory*. In this condition (a form of amnesia) the person taking the drug has a reduced capacity for learning and retaining new information that is presented after taking a therapeutic dose.[18] Older people are more susceptible to this phenomenon than younger individuals are.

The danger of *benzodiazepine dependence* is very real, although these drugs are not as powerful reinforcers as are the barbiturates and opioids. Even in therapeutic doses, all minor tranquilizers can cause psychological dependence with continued use. While there is very little tolerance to the antianxiety effects of benzodiazepines, tolerance to the hypnotic effects of these drugs usually develops after just one to two weeks. The withdrawal reaction, evidence of a physical dependence, may occur at both therapeutic as well as very high doses, and may include the following symptoms:[19] anxiety, numbness in the extremities, unpleasant feelings, intolerance for bright lights and loud noises, nausea, sweating, muscle twitching, and even convulsions. However, withdrawal does not typically involve a craving for the drug.

Controversial aspects of the antianxiety drugs have been publicized widely. Critics of America's "tranquilized society" claim that many physicians have been slow to recognize the addictive qualities of Valium. The lax prescribing habits of some physicians have been assailed for giving the impression that Valium is a "benign little anxiety-reducer" capable of abolishing tension and even environmental stressors.

In her autobiography, *I'm Dancing as Fast as I Can*, filmmaker Barbara Gordon describes her valium addiction.[20] She addresses the problem of easy tranquilizer availability in the United States during the 1960s and 1970s, and refers to the antianxiety medications as "anesthetics of the emotions." Gordon further cautions the general public about the potential seriousness of withdrawal from Valium and the problems of Valium abuse.

In response to such charges and allegations, the American medical community has significantly reduced the prescription of the benzodiazepines. Recognizing the major problems resulting from the use of minor tranquilizers, physicians now prescribe these drugs much more cautiously. The wider application of nondrug stress reduction techniques, such as biofeedback, self-hypnosis, meditation, and relaxation exercises, has also contributed to the declining use of the minor tranquilizers.

Factors influencing the use of minor tranquilizers have been identified through analyses of drug-use patterns in various populations. Such investigations suggest that the major factor in the widespread use and misuse of the "minor tranquilizers" is anxiety itself, the mental uneasiness caused by the anticipation of danger or misfortune. Whether at work, at home, in school, or in relationships with others, life is filled with tension and stressors—the agents of internal stress. Some people, perceiving the need for a "chemical

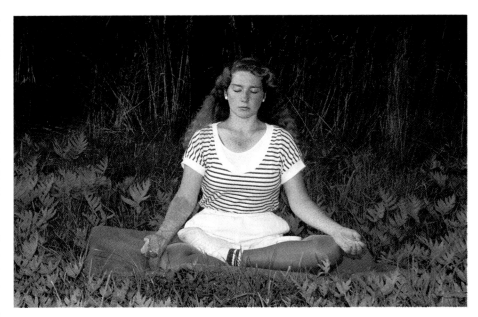

Increasing adoption of nondrug stress reduction techniques, including relaxation exercises has contributed to the declining use of anti-anxiety medications, such as Valium.

© *Ann Marie Rousseau/The Image Works*

crutch" or a "bridge over troubled waters," turn to the antianxiety drugs to ease their feelings of dread and nervousness.

Many factors have propelled people into using the antianxiety drugs: job pressures, changing social roles, feelings of worthlessness, boredom resulting from too much leisure time, problems of child rearing, and the "empty nest" syndrome experienced by parents when their grown children finally leave home. Some of these circumstances have been proposed to explain why more women than men take antianxiety drugs and become dependent on them.

For many years, the connection between female drug use and the "minor tranquilizers" was assumed to be women's tendency to seek medical assistance more often than men do. Once with their physicians, they reported more symptoms of emotional discomfort and discussed their emotional life and frustrations more openly than men. Thus women were more likely to be prescribed antianxiety drugs than were men. However, further analysis of the situation has revealed that drug companies' promotional ads to physicians often suggest that life problems can be made more tolerable by drugs and that women are more likely than men to need antidepressant therapy. Could it be that the physician's own perception of problems affecting male and female patients is the important determining factor in prescribing any drug?

Other Antianxiety Medications

In addition to the benzodiazepines, there are three other classes of drugs sometimes used to relieve anxiety—the so-called beta-blockers, the antidepressants, and buspirone.

Beta-blockers (Oxprenolon and Propranolol) are often used in the treatment of angina, hypertension, and irregular heart rhythms. Occasionally, these drugs are also given to reduce anxiety, such as "stage fright" and "butterflies in the stomach," as well as the shaking and palpitations (extremely rapid actions of the heart) related to anxiety. By blockading the stimulating action of the norepinephrine neurotransmitter, beta-blockers produce a wide variety of effects, including a slowing of heart rate, lowering of blood pressure, and reduction in muscle tremor as seen in anxiety states.

Certain antidepressant drugs, described in more detail in chapter 8, may also be prescribed for anxiety arising out of depressive illness. Although the *tricyclics* and *fluoxetine* (Prozac) are marketed as treatments for serious depression, some physicians might use them to relieve anxiety conditions. Antidepressants work by increasing the level of one or more excitatory neurotransmitters.

Another antianxiety medication, *buspirone* (BuSpar), has been introduced recently for medical use. This drug is not a member of the benzodiazepines and is chemically unrelated to other antianxiety compounds. Although the precise mechanism of its action is unknown, buspirone likely affects neurotransmitter functions. A prescription drug not scheduled as a controlled substance, BuSpar relieves anxiety and nervous tension without causing significant sedation. Moreover, buspirone does not exert anticonvulsant or muscle relaxant effects typically associated with use of benzodiazepines.[21]

In both human and animal studies, this antianxiety drug has shown no potential for abuse or diversion from legitimate sources, and there is no evidence that its use results in tolerance or either physical or psychological dependence. While buspirone has not been used by large numbers of people for extended periods of time, this drug has been particularly effective among the elderly, alcoholics, and addiction-prone individuals.[22]

Inhalants

According to the National Institute on Drug Abuse, **inhalants** are a diverse group of breathable chemicals that produce mind-altering vapors. Representative inhalants include various commercial products used as cleaners, cosmetics, paint solvents, glues, motor fuels, and aerosol sprays. Hundreds of such volatile substances are present in the home and available in the marketplace. Because they were never meant to be inhaled for either medical or recreational use, many people do not even think of these products as drugs.

Although inhaling volatile substances (chemicals that evaporate easily and are breathable) is an ancient method of achieving intoxication, this behavior has seldom generated the public interest and professional concern surrounding other abused substances. Such general reluctance to approach inhalant abuse in a systematic way has persisted despite the numerous abused medicinals that have been inhaled or sniffed for centuries. Often considered a minor problem, the abuse of certain solvents might be even more prevalent than the "common" drugs of abuse. It is certain that the toxicity of some inhalants exceeds that of other abused substances.

Commercial solvents, including gasoline, tend to be the intoxicants of young adolescents, and more often of males than females.[23] These substances are sometimes the very first psychoactive agents that young people use nonmedically, often before either tobacco or alcohol.

Recently, though, increasing numbers of male and female adults looking for a quick and inexpensive high have been engaging in sniffing certain aerosols and anesthetics. Although not aphrodisiacs, amyl nitrite and butyl nitrite seem to intensify sexual orgasm when inhaled close to the peak of passion. These chemicals rapidly gained favor as "love drugs," particularly among homosexual males who discovered that both amyl and butyl nitrite help relax the anal sphincter, making penetration easier.[24] For the past several years, nitrogen oxide, or "laughing gas," has become a popular intoxicant among high school and college-age persons, as well as among some young urban professionals.

Reasons for Use

Most people find it difficult to comprehend why anyone would deliberately breathe in strange compounds whose toxic potential has either remained uncertain or been considered a major threat to health and life. Surveys of juveniles who had developed a dependence on solvents suggested several categories of justification for use of inhalants. According to the National Institute on Drug Abuse, the categories are these:

Peer-group influence—This is perhaps the strongest factor in beginning and continuing the use of a particular inhalant.

Cost effectiveness—This is a prime factor in determining whether to use one of the inhalants, especially if the abuser is from a low-income family. A seventy-five cent can of varnish remover can intoxicate more people than a gallon of cheap wine.

Easy availability—Industrial and household substances can be found easily, even in places where alcoholic beverages are not present. Gasoline, paints, and various aerosols are more prevalent than liquor, and they can be found at service stations, convenience stores, supermarkets, hardware stores, and pharmacies. If they cannot be purchased, they can be shoplifted.

Convenient packaging—Many inhalants come in small, compact packages that permit concealment as well as mobility. A bottle of nail polish remover can be hidden more easily than a pint of wine. Such convenient packaging permits the abuser to bring the inhalant to school for between-class sniffs.

Mood elevation—Similar but not identical to alcohol intoxication, the inhalant-induced high is a major attraction or thrill of the volatile substances. Users describe the high as a floaty euphoria and a blotting out of unpleasant aspects of their lives.

Course of intoxication—Inhalation produces a more rapid onset of the high than does drinking alcohol or eating other drug substances. Effects subside after just one or two hours, and the hangover is regarded as less unpleasant than that of alcohol. Inhalants are considered more reliably intoxicating than marijuana.

Legality—Inhalants are usually legal compounds, at least for adults, and most of the volatile substances are produced, distributed, and sold for legitimate purposes.

Thus, from the consumer's viewpoint the use of inhalants is more understandable. As indicated, the volatile substances have certain advantages over other psychoactive substances.

General Effects

The volatile substances are CNS depressants and tend to slow down the function of the brain and spinal cord. When inhaled, the vapors soon produce a state of intoxication or a dreamlike high closely resembling drunkenness. At low doses, users might experience a relaxed, somewhat light-headed giddy feeling with reduced inhibitions; at higher doses, they might undergo a numbing of senses, sustain hallucinations, and eventually lose consciousness. Headache, nausea, dizziness, slurred speech, shakiness, uncoordinated actions, double vision, and muscle spasms often accompany the sniffing of these chemicals.

Categories of Abused Inhalants

The inhalants are generally classified into three major groups, all of which are potentially hazardous to users.

1. *Commercial solvents*, such as toluene (a popular and preferred inhalant), xylene, benzene, naphtha, acetone, and carbon tetrachloride are components of commercial products, such as airplane glue, plastic cement, paint thinner, gasoline, cleaning fluids, nail polish remover, cigarette lighter fluid, and typewriter correction fluid.

2. *Aerosols* are suspended particles in a gas. These foglike mixtures are the propellant gases in many household and commercial sprays. Containing various hydrocarbons, these propellants are abused in products such as cooking sprays, glass chillers, spray paints, and hair sprays. Also in this category are Freon gas, used in refrigerators and air conditioners, and propane gas, a widely used fuel.

Amyl nitrite, an inhalant prepared in cloth-covered glass capsules (ampules), has a legitimate medical use in treating heart patients. This prescribed drug relieves the suffocation effect and associated fear common in angina pectoris. In addition, it produces a dilation (expansion) effect on the brain's arteries and thus induces a flushing sensation with feelings of light-headedness. Upon breaking, the amyl nitrite capsules make a snapping or popping sound that has given rise to their common street names, *snappers* and *poppers*.

Butyl nitrite, a substance legally manufactured and formerly sold as a room odorizer or liquid incense, produces a short high when sniffed. A clear yellow liquid, sometimes packaged in ampules, this frequently abused product was commonly known as "Rush," "Locker Room," "Super Bullet," and "Jacaroma." The odor of butyl nitrite was comparable to the smell of rotting apples or dirty sweatsocks and other athletic gear affected by mildew.

3. *Anesthetics*, such a chloroform, ether, and halothane (all volatile liquids), and nitrous oxide and cyclopropane gases are abused inhalants. When tanks of nitrous oxide (laughing gas) cannot be diverted from medical sources, the intoxicating gas can be obtained from whipped-cream propellants, pressurized pellets, and tracer gas used to detect pipe leaks.

Health Hazards

The shared effect of these volatile chemicals, the euphoria of intoxication, is also the common danger, with the impairment of judgment and motor functioning. Acute intoxication may be relatively short—a matter of several seconds to several minutes—or it may last up to an hour or two, depending on the substance used and the dosage. Similar to that of clinical anesthesia, the high may be characterized by delirium, impulsive behavior, sedation, hallucinations, and delusions. Tolerance can develop with regular use, although physical dependence has not been established.

Although some of the dangers associated with inhalant use have been exaggerated, excessive intake presents definite hazards. Overdoses can result in nausea, vomiting, loss of motor coordination, paralysis and coma. Even more serious problems should not be underestimated.[25] Fatal accidents do occur; for example, inhaling vapors from a plastic bag held over the head or from a balloon can result in a lack of oxygen or suffocation. Lead poisoning may develop from inhaling vapors of lead-based paints, transmission fluid, and various petroleum products. When inhaled, Freon gas is so cold that it can freeze the throat and larynx and cause suffocation. Oily sprays can coat the inside of the lungs, interfere with proper exchange of oxygen and carbon dioxide, and result in asphyxiation.

Long-term or frequent users of amyl and butyl nitrite run the risk of developing glaucoma (increased pressure within the eyeball), red blood cell damage, and Kaposi's sarcoma—a rare form of cancer associated with impairment of the immune system and often seen in AIDS patients.[26] And when users of "laughing gas" tap the pressurized tanks of nitrous oxide, there is an increased risk of sustaining brain injury and suffocation (from lack of oxygen), freezing of the lips and throat (due to the cold temperature of the gas), and ruptured blood vessels in the lungs as well as collapsed lungs.

Certain volatile substances are extremely poisonous. Because of carbon tetrachloride's toxicity to the kidneys and liver, the product has been removed from commercial trade. Leaded gasoline—rapidly disappearing from the marketplace—can cause serious inflammation of the peripheral nerves. Toluene has been involved in instances of kidney, nervous system, and bone-marrow disorders. Sudden sniffing death can occur when a solvent or aerosol propellant is inhaled while the abuser engages in strenuous activity. The reduced oxygen content of the blood results in ventricular fibrillation (uncoordinated heart contractions) or other irregularities of heart action, ending in abrupt death.

Prevention of Inhalant Abuse

Various measures have been undertaken with only minimal success in the prevention of inhalant abuse. Most of these substances have valid nonmedical uses and are legally purchased, at least by adults. However, reducing the availability of supplies of certain volatile substances has decreased the numbers of new users and discouraged certain established users from continuing their practice. For instance, some states and cities have outlawed the sale of airplane glue to minors. Perhaps more effective is the Testor Corporation's practice of adding artificial oil of mustard to model airplane cement. Inhalation of the glue's vapors produces nausea. Legislation has also been used in some states to ban the sale of butyl nitrite. However, federal law now forbids the manufacture and retail sale of "Rush" as a dangerous and hazardous substance.

Environmental concerns have already resulted in a reduction in the use of Freon gases as these propellants and working fluids in refrigeration and air conditioning are being phased out of production. With the eventual elimination of tetraethyl lead from gasolines, morbidity due to lead poisoning from chronic inhalation of gasoline vapors will likely decline.

Other prevention approaches include changes in product composition to lessen the euphoric effects of inhalation; reformulation of volatile substances to reduce their toxicity; modification of warning labels to better identify potential dangers; and more-effective educational campaigns, including radio and television as well as school-based drug-information programs. One of the best educational messages about volatile substances is to caution individuals about the dangers of prolonged inhalation, whether by accident or on purpose.

However, school-based programs concerning inhalants must be designed to avoid becoming a "how to" primer for experimenters. Just as importantly, schools ought not send mixed messages about inhalants and then allow students at social functions to inhale helium from balloons. Although small amounts of this gas might not be harmful, this action is "only one step removed from huffing whippets (nitrous oxide)."[27]

Chapter Summary

1. Sedative-hypnotics are psychoactive drugs that have a depressant effect on the central nervous system. They are prescribed to produce a calming effect and to induce sleep.

2. Major sedative-hypnotics include the barbiturates, nonbarbiturate sedative-hypnotics, minor tranquilizers, and abused inhalants. All of these drugs tend to be widely misused and abused.

3. Recreational use of these drugs is often related to the enjoyment of pleasurable responses (appetitive use) or the relief from worry or unpleasant sensations (escape-avoidance use).

4. In general, the sedative-hypnotics tend to produce a CNS depression, a continuum of sedation, additive and potentiating or synergistic drug interactions, tolerance, psychological and physiological dependence, and even cross-tolerance and cross-dependence.

5. Barbiturates are classified as ultrashort-acting (Pentothal and Surital); short-intermediate acting (Seconal and Nembutal); and long-acting (Luminal and Mebaral).

6. Barbiturate withdrawal is extremely serious and dangerous, and can lead to death.

7. Before its production stopped in 1983, methaqualone (Quaalude) was one of the most frequently abused sedative-hypnotics.

8. Technically antianxiety drugs or "minor tranquilizers," flurazepam (Dalmane), triazolam (Halcion), and temazepam (Restoril) are benzodiazepines promoted as hypnotics.

9. Self-care for inducing sleep includes establishing a consistent sleep pattern and a favorable sleeping environment, drinking a mixture of warm milk and malt, exercising daily, taking an unhurried bath about three hours before bedtime, and practicing systematic desensitization.

10. Sleep normally consists of two distinct phases: rapid eye movement (REM) or dreaming sleep, and non-REM or slow-wave sleep.

11. So-called minor tranquilizers act like sedative-hypnotics and are appropriately described as having an antianxiety effect.

12. Minor tranquilizers include meprobamate and the widely prescribed benzodiazepines (Xanax, Valium, and Serax). Extensive use of these antianxiety drugs has led to their misuse and abuse.

13. Dependency-producing with prolonged use, antianxiety medications can prove to be deadly when used in combination with alcohol or another CNS depressant.

14. Abused inhalants—chemicals that produce mind-altering vapors—slow down CNS function and produce a dreamlike high resembling drunkenness.

15. There are significant health hazards associated with using inhalants, such as commercial solvents, aerosols, and anesthetics. Physical dependence is not observed.

Review Questions and Activities

1. What is a sedative-hypnotic psychoactive drug?

2. What drug families, or groupings of psychoactive drugs, are considered to be sedative-hypnotics?

3. How do the sedative-hypnotics differ from the narcotic analgesics?

4. What factors account for the medical use and recreational abuse of the sedative-hypnotics?

5. How does the combination use of sedative-hypnotics contribute to drug overdose and death?

6. Do you believe that sedativism is prevalent in America today? What psychoactive drugs other than the sedative-hypnotics contribute to sedativism?

7. Trace the major historical factors in the evolving development of sedative-hypnotic drugs and their use.

8. What factors make the recreational use of barbiturates particularly hazardous?

9. What factors contributed to stopping the production of methaqualone?

10. Describe the normal phases and stages of sleep.

11. What effects, if any, do the sedative-hypnotics have on the normal sleep pattern?

12. Explain why the major tranquilizers are rarely abused as recreational drugs.

13. Why have the benzodiazepines largely replaced the barbiturates in the practice of medicine?

14. Do you believe that America is really a "tranquilized" society? What evidence might you offer to support your response?

15. Explain why women are alleged to use minor tranquilizers more frequently than men.

16. Which prevention activity is the most effective in reducing the abuse of inhalants? Explain.

References

1. Lester Grinspoon and James Bakalar, *The Harvard Medical School Mental Health Review: Drug Abuse and Addiction* (Boston: Harvard Mental Health Letter, 1993), 22.

2. Avram Goldstein, *Addiction: From Biology to Drug Policy* (New York: W. H. Freeman, 1994), 124.

3. Grinspoon and Bakalar, *The Harvard Medical School Mental Health Review,* 23.

4. Anthony J. Trevor and Walter L. Way, "Sedative-Hypnotics," chapter 21 in *Basic and Clinical Pharmacology,* 4th ed., ed. Bertram Katzung (Norwalk, Conn.: Appleton & Lange, 1989), 264–77.

5. Gail Winger, Frederick Hofmann, and James Woods, *A Handbook on Drug and Alcohol Abuse: The Biomedical Aspects,* 3d ed. (New York: Oxford University Press, 1992), 78–81.

6. Jim Parker, *Downers: A Guide to Depressant Drugs* (Tempe, Ariz.: Do It Now, 1993), 4–6.

7. Drug Enforcement Administration, U.S. Department of Justice, *Drugs of Abuse* (Washington, D.C.: U.S. Government Printing Office, 1989), 26.

8. Barry Stimmel and the Editors of Consumer Reports Books, *The Facts about Drug Use: Coping with Drugs and Alcohol in Your Family, at Work, in Your Community* (New York: Haworth Medical Press, 1993), 97–99.

9. Theodore Rall, "Hypnotics and Sedatives: Ethanol," chapter 17 *Goodman and Gilman's The Pharmacological Basis of Therapeutics,* 8th ed., ed. A. G. Gilman, T. W. Rall, A. S. Nies, and P. Taylor (New York: McGraw Hill, 1990), 361–62.

10. Parker, *Downers,* 2.

11. Robert Julien, *A Primer of Drug Action* (New York: W. H. Freeman, 1992), 65.

12. *Physicians' Desk Reference,* 48th ed. (Montvale, N.J.: Medical Economic Data Production Company, 1994), 1959.

13. "The Halcion Story: What You Need to Know, but the FDA Won't Tell You," *Public Citizen Health Research Group Health Letter* 6, no. 1 (January 1990): 1–3, 8.

14. "Halcion and Other Sleeping Pills," *University of California at Berkeley Wellness Letter* 8, no. 10 (July 1992): 3.

15. Quentin Regestein, David Ritchie, and the Editors of Consumer Reports Books, *Sleep: Problems and Solutions* (Mount Vernon, N.Y.: Consumers Union, 1990), 182–85.

16. Grinspoon and Bakalar, *The Harvard Medical School Mental Health Review,* 22.

17. United States Pharmacopeia, *Complete Drug Reference* (Yonkers, N.Y.: Consumer Reports Books, 1994), 226–27.

18. Harold Doweiko, *Concepts of Chemical Dependency,* 2d ed. (Pacific Grove, Calif.: Brooks/Cole, 1993), 63.

19. Lester Grinspoon and James Bakalar, "Substance Use Disorders," chapter 19 in *The New Harvard Guide to Psychiatry,* ed. Armand M. Nicholi, Jr. (Cambridge: Belknap Press/Harvard University Press, 1988), 425.

20. Barbara Gordon, *I'm Dancing as Fast as I Can* (New York: Harper & Row, 1979).

21. *Physicians' Desk Reference,* 1384.

22. James Long and James Rybacki, *The Essential Guide to Prescription Drugs* (New York: HarperPerennial, 1994), 281.

23. H. Thomas Milhorn, *Drug and Alcohol Abuse* (New York: Plenum Press, 1994), 313, 321.

24. Ibid., 314.

25. Isabel Burk, "Huffing: Invisible Substances Right Under Our Noses," *Student Assistance Journal* 7, no. 3 (November–December 1994): 20–23.

26. Samuel Irwin, *Drugs of Abuse: An Introduction to Their Actions and Potential Hazards* (Phoenix, Ariz.: Do It Now, 1989), 15.

27. Burk, "Huffing," 23.

part
three

The Stimulants

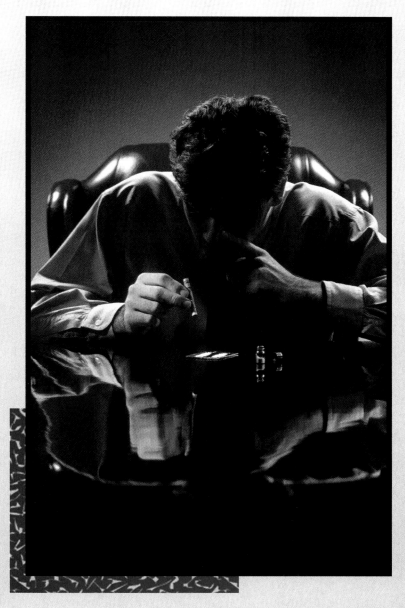

Questions of concern

1. What is the likelihood that America will eventually become a tobacco-free society?

2. While cocaine has assumed the status of a life-threatening drug, why is there still a crack cocaine epidemic?

3. Despite all the personal and social problems related to the use of stimulants, wouldn't many Americans benefit from such drugs if they counteract the depressing and monotonous aspects of daily living?

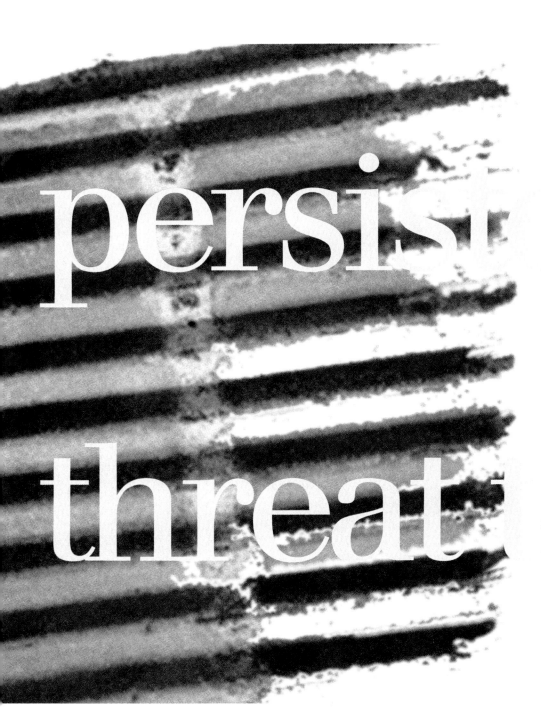

chapter

7

tobacco: a persistent threat to health

Bronchogenic Carcinoma
Carbon Monoxide
Carcinoma *in situ*
Cardiovascular Disease
Chewing Tobacco
Chronic Bronchitis
Chronic Obstructive Lung Disease
  (COLD)
Cigarette
Ciliary Function
"Cold Turkey"
Coronary Heart Disease
Craving
Environmental Tobacco Smoke
Hyperplasia
Involuntary Smoking
Lower-Yield Cigarette
Lung Cancer
Mainstream Smoke
Nicotiana tabacum
Nicotine
Nonsmokers' Liberation Movement
Oral Gratification
Particulates
Passive Smoke
Polycyclic Aromatic Hydrocarbons
Pulmonary Emphysema
Sidestream Smoke
Smokeless Tobacco
Snuff
Snuff Dipping
"Tar"
Tobacco
Tobacco Additives

chapter objectives

After you have studied this chapter, you should be able to do the following:

1. Describe the origins of tobacco use.

2. Estimate the number and percentage of Americans who smoke and use smokeless tobacco.

3. Identify several patterns and trends in the use of tobacco products.

4. Explain why smoking less-hazardous cigarettes can sometimes increase health risks.

5. Define the following terms: *lower-yield cigarette, snuff, smokeless tobacco.*

6. Explain the meaning of the nonsmokers' liberation movement.

7. Describe smoking as a learned behavior.

8. Identify several psychosocial predictors of smoking among American adolescents.

9. Classify smokers according to the following factors: stimulation, handling, pleasurable relaxation, tension reduction, craving, and habit.

10. Name the major phases and constituents of cigarette smoke.

11. Explain the role of nicotine in the maintenance of smoking behavior.

12. Explain what is meant by the term *dose-related* as it pertains to cigarette smoking and excess mortality.

13. Identify several significant findings of research that relate to the health consequences of smoking.

14. List several complications resulting from maternal smoking during pregnancy.

15. Define the following terms: *involuntary smoking, sidestream smoke, mainstream smoke.*

16. Identify at least five major health consequences associated with passive smoking.

17. Name two specific undesirable smoking-drug interactions that can occur in the human body.

18. Explain the probable actions of nicotine and carbon monoxide in the development of cardiovascular disease associated with cigarette smoking.

19. Distinguish each of the following from the others: hyperplasia, loss of ciliary function, and carcinoma *in situ.*

20. Define the terms *bronchogenic carcinoma, chronic obstructive lung disease,* and *alveoli.*

21. Distinguish between pulmonary emphysema and chronic bronchitis.

22. Compare the health hazards associated with smoking with those now related to smokeless forms of tobacco.

23. Explain why people continue to smoke in spite of scientific evidence that smoking is harmful to health.

24. Describe five techniques for reducing the risks of smoking for those who cannot or will not stop.

25. Name at least five benefits of smoking cessation.

Introduction

Since the U.S. surgeon general's first warning about smoking and cancer, heart disease, and other health problems, the nation's smoking rate has fallen dramatically. In the mid 1960s, an estimated 40 percent of the adult population smoked—53 percent of men and 32 percent of women.

Now the rate of cigarette smoking is the lowest ever reported, with just 28 percent of men and 23 percent of women classified as regular smokers. Only 20 percent of these regular cigarette users are estimated to smoke every day. Nevertheless, between 46 and 50 million American adults continue to smoke, and another 12 million—mostly adolescent males and young adults—use smokeless tobacco. Of the various forms of tobacco use, cigarette smoking remains the most popular and potentially the most dangerous.

Although the recent increase in popularity of smokeless tobacco has been related to its perceived harmlessness, the persistent use of any tobacco product carries a major risk of endangering health. Continuing such life-threatening behavior is frequently related to the many psychological rewards associated with using tobacco, the influences of marketing campaigns, the impact of peer pressure and role models, and the addictive nature of nicotine.

This chapter begins by examining the patterns and trends in using tobacco products and provides an analysis of the psychosocial aspects of this behavior. Then the serious health consequences of smoking, including passive smoking, and using smokeless tobacco are detailed, with a focus on cardiovascular diseases, lung cancer, and chronic obstructive lung disease. However, reflecting the health promotion and disease prevention theme of the text, the benefits of smoking cessation are included for those smokers who are convinced that there is no safe cigarette and no safe level of smoking.

Use of Tobacco: Questions and Issues

Although smoked by native Indians for centuries before the European settlers arrived in the New World, **tobacco** is often considered a newcomer to the American drug scene. One of the nightshade family of plants native to the Western Hemisphere, tobacco leaves have been smoked, chewed, and sniffed in the Western world for only four hundred years. Supposedly introduced to Europe by Columbus and his crew of explorers, tobacco was popularized by Jean Nicot, a French diplomat. At first, tobacco was valued for its assumed sanitary and curative properties. However, it was not long before kings and popes denounced tobacco and the practice of smoking as offensive.

While the prepared leaves of *Nicotiana tabacum* have become a popular source of mood modification throughout the modern world, **cigarette** smoking is frequently described as the major cause of preventable illness and premature deaths in the United States. Increasingly, the use of cigarettes and other tobacco products is seen as addictive suicide.[1] By contrast, stopping smoking is "the single most important step that smokers can take to enhance the length and quality of their lives."[2]

Smoking tobacco cigarettes and cigars, chewing plugs of tobacco, and sniffing powdered tobacco are potentially dangerous practices. Such behaviors can and do lead to various ailments and severe disorders, from discolored teeth and impaired breathing to debilitating and fatal illnesses, especially heart disease and cancer. These facts are widely known and even accepted by most Americans, including many who smoke. Since the first surgeon general's report on smoking and health was issued in 1964, millions have quit smoking. Nevertheless, millions of people continue to smoke, although nearly 70 percent of them claim they want to quit. And more than 1,000 Americans die each day from smoking-related diseases; that is nearly 450,000 each year. In the United States, smoking is now responsible for more than one of every six deaths. And according to the World Health Organization (WHO), approximately 2.5 million people die worldwide each year as a result of using tobacco. The immediate question one might ask is, Why? Why do so many start to smoke and then continue to smoke?

Countless individuals have made personal decisions about smoking—to start, to change brands, to stop, and to start again after a period of abstinence. Why don't more people stop smoking?

Once a person starts to smoke, his or her future choices about smoking are less freely made, because smoking tobacco is addictive.[3] The smoker almost innocently becomes "hooked" after thousands of puffs a year. Each day of smoking, the hundreds of puffs inhaled produce a well-established puff-inhalation dependency—a dependency that is extremely hard to break!

While an estimated 34 percent of all smokers have actually tried to quit, only 8 percent have succeeded in doing so. Cigarette smoking has, indeed, become the most widespread example of drug dependency in this country, similar in many ways to heroin addiction. It is becoming apparent that the addictive qualities of nicotine are sufficient to overpower a smoker's fear of premature death.[4]

More than individuals become tobacco dependent, however. Our society at large is "hooked"—burdened with a king-sized tobacco industry, a mammoth agricultural enterprise, a considerable source of governmental revenues, a significant customer of the print media, and a potent force in regional and national politics.

While public and private health agencies emphasize the serious health risks of both smoking and smokeless tobacco, the federal government continues to subsidize tobacco growers. Again the question is, Why? Why should taxpayers support growing a harmful product and then have to finance disease-prevention activities to discourage the use of the same product?

As a nation, we face a major public health problem and a persistent threat to health that costs an estimated $68 billion per year in lost productivity and the treatment of smoking-related diseases. The American Cancer Society claims this economic expense amounts to nearly $2.59 for each pack of cigarettes sold in the United States.[5]

Yet the major health problems associated with tobacco smoking are created largely by individuals who decide to risk well-being for a puff of smoke, a plug of chewing tobacco, or a pinch of snuff. Why?

The questions and issues raised here illustrate the complex problem of understanding a learned behavior that often develops into a dependency, and the difficulty in proposing and applying solutions. More than personal satisfaction is involved in using tobacco. Sociocultural, economic, political, pharmacological, and even moral factors are identified in the continuation of a legal, mood-modifying activity that is also a primary health risk.

Patterns and Trends of Tobacco Use

Though cigarette smoking has been a popular and widespread practice in the recent past, smokers are now in the minority. Although smoking was once perceived as an admired status symbol, current smoking activity is at its lowest level in more than forty years, and it appears to be heavily concentrated in America's lower socioeconomic classes. At present, the prevalence of smoking remains higher among those living below the poverty level. While overall consumption of cigarettes continues to fall, the decreases have not been uniform across all groups.[6] Less-educated people and minority groups have had smaller reductions in usage rates, and so have females in comparison with males. In addition, the highest proportion of smokers is still found among people between the ages of 25 and 44, while the lowest occurs among those 75 years or older.

With fewer smokers now than in the recent past and with the per capita consumption falling (see fig. 7.1), the U.S. production of cigarettes is an estimated 702 billion each year, an all-time high. The recent significant increase in domestic production is the result of foreign demand for U.S. tobacco and American manufacturers' offering discounted cigarettes and lower prices on premium brands to Japan, South Korea, Burma, and numerous third-world countries.[7]

Since its introduction into Western civilization by explorers returning from the New World, smoking until recently was viewed almost exclusively as a masculine activity. Before World War I, a woman who smoked was usually

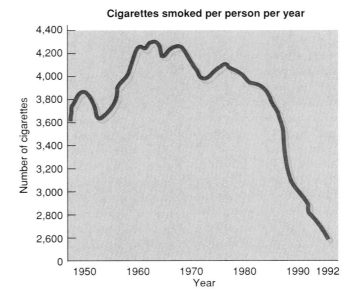

Cigarettes smoked per person per year

figure 7.1

Per capita consumption of cigarettes, 1950–1992.

Source: Office on Smoking and Health, Center for Health Promotion and Education, 1992; and the American Cancer Society, 1992.

considered unfeminine. During the past seventy years, however, women have gradually cast aside the moral and social stigmas surrounding cigarette use, and since World War II they have been smoking more and more like men—and dying like men! Due to the increase in beginning rates of smoking among less-educated young women, the prevalence of daily smoking has been higher among high school senior females than among males.

The proportions of both women and men smokers have declined over the past twenty years. But surveys indicate that the number of men smokers dropped more rapidly and to a much greater degree than the number of women smokers. Although some adult women are now beginning to quit at rates comparable to those for adult men, the rate of starting to smoke among younger women has not declined. By contrast, adolescent males have slowed their rate of smoking initiation.

Although the prevalence of smoking in the adult and adolescent populations has declined over the last decade, the average daily number of cigarettes consumed by those who continue to smoke has actually increased. Those who do smoke appear to be smoking more than

ever before—a condition some scientists relate to the introduction of filter-tipped and low-tar/low-nicotine cigarettes. The popularity of cigars and smoking tobacco for pipes has also declined somewhat in recent years, along with cigarettes.

Resisting this general downward trend is the rather sudden increase in the use of **"smokeless tobacco"—chewing tobacco** and **snuff.** Associated largely with an aggressive advertising campaign, smokeless tobacco has become a fad among junior high, senior high, and college athletes in particular, and younger males in general.[8] Rather than sniffing powdered tobacco, the individual usually inserts the substance between the gum and cheek, a practice known as **snuff dipping.** Though its popularity has increased significantly, smokeless tobacco should not be considered as a safe alternative to smoking. It isn't!

The Changing Cigarette

Currently at least 90 percent of all U.S. smokers use filter-tip brands, and more than half of all cigarettes consumed are "low-tar" cigarettes, which are defined as yielding 15 milligrams of "tar" or less per cigarette. (Tar is the particulate matter in

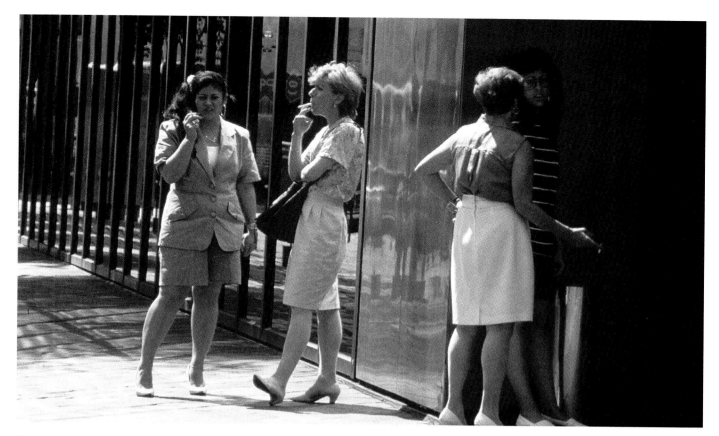

Since the end of World War II, women have been smoking more and more like men—and dying like men from tobacco-related diseases.

© Lee Snider/The Image Works

cigarette smoke.) Such preferences in product choice and cigarette use are often related to the public's increased concern about the dangers of smoking. Women smokers are more likely to use these **lower-yield cigarettes** than men are, and smokers of higher income and education also select lower-yield cigarettes in a higher percentage of cases.

Many health authorities approve of this switch from high-tar and high-nicotine cigarettes to lower-yield ones. In theory, such a change should be protective, because the danger of smoking is believed to be proportional to the dose of inhaled tar, nicotine, and carbon monoxide. Health risk generally is related to the amount of smoke as measured by the number of cigarettes consumed. Smoking these "safer" cigarettes, however, gives only limited reduction of the risks of lung and larynx cancer.

Cancer rates for smokers of such cigarettes are still much higher than those

for nonsmokers. In addition, there is insufficient evidence that the "safer" cigarettes reduce the excess risk of other smoking-related cancers, cardiovascular disease, bronchitis, emphysema, complications of pregnancy, and other disorders linked to smoking. Emphasizing that there is *no safe cigarette* and *no safe level of consumption,* the surgeon general's report on "the changing cigarette" suggested that smoking less-hazardous cigarettes can actually increase one's health risk!

While the foregoing statement appears contradictory, it is based on the common tendency of low-yield smokers to compensate for their decreased intake of nicotine. Compensation often takes the form of increasing the number of cigarettes smoked, shortening the interval between puffs, increasing the depth of inhalation, and smoking to a shorter butt. Such compensatory changes may

turn a nominally lower-yield cigarette into a higher-yield product. Thus the shift to lower-tar cigarettes may not result in reduced smoke exposure. Any advantage of the lower-yield product is canceled. In some instances, the health risks are even greater than if fewer of the higher-tar cigarettes were smoked on a daily basis.

An additional concern deals with health risks related to the design, filtering mechanisms, tobacco ingredients, and additives of the lower-yield products. The chief concern involves the increasing use of **tobacco additives** for processing or flavoring, as described in box 7.1. Some of these additives are either known or suspect cancer-causing substances or give rise to carcinogenic substances when burned. The use of these additives may cancel the beneficial effects of reducing the tar yield or might pose increased or new and different disease risks.

box 7.1

Tobacco Additives

Tobacco additives are nontobacco substances, including artificial tobacco substitutes and flavoring extracts, that are typically added to the tobacco mixture of low-tar and low-nicotine cigarettes. These additives are now included along with tobacco to speed up or slow down the burn rate of the cigarette, to promote cohesion of the ash, and to improve flavor and aroma.

Among the additives more frequently used in the manufacture of lower-yield cigarettes are the following:

Artificial tobacco substitutes

Tobacco stems

Flavor extracts of tobacco and other plants

Chemicals specified as "exogenous" enzymes—substances that can promote certain chemical changes

Powdered cocoa flavoring

Licorice

Sugar

Caramel

Freshness-preserving chemicals known as glycols

The precise identity, chemical composition, and potential harmfulness of these additives are not completely known at the present time. However, when burned, some of them are considered to be cocarcinogens—substances that increase the power or activity of cancer-causing chemicals, such as tobacco

tars. Until the Food and Drug Administration has the authority to supervise the manufacture of tobacco products, it is likely that many years of research will be required before scientists and smokers learn all of the hazards of the new, "milder" cigarettes.

Another additive, ground cloves, has been responsible for the recent popularity of "clove cigarettes," or kreteks. Imported from Indonesia, these products contain about 60 to 70 percent tobacco and 30 to 40 percent cloves. However, the smoker is exposed to twice as much tar, nicotine, and carbon monoxide from clove cigarettes as from regular American cigarettes. Typically, clove cigarette smoke is inhaled more deeply and retained in the lungs longer.

The major active ingredient in cloves is the chemical eugenol, which has an anesthetic effect. It is possible that eugenol anesthetizes the backs of smokers' throats and tracheas, thus permitting deeper inhalation and possibly encouraging smoking in some people who would otherwise be discouraged by the harshness of regular cigarettes.

Cloves may improve the fragrance of cigarettes and may produce a mild high, but they certainly do not make tobacco cigarettes less hazardous. Preliminary research indicates that ground cloves can produce serious lung damage and sudden respiratory distress. Accumulation of fluid in the lungs; spasms of the lungs' airways; spitting up or coughing up blood; and increased nausea, vomiting, angina, and respiratory infections have all been reported. Other medical problems related to smoking clove cigarettes include severe asthma attacks, difficulty in breathing, chronic coughing, and nosebleeds.

Personal Use Versus the Nonsmoker

Until the invention of the cigarette manufacturing machine after the Civil War, tobacco was principally consumed in pipes and cigars and in chewing and sniffing. Once mass production of cigarettes was a reality and production costs decreased, cigarettes became readily available. Their preeminence as a tobacco form has been traced to World War I, when they found the favor of the doughboys (soldiers).

Cigarettes became immensely popular because they provided the user with certain personal gratifications unobtainable in other tobacco forms. Cigarettes can be smoked easily and quickly; they can be

inhaled; they are readily available and still relatively inexpensive; and they had achieved limited social acceptance or toleration, until the nonsmokers' liberation movement became prominent and active in the 1970s.

Not to be overlooked as a factor in cigarette consumption are the persistent promotional activities of tobacco companies and their advertising agencies. Long ago, motivational research revealed that sales could be increased if products were linked with basic human desires and drives. Not content with assertions of mildness and good taste, advertisements soon depicted smokers as models of sophistication, eternal youth, handsome ruggedness, enduring beauty, alluring sexuality, and determined individualism, and with athletic prowess sufficient to walk at least a mile for a favorite cigarette.

To counteract declining numbers of both cigarette smokers and cigarette sales, manufacturers have introduced recently a record number of new brands in a frantic attempt to increase their own market shares. New entries include "designer smokes" for fashion-conscious females, full-flavor (high-tar) cigarettes aimed at Hispanic Americans, premium-priced brands for young upwardly mobile professionals, and even a special cigarette for smokers in the military service.

Several years ago, one major manufacturer test-marketed a "smokeless" or low-smoke cigarette that was advertised as relatively safer than its standard, traditional competition. While such a tobacco product actually reduced "sidestream" smoke—often offensive to nonsmokers—and lowered the smoker's own exposure

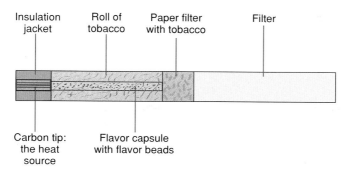

Insulation jacket · Roll of tobacco · Paper filter with tobacco · Filter

Carbon tip: the heat source · Flavor capsule with flavor beads

Rather than burning tobacco and providing nicotine-laden smoke as in conventional cigarettes, the "Premier" delivered nicotine to the smoker without actually burning tobacco. When a smoker lighted the carbon tip – the heat source – the aluminum insulation core got warm and set off a chemical reaction that released flavor, nicotine, and various other chemicals, which were inhaled into the smoker's lungs. This drug-delivery system provided nicotine to the smoker, while innovative "denicotinized" cigarettes still delivered tobacco tars to the smoker. Smokers, beware!

 7.2

Cross-section of the short-lived "Premier," test-marketed as a "smokeless" cigarette.

to tobacco tars, medical scientists generally describe this innovative cigarette as nothing more than a high-technology drug-delivery system (see fig. 7.2).

This smokeless device did not actually burn tobacco, but rather heated it along with unknown flavor-enhancing chemicals. Nevertheless, the new cigarette did deliver nicotine to the user in a dose sufficient to maintain a nicotine dependence, and provided as much carbon monoxide as regular low-tar cigarettes. Although this new smokeless product addressed some antismoking criticisms, it was withdrawn eventually from production because of poor consumer acceptance. Undaunted by such initial rejection, the same tobacco company later developed yet another cigarette product that gets nicotine to the smoker without filling the air with sidestream smoke. This new product, known as Eclipse, does not burn tobacco as conventional cigarettes do. Nevertheless, the U.S. Food and Drug Administration is likely to consider Eclipse as nothing more than a nicotine-delivery device. If such a determination is made, then the Food and Drug Administration may be able to regulate this new cigarette, because it is a drug.

Though federal laws ban their promotion on television and radio, cigarettes and smokeless tobacco products have been advertised heavily in newspapers, magazines, direct mail, billboards, posters in trains and buses, bus terminals, subways, and airports, and on small placards in taxis and on the backs of ski-lift chairs. Other tobacco products may still be promoted on radio and television in the United States, but not for long, if proposed antitobacco measures are enacted. Now under consideration is a total ban on all tobacco advertising in all electronic, print, and display media, and stricter enforcement of laws forbidding the sale of tobacco products to anyone under 18 years of age.

Smoking has long been considered an individual adult right. However, little thought or consideration has been given to what right the nonsmoker has to live and work in areas free from air polluted by smoke. It would seem as though the nonsmoker has a right to travel in an airplane, bus, or train; to listen to a lecture or attend a concert in an auditorium; to work; or to eat at a restaurant without being exposed to air filled with the smoke from cigarettes, pipes, or cigars. This consideration has resulted in major changes in public places, first as separate areas for smokers and nonsmokers, then as totally smoke-free areas, which are increasingly demanded.

Recently, the silent majority of nonsmokers has become assertive in its demands for plain, unpolluted air. Tired of tobacco smoke assaulting them, the vocal and visible nonsmokers now proclaim that the smokers' liberty ends where their noses begin. Organized groups of nonsmokers, such as Action on Smoking and Health (ASH) and the Group Against Smokers' Pollution (GASP), together with the American Lung Association, the American Cancer Society, and professional medical and dental associations, have been successful in restricting or banning smoking in both public and private areas, including work areas, and in establishing the legal right of nonsmokers to be free of others' cigarette smoke, now referred to as **"passive smoke."**

The **nonsmokers' liberation movement** has been successful in restricting smoking in hospitals, museums, and elevators, and in lobbying for laws and regulations that require health warnings on cigarette packages and for separate smoking and nonsmoking sections on commercial interstate buses and national airlines. Federal legislation now forbids smoking on most domestic flights, and some airlines are now prohibiting smoking on international flights as well.

Many states and cities have passed laws requiring either the separation of smokers and nonsmokers or the complete prohibition of smoking in public places, including educational institutions, restaurants, and retail establishments such as grocery and department stores. Some municipalities have even attempted to restrict tobacco smoking in private workplaces. A growing number of companies have adopted total smoking bans and even refuse to hire smokers. Some pay bonuses to employees who quit smoking.

As some companies move to restrict smoking both on and off the job, and thus influence what many consider to be an individual right, die-hard smokers have begun to fight back. Several states have now passed legislation that forbids the firing of employees who engage in legal off-duty behavior, including smoking. And with the full implementation of the federal "Americans with Disabilities Act," employers will be prohibited from asking job applicants if they smoke. The battle between smokers and nonsmokers continues!

Psychological Aspects of Smoking

Why do people begin and continue to smoke, when most smokers admit that smoking is harmful to personal health? Many smokers express a desire to quit, undertake a program of cessation, but just cannot manage to do so. Perhaps a consideration of the origins and functional aspects of smoking behavior will reveal some of the reasons and motivations involved in the use of cigarettes.

A Learned Behavior

Smoking is often viewed as a learned behavior. No one is born a smoker, although the new baby may interact with smokers and with smoke early in infancy—often on the way home from the hospital after delivery. Curiosity and the desire to imitate adults, especially smoking parents, probably encourage many children to experiment. The initial reaction, however, is likely to be unpleasant. It is not until adolescence that smoking becomes a real option for most young people. More time is now spent away from home with peers; there is increased freedom from authority figures who often discourage or forbid smoking; needs for security and acceptance through group conformity grow; and the demand for immediate need gratification flourishes. The psychological stage for smoking has been set and is fertile enough to produce nearly a million new young smokers each year. Other factors have also been recognized as predictors of tobacco use by young people, as noted in table 7.1.

According to the surgeon general's report *Preventing Tobacco Use among Young People,*[9]

- Nearly all first use of tobacco occurs before high school graduation. If adolescents can be kept tobacco-free, most will remain tobacco-free for the remainder of their lives.

- Male and female adolescents are now equally likely to smoke cigarettes, but males are more likely than females to use smokeless tobacco.

table 7.1 Summary of Factors Appearing to Increase the Risk of Tobacco Use by Young People

Sociodemographic Factors
Young people from families with lower socioeconomic status
Adolescents living in single-parent homes
Environment Factors
Peer influence in beginning experimentation
Peer-group approval of and support of tobacco use by providing experimentation, reinforcement, and cues for continuing use
Social Environment Factors
Adolescents who highly overestimate the number of young people and adults who smoke
Young people who perceive that cigarettes are easily accessible and generally available for use
Behavioral Factors
Perception that tobacco use assists in achieving physical maturity, a coherent sense of self, and emotional independence
Belief that smoking serves positive functions, such as bonding with peers, being independent and mature, and having a positive social image
Lack of confidence to be able to resist peer offers of tobacco
Intention to use tobacco
Experimental smoking

Source: *Preventing Tobacco Use among Young People: A Report of the Surgeon General, Executive Summary,* pages 7–8, Centers for Disease Control and Prevention, 1994.

- White adolescents are more likely to use tobacco than are African American and Hispanic adolescents, and whites are much more likely to be heavy or frequent smokers.

- Most young people who smoke are addicted to nicotine and report that they want to quit but are unable to do so.

- Tobacco is often the first drug used by young people who later use alcohol and other illegal drugs, especially marijuana.

- Among young people, those with poorer grades and lower self-images are most likely to begin using tobacco.

- Cigarette advertising appears to increase young people's risk of smoking by conveying the message that smoking has important social benefits and that smoking itself is far more common than it really is.

- Adolescent tobacco use is associated with involvement in fights, carrying weapons, and engaging in risky sexual behavior.

Psychological Rewards

There are many psychological rewards for the new smoker. Smoking may be the passport to acceptance among one's peers; it may represent freedom or independence from restrictive home life and passive, traditional sex roles, or revolt against parental authority; it may be the result of an unconscious desire to imitate esteemed smokers; it may be nothing more than a soothing and pleasurable way to counteract boredom.

Because of the ritualistic hand-to-mouth motions associated with lighting up, cigarette smoking may represent a convenient "psychological recycling center" that provides a peer-approved and refreshing activity between various problems and challenges of living. Of course, some people like the taste and smell of cigarettes, and a few enjoy watching the smoke. In essence, the cigarette provides a smoker with a readily available way to deal with a host of personal problems and needs.

Factors in Smoking Behavior

The reasons for beginning cigarette use are not always the same as those for continuing to smoke. Original motives are often replaced by powerful and seemingly irresistible factors, both psychological and biochemical. These factors are most apparent in a classification of experienced smokers according to the major satisfactions people believe they get from using tobacco cigarettes. Six "satisfaction" categories are detailed below to provide an understanding of why people smoke. This brief analysis also offers various alternatives to those who wish to quit.

1. **Stimulation.** Many smokers get a lift from smoking—they feel that it helps them wake up, organize energies, and keep them going. The perking-up effect is due to nicotine's temporary stimulation, which briefly relieves fatigue. If you try to give up smoking, you may want a safe substitute: a brisk walk or moderate exercise whenever you feel the urge to smoke.

2. **Handling—oral gratification.** Having something to handle, manipulate, or fondle can be very satisfying. Additionally, having something in your mouth to chew on, such as a toothpick, straw, or pencil can fulfill certain emotional needs. From a Freudian perspective, cigarette smoking may be seen as a satisfaction of infantile needs to suck or chew—a fixation of libidinal energy at the oral or mouth level.

   Why not toy with a pen or pencil? Try doodling or play with a coin, a piece of jewelry, or some other harmless object. If you must put something in your mouth, use candy cigarettes or even a real cigarette if you can trust yourself not to light it.

3. **Pleasurable relaxation.** Other smokers smoke for positive feelings of contentment, achievement, victory, and satisfaction—such as upon completion of a job well done or after a delicious mouth-watering meal.

   Those who do get real pleasure out of smoking often find that an honest consideration of the harmful effects of their habit is enough to help them quit. They substitute eating, drinking, social activities, and physical activities—within reasonable bounds—and find they do not seriously miss their cigarettes.

4. **Crutch—tension reduction.** Many smokers use the cigarette to manage negative effects, such as stressful situations, and feelings of anger, fear, and anxiety. Sometimes the cigarette is used as a tranquilizer or as an escape from cares and worries. Thus smoking represents a tension-reducing activity. When the going gets rough, cigarettes can be a crutch, a comfort, and a consolation.

   When it comes to quitting, this kind of smoker may find it easy to stop when everything is going well but may be tempted to start again in a time of crisis. Again, physical exertion, eating, drinking, or social activity—in moderation—may serve as useful substitutes in times of tension.

5. **Craving—psychological and physical addiction.** Quitting smoking is difficult for the person who has developed a **"craving"**. For such an individual, the overpowering desire for the next cigarette begins to build up the moment the old one is put out. A dependent or addicted smoker must have a cigarette after a short period of time or otherwise experience mild withdrawal symptoms—a "nicotine fit" with its uneasiness, restlessness, nervousness, anxiety, headache, digestive disturbances, and impairment of concentration, judgment, and psychomotor performance.

   Peculiarly, the dependent smoker craves a cigarette, as in chain-smoking, first to increase positive feelings and then to decrease negative feelings of withdrawal. In essence, the smoker satisfies a need to smoke—a physical need for more nicotine.

   The very first cigarette each day sends a burst of nicotine to the brain, which produces an immediate feeling of satisfaction and mild euphoria. During the remainder of the day, the smoker tries to maintain this feeling by manipulating the intake of tobacco smoke, inhaling more or less deeply, taking more or fewer puffs, and smoking at different intervals—all characteristics of a controlled, compulsive behavior.

   Contrary to popular belief, research now suggests that smoking does not reduce anxiety or calm nerves. Under stress, smokers consume cigarettes heavily because stress depletes the body's nicotine. Thus nicotine-deficient smokers smoke more under stress to maintain their usual nicotine level.

   Tapering off is not likely to work for dependent smokers. They must go **"cold turkey,"** that is, quit all at once. It may be helpful for them to smoke more than usual for a day or two, so that the taste of cigarettes is spoiled, and then isolate themselves completely from cigarettes until the craving is gone. Giving up cigarettes may cause so much discomfort that once these people quit, they will find it easy to resist a return to smoking. Otherwise, they know that someday they will have to go through the same agony again.

6. **Habit.** The habit smoker establishes a behavioral pattern almost involuntarily. This individual responds automatically to some cue—a cup of coffee, getting into a car, or nearing the

vicinity of an ashtray. Once regarded as psychologically significant, smoking loses its former functions of fulfilling status, relaxation, security, or other emotional needs. Such a smoker no longer gets much satisfaction from cigarettes.

This smoker may find that it is easy to quit and stay off cigarettes if he or she can break developed habit patterns. Cutting down gradually may be quite effective if there is a change in the way cigarettes are smoked and the conditions under which they are smoked. The key to success is becoming aware of each cigarette you smoke. Ask yourself, "Do I really want this cigarette?" You may be surprised at how many you do not want.

Health Consequences of Smoking

In the past, many people were willing to accept smoking as long as it did not injure the health of the smoker or cause harm to others. Unfortunately, smoking is a health threat to smoker and nonsmoker alike.[10] Even unborn children can be affected adversely by this multidimensional problem often leading to self-inflicted disease (morbidity) and premature death (mortality). The smoking problem also results in increased health and welfare costs, added irritating effects of cigarette-induced air pollution, and the persistent threat of home, commercial, and forest fires caused by discarded cigarettes.

Constituents of Tobacco Smoke

The starches, proteins, sugars, and hydrocarbons of the tobacco leaf, when burned, are converted into a complex aerosol mixture of *gases* and *particulate matter* (**particulates**) (see box 7.2). The lighted cigarette generates about two thousand compounds, many of which produce undesirable effects. At the burning zone, the temperature of the smoke is nearly 900°C, although that which reaches the smoker's mouth is in a temperature range from 30° to 50°C.

In the *gas phase* of cigarette smoke are *nitrogen, oxygen,* and *carbon dioxide,* and numerous toxic components, some of which cause cancer, initiate tumors, and damage the hairlike cilia that line the bronchial tubes in the lungs. Of course, **carbon monoxide** is a poisonous component of this smoke and combines with the hemoglobin in red blood cells, thereby reducing the oxygen-carrying capacity of the blood. Also isolated in this phase of smoke are various *nitrosamines, vinyl chloride, formaldehyde, nitrogen oxides, hydrogen cyanide, ammonia,* and *pyridine.*

The *particulate phase* of cigarette smoke is composed of tiny particles that irritate the respiratory tract. The major components are *nicotine* and **"tar."** Investigations have shown that more than 90 percent of these particles remain in the lungs of smokers who inhale. When condensed, the particles—regarded as lung-damaging in size—form a yellow-brown sticky mass known as tobacco tar. The tar contains several *carcinogenic* (cancer-producing) *hydrocarbons,* known as **polycyclic aromatic hydrocarbons** (PAH). Among these PAH are nonvolatile *nitrosamines, aromatic amines, pyrenes, benzo(a)pyrenes,* and *chrysenes.* Also included in the tar are *phenols, cresols, carboxylic acids, metallic ions, radioactive compounds, agricultural chemicals,* and various *additives* and *flavoring agents.*

Nicotine, the other major component of the particulate, is a colorless, oily compound in some commercial insecticides. It is generally accepted that nicotine is the principal component responsible for cigarette smokers' pharmacologic responses. Nicotine causes the *release of catecholamines* (excitatory neurotransmitters), and initiates a series of nervous and endocrine functions experienced as a *temporary stimulation* following smoking. Common bodily actions attributed to nicotine are increased heart rate, blood pressure, and cardiac output (the heart works harder); vasoconstriction (blood-vessel narrowing), which lowers skin temperature; increased gastrointestinal activity; increased respiration; and a release of glycogen from the liver, causing the brief "kick" and reduction of fatigue often reported by smokers.

These actions of nicotine soon become reinforcing, or rewarding. The most likely site of this reinforcing action is the brain. Inhaling smoke thus ensures rapid delivery of nicotine. (It takes about 13.5 seconds for an intravenous injection of nicotine in the arm to reach the brain, but by inhalation the delivery time is just 7.5 seconds.) An individual who smokes only one pack per day can average 70,000 such nicotine "injections" per year. As such, smoking has many potential conditioned stimuli, ranging from the taste, sight, and feel of the cigarette to the many social settings in which

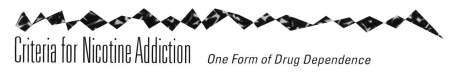

Criteria for Nicotine Addiction *One Form of Drug Dependence*

Primary Criteria

User's behavior is highly controlled by a drug substance

Drug has a psychoactive (mind-changing) effect

Presence of drug-reinforced behavior

Additional Criteria

Dependence-producing drug use often results in:

Tolerance

Physical dependence evidenced by withdrawal syndrome

Pleasant (euphoric) effects

Addictive behavior often involves:

Repetitive and stereotypic use patterns

Quitting episodes followed by resumption of drug use (relapse)

Compulsive use despite harmful effects

Recurring cravings or urges to use the drug, especially during drug abstinence

Note: The terms *drug addiction* and *drug dependence* are scientifically equivalent and are often used synonymously.

Source: Modified from *The Health Consequences of Smoking: Nicotine Addiction, A Report of the Surgeon General,* 7, 1988.

smoking takes place. It is easy to see, therefore, how smokers can become psychologically dependent on tobacco.

Nicotine Addiction

For many years, people have thought of tobacco use as merely habituating (habit-forming). This attitude prevailed despite the fact that many cigarette smokers, who had repeatedly failed in their attempt to stop smoking, probably realized that their tobacco use was something more than a simple little habit. Now the scientific community has recognized the addictive or dependency-producing nature of cigarette smoking and tobacco use. This formal recognition helps explain why so many people continue to use tobacco, despite its known health risks.

After observing smokers' behavior, scientists now believe that most cigarette users—perhaps as many as 90 percent—are physically dependent on smoking. And nicotine is the leading candidate for the addictive agent.[11] Moreover, recent allegations have been made that cigarette manufacturers have intentionally regulated the nicotine content of their products. Such a practice not only entraps new smokers, but also

keeps these smokers addicted. Addicted smokers are, after all, very reliable customers who continue to purchase cigarettes despite a strong desire to quit smoking.

The blood plasma half-life of nicotine is about 30 minutes, and the pack-a-day smoker lights up approximately every 30 to 40 minutes of the day. This activity suggests that the smoker is attempting to maintain a constant level of nicotine in the brain. When deprived of this regular dose, the nicotine-dependent smoker begins to suffer discomfort, jumpiness, irritability, craving for another smoke, nausea, and sometimes headache. Although individuals such as these may desire the pleasant, stimulated feeling provided by a rush of nicotine, they continue to smoke because they want to prevent the unwanted effects of withdrawal. With 200 to 300 practice puffs each day, most smokers become fairly proficient at regulating their intake of nicotine.

Upon thorough analysis of available evidence, the surgeon general concluded that cigarettes and other forms of tobacco, too, are indeed addicting.[12] And nicotine is the drug in tobacco that causes this addiction. Furthermore, the drug actions and

behavioral processes that determine tobacco addiction are similar to those that determine addiction to heroin and cocaine.

And in a comparison of tobacco cigarette dependence with other drug dependencies, 57 percent of drug-dependent individuals said that cigarettes would be harder to quit than their own problem substance.[13] Alcohol-dependent persons were about four times more likely than drug-dependent persons to say that their strongest urges for cigarettes were at least as great as their strongest urges for their problem substance. However, cigarettes were generally rated as less pleasurable than either alcohol or other mind-altering drugs.

The core or central element among all forms of drug addiction is that the user's behavior is largely controlled by a substance having a psychoactive effect. There is often compulsive use of the drug despite damage to the individual or to society, and drug-seeking behavior can take precedence over other important life priorities. In addition, the drug is reinforcing, that is, the drug's effect is sufficiently rewarding to maintain self-administration over and over again.

Another aspect of drug addiction is *tolerance,* a condition in which a given dose of a drug produces less effect, or increasing doses are required to achieve a desired response. *Physical dependence* on the drug can also occur and is characterized by a *withdrawal syndrome* (including craving for tobacco, irritability, anxiety, difficulty in concentrating, restlessness, headache, drowsiness, and gastrointestinal disturbances) that usually accompanies drug abstinence. After cessation of drug use, there is a strong tendency to *relapse* or restart using the drug again.

Research now demonstrates that tobacco use and nicotine in particular meet all of these criteria.

Research Findings

Human population studies, health surveys, animal experimentation, and clinical and autopsy studies have been the bases for the present knowledge of the health and disease effects of smoking cigarettes. Following are the significant findings of these research endeavors.

1. **Overall death rates.** Cigarette smokers have overall death rates that are substantially greater than those of nonsmokers. Estimates of excess deaths associated with cigarette smoking have ranged up to 450,000 per year. Heart and blood-vessel diseases, including stroke, along with lung cancer, chronic obstructive lung (respiratory) disease, and other cancerous conditions are the major contributors to this excess of smoking-related mortality.

2. **Other cancerous conditions.** In addition to the epidemic of smoking-caused lung cancer, cigarette smoking is also the major cause of cancer of the larynx (voice box), mouth, and esophagus, and a contributing factor in the development of cancer of the bladder, pancreas, and kidney. Use of tobacco cigarettes is now associated with increased risk of cancer of the stomach and uterine cervix as well as of the colon or rectum.[14,15]

3. **Life expectancy.** Expected life span at any given age is significantly shortened by cigarette smoking. An average drop of seven to nine years in smokers' life expectancy has been reported, although one study suggests that smokers may actually lose as many as 18 years of their life expectancy, in comparison with nonsmokers.[16]

4. **Dose-related mortality.** In both men and women smokers, excess mortality is dose related. That is, death rates increase with the *number of cigarettes smoked* and are proportional to the *duration of smoking,* an *earlier age of beginning cigarette smoking, inhalation of cigarette smoke,* and a *higher tar and nicotine content* of the cigarette.

5. **Pipe and cigar smoking.** Pipe and cigar smoking are also associated with elevated mortality for cancers of the upper respiratory tract, including cancer of the oral cavity (mouth and lip), the larynx (throat and vocal

cords), and the esophagus. Such smoking results in lower death rates than for cigarette smokers, but higher than for nonsmokers.

6. **Chronic (long-term) health conditions.** In general, male and female cigarette smokers tend to report more chronic health conditions, such as chronic bronchitis and/or emphysema, chronic sinusitis, peptic ulcer disease, and arteriosclerotic heart disease, than people who never smoked. Women who smoke also experience a higher risk of broken bones, because smoking tends to reduce bone density. There is a dose-response relationship between the number of cigarettes smoked per day and the frequency of reporting for most of the chronic conditions just cited.

7. **Acute (short-term) health conditions.** The occurrence of acute conditions (for example, influenza and the common cold) for males who had ever smoked was 14 percent higher, and for females 21 percent higher, than for those who had never smoked cigarettes.

8. **Lost workdays and disability.** Both male and female current cigarette smokers experienced an excess of workdays lost, days of bed disability,

and longer limitation of activity due to chronic diseases than did people who never smoked. Additionally, current and former smokers reported more hospitalization than nonsmokers in the year prior to being interviewed. Significantly, all measures of smoking disability were dose related; that is, the more smoking there was, the greater the likelihood of developing a disability or disablement.

9. **Smoking during pregnancy.** Babies born to women who smoke during pregnancy weigh an average of 200 grams less than babies born to comparable nonsmoking women. The more a woman smokes during pregnancy, the greater the reduction in infant birth weight. Moreover, maternal smoking during pregnancy may adversely affect the child's long-term growth, intellectual development, and behavioral characteristics. The risks of spontaneous abortion, fetal death, neonatal death, placental disorders, bleeding early or late in pregnancy, premature and prolonged rupture of amniotic membranes, and pre-term delivery all increase directly with increasing levels of maternal smoking during pregnancy. Research also suggests that maternal

SURGEON GENERAL'S WARNING: Smoking Causes Lung Cancer, Heart Disease, Emphysema, and May Complicate Pregnancy.

SURGEON GENERAL'S WARNING: Quitting Smoking Now Greatly Reduces Serious Risks to Your Health.

SURGEON GENERAL'S WARNING: Smoking by Pregnant Women May Result in Fetal Injury, Premature Birth, and Low Birth Weight.

SURGEON GENERAL'S WARNING: Cigarette Smoke Contains Carbon Monoxide.

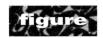 **7.3**

Warning labels.

Source: Surgeon General's Public Health Service, Office of the Assistant Secretary for Health.

smoking during pregnancy may biologically prime the fetal brain of daughters, predisposing them to smoke years after their birth.[17]

10. **Reproductive problems and male erectile dysfunction.** Studies in women and men suggest that cigarette smoking may impair fertility—the capability of reproducing—by interfering with the production of eggs, sperm, or the conception process. Women who smoked more than a pack of cigarettes a day had two-and-one-half times the chance of developing an ectopic pregnancy—implantation of a fertilized egg outside the lining of the uterus—as women who did not smoke.[18] Those who smoked only a half pack a day were one-and-one-half times as likely to have such a pregnancy. And among men, the more cigarettes smoked over time, the higher the risk of developing male erectile dysfunction. It is thought that nicotine damages the penile arteries, which become narrowed and eventually block the flow of blood, leading to impotence.

11. **Sudden infant death syndrome.** An infant's risk of developing sudden infant death syndrome (SIDS) is increased by maternal smoking during pregnancy. Smoking tends to double the risk in what appears to be a dose-response relationship, that is, the more the mother smokes while pregnant, the greater the likelihood the infant will experience a stoppage of breathing while asleep.[19]

12. **Depression.** Research now indicates that mental depression plays an important role in the dynamics of cigarette smoking. Individuals with a history of major depression may be "self-medicating" their psychic pain by smoking tobacco cigarettes. In addition, smokers are more likely than nonsmokers to be depressed, and smokers who are depressed usually find it more difficult to quit smoking than smokers who are not mentally depressed.[20,21]

13. **Decreased oxygen uptake and exercise tolerance.** Elevated carbon monoxide levels in the blood—a consequence of using tobacco cigarettes—have been shown to decrease maximal oxygen uptake in healthy people, as well as decrease the exercise tolerance of persons with heart disease. Additionally, cigarette smoking tends to impair exercise performance, especially in some types of athletic events and activities involving maximal work capacity.

14. **Smoking and other unhealthy behaviors.** A national research study revealed that smokers tend to display several unhealthy behaviors that may increase the probability of their developing serious illness and disability and experiencing premature death.[22] Compared with nonsmokers, smokers are more likely to get little sleep (six hours or less per night), skip breakfast, not exercise actively, and drink alcohol heavily (two drinks or more daily). In contrast, smokers were less likely to be overweight and less likely to snack daily than were nonsmokers. The more favorable weight status and snacking behavior tended to be most characteristic of lighter smokers.

15. **Premature facial wrinkling.** Cigarette smoking has been identified recently as an independent risk factor for the development of premature facial wrinkling.[23] This risk for excessive wrinkling is dose dependent to smoking exposure measured in "pack years" (1 pack year equals smoking one pack a day per year), and doubles for pack years between 1 and 49. For heavy smokers with more than 50 pack years (1 pack a day for 50 years, 2 packs a day for 25 years, or 3 packs a day for 17 years), the risk is 4.7 times greater than for nonsmokers. When excessive sun exposure and cigarette smoking occurred together, the risk for developing excessive facial skin wrinkling is multiplied by 12.

16. **Source of drug interactions.** Smoking of tobacco should be considered as one of the primary sources of drug interactions in the human body. For certain drugs, smokers may need a larger dose or may have to take the drug more often than nonsmokers. Smoking may also result in increased risks with drug use, affect an individual's response to certain common diagnostic tests, and interact with certain food constituents.

One specific smoking-drug problem is the increased risk of heart attack, stroke, and other circulatory diseases among those women who smoke and also use oral contraceptives. This risk is even higher in women older than 37 years and among heavy smokers. The official Food and Drug Administration's warning is loud and clear: "*Women who use oral contraceptives should not smoke.*"

Another such smoking-drug interaction is apparent in alcohol usage. Beverage alcohol and cigarette smoking show synergistic effects in causing cancer of the upper digestive tract.

Passive Smoking

Inhaling tobacco smoke from another person's cigarette, cigar, or pipe can be more than annoying. In some cases, it can be deadly. There is now considerable evidence that nonsmokers are exposed to the elements and hazards of tobacco smoke when they are around people who are smoking.[24] It is also clear that the tobacco smoke left in the air by smokers can produce some very serious diseases in nonsmokers who must breathe the very same air.[25]

Secondhand **sidestream smoke** from the burning tobacco products of others, smoke that escapes from the nonburning ends, and **mainstream smoke** that has been inhaled by smokers and then exhaled—all mix with air in an enclosed

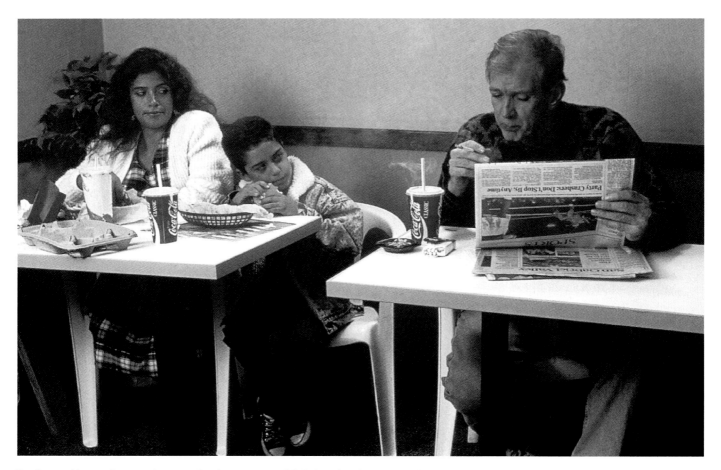

Passive smoking can be more than annoying. In some cases, inhalation of environmental tobacco smoke increases the risk of lung cancer, heart disease, and other cardiac, blood vessel, and blood disorders.

© Stephen McBrady/Photo Edit

space to form **environmental tobacco smoke,** or ETS. Passive smoking involves the involuntary inhalation of ETS. This environmental tobacco smoke is basically the same, though lower in concentration, as the mixture to which smokers are exposed. It is this ETS that tends to cause a large proportion of healthy nonsmokers to experience irritation of the eyes, nose, and throat.

Sidestream smoke is not filtered (as the smoker's is) and often has higher concentrations of hazardous substances than does mainstream smoke. In fact, concentrations of at least seventeen cancer-causing chemicals are higher in sidestream smoke than in mainstream smoke. For example, the concentration of highly carcinogenic N-nitrosamine is so much higher in sidestream smoke

that nonsmokers in very smoky rooms for just one hour would inhale as much of this chemical as they would by smoking ten to fifteen cigarettes.

Passive cigarette smoke can make a significant and measurable contribution to the amount of indoor air pollution at levels of smoking and ventilation common in the indoor environment. Exposed to an atmosphere of environmental tobacco smoke (ETS) in a confined space, the nonsmoker may also develop varying degrees of stress, discomfort, coughing, wheezing, and allergic reactions. People with certain heart and lung diseases and allergies may also suffer a worsening of their symptoms as a result of exposure to tobacco smoke-filled environments.

Recent studies summarized below indicate that secondhand tobacco smoke is

more than just an irritant or a contaminant that merely aggravates the symptoms of those who suffer respiratory diseases (box 7.4).

1. The National Academy of Sciences and the surgeon general of the United States have concluded that passive smoke increases the risk of lung cancer among nonsmokers by up to 34 percent, particularly for spouses of smokers. Furthermore, 20 percent of lung cancer deaths among nonsmokers can be attributed to passive smoke—the residue of vapors and particles in the air from burning cigarettes and other tobacco products.

2. The Environmental Protection Agency (EPA) has identified passive

Health Consequences of Involuntary (Passive) Smoking

Lung Cancer in Nonsmoking Adults

1. Passive smoking is causally associated with lung cancer in adults.
2. Approximately 3,000 lung cancer deaths per year among nonsmokers (never smoked and former smokers) of both sexes are estimated to be linked to environmental tobacco smoke (ETS) in the United States.

Noncancer Respiratory Diseases and Disorders

1. Exposure of children to ETS from parental smoking is now causally associated with
   a. increased prevalence of respiratory symptoms of irritation, such as coughing, sputum production, and wheezing;
   b. increased prevalence of middle-ear effusion, a sign of middle-ear disease; and
   c. a small but statistically significant reduction in lung function.
2. ETS exposure of young people and particularly infants from parental (and especially mother's) smoking is causally associated with an increased risk of lower respiratory infections (LRIs), including pneumonia, bronchitis, and bronchiolitis. An estimated 150,000 to 300,000 LRIs occur annually in infants and children less than 18 months of age, resulting in 7,500 to 15,000 hospitalizations annually.
3. Additional episodes and increased severity of asthma in children who already have the disease. It is estimated that ETS exposure worsens symptoms in approximately 20 percent of this nation's 2 million to 5 million asthmatic children and is a major aggravating factor in approximately 10 percent.
4. Evidence is suggestive, but not conclusive, that ETS exposure increases the number of new cases of asthma in children who have not previously exhibited symptoms.
5. Passive smoking has subtle but significant effects on the respiratory health of nonsmoking adults, including coughing, phlegm production, chest discomfort, and reduced lung function.

Source: U.S. Environmental Protection Agency and the U.S. Department of Health and Human Services.

smoke as a "class A carcinogen"—a cancer-causing substance that can be as deadly as radon and benzene in humans. As such, environmental tobacco smoke causes nonsmokers to develop an estimated three thousand cases of lung cancer each year.

3. Yale University scientists have found that approximately 17 percent of lung cancers among nonsmokers can be traced to exposure to high levels of cigarette smoke during childhood and adolescence. The apparent risk for getting lung cancer as adults doubled with exposure to twenty-five or more "smoker years"—the number of years a child or adolescent lived in a household multiplied by the number of smokers in the household.[26]

4. For nonsmoking women with spouses who smoke, the risk for developing lung cancer is about 30 percent higher over a lifetime than for those with nonsmoking spouses. This study confirms preliminary data that suggested exposure to ETS during adult life increases risk of lung cancer in lifetime nonsmokers.[27]

5. Other researchers have claimed that heart disease is an important consequence of being exposed to environmental tobacco smoke, and that ETS actually causes heart disease.[28,29] The increase in risk translates into nearly ten times as many deaths from ETS-induced heart disease as from lung cancer. Such

deaths contribute greatly to the estimated 53,000 deaths each year from passive smoking.

Still other harmful effects are now associated with ETS. Carbon monoxide levels occasionally reached in some **involuntary smoking** situations have resulted in impaired psychomotor function, especially attentiveness and cognitive skills. And recent data indicate that even fetal growth can be adversely affected when the mother is passively exposed to tobacco smoke during pregnancy.[30]

It has also been recognized that long-term exposure to tobacco smoke in the work environment is deleterious to the nonsmoker and significantly reduces small airway function in the lungs. Based upon tests of the lungs' ability to hold and expel air, research has concluded that passive smoking causes a measurable loss in breathing capacity. Apparently, tiny air tubes and sacs in the airways of the lungs become scarred and permanently damaged.

Smoking and Cardiovascular Diseases

Cigarette smoking is now recognized as a major risk factor in the development of specific **cardiovascular** (heart and blood vessel) **diseases,** namely, **coronary heart disease,** *atherosclerosis* (the buildup of blood fats inside the arteries), and *abnormal conditions of the blood vessels in the arms and legs.* The risk of heart attack due to coronary heart disease is more than twice that of nonsmokers.[31] Significantly, cigarette smoking is the biggest risk factor for sudden cardiac death—smokers have two to four times the risk of nonsmokers. And smoking is thought to be responsible for an estimated 30 percent of all deaths in the United States each year that are caused by heart disease.

Cigarette use has also been associated with increased mortality from cerebrovascular accidents (strokes) and non-syphilitic aortic aneurysms (balloonings of the major artery of the body). Though smoking is considered a secondary risk factor in this instance, it affects the risk of stroke indirectly by increasing the risk of heart disease—a primary risk factor for stroke. Compared with nonsmokers, male cigarette smokers have two to three times greater risk of stroke, even when other stroke risk factors are controlled.

The exact mechanisms of cigarette-related cardiovascular diseases are not fully known, but they are thought to involve *nicotine and carbon monoxide as principal malefactors*. Smoking may initiate a disease process by causing irreversible damage; it may enable or provide positive support to the development of an abnormal condition; it may interfere with and thereby reduce the normal ability of an organism to cope with a disease process; or it may produce temporary conditions that increase the likelihood that some critical event will occur with possibly fatal consequences, such as a heart attack. One or more of these mechanisms may be operable independently or in conjunction with other factors often associated with cardiovascular diseases: obesity, high serum cholesterol, high blood pressure, and physical inactivity.

It is an established fact that nicotine is responsible for the near-instantaneous increase in heart rate, blood pressure, cardiac output, heart contractions, and consumption of oxygen by heart muscle. Because of its blood-vessel narrowing effect, nicotine can also decrease peripheral blood flow, thus placing added stress on the smoker's heart.

Since the smoker's heart is working harder now, it requires more oxygen to function in its adaptive response to smoking. But carbon monoxide from cigarette smoke tends to displace oxygen from hemoglobin (the substance in red blood cells that carries oxygen and gives blood its red color), thus interfering with the transportation of oxygen and depriving heart muscle of its needed oxygen supply. Such sudden, though temporary, burdens placed on a heart already diseased with clogged coronary (heart) arteries can result in death.

In a compensatory action of adaptation, the body produces more red blood cells, which are associated with increased clotting as the blood becomes viscous or gummy. The body is slowly starved for oxygen, particularly the brain, which is dulled. Reaction time is lengthened and may be a factor in causing auto accidents in rush hour traffic.

It is also possible that carbon monoxide causes damage by injuring the walls of arteries, enhancing the buildup of cholesterol in the development of atherosclerosis, which narrows the arteries, and reducing the supply of oxygen and other nutrients to various body cells. Such actions may explain why young males who smoke or have high blood-cholesterol levels are more likely than others to show signs of heart disease before they reach 35 years of age.

Recent evidence suggests that absorbed nicotine and carbon monoxide jointly contribute to the development of atherosclerosis. Cigarette smoking may also be a factor in increased platelet adhesiveness, which predisposes to blood-clot formation.

Smoking and Lung Cancer

In **lung cancer** victims, cures are rare, and 87 out of every 100 people who develop lung cancer will be dead within five years. In fact, the survival rate for the first year after diagnosis of lung cancer is only 25 percent.

Studies of the frequency, distribution, causes, and control of cigarette-related diseases have led an overwhelming number of scientists to conclude that *smoking is the major cause of lung cancer* in both men and women. Since 1987, more women have died of lung cancer than of breast cancer, which for over forty years was the major cause of cancer deaths in females.

At present, lung cancer is the leading cause of cancer deaths in the United States, with a yearly toll in excess of 153,000 victims.[32] The incidence or occurrence rate of lung cancer, which had been increasing steadily in both men and women for several decades, has begun to decline in men, but not in women.

This form of cancer, uncontrolled cellular growth, or malignant neoplasm, in the lungs is termed **bronchogenic carcinoma** because it arises in the lining of the bronchial tubes, through which air passes inwardly to various parts of the lungs. The chances of sustaining lung cancer are enhanced with increased numbers of cigarettes smoked per day, with the duration or length of smoking, and with earlier initiation of use. The risks are reduced when smoking ceases. Apparently, cigarette smoking triggers a disease process (via the *tobacco tars*) in which continual repair and recovery are possible up to some "hazardous point." Beyond this critical point, the process is not reversible in most cases.

Laboratory Experiments

In laboratory experiments involving dogs, hamsters, and mice, the cancer-producing (carcinogenic) nature of the tobacco tars, whole cigarette smoke, and filtered smoke has been demonstrated. When applied to test animals by skin painting, tracheal installation or implantation, and inhalation, the components of cigarette smoke were capable of producing cancerous growths similar to those found in the lungs and larynx of smokers.

Autopsy Studies

However, the most incriminating evidence against cigarettes has been derived from detailed autopsy studies conducted on patients who died of lung cancer in comparison with noncancer patients. Lung cancer victims were found to have increased presence of bronchial tissue changes considered by investigators to be the precursors (forerunners) of invasive cancer. Additional studies then compared the frequency of these cancer-related changes in the lungs of smokers and nonsmokers. In nearly every case, there was noted an increased prevalence of these cellular alterations or adaptations among smokers as compared with nonsmokers. Such changes in the lungs generally occur before cancer cells break through the basement membrane of the bronchial lining and spread throughout the lungs and to other parts of the body. The changes are (1) **hyperplasia,** (2) *loss of* **ciliary function** *in columnar cells,* and (3) **carcinoma *in situ.***

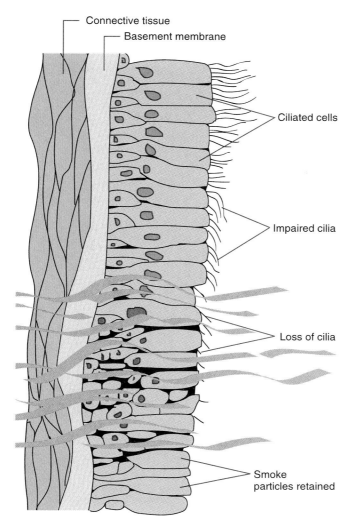

Connective tissue
Basement membrane
Ciliated cells
Impaired cilia
Loss of cilia
Smoke particles retained

 7.4

The effect of tobacco smoke on ciliary function within the bronchial tubes of the lungs.

Source: National Advisory Cancer Council.

Hyperplasia

Hyperplasia, an increase in the number of layers of basal cells that underlie the inner surface of the bronchial tubes, was the first major effect observed. This condition was prevalent in 95 percent of heavy smokers and in 80 percent of light smokers. It was rarely found in nonsmokers. A typical reaction of surface tissue to irritation, hyperplasia probably results from the constant bombardment of tobacco smoke products that under certain conditions accumulate on the lining of the bronchial tubes.

Loss of Ciliary Function

Both particulate matter and gaseous components of cigarette smoke have been shown to retard greatly and eventually stop the sweeping movements of cilia, tiny hairlike projections extending from the surface of the columnlike cells of the bronchial tubes (fig. 7.4). Cilia sweep mucus and other debris out of the respiratory tree into the mouth, where it is swallowed or expectorated. Retarded ciliary function interferes with mucus removal and permits the deposit of smoke irritants on the bronchial tube lining, and it gives

rise to the smoker's cough. The remaining columnar cells undergo a flattening and enlargement, characteristic of smokers' lung tissue.

Carcinoma in Situ

Characterized by the development of disordered cells with atypical nuclei, carcinoma *in situ*—literally, a cancerous growth remaining at the site of its origin—describes a noninvasive cancer. A major change noted in the lung tissue of smokers, this condition of cancer is confined to the lining (epithelium) layer of the lungs (fig. 7.5). Such a phenomenon usually precedes *metastasis*—the spreading of uncontrolled cell growth throughout an individual's body. Nicotine may actually promote or enhance the spread of cancer cells.

Significantly, the number of cells with abnormal nuclei decreased noticeably in the bronchial lining of ex-cigarette smokers, depending upon the length of time between cessation of smoking and death. There are advantages to giving up cigarettes!

Chronic Obstructive Lung Disease

Pulmonary emphysema and **chronic bronchitis,** two diseases that until recently were infrequently reported in the population, today are reaching epidemic proportions. Often seen together in the same patient, the two diseases are jointly referred to as **chronic obstructive lung disease (COLD),** which is characterized by slow, progressive interruption of the airflow within the lungs. COLD is now one of the leading causes of death in the United States. COLD is also an adaptive response to inhaled irritants and a maladaptation to smoking tobacco.

Cigarette smoking has been identified as the most important cause of COLD, and it greatly increases the risk of dying from pulmonary emphysema and chronic bronchitis. While other factors, including hereditary predisposition, may contribute to COLD, cigarette smoking is now recognized as the major factor in the promotion of "pulmonary cripples." When COLD morbidity is considered, there are more than one million more cases in America than there would be if all people had the same disease rate as those who never smoked.

Pulmonary Emphysema

In pulmonary emphysema, the *alveoli* (tiny air sacs of the lungs) lose the elasticity that ordinarily permits them to expand and contract. Air becomes trapped in the alveoli. Eventually, many of the air sacs are stretched abnormally, rupture, and are destroyed. In a vain attempt to accommodate the overstretched lungs, the chest cage enlarges, which unfortunately reduces the efficiency of the diaphragm. As this condition progresses, the ability of the lungs to exchange gases is so seriously impaired that the bloodstream becomes low in oxygen and retains carbon dioxide. Typically, the victim develops shortness of breath and an overworked heart, which speeds up to supply body cells with their oxygen requirements.

Chronic Bronchitis

Recurring inflammation of the bronchial tubes with excessive mucus production is common in chronic bronchitis. Invariably, a persistent cough develops in an attempt to dislodge the mucus from the narrowed airways. Deep coughing and thick mucus interfere with normal breathing and reduce normal lung function.

Chemicals in inhaled cigarette smoke irritate the bronchial tubes and alveolar sacs over and over again with each puff. In time, the tissues lining the bronchi thicken, the mucous glands enlarge, and the normal cleansing system of the lungs, especially ciliary function, is impaired. The smoker is now more predisposed to respiratory infections and aggravation of existing ones than is the nonsmoker.

People who sustain COLD as a result of smoking often spend many years of their lives incapacitated, gasping and struggling for breath, never moving more than a few feet away from a supply of oxygen.

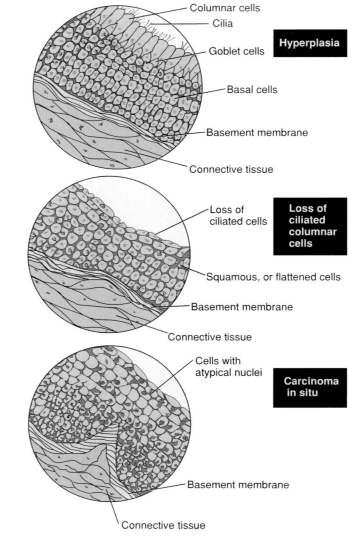

figure 7.5

Cellular changes or alterations in the bronchi of cigarette smokers.

Source: National Advisory Cancer Council.

While the relative importance of air pollution in the development of COLD remains controversial, clearly air pollution is a less significant factor under most circumstances than cigarette smoking.

In addition to an increased risk of COLD, cigarette smokers are more frequently subject to, and require longer convalescence from, other respiratory infections than are nonsmokers. Also, if they require surgery, smokers are more likely to develop postoperative respiratory complications.

Smokeless Tobacco

Smokeless tobacco products include both **chewing tobacco** and **snuff**—mixtures of tobacco leaves and various sweeteners, flavorings, and scents.[33] In chewing tobacco, the leaves are shredded, pressed into bricks or cakes (plugs), or dried and twisted into ropelike strands. A portion of a plug or strand is either chewed or held in place in the cheek or between the lower lip and gum. Made from powdered or finely cut

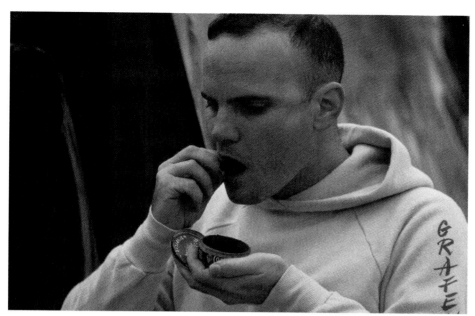

The recent upsurge in use of smokeless tobacco among younger American males has been traced to advertising campaigns featuring athletes and entertainers who engage in chewing, dipping and spitting as macho art forms.

© M. Edrington/The Image Works

tobacco leaves, both dry and moist snuff are used in the mouth, or "dipped." A small amount of snuff is usually held in place between the lip or cheek and the gum.

Historically, smokeless tobacco was widely used in the United States before the introduction and social acceptance of cigarettes. During the early part of the twentieth century, the use of smokeless tobacco declined sharply, until the early 1980s. Now there is ample evidence that chewing tobacco and snuff are gaining in popularity once again.

Original estimates indicated that over 12 million people used some form of smokeless tobacco each year. Recently, the National Institute on Drug Abuse estimated that as many as 22 million Americans have used smokeless tobacco products. However, "dipping" and "chewing" appear to be concentrated among young American males—teenagers and college-age youths, and especially those who are athletes. Nevertheless, smokeless tobacco use is prevalent in women in certain geographic areas as well as within some cultures and populations. For instance, in some Native American tribes, smokeless tobacco use rates among adolescent females approach 45 percent.

Studies of professional baseball players revealed that as many as 39 percent of major and minor league players used smokeless tobacco, mostly snuff, during spring training.[34] And surveys of 2,200 National Collegiate Athletic Association (NCAA) varsity athletes indicated that use of illegal drugs was actually declining, but smokeless tobacco use increased by 8 percent over a four-year period.[35] Among males, six of ten baseball players chewed, and 40 percent of football players chewed, while 9 percent of female softball players also chewed tobacco. The overall use of snuff had increased in every racial and ethnic group studied.

Several factors have likely contributed to the renewed acceptance of smokeless tobacco, especially the physical effects of absorbed nicotine. The absorption process results in a gradual release of nicotine over a period of hours, which is felt in a "time-release" action. Particularly appealing are the increase in blood pressure and heart rate, a reduction in one's appetite, a calming action, and a reduced sensitivity to pain and stress for several hours.[36]

Significantly, powerful advertising campaigns that use professional athletes and entertainers to promote smokeless tobacco

have established chewing and dipping as art forms and spitters as ultramacho. Not to be overlooked are the clever marketing strategies that display smokeless tobacco products in locations removed from smoking tobacco in grocery and convenience stores, and promotional giveaways on college campuses and at state fairs and sporting events. In addition, the health effects of smokeless tobacco are not so well recognized as is the causal link between cigarette use and harmful health conditions.

Cancer and Smokeless Tobacco

Chemical analysis of various types of smokeless tobacco has revealed the presence of several carcinogenic (cancer-causing) compounds, including polonium–210, polycyclic aromatic hydrocarbons, and the tobacco-specific nitrosamines. These carcinogens are part of the strong scientific evidence that the use of smokeless tobacco can cause cancers in humans.

The actual association between cancer and use of such products is strongest for cancers of the oral cavity (mouth). Oral cancer has been shown to occur several times more frequently among snuff dippers than among nontobacco users, and the excess risk of cancers of the cheek and gum may be nearly fifty times greater among long-term users. Some investigations also suggest that the use of chewing tobacco also may increase the risk of oral cancer.

Noncancerous and Precancerous Oral Effects and Smokeless Tobacco Use

Smokeless tobacco use is responsible for the development of a portion of oral *leukoplakias* in both teenage and adult users. Leukoplakias are the "white patches" that develop on the mucous membrane surface that lines the inside of the mouth. These white patches occur frequently with smokeless tobacco use. With continued use, the leukoplakias can undergo a transformation to malignant conditions, that is, cancerous tumors.

The degree to which the use of smokeless tobacco affects the tissues of the mouth is variable, depending on the site of action, type of smokeless tobacco product, frequency and duration of use,

box 7.5

A Common Question; an Uncommon Answer

CHEW or SNUFF is REAL BAD STUFF.

bad breath. mouth sores. cancer.

Some of the things the ads don't tell you about chew & snuff.

QUESTION

What can cause cancer, gum disease, and mouth sores, cost a bundle, ruin your looks, and make your blood pressure go up?

Smokeless tobacco comes in different forms.

You may know it as chewing tobacco or snuff.

Some kids use it because they think it looks cool.

Others may because their friends, coach, or relatives do.

But your doctor or dentist can tell you that using tobacco in any form—dipping, chewing, or smoking—is very bad for your health and can turn off friends.

ANSWER

This can.

CANCER AND OTHER MOUTH PROBLEMS. Using smokeless tobacco can cause cancer—especially in your cheeks, gums, and throat. But even before cancer develops, changes can occur in your mouth—sometimes after only a few weeks of dipping. Your gums and lips can sting, crack, bleed, wrinkle, and get sores and white patches. These white patches may become cancerous. Stopping use of smokeless tobacco can make the white patches go away.

IT ADDS UP. Kids who dip or chew often use a can of snuff or a pouch of chew every day or two. The cost adds up by the week, month, and year. Why would anyone want to pay to hurt his looks and health?

TOBACCO ADDICTION. Tobacco contains a drug called nicotine that can get you addicted or hooked. After using tobacco for a short time, you need another dip every 20 to 30 minutes to keep the tobacco buzz or high from ending. You can become dizzy, shaky, and grouchy when trying to quit. Many kids who have used smokeless tobacco for some time have said that it was hard to quit.

HEART EFFECTS. Chewing and dipping may make you feel relaxed. But the nicotine in tobacco causes your heart to beat faster and your blood pressure to go up—bad news for anyone.

A SPITTIN' IMAGE. Tobacco juices can damage your gums and expose the roots of your teeth. Chewing or dipping may stain your teeth, give you bad breath, affect your ability to taste, and cause worn spots on tooth enamel—nothing to smile about! Snuff and chewing tobacco make your mouth water all the time, so you have to spit constantly wherever you are.

Source: National Cancer Institute, U.S. Department of Health and Human Services.

possible predisposing factors (including smoking), and other factors not yet determined. For example, among snuff users, oral lesions (abnormalities of tissue) were found in 67 percent of baseball players who were year-round users, but in only 32 percent of baseball players who used snuff only during the baseball season.

Although research is not yet complete, there is some evidence that now supports the association of smokeless tobacco use with gingival recession, or receding gums, especially where the tobacco is placed repeatedly. Negative health effects from long-term use of smokeless to-bacco also include tooth discoloration, tooth decay and loss, bad breath, and gingivitis (inflammation and destruction of the gums).

Nicotine Exposure and Smokeless Tobacco

The use of smokeless tobacco products can and does lead to nicotine dependence. Yes, tobacco chewers and snuff dippers can become addicted! An examination of nicotine absorption, distribution, and elimination that results from both smoking and smokeless tobacco use indicates that the extent of nicotine exposure is similar for both.

As is the case with most other drugs of abuse, nicotine produces effects in the user that are considered desirable to the user. These effects are caused by the nicotine and not simply by the tobacco leaf or tobacco smoke.

Since the exposure to nicotine from both cigarette smoking and smokeless to-bacco is similar, the health consequences of smoking that are caused by nicotine also

Should advertising of tobacco products be banned?

Point: Although many "social engineers" favor a prohibition on all advertising of tobacco products, such a ban would be a major infringement on the First Amendment right to free speech. After all, advertising is the voice of free choice in a democratic society. Besides, there is insufficient proof that advertising any tobacco product has ever induced or seduced people to begin using that product. Moreover, in those countries with tobacco advertising bans, such as Canada and Finland, youth smoking rates have not declined. Kids don't begin smoking because of advertising; they smoke because they associate the behavior with being adult. Tobacco advertising is merely an attempt to inform consumers of various brand comparisons and to increase the market share of specific products among the tobacco-using population. As long as tobacco is legal, then advertising tobacco products is just as legal. After all, this is still America!

Counterpoint: Many people would agree with a recent Health and Human Services Secretary who said that while tobacco advertising may be legal, it is medically and morally wrong to promote a product that when used as intended, causes death, disease, and addiction. Yes, such ads should be banned! The major concern is not the legality of tobacco advertising, but the health of users and those who come into contact with users' smoke. It is no secret that women, youth, and minority citizens have been targeted with advertising and promotional campaigns aimed at increasing these individuals' consumption of tobacco products. Cigarette advertising typically portrays attractive, healthy people using tobacco in beautiful, pleasant settings that may be interpreted as suggesting a compatibility between smoking and good health. In fact, the two are mutually exclusive and actually incompatible. The use of young, attractive models conveys the wrong message to our youth who are being actively recruited to replace the 400,000 smokers the industry loses each year due to death.

would be expected to be hazards of smokeless tobacco use. Areas of particular concern in which nicotine may play a contributing or supporting role in the origin of disease include coronary artery disease, peripheral blood-vessel disease, hypertension, peptic ulcer disease, and fetal mortality and morbidity among pregnant women.

Rewards Versus Risks

The serious health risks just discussed should be sufficient to discourage smokers and users of smokeless tobacco from continuing their life-threatening forms of adaptive behavior and to discourage new tobacco users. However, the mere presentation of facts has little effect upon smokers,

tobacco chewers, and snuff dippers, except those who are highly motivated to reduce their exposure to tobacco or to quit using it entirely.

Persistence in smoking might seem contradictory in this enlightened, scientific era, but it is due in part to the effectiveness of early learning that is reinforced thousands of times, puff after puff. As a result of so many rewarding interactions with cigarettes, smoke, and other smokers, the individual's personal values and basic attitudes about life become so ingrained and inflexible that they cannot be cast aside, even when the person recognizes and openly admits the errors of prior learning. In time, tobacco users continue their habits because they have become addicted to nicotine.

Other considerations play a role in maintaining the conflict between smoking behavior and possible health hazards. One, of course, is the fact that not everyone who smokes becomes ill, incapacitated, or dies. Indeed, certain of the cigarette-related diseases may require some genetic, biological, chemical, or physical factor to be operable before smoking takes its toll.

Then, too, rationalization is commonly employed to justify the smoker's action. We often hear these replies to probing inquiries: "Just one cigarette never hurt anybody." "It won't happen to me because I'm lucky." "Why should I quit since I don't feel sick?" "Why worry? They will find a cure for cancer before I die." Do any of these excuses sound familiar? Many of them are based on the remoteness, the delayed action of the possible harmful effects of smoking. If one cigarette caused serious, immediate illness or instant death, smoking would rapidly decline or become extinct.

Risk taking, a necessary component of daily living, compounds the smoking problem. Certainly people should avoid certain risks, but sometimes risks are taken if they seem negligible or remote in anticipation of the possible, immediate rewards. Not to be overlooked as a further explanation for perpetuating a disease- and death-inducing adaptive behavior is the very real reluctance of individuals to acknowledge that their actions are stupid, irrational, or injurious to themselves.

Still another dimension of the cigarette problem is raised by Norman Cousins, who inquires about the significance of life in an affluent society. His classic essay suggests that some smokers really do not care if their life expectancy is reduced.[37] Such dangerous indifference may reflect an insensitivity to the "fragility and preciousness of life" and may correlate with the spread of violence and our lifestyle of abundance. In essence, the real danger beyond smoking may be a crisis in basic human values.

Recognizing that people have been rewarded with feelings of relaxation, well-being, and stimulation through smoking, the American Lung Association has devised a unique program of helping smokers quit. Known as "Freedom from Smoking in Twenty Days," the program is based upon establishing a system of personal rewards for quitting smoking. Although the idea may appear strange, a system of self-rewards greatly improves an individual's chances of becoming a permanent nonsmoker. The rewards should be enjoyable, easy to obtain, occasionally expensive, material as well as immaterial, in proportion to what has been achieved, and administered as soon as possible after completing some activity in the program. Suggested self-rewards include reading in bed on a weekend morning, buying and wearing a new piece of clothing, talking with a friend on the telephone, eating a special food, having someone else clear the table, getting a back rub, and going bowling. By devising a system of similar rewards, a person will have an incentive for modifying smoking behavior.

Reducing the Risks

Almost every type of study has led scientists to conclude that increased exposure to cigarette tars, nicotine, carbon monoxide, and other smoke components leads to increased health risks among the smoking and nonsmoking population. Elimination of the exposure to cigarettes is the best and quickest way to reduce both dosage and related risks. And the benefits of eliminating smoking for the individual smoker are enormous! People who quit smoking live longer because smoking cessation at all ages reduces the risks of premature death. Quitting smoking carries major and immediate health benefits even to those in older age groups and applies not only to healthy people, but to those already suffering from smoking-related diseases.[38] The longer people refrain from smoking after once stopping, the more probable it is that their health condition will approach that of their nonsmoking counterparts. For instance, after fifteen years of nonsmoking, the risk of coronary heart disease is similar to that of persons who have never smoked (see box 7.6).

There are some apparent consequences of quitting. Many former smokers report a reduction in smoker's cough, nasal stuffiness and discharge, and sputum production. Shortness of breath usually improves within a few weeks. In time, food tastes better, sleep is sounder, fatigue diminishes, taste in the mouth improves, and yellowish stains on teeth and fingers disappear. The economics of giving up cigarettes should not be discounted. Giving up smoking one $1.90 pack of cigarettes a day over a 30-year period will result in a savings of more than $20,800!

Although the development of a cigarette that is absolutely safe with respect to all presently associated diseases is not likely, tobacco companies have been successful in reducing the tar and nicotine content of their products. Reconstituted tobaccos and improved filters have met with considerable acceptance by the smoking population. These measures have helped to reduce exposure to potentially harmful substances. The risk to a filter-cigarette smoker, however, still remains above that of the nonsmoker. Unfortunately, the popular 100- and 120-millimeter cigarettes increase both the dosage and risk. Moreover, the addition of menthol may improve the taste, but it does not reduce the health hazards.

While *there is no safe way to smoke,* there are some suggestions that smokers can follow if they wish to make their cigarette use less hazardous. The following recommendations are offered by the Public Health Service.

1. *Inhale less.* Cigarette smoke that enters the lungs is the disease-causing agent in pulmonary and cardiovascular disorders. Death rates and morbidity rates increase with the degree and frequency of inhalation. Some smokers may wish to switch to pipes or cigars, in which smoke usually is not inhaled. Having switched, they may reduce their risks of having lung cancer, COLD, and cardiovascular diseases, but they may increase their risks of developing cancer of the larynx, lip, and esophagus.

2. *Smoke fewer cigarettes.* The exposure to health risks is in direct proportion to the number of cigarettes smoked. The fewer smoked, the lower the risks. This procedure can be promoted by making a conscious effort to stretch the existing supply, by postponing smoking, by placing cigarettes in an out-of-the-way location, and by promising oneself not to smoke during a particular time of day.

3. *Take fewer puffs.* Although a smoker may not be able to reduce the total number of cigarettes used, puffing less on each one will reduce the exposure to the total dose of tars, gaseous components, and toxic chemicals inhaled. While this procedure might seem expensive in the purchase of more cigarettes, it is cheaper in the long run as expressed in personal health, working ability, and longevity.

4. *Smoke one-third down.* Regardless of the brand smoked, the major amounts of tars and nicotine are found in the last few puffs of a cigarette. Tobacco acts as a filter and screens out a portion of the tars and nicotine as they pass through it. As a consequence, smoke from the first third of a cigarette contains approximately 2 percent of the total tars and nicotine, while the last third yields nearly 50 percent. Do not smoke all the way down on cigarettes. Those extra puffs can be perilous puffs!

5. *Choose a low-tar and low-nicotine cigarette.* By reducing one's exposure to these constituents of cigarette smoke, health risks are likely reduced but not eliminated. No minimum levels of these substances have as yet been determined risk-free or safe. Because of governmental action and increased public interest, cigarette manufacturers now reveal the tar and nicotine content of their products. Choosing a less harmful cigarette may be as easy as switching to another brand or to another version of the same brand. In every instance, the buyer should beware!

Anything short of quitting completely is only a compromise, however. While most successful quitters stop smoking immediately and permanently, others—particularly heavy, addicted smokers—find participation in a smoking withdrawal program to be helpful.[39,40] Stop-smoking programs have been particularly effective, especially those conducted by the American Lung Association, the American Cancer Society, the American Heart Association, Seventh Day Adventist Breathe-Free Plan to Stop Smoking, Smoke Stoppers, and Smokers

box 7.6

Benefits of Smoking Cessation

Key

"CS" refers to continuing smokers,

"NS" refers to never smokers.

Stroke risk reduced to that of "NS" 5 to 15 years after quitting.

Cancers of the mouth, throat, and esophagus risk halved compared to "CS" 5 years after quitting.

Cancer of the larynx risk reduced compared to "CS" after quitting.

Coronary heart disease excess risk halved compared to "CS" 1 year after quitting; risk returns to that of "NS" after 15 years.

Chronic obstructive pulmonary disease risk of death reduced compared to "CS" after long-term quitting.

Lung cancer risk as much as halved compared to "CS" 10 years after quitting.

Pancreatic cancer risk reduced compared to "CS" 10 years after quitting.

Ulcer risk reduced compared to "CS" after quitting.

Bladder cancer risk halved compared to "CS" a few years after quitting.

Peripheral artery disease risk reduced compared to "CS" after quitting.

Cervical cancer risk reduced compared to "CS" a few years after quitting.

Low birthweight baby risk reduced to that of "NS" for women who quit before pregnancy or during first trimester.

Source: *The Health Benefits of Smoking Cessation: A Report of the Surgeon General, 1990—At a Glance,* U.S. Department of Health and Human Services, publication no. (CDC) 90-8419.

Anonymous. Local smoking control programs are usually listed under "Smokers' Information and Treatment Centers" in the telephone company's Yellow Pages. Community hospitals, counseling programs, health agencies, and health promotion centers often sponsor support groups that prove helpful to some smokers.

For many individuals who are not successful in their own attempts to quit smoking via self-help books, videotapes, E-Z Quit simulated cigarettes, quit-smoking computers, and various other techniques, a recently formulated prescription drug is now available. Known as *Nicorette,* this nicotine chewing gum decreases the smoker's desire for nicotine and relieves withdrawal symptoms. More effective, practical, and safer than injected and capsule or pill forms of nicotine, the chewing gum allows the nicotine to be absorbed through the mouth's lining directly into the bloodstream.

Developed as a temporary aid to smoking cessation, nicotine chewing gum is most effective in the early phase of withdrawal. However, *Nicorette* is no panacea. Studies of the gum's effectiveness have found mixed results. Successful quitting appears to depend on more than just chewing the nicotine gum. The smoker's motivation to quit, presence or absence of contraindications, awareness of and willingness to tolerate possible side effects of the gum, physician support, and participation in a professionally supervised behavior modification program influence the success or failure of this technique. It appears that group-based behavioral programs that rely on social reinforcement and follow-up support, in combination with nicotine gum, will likely prove the most effective strategy for most smokers. However, drinking coffee and carbonated beverages tends to interfere with the effect of the prescription gum. Those who use *Nicorette* are well-advised not to chew the gum on their coffee breaks or to eat or drink anything during or immediately before *Nicorette* use.[41]

An even newer form of medical nicotine is also marketed as the *nicotine patch*. Similar to *Nicorette* chewing gum, the patch provides a dose of nicotine that can help relieve the body's craving for this addictive substance. Available only by prescription, *Nicoderm* and *Habitrol* are small, thin, 24-hour patches that go on a person's upper body and deliver a continuous flow of nicotine through the skin. This new nicotine patch—a transdermal (across the skin) system—can reduce nicotine withdrawal symptoms that usually develop with quitting smoking. In order to reduce the risk of heart attack, however, patients are warned not to smoke while wearing the patches.

What You Should Know about Quitting Smoking

box 7.7

Smokers often try to quit more than once before they succeed. Nearly 70 percent of ex-smokers make one or two quit attempts, while 9 percent quit six or more times before succeeding. So far, more than 38 million Americans have succeeded! About 90 percent of successful quitters eventually do so on their own, but with good cessation programs, 20 percent to 40 percent of participants are able to quit smoking and stay off cigarettes for at least one year.

Some Consequences of Quitting Are . . .

- Nearly 80 percent of those who quit smoking gain weight, compared to 56 percent of continuing smokers.

- Short-term consequences of nicotine withdrawal include anxiety, irritability, frustration, anger, difficulty in concentrating, and restlessness. Possible long-term consequences are urges to smoke and increased appetite.

But at the Same Time . . .

- The average weight gain after quitting is just 5 pounds, and only 3.5 percent of those who quit gain more than 20 pounds after quitting.

- Nicotine withdrawal symptoms peak in the first 1 to 2 days after quitting and subside rapidly during the following weeks. With long-term abstinence, ex-smokers are likely to enjoy favorable psychological changes such as enhanced self-esteem and increased sense of control.

- People who quit smoking are more likely than current smokers to exercise regularly. Exercise may help new quitters to stay off cigarettes and avoid or minimize weight gain.

The Bottom Line . . .

The health benefits of quitting far exceed any risks from the average 5-pound weight gain or any adverse psychological effects that may follow quitting. To help limit any weight gain after quitting, eat a well-balanced diet and avoid the excess calories in sugary and fatty foods; satisfy cravings for sweets by eating small pieces of fruit; have low-calorie foods on hand for nibbling; drink six to eight glasses of water per day; and build exercise into your life by walking 30 minutes a day or doing the physical activity of your choice.

Source: *The Health Benefits of Smoking Cessation: A Report of The Surgeon General, 1990—At A Glance*, U.S. Department of Health and Human Services, publication no. (CDC)90-8419.

Chapter Summary

1. A plant native to the New World, tobacco has become a popular source of mood modification. However, the smoking of tobacco cigarettes is now considered the largest single preventable cause of illness and premature death in the United States.

2. Both individuals and the American society are "hooked" on tobacco products. While the federal government supports antismoking programs and research, it also subsidizes tobacco growers.

3. About 25 percent of the adult population smokes. This number represents a declining minority, but there is evidence that females are increasing their use of tobacco products, while males are slowing their rate of beginning smoking.

4. Recently, more people are smoking low-tar and low-nicotine cigarettes. However, any such protection from diseases offered by these new tobacco products is negated by compensatory practices—increasing the number of cigarettes smoked, shortening the interval between

puffs, increasing the depth of inhalation, and smoking to a shorter butt.

5. Although cigarettes have provided the user with certain personal gratifications, the nonsmoking majority has become assertive in demanding plain, unpolluted air. The nonsmokers' liberation movement has resulted in many restrictive practices on smokers' behavior.

6. Smoking is a learned behavior with many psychological rewards, especially for maturing adolescents. Factors in smoking behavior are

classified as stimulation, handling/oral gratification, pleasurable relaxation, tension reduction, psychological and physical addiction, and habit.

7. The health consequences of smoking are related to the constituents of tobacco smoke: gases, tar, and nicotine, the physical dependency-producing component. Additionally, excess mortality and morbidity associated with smoking are dose related; that is, death and disease rates increase with amount smoked, duration of smoking, earlier age of initiation, inhalation of smoke, and higher tar and nicotine content.

8. Passive smoking, the inhalation of environmental tobacco smoke by a nonsmoker, is now recognized as having several adverse health effects on the nonsmoking population. Secondhand smoke can cause heart disease, lung cancer, and the increased occurrence of respiratory disability and diseases.

9. Cigarette smoking contributes to coronary heart disease, lung and various other cancers, chronic obstructive lung disease, a variety of chronic and disabling conditions, lower birth weight of infants, increased risk of spontaneous abortion, sudden infant death syndrome, impaired oxygen uptake and exercise tolerance, premature facial wrinkling, and undesirable drug interactions.

10. Nicotine and carbon monoxide are the culprits in coronary heart disease and other cardiovascular diseases; tobacco tars are responsible for triggering lung cancer and its precursors of tissue changes: hyperplasia; loss of ciliary function in columnar cells; and carcinoma *in situ*. Chronic obstructive lung disease is a response to inhalation of smoke irritants and is manifest as pulmonary emphysema and chronic bronchitis.

11. Use of chewing tobacco and snuff represents a significant health risk. Smokeless tobacco is not a safe substitute for smoking cigarettes. It

can cause cancers of the mouth and throat, gum damage, loss of teeth, and can lead to nicotine addiction and dependence.

12. Smoking of tobacco is often portrayed as a reward vs. risk practice. The psychosocial and short-term rewards of smoking are perceived as more important than the long-term risks of diseases and premature death. Perhaps the danger beyond smoking is a crisis in human values.

13. Although there is no safe, risk-free cigarette and no safe level of smoking, a smoker can reduce the risks associated with tobacco use by inhaling less smoke, smoking fewer cigarettes, taking fewer puffs, smoking only one-third down on each cigarette, and choosing a low-tar, low-nicotine, and low-carbon-monoxide yielding product.

14. The benefits of smoking cessation via the self-initiated "cold-turkey" approach, group-based smoking withdrawal programs, or the use of *Nicorette* or the nicotine skin patch are significant. Quitting smoking reduces the risk of heart disease, lung cancer, and various other cancerous diseases, stroke, chronic obstructive pulmonary (lung) disease, and low-birth-weight babies.

Review Questions and Activities

1. Where did smoking of tobacco leaves first begin?

2. Why is smoking considered as "suicide in slow motion"?

3. What contradictions are apparent in the puzzling phenomenon known as tobacco smoking?

4. Survey your class, friends, and/or neighbors to determine the prevalence of smoking. How do these results compare with national statistics cited in the text?

5. What factors may be responsible for the continuing increase in smoking among young females?

6. Determine if chewing tobacco or "snuff dipping" is popular among your friends and acquaintances. What reasons do they give for such practices?

7. Why is smokeless tobacco not considered a safe substitute for smoking cigarettes?

8. Explain how compensatory smoking can negate the benefits of low-yield cigarettes.

9. What motivational appeals do cigarette advertisers use to promote smoking?

10. What are some of the psychological rewards associated with smoking?

11. What factors likely influence teenagers to begin smoking?

12. If you do not smoke, explain the following terms in relation to cigarette smoking: *stimulation, handling/oral gratification, relaxation, tension reduction, craving,* and *habit.*

13. What components of tobacco smoke are thought to be responsible for the major diseases associated with smoking?

14. In what way is *nicotine* responsible for the continuation of smoking?

15. Is tobacco use psychologically or physically dependency producing? What do you think?

16. Summarize the major research findings linking cigarette smoking and passive smoking with excess mortality and morbidity.

17. Define the terms dose-related, involuntary smoking, smoking-drug interaction, nicotine, carbon monoxide, and tobacco tars.

18. How is smoking thought to contribute to heart and blood-vessel diseases?

19. What are three smoking-induced cellular changes that are considered as precursors of lung cancer?

20. How does smoking contribute to chronic obstructive lung disease?

21. Contrast pulmonary emphysema with chronic bronchitis.

22. Explain smoking behavior in terms of a rewards vs. risks phenomenon.

23. In what ways can a smoker reduce the health risks often linked with tobacco use?

24. What specific resources are available in your community to help smokers quit their use of tobacco products?

References

1. Avram Goldstein, *Addiction: From Biology to Drug Policy* (New York: W. H. Freeman, 1994), 101–17.

2. Antonia C. Novello, "Preface," in *Health Benefits of Smoking Cessation,* a report of the Surgeon General, executive summary, USDHHA Publication No. CDC-90-8416 (Washington, D.C.: U.S. Government Printing Office, 1990), xi.

3. H. Thomas Milhorn, *Drug and Alcohol Abuse* (New York: Plenum Press, 1994), 293.

4. David Krogh, "Smoking: Why Is It So Hard to Quit?" *Priorities,* spring 1992, 29–31.

5. American Cancer Society, *Cancer Facts and Figures—1994* (Atlanta: American Cancer Society, 1994), 22.

6. Institute for Health Policy, Brandeis University, *Substance Abuse: The Nation's Number One Health Problem* (Princeton, N.J.: Robert Wood Johnson Foundation, 1993), 13.

7. American Cancer Society, *Cancer Facts and Figures—1994,* 22.

8. Barry Stimmel and the Editors of Consumer Reports Books, *The Facts about Drug Use: Coping with Drugs and Alcohol in Your Family, at Work, in Your Community* (New York: Haworth Medical Press, 1993), 216–18.

9. U.S. Department of Health and Human Services, *Preventing Tobacco Use among Young People,* a report of the Surgeon General, executive summary (Atlanta: U.S. Department of Health and Human Services, Public Health Service, Centers for Disease Control and Prevention, Office on Smoking and Health, 1994), 5–6.

10. This section is based on the following Public Health Service (USDHHS) reports of the Surgeon General (all available from the U.S. Government Printing Office): *Smoking and Health; The Health Consequences of Smoking for Women; The Health Consequences of Smoking; The Changing Cigarette;* and *The Health Consequences of Smoking: Cancer.*

11. Robert Julien, *A Primer of Drug Action* (New York: W. H. Freeman, 1992), 142–43.

12. C. Everett Koop, *The Health Consequences of Smoking: Nicotine Addiction,* a report of the Surgeon General (Washington, D.C.: U.S. Government Printing Office, 1988), 9.

13. Lynn Kozlowski, Adrian Wilkinson, and others, "Comparing Tobacco Cigarette Dependence with Other Drug Dependencies," *Journal of the American Medical Association* 261, no. 6 (10 February 1989): 898–901.

14. Edward Giovannucci and others, "A Prospective Study of Cigarette Smoking and Risk of Colorectal Adenoma and Colorectal Cancer in U.S. Women," *Journal of the National Cancer Institute* 86, no. 3 (2 February 1994): 192–99.

15. Edward Giovannucci and others, "A Prospective Study of Cigarette Smoking and Risk of Colorectal Adenoma and Colorectal Cancer in U.S. Men," *Journal of the National Cancer Institute* 86, no. 3 (2 February 1994): 183–91.

16. "The Eighteen-Year Gap," *University of California at Berkeley Wellness Letter* 7, no. 4 (January 1991): 2.

17. Denise Kandel, Ping Wu, and Mark Davies, "Maternal Smoking during Pregnancy and Smoking by Adolescent Daughters," *American Journal of Public Health* 84, no. 9 (September 1994): 1407–13.

18. Joel Coste, Nadine Job-Spira, and Herve Fernandez, "Increased Risk of Ectopic Pregnancy with Maternal Cigarette Smoking," *American Journal of Public Health* 81, no. 2 (February 1991):199–201.

19. Bengt Haglund and Sven Cnattingius, "Cigarette Smoking As a Risk Factor for Sudden Infant Death Syndrome: A Population-Based Study," *American Journal of Public Health* 80, no. 1 (January 1990): 29–32.

20. Alexander Glassman and others, "Smoking, Smoking Cessation, and Major Depression," *Journal of the American Medical Association* 264, no. 12 (20 September 1990): 1546–49.

21. Robert Anda, David Williamson, Luis Escobedo, Eric Mast, Gary Giovino, and Patrick Remington, "Depression and the Dynamics of Smoking," *Journal of the American Medical Association* 264, no. 12 (26 September 1990): 1541–45.

22. National Center for Health Statistics, "Relationships between Smoking and Other Unhealthy Habits: United States, 1985," *Advancedata* 154 (27 May 1988): 6.

23. Donald Kadunce, Randy Burr, Richard Gress, Richard Kanner, Joseph Lyon, and John Zone, "Cigarette Smoking: Risk Factor for Premature Facial Wrinkling," *Annals of Internal Medicine* 114, no. 10 (15 May 1991): 840–44.

24. Public Health Service, *The Health Consequences of Involuntary Smoking,* a report of the Surgeon General (Washington, D.C.: U.S. Government Printing Office, 1986).

25. U.S. Environmental Protection Agency and U.S. Department of Health and Human Services, *Respiratory Health Effects of Passive Smoking: Lung Cancer and Other Disorders,* a report of the EPA, NIH Publication No. 93-3605 (Bethesda, Md.: National Institutes of Health, 1993), 3–17.

26. Dwight Janevich and others, "Lung Cancer and Exposure to Tobacco Smoke in the Household," *New England Journal of Medicine* 323, no. 10 (6 September 1990): 632–36.

27. Elizabeth Fontham and others, "Environmental Tobacco Smoke and Lung Cancer in Nonsmoking Women," *Journal of the American Medical Association* 271, no. 22 (8 June 1994): 1752–59.

28. Stanton Glantz and William Parmley, "Passive Smoking and Heart Disease: Epidemiology, Physiology, and Biochemistry," *Circulation* 83, no. 1 (January 1991): 1–12.

29. "Is Secondhand Smoke a Hazard?" *Consumer Reports* 60, no. 1 (January 1995): 27–33.

30. Fernando Martinez, Anne Wright, and Lynn Taussig, "The Effect of Paternal Smoking on the Birthweight of Newborns Whose Mothers Did Not Smoke," *American Journal of Public Health* 84, no. 9 (September 1994): 1489–91.

31. American Heart Association, *Heart and Stroke Facts* (Dallas: American Heart Association, 1994), 19.

32. American Cancer Society, *Cancer Facts and Figures—1994* (Atlanta: American Cancer Society, 1994), 9.

33. Unless otherwise indicated, the information in this section is derived from the following sources: Public Health Service, *The Health Consequences of Using Smokeless Tobacco,* a report of the Advisory Committee to the Surgeon General (Washington, D.C.: U.S. Government Printing Office, 1986); and U.S. Department of Health and Human Services, Public Health Service, *Smokeless Tobacco or Health: An International Perspective,* NIH Publication No. 93-3461 (Bethesda, Md.: National Institutes of Health, 1993).

34. Virginia Ernster and others, "Smokeless Tobacco Use and Health Effects among Baseball Players," *Journal of the American Medical Association* 264, no. 2 (11 July 1990): 218–24.

35. "College Athletes," *Monday Morning Report* 14, no. 23 (25 March 1991): 1.

36. *Smokeless Tobacco,* Datafax Information Series (Tempe, Ariz.: Do It Now, 1990), 2.

37. Norman Cousins, "The Danger beyond Smoking," *Saturday Review,* 25 January 1964, 22. *Saturday Review* was one of the first national publications to refuse cigarette advertising.

38. Antonia C. Novello, "Preface," in *Health Benefits of Smoking Cessation,* v–xii.

39. Thomas Glynn, "Methods of Smoking Cessation—Finally, Some Answers," *Journal of the American Medical Association* 263, no. 20 (23–30 May 1990): 2795–96.

40. Michael Fiore and others, "Methods Used to Quit Smoking in the United States," *Journal of the American Medical Association* 263, no. 20 (23–30 May 1990): 2760–65.

41. Jack Henningfield, Aleksandras Radzius, Thomas Cooper, and Richard Clayton, "Drinking Coffee and Carbonated Beverages Blocks Absorption of Nicotine from Nicotine Polacrilex Gum," *Journal of the American Medical Association* 264, no. 12 (26 September 1990): 1560–64.

chapter

8

cocaine and other "chemical uppers"

chapter objectives

After you have studied this chapter, you should be able to do the following:

1. Identify psychoactive drugs that are central nervous system stimulants.

2. Describe several general effects of behavioral stimulants, such as cocaine and the amphetamines.

3. Explain why using CNS stimulants frequently becomes a compulsive drug-taking behavior.

4. Discuss the historical influences that have been responsible for cocaine's initial popularity as a recreational drug.

5. Distinguish among the various use patterns of cocaine consumption.

6. Compare the relative hazards involved in snorting, injecting, and freebasing cocaine.

7. Describe the unique features of "crack," including its addictive nature.

8. Explain both the attraction and the dangers of combining cocaine with CNS depressants or sedatives.

9. Describe the probable effects of cocaine use in relation to light or moderate use, to use of relatively high doses, and to long-term use.

10. Define the following terms associated with prolonged use of cocaine: *cocaine psychosis, formication,* and *cocaine dependence.*

11. List the similarities and differences between cocaine and the amphetamines in terms of origin, specific effects, duration of effects, reasons for abuse, and frequently associated risks to health.

12. Compare and contrast the effects of "crack" with those of "ice"—the smokable form of methamphetamine.

13. Name three current medical uses of the amphetamines.

14. Describe the general effects and therapeutic uses of MAO inhibitors, tricyclic compounds, and fluoxetine (Prozac).

15. Identify the commonly experienced drug effects of caffeine.

16. Distinguish the condition of caffeinism from the phenomenon of caffeine dependence.

17. Explain how individuals can protect themselves from potential health risks associated with caffeine-based beverages and medications containing caffeine.

18. Compare and contrast the origins, motivations for use, and effects of methcathinone and ephedrine.

Introduction

In chapter 7 we considered one powerful, toxic stimulant—nicotine. In this chapter the focus is on the other "chemical uppers"—cocaine, amphetamines, caffeine, and various plant stimulants, including khat. These psychoactive drugs tend to speed up, excite, and activate various body functions and parts.

The underlying reasons for using "chemical uppers" are complex. On occasion, most people have sought some type of physical or mental "uplifting"—an energizing experience of pleasurable satisfaction or psychic renewal. Perhaps such a desire originated in the fatigue due to overexertion, the depression resulting from disappointment or rejection, the need to stay awake in preparation for a final examination, or the necessity to drive

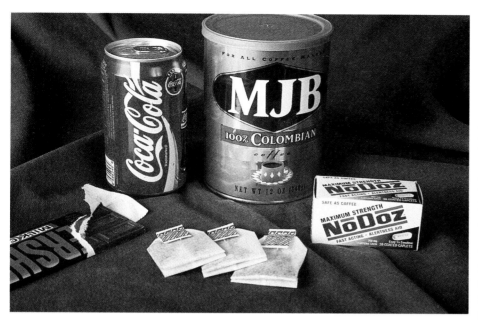

All of these products contain a legal stimulant, caffeine.
© Jonathan Nourok/PhotoEdit

a motor vehicle for a long distance without stopping for sleep. To some extent, the reduction of fatigue, the prevention of sleep, and the elevation of mood have all been achieved temporarily through the use of drugs called central nervous system (CNS) stimulants.

There are several types of CNS stimulants. In this chapter the major emphasis will be on the so-called behavior stimulants (such as cocaine and the amphetamines) that increase mental and physical activity and elevate mood in "normal" individuals. The clinical antidepressants that have no pharmacological effects in "normal" people will then be explained, as well as the common stimulant found in coffee, tea, chocolate, and certain medications.

Chemical Uppers

Of all the abused drugs, *cocaine,* the *amphetamines,* and *caffeine* are among the most powerfully reinforcing. That is, the pleasurable effects experienced from taking these central nervous system (CNS) stimulants compel the users to engage in repeated, compulsive consumption of such substances. As addiction to these drugs occurs—especially cocaine and the amphetamines—the repeated

use of these psychoactives will likely continue, despite many harmful and self-destructive consequences.

Drugs classified as central nervous system (CNS) **stimulants** increase alertness, physical activity, and excitement by speeding up the body's processes. Because these stimulating drugs increase behavioral activity and psychomotor functions, they are often called "uppers" or "ups."

Unlike the depressant-type drugs, or "downers," all of which cause a general sedation, the stimulants display a very diverse pharmacology. For instance, the convulsions produced by strychnine—a CNS stimulant better known as a rat poison ingredient—are quite different from the euphoria and improved performance induced by an amphetamine, another common stimulant drug.

Among the most widely used stimulants are **caffeine** and **nicotine**—two substances rarely perceived as drugs until recent times. Use of either can result in a drug dependency (classified as a "disorder" by the American Psychiatric Association), but neither causes acute intoxication, serious psychiatric symptoms, or serious impairment of work and family life—except for the adverse consequences of long-term tobacco use.[1]

The active ingredient in coffee, tea, and cola-based soft drinks, caffeine is often used as a mild "pick-me-up" or "wake-me-up" substance as well as a component of nonprescription sleep preventives.

Nicotine, one of several chemical compounds in tobacco, tends to relieve fatigue and increase alertness. Numerous health-threatening effects are also associated with nicotine, as noted in chapter 7. As a result of their legality and widespread use, however, both caffeine and nicotine have become somewhat accepted parts of American culture.[2]

Other CNS stimulants are more potent and have an even greater potential for producing a drug dependency. Available by prescription or only for medical research, drugs such as cocaine and amphetamines are controlled medications (Schedule II) under provisions of the Controlled Substances Act. Of course, cocaine and various amphetamines are also available on the illicit street market, especially since their medical uses have been curtailed in the United States.

General Effects of Behavioral Stimulants

Use of "chemical uppers," especially stronger stimulants like cocaine and amphetamines, forces the body to release its own natural stimulants—neurotransmitter substances, such as epinephrine (adrenalin). This sudden release of neurotransmitter-based energy produces a feeling of exhilaration, a surge of energy, and the enhancement of self-confidence.[3]

Other stimulating actions include an increased heart rate and blood pressure, energized muscular activity, and a decreased blood supply to the skin, arms, and legs. Overstimulation may surface as irritability, restlessness, and insomnia. When long-term or excessive high-dose use of stimulants depletes the body's natural supply of energy-producing neurotransmitters, various body systems begin to shut down, resulting in physical collapse and mental depression.

Psychological reliance upon the stimulants is quite common because they tend to make users feel stronger, more decisive, and self-possessed. These stimulants also produce a euphoria along with a decreased perception of fatigue, a decreased need for sleep, and a decreased appetite. Some nonmedical users also believe stimulants increase the desire for and pleasurable aspects of sexual behavior.

Due to the cumulative effects of these drugs, long-term users sometimes develop a pattern of stimulant use during the day and depressant (alcohol and sleeping pills) use at night. This chemical rotation—"speeding up" followed by "slowing down"—interferes with normal body processes, which can lead to serious illness.

At very low doses, behavioral stimulants bring about an alerting arousal or behavior-activating response, similar to a person's typical reaction to an emergency or stressful situation.[4] This effect closely resembles the action of norepinephrine, another chemical neurotransmitter associated with arousal reactions and moods, as noted in chapter 3. Both the amphetamines and cocaine, as well as the antidepressants, such as Parnate and Elavil, potentiate the action of this neurotransmitter substance.

However, while cocaine, amphetamines, and plant stimulants such as methcathinone and ephedrine tend to elevate mood and stimulate the behavior of "normal" people, the antidepressants have no significant effect on healthy people. Reflecting their unusual pharmacological characteristics, the antidepressants produce their desirable effects only in those individuals who are psychologically depressed.

The chemical "eye openers" are used in various recreational or nonmedical ways to achieve a feeling of well-being and increased alertness. Until recently, the most common patterns involved periodic oral use of stimulants, such as swallowing amphetamine capsules and inhaling (snorting) cocaine. Occasionally, these stimulants have been used in combination with depressant drugs, including alcohol, barbiturates or other sleeping pills, tranquilizers, marijuana, and various psychedelics.

When used alone in large doses, stimulants often induce a temporary sense of exhilaration with superabundant energy, increased activity, extended wakefulness, and loss of appetite. At this dosage level,

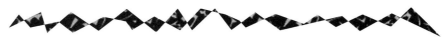

Cocaine, Amphetamines, Caffeine, and Driving   *Why Take the Risk?*

box 8.1

Cocaine, amphetamines, and other stimulants including phenylpropanolamine, ephedrine, and caffeine (found in specific nonprescription medicines) all stimulate the central nervous system. Small amounts of these drugs generally make people who are tired feel more alert.

In fact, studies reveal that small doses of amphetamines, given to subjects for a limited period of time, generally improve performance of several driving skills. However, these subjects tend to overestimate their performance and take more risks. Actual driving records indicate that people who take amphetamines are slightly more accident prone, probably for these reasons.

While heavy amphetamine use and repeated use of other stimulants to combat fatigue will tend to keep drivers awake and active for long stretches of time, these stimulants will also make the drivers edgy, less coordinated, and more likely to be involved in traffic accidents. One accident study found that amphetamine users were four times more likely to be involved in car crashes than nonusers.

Presently, there is only limited information about cocaine's effects on psychomotor driving skills. Research does show that typical so-called social amounts of inhaled cocaine can produce lapses in attention and concentration. Although users often report that cocaine,

like other stimulants, increases their concentration and improves performance on a variety of tasks, there is no objective evidence supporting these reports. Moreover, cocaine is a short-acting drug, and within an hour the user feels not only less alert but more anxious, tired, or depressed than before.

Regular users sometimes report feelings of restlessness, irritability, and anxiety, but even low doses may create psychological problems. These adverse effects are minor in comparison with the consequences of combining alcohol with cocaine, a practice known as "speedballing." Used in such a combination, cocaine tends to mask alcohol's effect, so that an individual who feels sober enough and sufficiently alert to drive will become intoxicated as the effects of cocaine wear off.

Although caffeine can help the drowsy driver stay alert, coffee can't make the drunk driver sober. Studies show that ordinary amounts of caffeine do not improve an inebriated person's driving skills.

Driving requires a combination of thought and motor skills, a great deal of common sense, and a concern for the safety of everyone on the road. Safe driving requires an observant eye, a steady hand, and a clear head. By mixing drugs with driving, you are only asking for trouble. Why take the risk?

Source: Modified from the National Institute on Drug Abuse.

the user may also experience dizziness, tremors, confusion, headaches, flushing or sweating, nausea, chest pain, and the sensation of a racing heart. With only infrequent use of stimulants, however, the condition of tolerance does not usually develop. Such use is typical of those who obtain stimulants by prescription and use them under close medical supervision.

Another major pattern of stimulant use is intravenous injection, usually of a specific amphetamine (methamphetamine,

or "speed") or cocaine. Such a use pattern often develops after extended oral use of amphetamine or cocaine inhalation. After the injection, users typically report an initial **"flash"** or **"rush" reaction.** This "flash" effect is a short, intense, generalized sensation similar to a sudden splash of cold water or a total body orgasm. Almost instantaneously, total well-being is experienced and feelings of boredom and depression vanish. Users also perceive a marked enhancement of their physical strength and mental abilities.

Sometimes, though, CNS stimulant abusers also experience irritability, anxiety, and apprehension, and some even display hostile, aggressive behavior.

Yet another form of stimulant use was introduced in the late 1970s with the appearance of freebase, a form of cocaine that could be smoked. This first form of smokable cocaine involved a rather dangerous process of converting "street cocaine" to freebase crystals that were then smoked through a water pipe. Then, in the mid 1980s, a newer form of cocaine, called "crack," emerged. Relatively low in cost and now available in ready-to-smoke form without fancy paraphernalia, crack is considered to be the most addictive form of cocaine. In reality, crack is intensified cocaine. Its effects are amplified, sharper, meaner, and uglier than those of plain cocaine. Many experts now believe that crack accounted for much of the cocaine-abuse epidemic that began in the United States in 1985 and still continues today.

Tolerance to both the euphoric and the appetite-suppressant effects develops quite rapidly with intravenous injection. Extremely high dose levels are sometimes accompanied by paranoid feelings. In addition, the user may engage in endless compulsive activities of a nonsensical nature, such as grinding the teeth and touching and picking the face and extremities. These peculiar behaviors are often referred to as hypomania or knick-knacking.

There may also be a preoccupation with one's own thoughts, a general suspiciousness, and eventually a **toxic syndrome,** consisting of tremors, agitation, hostility, panic, headache, flushed skin, chest pain, excessive perspiration, vomiting, and abdominal cramps. If there is no medical intervention, high fever, convulsions, and heart and blood-vessel collapse may be followed by death.

A desire to reexperience the "flash" and to avoid the loss of the stimulant's effects and the onset of "withdrawal symptoms" compels some long-term users to engage in **speed runs.** These are days of continuous stimulant use during which a solution of amphetamine is injected at one- to two-hour intervals. In time, such chronic use leads to total exhaustion of the user, who is completely disorganized mentally and very tense. When this individual finally stops taking the drug—often to end an unpleasant "speed run"—he or she experiences a very disturbing period of depression. This sudden mental "low" is referred to as **crashing.** Such rebound depression is in sharp contrast with the mental "high" induced by the stimulant.

Now the person sleeps for as long as 48 hours, then awakens with a huge appetite. However, the individual feels quite lethargic for several days to several weeks. Panic reactions, continued depression, irritability, and assaultive and suicidal behavior are common. These reactions to discontinued amphetamine use are indicative of a withdrawal phenomenon.

In the past, scientists have disagreed about the capability of CNS stimulants to cause a true physical dependence. There is now a consensus that both cocaine and amphetamines are addictive, i.e., they are capable of producing both physical and psychological dependency. However, whether the withdrawal symptoms are physical or merely psychological in origin is somewhat academic, since amphetamines and cocaine are among the most powerful agents of the reward and reinforcement that underlie the basic problem of dependence.[5]

Cocaine

The major psychoactive ingredient extracted from the leaves of the coca plant (*Erythroxylon coca*), **cocaine** is the most powerful CNS stimulant of natural origin. The U.S. Pharmacopeia compound consists of white, odorless crystals or crystalline powder derived from a coca leaf paste. A vegetable alkaloid chemically labeled *benzoylmethylecgonine (methylbenzoylepgonine)*, cocaine is better known as "coke," "C," "snow," "blow," "toot," "leaf," "flake," "freeze," "happy dust," "Peruvian lady," and "white girl." Sold on the street, this drug is a mixture of the pure cocaine substance (cocaine hydrochloride) and various adulterants added to increase the quantity, typically for the seller's profit. Common adulterants include various sugars (lactose, inositol, and mannitol) and local anesthetics such as lidocaine.

The purity of cocaine varies from a low of about 15 percent to a high of nearly 95 percent, depending upon the amount of adulterants in any particular sample. Usually, samples of cocaine powder are about 66 percent pure cocaine or higher today, whereas comparable samples several years ago were only about 27 percent pure cocaine. And smokable crack cocaine now averages from 75 to 90 percent pure, up significantly from only 34 percent purity in the late 1980s.

Since enactment and enforcement of the Harrison Narcotic Act of 1914 and its amendments, cocaine has been classified with the narcotics and subjected to the same controls as opium, morphine, and heroin. In 1922, the coca leaf derivative was defined legally as a narcotic drug, although cocaine is not a narcotic in the pharmacological sense. This narcotic definition still applies today, despite cocaine's differing drug effects.

One of the most effective euphoriants ever discovered or experienced, cocaine became an "in" drug among nearly all socioeconomic, racial, and ethnic groups in the United States. Its popularity is related to the almost universal guarantee of immediate pleasure, well-being, and alertness. Greatly feared earlier in this century, cocaine soon achieved a status as a luxury drug with an unjustified reputation of having no undesirable health effects.

Originally a favorite "upper" among entertainers, cocaine eventually became prevalent among all age groups and regions of the country. Because of its low purchase price, crack cocaine has become popular among adolescents and residents of inner cities, where its use appears to be concentrating and where the supply is often controlled by teenage dealers and drug gangs.

Business executives, physicians, lawyers, politicians, and millions of upwardly mobile citizens of various occupations were the major users of cocaine in the 1980s. However, now that cocaine has replaced heroin in the public's perception as the hardest of hard drugs, the primary users tend more and more to be blue-collar workers, the homeless, high school dropouts, criminals, young males in search of machismo, the unemployed, and heroin addicts. Nevertheless the impact of cocaine on the American economy is staggering. The extent to which illegal cocaine trade has touched our mainstream commerce is illustrated by the fact that in most urban centers of the United States, more than three dollar bills in four, most notably twenties, will test positive for contamination with cocaine.

Medical Uses

For hundreds of years, the Inca tribes of South America have chewed coca leaves for mild refreshment and relief from fatigue. During the last quarter of the nineteenth century, cocaine was a recommended therapy for depression and other mental illnesses, digestive disorders, degeneration of tissues, morphine and alcohol addiction, and asthma, and as an aphrodisiac and local anesthetic.

Presently, cocaine has only limited therapeutic uses.[6] One clinical application is related to its unique characteristics as a local anesthetic. When applied to the surface of mucous membranes, cocaine produces both anesthesia and vasoconstriction (a narrowing effect on blood vessels). This vasoconstriction action reduces bleeding during surgery. As such, cocaine has been a valuable drug to both patient and surgeon when applied to the nose, throat, larynx, or lower respiratory passages in intranasal surgery. However, even this use may be accompanied by severe toxicity. At one time, cocaine was used extensively in eye surgery, but even this therapeutic application has become obsolete with the introduction of safer drugs as local anesthetics.

Another therapeutic use, until quite recently, has been in conjunction with *Brompton's cocktail.* A solution of cocaine, methadone, and alcohol, the special "cocktail" was first used for the relief of pain in terminally ill patients. The legal use of cocaine in Brompton's cocktail increased, especially in England, due to the proliferation of hospice services in which controlling patients' pain without causing stupor or unconsciousness is highly desirable. This liquid analgesic was administered in low doses at regular intervals or upon demand by patients. Thus, the dying

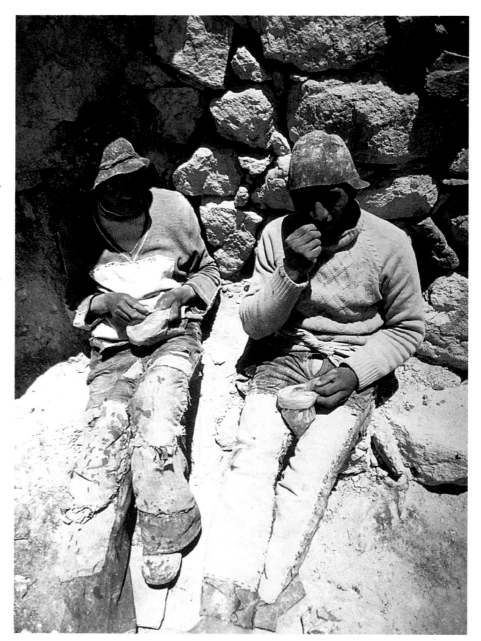

In Bolivia, these miners are chewing coca leaves as a social ritual and for mild stimulation during a workbreak.

© *Jeffrey L. Rotman/Peter Arnold, Inc.*

were maintained as pain-free as possible, awake, alert, and fully conscious until the final moments of their lives.[7] However, nearly all hospices reformulated their painkillers without cocaine and now rely instead upon a combination of morphine and alcohol, the standard in such caregiving institutions in the United States.

Historical and Legal Aspects

Although the precise origin of chewing coca leaves for euphoric effects has not been determined, many authorities date its widespread practice to the pre-Colombian South American Indians who inhabited the Andes Mountains.[8] Early myths

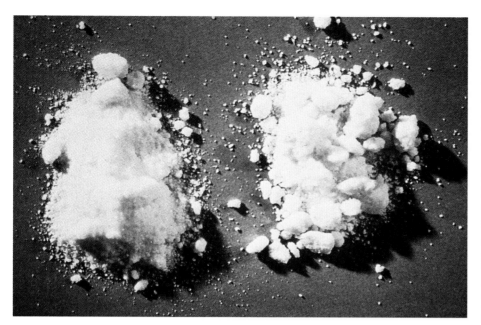

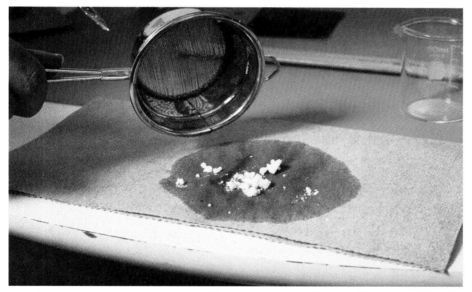

(Top): Pure cocaine, known as cocaine hydrochloride, appears as a white crystalline powder. (Bottom): Crack cocaine, the most addictive form of cocaine, appears as white gravel, slivers of soap, or tiny chunks known as "crack rocks."

Drug Enforcement Agency

of political authority or social status. Nevertheless, the Spanish soon realized the profit potential of trading coca leaves with the Incas for their gold and silver. After their conquest, the Incas increased their coca leaf chewing, possibly because of a decline in the food supplies, the institution of formal labor by the Spanish, and the euphoric feeling induced by the drug.

Although the chewing of coca leaves never became popular in either Europe or North America, various drinks made from the coca leaf were introduced into Europe. One of them, **Mariani's wine,** became most successful with endorsements from notable artists and religious leaders. In the United States, John Styth Pemberton introduced a product similar to Angelo Mariani's wine in 1885, and promoted the new French Wine Cola as a nerve and tonic stimulant.

The very next year, Pemberton concocted another coca product, a syrup that he named Coca-Cola. This new "remarkable therapeutic agent" and "sovereign remedy" contained both coca leaf flavoring (cocaine) and caffeine, an extract of the kola nut. Eventually, all references to Coca-Cola's medicinal properties were dropped, and by the time the Pure Food and Drug Law was passed in 1906, Pemberton's successors had removed the cocaine. The reformulated refreshing, exhilarating drink was flavored with decocainized coca leaves and caffeine.

It was not until 1844 or later that cocaine was first isolated in pure form from coca leaves. Early investigations by European and American physicians suggested that cocaine had great potential as a therapeutic agent. One of the stimulant's most noted advocates was Dr. Sigmund Freud, who used cocaine presumably to cure his own depression and promoted its use for numerous physical and mental disorders. Such initial enthusiasm supporting the therapeutic applications of cocaine soon diminished with mounting evidence of its health liabilities. Nevertheless, between 1890 and 1906—the "golden age of patent medicines"—cocaine was a basic ingredient of numerous ointments, powders, lozenges, and wines. These products were advertised as cures for asthma, colds, corns, eczema, neuralgia, opiate and alcohol addiction, and even venereal disease.

and legends suggest that the coca plant was of divine origin and was frequently associated with sexual behavior.

It is likely that some South American tribes chewed coca leaves as early as A.D. 600 to 800. However, by the thirteenth century a definitive role had been established for the coca plant in the religious and political structures of the early Inca Empire. To guarantee a safe crossing of the Andes Mountains, individuals offered coca leaves to the gods. Later, the Incas employed the leaves in their sacrificial rituals. The cultivation of the coca bush eventually became a state monopoly, and the use of coca leaves evolved as an exclusive privilege of the ruling class.

At the time of the Spanish conquest of the Inca Empire in the sixteenth century, coca leaves were no longer a symbol

By the turn of the century, both the federal government and the medical profession became very concerned with the widespread misuse and abuse of proprietary medicines. Influenced by horrible tales of cocaine-crazed individuals committing mass rapes and murders, public opinion also turned against cocaine. The national hysteria resulted first in the Pure Food and Drug Law of 1906 (which regulated labeling the patent medicines) and later in the Harrison Narcotic Act of 1914, which ended cocaine's use in patent medicines and established penalties for violations of regulated uses. This loss of respectability, together with the high cost of illegal cocaine, led to reduced cocaine use among Americans.

The reemergence of cocaine as a recreational drug in the mid 1960s began when the federal government initiated a campaign to crack down on the production and use of amphetamine, another CNS stimulant. Physicians were warned about overprescribing stimulant drugs, and the battle against illicit "speed" labs was stepped up. As the supply of one stimulant decreased, the smuggling of illicit cocaine suddenly became profitable.

Portrayed as the "caviar of drugs," in the 1970s, cocaine developed its appeal based on both pharmacologic effect as well as symbolism. Indeed, cocaine became an emblem of wealth and status, and a "black market" for the stimulant evolved rapidly and continues to flourish today as a profitable enterprise. But cocaine's initial acceptance was also related to the intense "high" it produces, the false perception that cocaine is not dangerous, and the mistaken belief that the drug is not addictive.

Most of the world's coca leaves come from the mountainous regions of Peru and Bolivia. Coca paste is refined in Colombia, and the final product is then smuggled into the United States, typically by either plane or boat. For several years, the main port of entry was south Florida. Now there are several others, especially on the East and West Coasts and along the Mexican border with the United States.

Although Americans are continuing their romance with cocaine at a somewhat lower level, exposure to the drug's risks

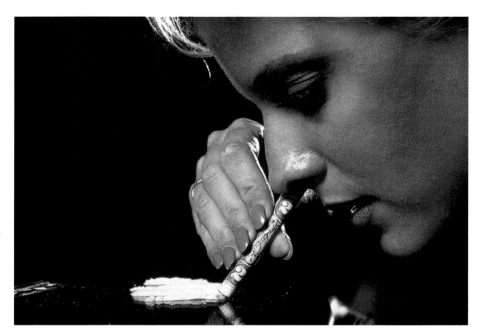

In this photo, the drug user is engaged in "snorting," which involves sniffing cocaine powder directly into the nostrils, where it is absorbed into the bloodstream through the nasal lining.

© 1986 Andy Levin/Photo Researchers, Inc.

still results in more than 100,000 emergency room episodes of cocaine abuse each year. Because of the numerous instances of overdose and the widely publicized deaths of prominent athletes due to cocaine's effects, Americans are becoming convinced that things really can go better without "coke."

Patterns of Using Cocaine

Several distinct use patterns have developed among those who consume cocaine. Some of these patterns, such as chewing and snorting, may be considered traditional, whereas the somewhat newer techniques involve injecting and smoking cocaine derivatives. The use patterns described below reflect the various methods of administering cocaine—the most powerful of the stimulant-type drugs.

Oral Use

Oral use of cocaine can still be found, especially in Peru, where Andean Indians chew coca leaves as a social ritual and for mild stimulation. Used in this way, cocaine evidently causes no serious health hazards or social problems.

Members of the upper socioeconomic classes in Peru also brew tea made from coca leaves. While not a typical use pattern in the United States, recent expanded interest in coca leaf chewing among counterculture groups has occurred as part of a trend toward organic or natural drugs.

Snorting

When extracted from other chemicals in the coca leaf, cocaine is isolated as a hydrochloride salt, known as cocaine hydrochloride. This form of cocaine usually appears as a white, crystalline powder. Dissolved in water, the cocaine can be mixed easily with other fluids and sold as "refreshing beverages" or injected directly into the veins.

Nevertheless, the modern epidemic of cocaine use featured neither drinking nor injecting, but a procedure referred to as **snorting.** Sometimes known as tooting or blowing, snorting involves sniffing

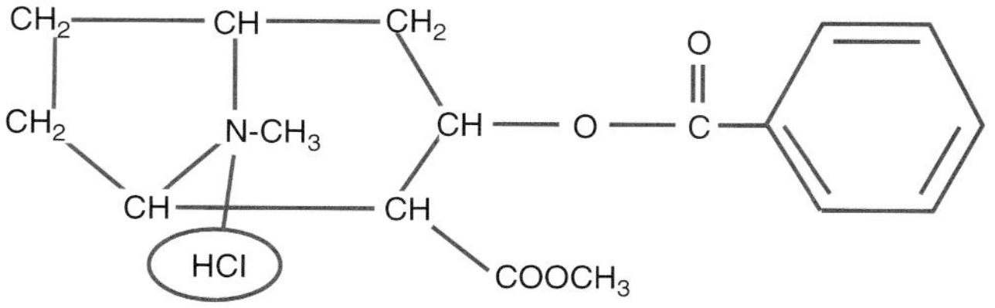

Cocaine hydrochloride

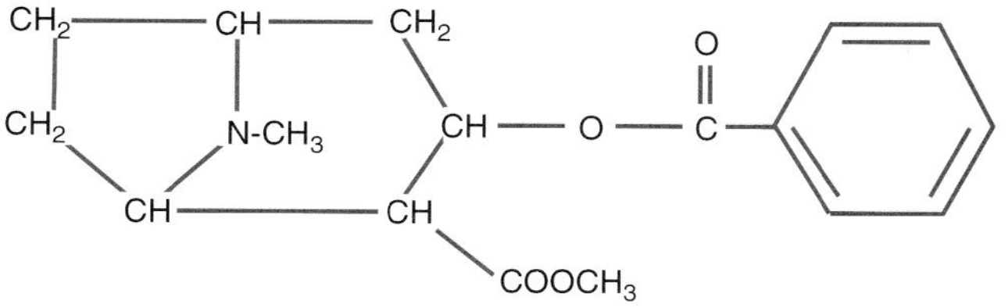

Freebase cocaine – without the HCI or hydrochloride molecule, also known as a "base." Consequently this is cocaine without the "base."

figure 8.1

Comparative molecular structures of cocaine used in snorting and injection with freebase cocaine.

cocaine powder directly into the nostrils, where it is absorbed into the bloodstream through the nasal mucosa (lining).

Typically, the user finely chops the "coke" powder with a razor blade on a hard, flat surface and then arranges the powder into thin lines or columns, approximately three to five centimeters long. The user than inhales intranasally a line of cocaine, often through a rolled dollar bill or a straw, or from a "coke spoon." The inhaled cocaine penetrates the mucous membranes of the nasal lining, enters the bloodstream, and is circulated to the brain within three to five minutes. One line usually provides the user with twenty to forty minutes of stimulation and mild euphoria.

Absorption through other mucous membranes is an alternative use pattern employed by a minority of cocaine users. Some people rub cocaine on their gums, palates, or the underside of their tongues, or have the powder blown from a straw onto the mucosal surface of the back of the throat. Another uncommon absorption technique involves the topical application of the powder to the mucosa of the vagina or the male genitalia. Some users report that this prolongs intercourse and intensifies orgasm. However, some males claim that using cocaine by any route of administration causes temporary impotence.

A number of cocaine users "snort" almost on a daily basis but manage to avoid tolerance. They claim that they can stop anytime. While the phenomenon of psychological dependence is not yet fully understood, regular cocaine use often produces the compulsive user, the cocaine addict.

Intravenous Injection

Intravenous injection of a cocaine solution, whether alone or in combination or alternation with another euphoriant, usually induces an intense, initial "rush" or "flash" not often experienced when cocaine is taken orally or snorted. A relatively short-lived experience of pure pleasure, the "rush" lasts about ten minutes. After this phenomenon, described as being like having electricity run through one's brain, the user craves yet another shot before undergoing the unpleasant experience of "crashing."

Recently, some cocaine "injectors," as well as addicted heroin "injectors," have switched to smoking a cocaine derivative, because of the very real danger of contracting AIDS (acquired immune deficiency syndrome) from needle-using "cokeaholics" and "junkies." Injecting cocaine carries additional hazards of other serious infections, formation of blood clots, and possible adverse reactions to impurities in the injected mixture.

Combined Use with Depressants

Combined use of cocaine with certain depressant drugs is a growing practice, especially among long-term compulsive users. Sometimes a mixture of cocaine and heroin—referred to as a **speedball**—is taken. Such combined or even sequential use of cocaine and a depressant smooths out the stimulant's effects, reduces nervousness and excitability, and softens "crashing" after an extended cocaine binge. Nonetheless, speedballing does increase the risks of drug dependency, toxic overdoses, and financial disaster, as well as deeper involvement with the law. John Belushi, a famous comedian, allegedly died because of speedballing—multiple injections of a cocaine-heroin mixture—which resulted in a sudden buildup of either or both drugs to toxic (poisonous) levels that proved deadly.

Contrary to widespread belief, CNS stimulants and depressants both reduce respiratory activity and produce a temporary lapse of breathing. Furthermore, the combination stimulant-depressant speedball is not an antidote for either drug. Though a small amount of cocaine reduces the depressant effect of heroin, equal amounts of the two drugs potentiate the effects of heroin. When heroin is not available, alcohol or barbiturates are sometimes substituted for the opioid after snorting or intravenous injection of cocaine.

Freebasing

A new cocaine danger called **freebasing** surfaced in the 1970s. Through an elaborate "do-it-yourself" chemical process, cocaine hydrochloride powder is changed into a smokable and more potent substance called "base" or "freebase." The actual procedure, which is extremely dangerous, involves treating the cocaine powder with a strong alkali and then ether. Comedian Richard Pryor apparently was involved in a freebasing accident that set fire to his clothing and left him with third-degree burns on the upper half of his body.

The "freebase" is then smoked in a water pipe or sprinkled on a marijuana or tobacco cigarette. Within a few minutes, the stimulant reaches the brain and produces a sudden and intense high. This euphoria subsides quickly and is often followed by a very uncomfortable restlessness, irritability, and depression. In order to maintain the high and avoid the crash, freebase smokers sometimes continue smoking until they are either exhausted or have run out of cocaine.

During the early 1980s, more cocaine users began freebasing and injecting intravenously. Both of these routes of administration result in quicker and more direct absorption of the drug and, therefore, provide a more immediate and intense euphoria. At the same time, though, freebasing and intravenous injection increase the possibility of acute toxic reaction—visual disturbances, nervousness, tremors, convulsions, irregular heartbeat, and stoppage of breathing. Increasing prevalence of freebasing also resulted in greater incidence of lung damage, psychosis, chemical poisoning, and explosion-type burns.

Crack Smoking

In 1985, another form of smokable cocaine emerged and dramatically changed the drug scene in America. **Crack cocaine** is also derived from cocaine hydrochloride. But unlike the dangerous ether procedure used in making freebase, the conversion process for making crack is somewhat safer and uses ammonia or baking soda and water. The name *crack* actually describes the sounds that occur when this form of processed cocaine is smoked.

Crack resembles hard shavings that are similar to slivers of soap, and it is often sold in small vials, in folding papers, or in heavy tinfoil. Sometimes the crack material is broken into tiny chunks that are sold as "crack rocks." Unlike freebase, which requires the use of elaborate paraphernalia, crack can be smoked either in a pipe or mixed with marijuana. On occasion, crack cocaine also contains a small amount of PCP, a particularly hazardous "dissociative anesthetic" known as "angel dust."

An intensified form of cocaine, crack is now considered one of the most addictive

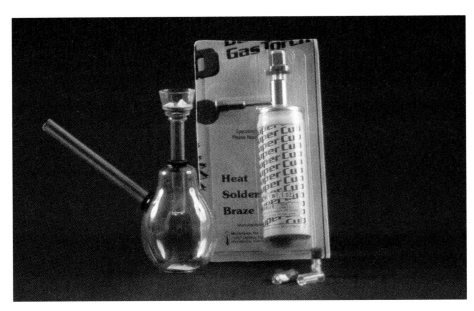

In this photograph of drug paraphernalia is a glass-bowled pipe used for smoking crack cocaine.
Drug Enforcement Agency

substances ever known, more so than heroin, barbiturates, and alcohol. Because its vapors are inhaled, crack is quickly absorbed through the lungs into the bloodstream and reaches the brain within a matter of seconds. This action is even faster than when cocaine is snorted or injected. Once within the brain, crack produces a short, intense, electrifying feeling of euphoria.

Then, within several minutes of the pleasant high, a smoker generally develops a severe crisis-like "hangover" characterized by a deep depression, extreme sadness, irritability, occasional feelings of paranoia, and an overwhelming craving for more of the drug. However, it is the withdrawal hangover, not the euphoric high, that makes crack so addictive.

Inhaling crack vapors rapidly bankrupts the brain of neurotransmitters—substances that enable the transfer of nerve impulses between nerve cells and thus control mood and behavior. This sudden release of neurotransmitter substances causes the intense euphoria, an extremely pleasant feeling. But cocaine also prevents the return of the neurotransmitters, including norepinephrine, dopamine, and serotonin, for reuse in the nerve cells. Consequently, the loss of neurotransmitters produces an emergency craving to replenish these natural chemicals of the

brain. The crack abuser mistakenly interprets this craving as a need for more cocaine. Soon, getting crack, smoking crack, and experiencing crack become more important than anything else.

Crack users have become innovative in their simultaneous use of smokable rock with other psychoactives. Sometimes crack smokers place rocks of freebase in marijuana to produce "champagne" or "caviar"—crack-laced joints. Smokable speedballs ("hot rocks") are combinations of crack and "tar" heroin. To concoct "space base," some users mix PCP (phencyclidine) with crack, while others prepare "crack coolers" by adding crack or regular cocaine to wine coolers.

More recently, still another form of smokable cocaine, *basuco,* surfaced in Miami, Florida, and then in New York City. Cocaine basuco (or "bazuko") is sometimes called cocaine sulfate, coca paste, or just simply "base." A crude form of cocaine, basuco is highly contaminated with lead and petroleum by-products. The drug is typically mixed with tobacco or marijuana and smoked as a cigarette. Relatively cheap in comparison with crack, basuco has sold for about $1 per dose. This low price and its high potency and rapid, addictive effect make basuco a "triple threat" among abused drugs.

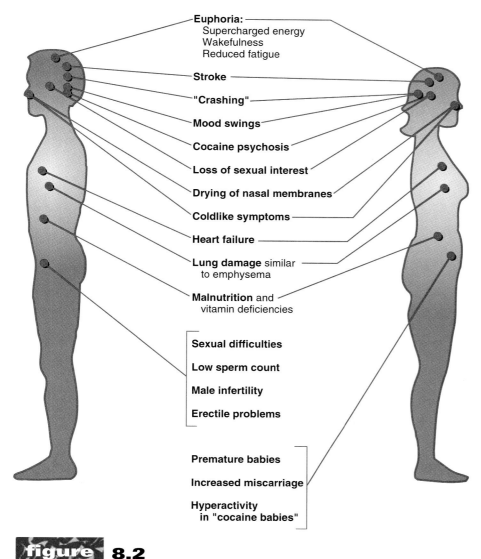

Euphoria:
Supercharged energy
Wakefulness
Reduced fatigue

Stroke

"Crashing"

Mood swings

Cocaine psychosis

Loss of sexual interest

Drying of nasal membranes

Coldlike symptoms

Heart failure

Lung damage similar
to emphysema

Malnutrition and
vitamin deficiencies

Sexual difficulties

Low sperm count

Male infertility

Erectile problems

Premature babies

Increased miscarriage

Hyperactivity
in "cocaine babies"

figure 8.2

Effects of cocaine use. Effects depend on dosage, frequency of use, and method of self-administration.

Effects of Cocaine

As with other drugs, the effects of this CNS stimulant are dependent upon the dose, the drug's purity, the user's mind-set, the psychosocial setting, and the route of administration. The initial euphoric effects are intense but subside quickly. Users report an increased feeling of self-confidence and supercharged energy. They also experience wakefulness, talkativeness, increased heart rate and blood pressure, dilation of the pupils of the eyes, a rise in body temperature, constriction of blood vessels, and a reduction of appetite. Other responses include a reduction of fatigue (masked by stimulation of the central nervous system), enhanced mental alertness, and increased sociability.

Occasional light use is associated primarily with pleasurable psychological effects. However, researchers familiar with the cocaine "street scene" have concluded that laboratory experiments and surveys of users often underestimate both the number and the severity of the undesirable effects, especially the depression and irritability of crashing, and the overwhelming desire for more of the drug.

Regular users sometimes report feelings of restlessness, irritability, anxiety, and even sleeplessness. In addition, even low doses of cocaine can create various psychological problems and "mood swings," while long-term use can result in hallucinations of touch, sight, taste, or smell. *Prolonged snorting* tends to dry out the mucous membrane linings of the nose until they crack, bleed, and develop ulcerlike sores. *Long-term use* also produces coldlike symptoms, with a runny nose; results in a dull headache; and may erode the cartilage separating the nostrils.

Regardless of the route of administration, prolonged use of cocaine often results in malnutrition because appetite is impaired. In time, chronic abusers often lose weight and develop a variety of vitamin deficiencies. Long-term use also contributes to a variety of sexual problems, including a loss of interest in sexual interaction, erectile difficulties, and greater insensitivity.[9] Moreover, it appears that prolonged use of cocaine is also linked with low sperm count and infertility in males.

Among the more alarming effects of prolonged cocaine use are confusion, anxiety, and **cocaine psychosis,** characterized by paranoia and hallucinations of a tactile, visual, olfactory, and auditory nature. This severe psychotic reaction can occur while the user is still taking cocaine. One hallucination that is particularly frightening is referred to as **formication.** Also known as parasitosis, formication is the false perception that bugs (insects such as ants) or snakes are crawling under one's skin. This feeling may be so intense that some individuals may scratch and pick their own skin into open sores and gouge themselves with a knife to cut out the imaginary invaders.[10]

Continued use of cocaine may also make the brain more sensitive to the drug (the so-called *kindling effect*), so that even low doses of cocaine may bring on seizures and eventually sudden death. In this case, no dose can be considered safe.

In addition to the most serious health effects associated with snorting and injecting, freebasing and crack-smoking can also lead to lung damage that is similar to emphysema and interferes with efficiency of lung function and breathing.

box 8.2

Cocaine Addiction and Drug Dependence

As defined by Dr. Mark Gold, founder of the national drug hotline "800–COCAINE," *addiction* is the irresistible compulsion to use a drug at increasing doses and frequency despite serious physical and/or psychological side effects and the extreme disruption of the user's personal relationships and value system.[a] According to this widely held interpretation of the *addicted state,* most psychoactive drugs are addictive, particularly *heroin, tranquilizers, barbiturates, alcohol, marijuana, amphetamines, and cocaine.* Though this is less common, psychedelic drugs and phencyclidine (PCP) can also be addictive.

Many scientists and physicians, including Dr. Gold, now believe that cocaine is the most addictive drug of all. They contend that the compulsive desire to repeat the sensation of euphoria is so great that "individual survival becomes irrelevant. No other drug does this."[b] In essence, the persistent need to take cocaine threatens the physical, psychological, social, and spiritual existence of the cocaine user. Foregoing food, basic personal hygiene, social interaction, and even sexual behavior, some cocaine abusers use the drug almost continuously, until their supply of coke has been exhausted. This pattern of use is called "binging" and signals loss of control over drug use.

Because the *four stages of the addictive process*—undergoing the euphoric high; occurrence of psychic depression and fatigue; development of irritability, insomnia, and paranoid feelings; and experience of cocaine-induced psychosis—can progress so rapidly with *crack,* this new smokable cocaine is considered the most addictive form of the CNS stimulant.

While there has been general agreement that cocaine is addictive and capable of producing a rapid psychological dependence, some authorities and many laypersons have doubted the ability of cocaine to cause a *physical dependence.* Indeed, when a person stops using cocaine, he or she does not experience a physical withdrawal crisis comparable to the alcoholic's delirium tremens. However, with the recent accumulation of clinical data on victims of the cocaine epidemic, the existence of a true withdrawal syndrome following cocaine use seems compelling.[c]

The severe feelings of depression, irritability, social withdrawal, intense craving for more cocaine, muscle pain, eating disturbances, tremors, electroencephalographic (brain-wave recordings) alterations, and changes in sleep patterns must be more than the simple consequences of traditionally defined psychological dependence. The experience of such withdrawal symptoms is evidence that a physical dependency to cocaine does indeed occur.

Tolerance, the need to use more cocaine to get the "high" once experienced with smaller doses, is a common occurrence among those who engage in intravenous injection, freebasing, and crack-smoking. Though tolerance does not usually develop with infrequent snorting, a switch to freebase or crack may indicate the development of tolerance. Some chronic users even report a *reverse tolerance,* in which they undergo an increased sensitivity to the effects of cocaine—evidence of the "kindling effect" in the brain.

Even the prestigious American Psychiatric Association (APA) now defines cocaine dependence as one of the major substance-use disorders. According to the APA findings, cocaine dependence is characterized by common mental or physical complications of long-term chronic use, such as paranoid ideas (feelings that others are hostile or persecutory), aggressive behavior, psychic depression, and weight loss.[d] Regardless of the route of cocaine administration, tolerance occurs with repeated use. Withdrawal symptoms, especially a dysphoric mood consisting of anxiety, depression, and restlessness, can be observed, but these are usually short-lived.

However, there are four significant reasons why the cocaine user continues to use cocaine,[e] and none of these has any relation to physical dependence:

1. The feelings with which cocaine provides the user— euphoria, enhanced power, elation, and brilliance—are extremely compelling.
2. Severe sadness, apathy, and dysphoria set in after a cocaine "run" has ended.
3. The drug provides temporary relief from the deep depression and the occasional suicidal cocaine psychosis that follow a "run."
4. Cocaine use can produce *anhedonia,* the inability to feel what happens during cocaine-free periods. Anhedonia is a condition in which nothing is perceived as enjoyable, pleasurable, or fun. Sooner or later, the only possible enjoyment is derived from cocaine.

Thus, cocaine use tends to become a persistent behavior to escape dysphoria, depression, and anhedonia.

References

a. Mark S. Gold, *800–COCAINE* (New York: Bantam Books, 1984).
b. Mark S. Gold, "A Psychiatrist's View of Addiction," *USA Today,* 16 September 1986, p. 4D.
c. Reese T. Jones, "The Pharmacology of Cocaine," in *Cocaine: Pharmacology, Effects, and Treatment of Abuse* [National Institute on Drug Abuse Monograph 50], ed. John Grabowski (Washington, D.C.: U.S. Government Printing Office, 1984), 47.
d. American Psychiatric Association, *Diagnostic and Statistical Manual of Mental Disorders,* 4th ed. (Washington, D.C.: American Psychiatric Association, 1994), 222.
e. Sidney Cohen, "Drug Abuse: The Coming Years," in *Substance Abuse Problems: New Issues for the 1980s* (New York: Haworth Press, 1985), 263–64.

Cocaine Babies

Sometimes cocaine abuse can have adverse effects on nonusers as well. For instance, if women use cocaine heavily during pregnancy, there is the distinct possibility that their children will be born as "cocaine" or "crack" babies. The mothers themselves tend to experience higher rates of premature births and miscarriages, while their babies are typically small at birth. In addiction, such prenatally cocaine-exposed infants tend to have a higher than average rate of minor congenital abnormalities. Some may suffer brain damage due to cocaine's constriction of blood vessels that supply fetal oxygen. However, there is no clear evidence of a crack baby syndrome as serious or as common as fetal alcohol syndrome.[11]

Early reports indicated that cocaine's effects on the developing fetus and the newborn could be devastating. Such accounts were eventually proved to be flawed. While it is true that many children of heavy cocaine users do suffer from attention deficit disorder (hyperactivity) and experience signs of tension, muscle stiffness, poor reflexes, and delayed motor development, most of the symptoms disappear by age 3. Though mothers' cocaine use during pregnancy is only one of many undesirable influences on their own children, in most cases it seems to have caused no serious, lasting brain injury.[12]

Life-Threatening Consequences

Although many physicians have long recognized the deadly potential of using cocaine, until recently the general public has been largely unaware of this drug's lethal characteristics. Contrary to the once-held belief that using cocaine was safe, it should be emphasized that this psychoactive drug is highly dangerous and in pure form can kill in just minutes.

And, it should be noted, with the smoking of freebase and crack, *the very first dose of cocaine can cause strokes, heart attacks, and sudden death.* Cocaine can kill through various physiological mechanisms.[13]

- Regardless of the dosage level, the livers of some users cannot produce an essential enzyme necessary to

detoxify cocaine. The continuing presence of unmetabolized cocaine might result in fatal complications, detailed below, that would not otherwise occur in individuals with normal functioning livers.

- Even when cocaine can be detoxified by the liver, death might result from uncontrolled body seizures following use or from paralysis of breathing muscles, due to sudden stimulation of the central nervous system.

- Cocaine can cause such a rapid elevation of blood pressure that a weakened blood vessel in the brain may rupture, resulting in a stroke (cerebrovascular accident) that might kill or paralyze.

- Death through heart failure is now related to cocaine's ability to cause damage to the heart muscle by disrupting the blood supply to cardiac muscles, resulting in a myocardial infarction, or heart attack.

- Injected, snorted, and smoked cocaine can cause irregularities in the heartbeat, which can be fatal, as well as heart attacks and even sudden death from cardiac arrest. There might develop a pattern of abnormally fast contractions of the heart's lower chambers—the ventricles—often in excess of 150 contractions per minute, which can rapidly prove deadly.

Amphetamines

Commonly referred to as "uppers," "pep pills," "bennies," "whites," "dexies," "hearts," **"speed,"** "meth," "crystal," "crank," and "ice," the **amphetamine drugs** are powerful CNS stimulants with cocainelike effects. Unlike naturally occurring cocaine, the amphetamines are synthetic, chemically manufactured substances. But like cocaine, amphetamines also affect those areas of the brain that control blood pressure, heart action, breathing, and metabolic rate, all of which are increased.

When amphetamines are used, appetite is markedly decreased and fatigue is effectively, though artificially, masked. In general, the human senses are hyperalert and the body is in a state of stress. These stimulant drugs enable the users to work harder than necessary and last longer than expected. Unlike those of cocaine, the effects of amphetamines typically last for several hours after taking the drug.

Amphetamine is actually a collective term for at least four closely related drugs:

1. *Amphetamine* or levoamphetamine (Benzedrine);
2. **Dextroamphetamine** (Dexedrine);
3. **Methamphetamine** (crystal, "meth" or "speed"); and
4. *Dextromethamphetamine* ("ice")

For oral use, these stimulants are manufactured as tablets or capsules that come in various decorator colors as well as basic white. Powdery or crystalline amphetamine can be snorted or, after being mixed with water, injected intravenously (see box 8.3). And recently, a smokable and purified form of crystal methamphetamine—known as **"ice"**—emerged as the latest variety of amphetamine drugs.

Effects of Amphetamines

The several amphetamine "chemical cousins" are very similar in the effects they induce. In typical therapeutic doses, the amphetamines produce wakefulness and alertness, elevate mood and self-confidence, reduce feelings of fatigue, depress the appetite, enhance concentration powers, induce a mild euphoria, and increase the desire and capacity to work. There is also a noticeable increase in motor and speech activity, along with an elevation of heart rate, respiration, and blood pressure.[14]

Amphetamines tend to be a favorite of those who wish to exert themselves beyond their normal physiological limits. Workers trying to maintain alertness during the night shift, truckers attempting to drive a long distance without stopping for sleep, students cramming all night for an examination, and athletes—including bikers—desiring to enhance their performance often fall into this category of drug

box 8.3

Speed: Yesterday and Today

During the 1960s, a new form of amphetamine abuse developed when massive-dose, intravenous injections of methamphetamine ("meth" or "speed") became popular. The sudden electrifying impact of speed—or "crystal," as it is often called today—was usually felt before the needle was removed from the arm of the user. Even today, those who inject crystal compare the "rush" or "flash" effect with the intense pleasure of physical and psychological exhilaration. In addition to this full-body feeling of well-being, some users also report an awareness of more rapid thinking, an experience of more efficient thought and action, and marked enhancement of sexual performance.

Currently manufactured in tablet form as the prescription drug Desoxyn,[a] methamphetamine is still available as "street crystal," but in greatly reduced amounts. This form of speed is a powder that can be injected, inhaled, or swallowed. Illegal "street crank," another form of methamphetamine, comes packaged in pill form. Regardless of its nickname or street preparation, methamphetamine is still dangerous and potentially lethal. Continued use places the abuser at risk for all the hazards associated with amphetamines. And needle users are especially vulnerable to skin abscesses, hepatitis, tetanus, and even AIDS—common penalties for injecting dirty or shared needles.

When a smokable form of methamphetamine first emerged in Hawaii in the late 1980s and then on the West Coast of the mainland United States, there was great concern that ice would soon become the latest drug menace to sweep across the nation. Highly addictive, "ice" is smoked like crack cocaine and provides a high lasting several hours. Tolerance develops so abruptly that users often smoke massive amounts during an ice run, a prolonged period of heavy drug use.

Although many predicted that ice would become the "drug of the 1990s," results of the ongoing Drug Use Forecasting (DUF) program suggest that many stimulant users are steering clear of it. While smokable methamphetamine has spread beyond the West Coast, the anticipated epidemic—the "ice storm"—has not yet materialized nationwide. The trafficking of ice appears to be tightly controlled, however, by a small group of Asians and affiliated gangs. As such, states having large Asian communities are likely to be among the first to report widespread availability and use.

The once popular slogan "Speed kills," originally described the death of the personality or spirit of the user who entered a state of limbo, neither physiologically dead nor psychologically alive. But speed can kill physically, because prolonged use can seriously wear out and tear down the human body through vitamin and mineral deficiencies—resulting from poor nutrition—and lowered resistance to disease.[b] Under a general state of stress, the speed freak's body literally begins to burn itself up. Highly energized and denied the benefits of rest, recovery, and even food, the individual undergoes a rapid deterioration of both physical and psychological health. Eventually, damage to major organs of the body (lungs, liver, and kidneys) occurs. In this sense, speed can kill!

Since controls on the production and distribution of legally produced amphetamines reduced their availability, the speed scene became dominated first by *look-alikes* and then by *act-alikes*. Look-alikes are drugs that are manufactured to look like real amphetamines and mimic their effects. However, the amphetamine look-alike tablets and capsules contain varying amounts of legal nonprescription stimulants, decongestants, and antihistamines, such as caffeine, phenylpropanolamine, and ephedrine. These three legal substances are relatively weak stimulants often found in over-the-counter drugs.

More recently, new single-ingredient drugs called act-alikes have been produced to circumvent state laws that prohibit look-alikes. These act-alikes contain the same ingredients as the look-alikes, but they do not physically resemble any prescription or over-the-counter drugs. Sold on the street as speed and uppers, these drugs are expensive even though they are not as strong as amphetamines. They are typically sold to young people, who are told they are legal, safe, and harmless. This is a major reason why they are abused.

Effects of look-alikes and act-alikes. When taken in large doses, these drugs are similar to amphetamines in their effects, which include anxiety, restlessness, weakness, throbbing headache, difficult breathing, and a rapid heartbeat. Severe high blood pressure can occur and lead to cerebral hemorrhaging (stroke) and death.

Dangers of look-alikes and act-alikes. Because look-alikes and act-alikes are not as strong as real amphetamines, they are extremely dangerous for people who, deliberately or accidentally, take the same amount of real amphetamines as act-alikes. For example, people who buy act-alikes on the street might unknowingly buy real amphetamines and take enough to cause an overdose. On the other hand, people who have abused amphetamines might underestimate the potency of the act-alike drugs and take excessive amounts that can result in a toxic reaction.

a. United States Pharmacopeia. *Complete Drug Reference*, 1994 ed. (Yonkers, N.Y.: Consumer Reports Books, 1993), 53–56.
b. Jim Parker, Crystal, Crank, and Speedy Stuff (Tempe, Ariz.: Do It Now, 1994), 4.

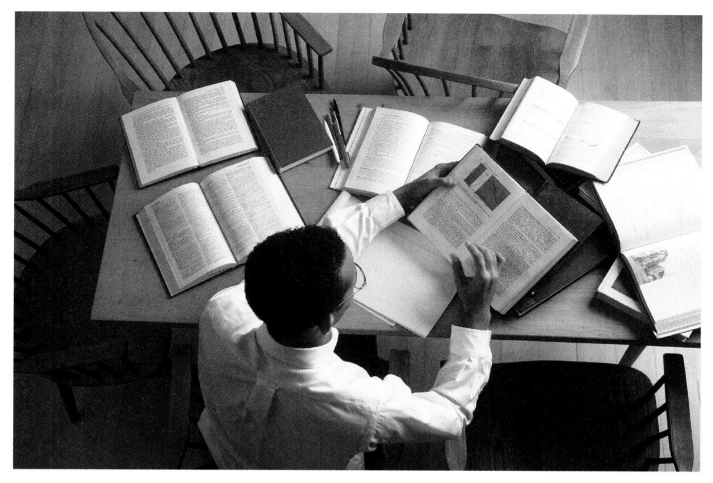

Cramming all night for an exam may be a sufficient, though hardly necessary, reason for using amphetamines.

© Llewellyn/Uniphoto Picture Agency

abuse. They all have discovered that the length of adequate performance is prolonged, while the effects of fatigue are at least partially reversed. (Although the need for sleep can be postponed, it cannot be avoided indefinitely.) Amphetamines are also used on occasion by sexually active people, including the gay population, who believe that "chemical uppers" enhance the pleasure and performance of various sexual behaviors.

Sporadic or infrequent use rarely leads to major health problems, although an amphetamine injection tends to produce a sudden increase in blood pressure that can cause death from stroke, high fever, or heart failure. In such a case, the entire cardiovascular system (heart and blood vessels) is stressed. Of course, injectors also risk the consequences of using contaminated needles.

Users might also experience dryness of the mouth, sweating, headaches, blurred vision, dizziness, sleeplessness, and anxiety. Higher doses intensify these effects, while long-term heavy use can lead to mood swings, mental confusion, delusions, hallucinations, skin disorders, ulcers, and various diseases that come from vitamin deficiencies. Lack of sleep, weight loss, and depression can also result from persistent use.

When "crystal meth" or "ice" is smoked, users often claim that the drug's euphoric effects are similar to those of cocaine, but without the distortion of mental states. Since ice is absorbed through the lungs, the effects are felt intensely and rapidly—a flash of euphoria followed by an extended period of energized alertness. These effects are identical to those produced by injecting speed, but are delivered without the hazards of using needles.[15] As the high fades, some ice-smokers seek to reexperience the euphoria by increasing their intake. This might involve repeated smoking for days or weeks with only a minimum of food and sleep—not unlike a "run" or binging period of persistent heavy use of speed by meth injectors. In both instances, tolerance tends to build rapidly as huge dosages are consumed.

Whether as extensions of therapeutic action or as a result of overdose, toxic effects can also include involuntary shaking of the body, tenseness, hyperactive reflexes, and assaultiveness. Panic states are common, and suicidal or homicidal tendencies sometimes develop, especially in mentally ill patients. Heavy, frequent doses can even produce brain damage that can result in speech disturbances and difficulty in turning thoughts into words.

Perhaps the most dramatic consequence of amphetamine abuse is the experience of stimulant-induced toxic psychosis. This bizarre phenomenon is characterized by feelings of persecution, delusions, and hallucinations, similar to the cocaine-induced paranoid schizophrenia-like state. During such an episode, the amphetamine abuser is quite capable of thinking clearly and can recall relevant and extraneous facts. However, such an individual is often preoccupied with *formication*—the perceived sensation of having "crank bugs" crawling under one's skin. Compulsively, the abuser begins picking at his or her own skin and, in doing so, creates multiple ulcerations. People sustaining *amphetamine psychosis* frequently exhibit other forms of equally strange and even violent behavior.[16]

Amphetamine Dependence

There is a great similarity in the patterns and symptoms of amphetamine and cocaine dependency. Taking large amounts of amphetamine on a continuing basis—to keep going, to feel "high," to counteract depression, and to deal with problems of living and emotional inadequacies—typically leads to drug dependence or addiction. Tolerance to the euphoric and appetite-suppressant effects of amphetamines usually develops rapidly after repeated oral, smoked, and injected doses, necessitating increased dosage levels to obtain the desired effects.

When the regular use of amphetamines is stopped suddenly, the individual commonly experiences severe mental depression, fatigue, irritability, long periods of sleep, and extreme hunger. These withdrawal symptoms are now considered as evidence of physical dependency by medical authorities. There is no doubt, moreover,

that amphetamines are capable of producing a psychological dependence even at low dose levels.

Because amphetamine-induced power, self-confidence, and artificial exhilaration are so pleasant, and because of the fear of experiencing the depression and fatigue of "crashing," amphetamine abusers, even though they may stop for a while, normally revert to continued abuse. Typically, such people are unable to pull themselves out of amphetamine abuse voluntarily, except through heated argumentation or wrangling, imprisonment, or having a psychotic experience.

Historical and Legal Aspects

Amphetamines were first synthesized in Germany in 1887. However, it was not until 1927 that physicians discovered the drugs' ability to stimulate the central nervous system, alleviate fatigue, and relieve congested nasal passages. Then in 1935 the first clinical use of the stimulant was in the treatment of **narcolepsy,** a condition of uncontrolled sleeping. In 1937, amphetamines were found to have a paradoxical calming effect on children with hyperkinetic disorders (extreme activity and impulsivity).

During World War II, the military services of both the Axis and the Allies used amphetamines to combat soldiers' fatigue, elevate mood, and prolong endurance.[17] In combat situations, amphetamines proved superior to cocaine because they could be taken by mouth rather than by sniffing, and their effect lasted for several hours, not just several minutes.

After World War II, **methamphetamine** or methedrine was introduced, and nonprescription Dexedrine inhalers for nasal decongestion became almost a fad among the American population. Eventually, the inhalers were removed from the market, but the nonmedical use of amphetamines spread like wildfire.

The modern day "speedball"—an injectable combination of amphetamine and heroin—was originated by military servicemen stationed in the Far East in the early 1950s. (Today the meaning of the

term *speedball* has been expanded generally to include the combination of any CNS stimulant and depressant.)

For the next twenty years, amphetamines were prescribed widely for the control of depression and as an aid in dieting. They were also used in treating epilepsy, asthma, sedative overdose, and nausea in association with pregnancy.

In 1970, the Controlled Substances Act placed amphetamines under Schedule II and thus restricted severely the manufacture and distribution of these CNS stimulants. Within a short period of time, legitimate production of these drugs fell by an estimated 80 percent. Many amphetamine tablets and capsules were then diverted from legitimate manufacturers, and continue to be even today. What could not be obtained by subterfuge or from "script doctors," in exchange for a fee, was often manufactured in secret "speed" labs and sold illegally on the street market.

Today, illicit amphetamine is still available "on the street" and is known as "crystal" and "crank" methamphetamine. When injected, *crystal* (the most powerful of all the different forms of speed) produces an intense wave of physical and psychic exhilaration—the "rush" or "flash" reaction. The rush associated with crystal is a potent reinforcer that induces people to continue using the drug, in spite of serious physical and psychological damage that can result from long-term abuse.

Crank is a common nickname for another form of methamphetamine, usually of the pill variety. However, *crank* can also refer to pharmaceutical amphetamine and various bootleg amphetamines.

In 1988, the most recent version of speed surfaced in Hawaii as smokable methamphetamine, or "ice." Originally smuggled into the United States from South Korea, Hong Kong, and the Philippines, ice is now made cheaply and easily in the same secret labs that produce illegal crystal and crank. Although ice provides a rapid feeling of intense pleasure that lasts for several hours, in comparison with crack cocaine's fifteen-minute high, this smokable methamphetamine is also responsible for a deep, post-use depression, with symptoms of severe paranoia, hallucinations, and delusions. These unfavorable experiences might actually prevent the expected epidemic of ice use, and contribute to a decline of the drug's initial popularity, before it spreads too far beyond the West Coast.

Medical Uses of Amphetamines

The use of prescribed amphetamines for the control of obesity has been one of the more popular applications of these CNS stimulants. In the medical world, amphetamines and amphetaminelike drugs that tend to curb the appetite are referred to as **anorectics.**

In an extensive review of anorectics, the U.S. Food and Drug Administration concluded that patients receiving such drugs will indeed lose more weight than those who are not treated with them. But patients who take these drugs and also diet will lose only a fraction of a pound more each week than those who rely only on dietary restriction. Thus anorectics were found to have only a very limited usefulness in treating obesity. Moreover, the rate of weight loss was found to be greater during the early stages of taking diet pills, and combinations of anorectics with barbiturates and tranquilizers were no better than anorectic drugs alone.

While the usefulness of amphetamines in treating obesity was being challenged, it also became apparent that the nonmedical use of prescribed anorectics was skyrocketing. Patients soon discovered the "pep-pill" effect of the amphetamines and increased their use as tolerance and dependence developed. Some people also experienced bizarre and even psychotic behavior as amphetamine anorectics were abused with alarming frequency.

For these reasons, the Food and Drug Administration began urging physicians in the late 1960s to exercise extreme caution in prescribing anorectics, and the FDA was instrumental in decreasing the legitimate production of these stimulants. Since obesity contributes so significantly to mortality, the selective and discriminating use of anorectics has been considered as preferable to a total ban on such drugs. Nevertheless, many physicians generally reject these medications for treating obesity, because they tend to increase the risk for addiction, sometimes accompanied by paranoid delusions. Concurrently, there was also a noticeable decline in the prescription of amphetamines for improving mood, increasing attention, and overcoming fatigue.

Recently, several other appetite-suppressant drugs have been developed as replacements for the amphetamines. Known collectively as *amphetamine congeners* or *surrogates,* two of these (fenfluramine and phentermine) proved remarkably effective when used as part of a weight-loss program that included a diet-and-exercise regimen and training in appetite control.[18] All of the amphetamine congeners produce amphetaminelike effects but are generally less potent than the amphetamines themselves. They are available by prescription only. However, like the amphetamines, none of these appetite suppressant drugs is a cure for obesity. They are useful only for the short-term management of obesity until patients adjust to various dietary restrictions and reform their eating habits.[19]

Somewhat less controversially, amphetamines are medically approved in the United States at the present time for treatment of two specific kinds of disorders:

1. **Narcolepsy** is a neurological disorder characterized by recurrent episodes or attacks of sleep. These episodes are usually induced by emotional excitement. Large doses of amphetamines prevent such attacks and help patients maintain wakefulness.

2. **Attention deficit-hyperactivity** (hyperkinetic) **disorders** in children are distinguished by extreme hyperactivity or motor restlessness, poor attention span, and impulsive and sometimes disorderly behavior. Dextroamphetamine and another related CNS stimulant, methylphenidate (Ritalin), are very effective in managing this disorder.

Aggressive and impulsive behaviors are reduced; the child begins to engage in greater goal-directed behavior and improves attention span. Why these CNS stimulants produce such calming and sedating effects in children is not fully known. Equally mysterious is the fact that amphetamines and methylphenidate do not induce euphoria or overstimulation in hyperkinetic children.

Caffeine

Usually considered a nondrug because it is taken invisibly into the body under the guise of various beverages, candies, and confections, caffeine is probably the most widely used social drug in the world. A bitter tasting, odorless compound, caffeine is a natural constituent of various plants that are the sources of coffee, tea, kola nut extracts, cocoa, and chocolate. Numerous medications also contain caffeine, including certain over-the-counter analgesics and stimulants.

The most important source of caffeine in the American diet is coffee, an extract from the fruit of the *Coffea arabica* plant and related species. It is estimated that the average American coffee drinker consumes about 1,000 cups of coffee each year. Another popular source of caffeine is the cola-flavored soft drinks people consume so heavily. Because of their physical size, children are more likely than adults to be affected by caffeine. Some people believe that the caffeine in cola drinks is responsible for hyperactivity in children.

People consume a surprising and alarming amount of caffeine. Depending upon product, brand, and method of preparation, each cup of coffee has an average caffeine dose of at least 70 milligrams (mg) and as much as 215 mg. Regular cola and pepper drinks range in caffeine content from 40 mg to 54 mg per twelve-ounce serving. Nonprescription alertness tablets contain from 100 mg to 200 mg each, and some analgesics deliver 32 to 65 mg per tablet.

Historical Aspects

The precise origin of caffeine use cannot be determined because of the drug's natural occurrence throughout the world. Nevertheless, it is assumed that in one form or another, caffeine has been consumed for thousands of years. It is probable that *coffee* was brought to Europe from Arabia and Turkey; *tea* was introduced into the Western world from China; the *kola nut* was used commonly in West Africa and later became an ingredient in cola drinks; the *cacao tree,* from which chocolate is derived, was found in Mexico and much of Central and South America; the *ilex plant,* source of maté, or Paraguayan tea, is native to Brazil; and *cassina,* the Christmas berry tree, was often used as the source of a caffeine beverage among Indians in colonial America.[20]

Opposition to caffeine beverages began early in history. Coffee was condemned as an intoxicant in certain cultures. Coffee sales were prohibited in Egypt when the beverage was first introduced in the sixteenth century. In Europe, attempts were made to outlaw the drink, while physicians attacked coffee as harmful. Despite all of these warnings and prohibitions, coffee eventually became an integral part of European and American culture. Today, coffee is a domesticated drug willingly consumed in vast quantities. Few people realize that coffee or caffeine is a drug; fewer yet consider caffeine as a potentially dangerous drug. As a poison, it is relatively safe, only because it is used typically in a very dilute form.

Effects of Caffeine

Caffeine is a "mild" CNS stimulant whose desirable effects are quite similar to those of the amphetamines and cocaine. The major pharmacological actions, due to caffeine-induced higher rates of cellular activity and increased synthesis of norepinephrine, are demonstrated primarily in the central nervous system, the kidney, and the cardiovascular system. Depending upon the individual user and the amount taken, effects typically include an immediate increase in body temperature, blood pressure, and general body chemistry.

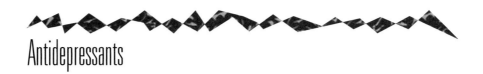
As a stimulant of the CNS, caffeine induces clearer thought, less drowsiness, shortened reaction time, improved intellectual effort, and increased motor activity, respiratory rate, and reflex excitability. Indeed, the first cup of coffee each day often functions as a morning "fix" that provides an initial uplifting eye-opener.

In the cardiovascular system, caffeine increases the rate and force of the heart's contraction, and it produces a general vasodilation of systemic blood vessels, including the coronary arteries, resulting in an increased blood flow. This vasodilation is short-lived and is accompanied by a vasoconstriction (narrowing) of the blood

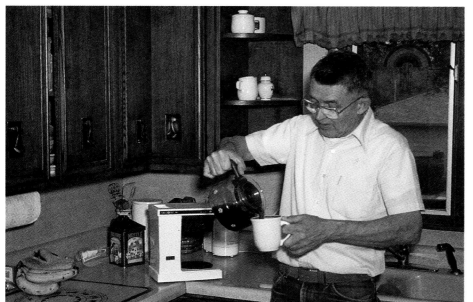

Many people drink coffee to "jump-start" their morning activities and to keep going throughout the day. Caffeine may be one of the most frequently used drugs in the world. So far, no study has related any significant health problems to drinking three cups of coffee or fewer per day.

© James L. Shaffer

vessels in the brain. Such vasoconstrictive action in the cerebral blood vessels provides some relief from hypertensive and certain types of migraine headaches.

In addition, caffeine speeds up the production of urine, increases the capacity for muscular work, and augments the volume and acidity of gastric secretions (pepsin and acid).

Caffeinism

The popularity of coffee and other products containing caffeine is related to their stimulating actions accompanied by a lessening of drowsiness, a reduction in fatigue, and a more rapid and clearer flow of thought.[21] The amount of such stimulation takes several forms and varies considerably from person to person. Some individuals are able to "sleep like a log" after drinking several cups of coffee, while others may experience a toxic response with just a single cup.

Overindulgence in caffeine can lead to a stimulated condition of chronic "caffeine intoxication" or poisoning known as

caffeinism. Common but often unrecognized, caffeinism is characterized by mood changes, anxiety, disruption of sleep, various bodily complaints, and sometimes the manifestation of other medical and psychological problems. Caffeinism often develops in individuals who consume five to seven cups of coffee (500 to 700 mg of caffeine) each day.

Frequent symptoms of this toxic condition include wakefulness, insomnia, restlessness, irritability, muscle twitching, tremulousness, headache, sensory disturbances (ringing in the ears and dry mouth), lethargy, depression, palpitations, irregularities in heartbeat, changes in blood pressure, diuresis, nausea, vomiting, stomach pain, gastric ulcers, and diarrhea. (By contrast, the tannin content of tea is likely to cause constipation rather than diarrhea.)

Fatal doses of caffeine are rare but have occurred in adults when doses of the stimulant have exceeded 5 to 10 grams—the equivalent of drinking fifty to a hundred cups of coffee in a very brief period of time!

Caffeine Dependence and Tolerance

The consumption of caffeine in various beverages and products is a culturally reinforced and socially encouraged practice. Surrounded by numerous coffee and tea drinkers, young people begin to associate consumption with taste, warmth, aroma, or some pleasant activity. However, it is possible that the drug's stimulating effects—the sense of well-being, the morning "lift," the alleged increase in efficiency—are the significant reinforcers for continuing use. Assuming that caffeine activates the brain's pleasure centers, it is not surprising that it is so difficult to "kick the caffeine habit."

There is no doubt that caffeine use can lead to psychological dependence, although until recently the existence of pharmacological tolerance has been disputed. Studies now indicate that in some people who report trouble staying away from caffeine, a definite chemical syndrome of caffeine dependence can be detected.[22] Criteria for such a diagnosis include continued use despite knowledge of a persistent physical or psychological problem that is likely caused or made worse by caffeine use, persistent desire or unsuccessful efforts to cut down or control use, a tolerance marked by increasing doses of this drug-beverage, and withdrawal. Common withdrawal symptoms include headache, irritability, lethargy, apathy, difficulty in concentration, decreased work efficiency, nervousness, restlessness, and mild nausea—all usually mild in intensity and tolerable until they subside.

Unfortunately, caffeine withdrawal headaches often lead to unnecessary use of pain relievers, some of which contain caffeine along with an analgesic. The treatment unwittingly contributes to the desire for more caffeine.

Caffeine, Pregnancy, and Birth Defects

Like many other psychoactive substances, caffeine is known to cross the placenta. Caffeine has also been detected in the milk of mothers who breast-feed their infants. Nursing mothers who drink large amounts of coffee on a daily basis report that their babies are often sleepless and irritable. In addition, the CNS stimulant has been proven capable of inducing chromosomal abnormalities in both plant and animal cells. Such findings have given rise to concern about caffeine's ability to endanger the human fetus and cause various birth defects.

Warnings about the possible link between caffeine and birth defects have been based largely on animal studies in which very large doses fed to pregnant rats caused birth defects in their offspring. Surprisingly, initial research suggested that there was no correlation between human birth defects and coffee drinking. Recently, scientists investigating women who engaged in heavy caffeine consumption beyond the sixth week of pregnancy found an increased risk for both retarded fetal growth and low birth weight of newborns.[23] This study concluded that women should reduce their caffeine intake to less than 300 mg daily early in pregnancy.

Additional research now reveals that caffeine intake before and during pregnancy is also associated with an increased risk of fetal loss (spontaneous abortion or miscarriage).[24] Consequently, most medical authorities advise women to be very cautious about using any drug, including caffeine and caffeine beverages, during pregnancy. Until further studies determine what precise role caffeine plays in causing birth defects and fetal loss, the U.S. Food and Drug Administration believes that pregnant women should also be alert to products other than coffee and tea that have caffeine in them, and avoid them entirely or use them only sparingly under medical supervision.

Caffeine and Diseases

In addition to the possible relationship between caffeine use during pregnancy, and birth defects, some scientists have expressed concern about the effects of the CNS stimulant on the occurrence of specific diseases, particularly cancer and heart disease. However, research indicating that coffee or caffeine has an adverse effect on health status is somewhat controversial and still hotly debated.

One area of study relates to *fibrocystic breast disease* (noncancerous breast lumps) in women. It has been alleged that dietary caffeine encourages the formation of lumpy breasts and that abstaining from products containing caffeine will shrink, reduce, or even eliminate the cysts. Indeed, some women report relief from such lumps when caffeine is excluded from their diets, but no consistent relationship between coffee consumption and fibrocystic breast disease has been demonstrated.

During the past twenty years, cancer of the pancreas—the body organ that produces enzymes vital to digestion and the hormone, insulin, for sugar utilization—has become a significant cause of death. More than 27,000 lives are claimed annually. In what has proved to be something of a false alarm, one large-scale investigation revealed a weak positive association between pancreatic cancer and coffee consumption. However, since this research was first published, the original investigators now report that if there is any association between coffee consumption and cancer of the pancreas, it is not as strong as their earlier findings suggested.[25]

Studies indicating a possible link between *colorectal cancer* and the use of coffee have resulted in contradictory findings. According to the American Cancer Society, an estimated 153,000 people are expected to die of colorectal cancer, and another 172,000 new cases will be diagnosed, in the present year. Some reports suggest that cancer affecting the lowermost portion of the digestive system occurs two and one-half times more often in people who drink more than two cups of coffee a day than among those who consume fewer than two cups or none at all. Other researchers have found no correlation whatsoever, and some have reported a possible preventive effect.

Early research on the cardiovascular effects of caffeine concluded that men who drank five or more cups of coffee each day were two to three times more likely to have *heart attacks* or *angina*, or to *die suddenly of heart disease*, than were those who did not drink coffee. In addition, coffee intake exceeding two and one-half to three cups per day was related to *increased levels of blood cholesterol* among sedentary, middle-aged men. Cholesterol was identified as the likely culprit in increased heart disease risks.

Additional investigations, however, appear to have dissolved the suspected link between caffeinated coffee consumption and the risk of heart and blood vessel diseases in males. In a massive study of 45,500 healthy males in the United States, total coffee intake was not associated with an increased risk of coronary heart disease or stroke.[26] By contrast, though, a high consumption of decaffeinated coffee was related with a moderate and marginally significant increase in risk of coronary heart disease.

Where does all this conflicting research leave the American coffee drinker? A person who drinks only a few cups each day will probably not develop any serious health risks.[27] No study has yet related any significant health problem to drinking three cups of coffee or fewer per day.

While it is recognized that coffee can cause irregularities in heartbeat, especially in people with preexisting heart conditions, most studies to date have failed to demonstrate that very small amounts of coffee contribute to heart disease in healthy individuals. It is likely that cigarette smoking and consumption of saturated fats contribute more to the development of cancer and heart disease than does caffeine.

Defense Against Caffeine

Although the evidence presented so far does not condemn coffee and caffeine in relatively small amounts, there is sufficient concern to suggest that even a moderate intake of coffee might not always be good to the last drop. What, then, can informed consumers do to protect themselves from caffeine dependence and other potential health risks of both beverage and drug? Here are several suggestions:

1. Before switching from coffee to another beverage, be aware that caffeine is present in many other drinks, including tea, cocoa, and many carbonated soft drinks.

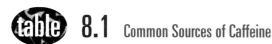

table 8.1 Common Sources of Caffeine

Beverages and Foods	Milligrams Caffeine Average	Milligrams Caffeine Range
Coffee (6-oz. cup)		
Brewed, drip method	100	70–215
Brewed, percolator	80	40–170
Instant	70	35–160
Decaffeinated, brewed	4	2–8
Decaffeinated, instant	4	2–8
Tea (5-oz. cup)		
Brewed, major U.S. brands	50	25–110
Brewed, imported brands	60	25–110
Instant	30	25–50
Iced (12-oz. glass)	70	67–76
Cocoa beverage (5-oz. cup)	5	2–25
Chocolate milk beverage (8 oz.)	5	2–7
Milk chocolate (1 oz.)	6	1–15
Dark chocolate, semisweet (1 oz.)	20	5–35
Baker's chocolate (1 oz.)	26	26
Chocolate-flavored syrup (1 oz.)	4	4
Soft Drinks		
Regular		
Cola, pepper		40–54
Decaffeinated cola, pepper		0–0.09
Cherry cola		18–23
Lemon-lime (clear)		0
Orange		0
Other citrus		0–32
Root beer		0
Ginger ale		0
Tonic water		0
Other regular		0–22
Juice added		less than 0.24
Diet drinks		
Diet cola, pepper		0.3
Decaffeinated diet cola, pepper		0–0.1
Diet cherry cola		0–23
Diet lemon-lime		0
Diet root beer		0
Other diets		0–35
Club soda, seltzer, sparkling water		0
Diet juice added		less than 0.24

Selected Medications	Per Tablet or Capsule
Prescription medicines	
Cafergot (migraine headache)	100
Norgesic Forte (muscle relaxant)	60
Norgesic (muscle relaxant)	30
Fiorinal (tension headache)	40
Fioricet (headache pain relief)	40
Darvon compound (pain relief)	32.4
Synalgos-DC (pain relief)	30
Synalgos-DC-A (pain relief)	30
Nonprescription medicines	
Alertness tablets	
NoDoz	100
Vivarin	200
Pain relief	
Anacin, Maximum Strength Anacin	32
Vanquish	33
Excedrin	65
Midol	32.4

Note: At present, all makers of nonprescription appetite suppressants and cold/allergy capsules have removed caffeine from their products.

Source: U.S. Food and Drug Administration.

2. While tolerance to caffeine apparently varies from one person to another, remember that the elderly generally have a decreased tolerance to drinks containing caffeine.
3. Aside from the nicotine in tobacco products, caffeine is the major nonprescription stimulant available in the United States today. An ingredient in nearly a thousand prescription drugs, caffeine is also added to numerous over-the-counter medicines, including aspirin and other analgesics.
4. Switch your coffee usage from beverages prepared by the drip and percolator methods to those that are prepared with instant and freeze-dried products (which contain less caffeine). Some brands of coffee—as well as tea—are decaffeinated and are 97 percent caffeine-free.
5. The amount of caffeine in "regular" coffee depends on how long the coffee is brewed (the longer it is brewed, the more caffeine), and how finely the beans are ground (the finer the grind, the greater the amount of caffeine). To cut back on caffeine, reduce the number of cups of coffee consumed daily, grind your coffee less finely, and do not brew your coffee for a long period of time.
6. Switch to soft drinks that are caffeine-free, including most root beers and caffeine-free versions of the popular cola drinks.
7. Become familiar with the caffeine content of various beverages and over-the-counter medicines as listed in table 8.1. Then, restrict yourself to less than 300 mg of caffeine per day. By limiting your caffeine intake, you can still enjoy that first cup of coffee in the morning.

Methcathinone

A relatively new drug of abuse in the United States, **methcathinone** has been spreading like wildfire recently in parts of northern Michigan, Wisconsin, Illinois, Indiana, and even Washington state. This home-made drug, known as "cat," is a powerful stimulant that resembles cocaine (in both appearance and potency) as well as amphetamine.

Methcathinone was originally investigated more than forty years ago by the drug manufacturing industry for possible use as a diet pill. Because of its destructive side effects—addictiveness, paranoia, and intense anxiety—methcathinone was dropped as a possible medication.[28] Chemically, this drug is derived from and similar to cathinone, a natural amphetaminelike substance found in the leaves of the East African **khat** or kat shrub, *Catha edulis*.[29] For many centuries, dried khat leaves have been chewed by native populations in the Middle East, Ethiopia, and Somalia as a stimulant and a social facilitator.[30]

Effects of Methcathinone

Typically snorted like cocaine, cat can also be smoked, liquefied and then injected by needle, or consumed orally in mixture with a beverage. The basic attraction of this drug is the burst of energy it produces, along with a lasting feeling of extreme well-being or euphoria. Users often report that they feel totally "hyper" and that everything they do is pure fun.[31] Such a high is often described as being greater than the high achieved through cocaine; it is so intense that users must sometimes combine cat with large doses of alcohol or marijuana in order to tolerate the intensity of energized feeling.

According to the Drug Enforcement Administration, some cat users binge on this drug for several days, during which they become engulfed in paranoia (delusions of persecution), experience excruciating nervousness, and suffer hallucinations.[32] Appetite decreases significantly or disappears entirely during such a binge, and this often leads to long-term weight loss. Dehydration can occur, along with severe pounding of the heart, headaches, stomach aches, and even the "shakes." When the binge is over, usually because the supply of methcathinone has been exhausted, a deep depression overwhelms the user, who becomes irritable and argumentative. This "crash" is often followed by a lengthy period of sleep, which does not always restore a sense of normal well-being.

Manufacture and Control of Cat

One of the more alarming concerns regarding home-made methcathinone is the easy availability and low cost of its chemical ingredients. The key component is ephedrine, a legal, over-the-counter asthma medication. Other easy-to-obtain components include drain cleaner, battery acid, paint thinner, Epsom salts, lye, and muriatic acid, which is sometimes used by construction workers to scrub dried mortar off the face of bricks. These basic ingredients when mixed together can produce fatally poisonous phosgene gas during the production process in secret backroom or basement labs.

Methcathinone has already been banned by the federal Drug Enforcement Administration and listed as a Schedule I controlled substance; other measures emphasize also limiting the availability of ephedrine.[33] Without ephedrine, there can be no cat. Persons who manufacture methcathinone or help others in doing so may now be prosecuted under various federal statutes. Manufacturing or possession with intent to distribute is a violation of the U.S. Code and is punishable by a prison term of up to twenty years and a fine of up to $1 million.

Ephedrine

A natural extract of the *Ephedra sinica* shrub, **ephedrine** is another close relative of the amphetamines. The leaves of the ephedra shrub have been used in stimulant teas and in centuries-old Chinese herbal medicines, such as Ma Huang. Because it helps to open or dilate bronchial tubes in the human respiratory system, ephedrine was originally used to treat asthma. The FDA has also approved its use as a decongestant. Some studies indicate that ephedrine in combination with caffeine can help overweight people lose unwanted pounds.

However, ephedrine is now advertised widely as a "thermogenic aid" that temporarily boosts the human body's metabolic rate.[34] Sold over the counter in health-food stores as well as at truck stops, ephedrine pills and capsules appear under the names of Diet Max, Diet Pep, Herb Trim, Escalation, and Mega Trim. Ephedrine is also an active ingredient in illicit drugs that are alleged to be amphetamines.[35]

Unsupervised use of this central nervous system stimulant as a pep pill or a diet pill has been linked with fatal strokes, because ephedrine increases heart rate and blood pressure and tends to constrict blood vessels. These drug actions create the conditions for a cerebrovascular accident (stroke) as well as a heart attack. Minor side effects include restlessness and insomnia, while serious adverse consequences now include nerve damage, rapid and irregular heartbeats, psychotic episodes, and loss of memory.

Although some states have attempted to restrict ephedrine, the FDA has not yet taken action to control the abuse of this common stimulant. This substance is banned for Olympic competition and international soccer because of its frequent use as an ergogenic aid to enhance athletic ability.

Other Plant Stimulants

Other stimulant drugs occasionally consumed in the United States are derived from numerous plants and have been used for centuries by millions of people either for recreation or medicine or both. Two of these plant derivatives are betel nuts and yohimbe.

Betel nuts are widely utilized in Asian countries and in the island nations of the Indian and Pacific Oceans. They are typically consumed as betel morsels—nuts from the areca palm tree, gum from the acacia tree, and burnt lime, all wrapped in a betel leaf. This small morsel is placed in the cheek or under the tongue and sucked for two or more hours.

A mild stimulation of the central nervous system is the primary drug effect, although a pleasant feeling and reduction of fatigue are often reported. Some people also chew betel nuts for their alleged aphrodisiac effect. Undesirable consequences of using the morsels include a dark-red staining of the teeth, mouth, and gums, a toxic condition in the body, and increased risk of cancer of the mouth and esophagus.[36]

Yohimbe, an extract from the tropical yohimbe tree found in West Africa, is used to brew a mildly stimulating tea often used for its aphrodisiac effect. A preparation of ground yohimbe bark can also be used as snuff for quicker results. A feeling of nausea is often the first effect; this is soon followed by a pleasant, euphoric state not unlike the initial stage of an LSD-induced hallucination.

Because the drug also affects the user's peripheral blood flow, penile erection is frequently reported. Both males and females claim enhancement of their sexual experiences. Similar to hallucinogenic drugs, yohimbe is used primarily for its stimulating effect. At present, yohimbe is available in the United States in various natural food and herbal stores.

Chapter Summary

1. CNS stimulants, such as cocaine and the amphetamines, generally increase mental alertness, physical activity, and excitement. They are known as "ups" or "uppers."

2. Cocaine and amphetamines—the more powerful stimulants—produce euphoria, decreased perception of fatigue, decreased need for sleep, a decreased appetite, and make users feel stronger, more decisive, and self-possessed.

3. Dependence on CNS stimulants is based upon the desire to experience repeatedly the intense pleasurable feelings of the "flash" or "rush" following injection, tolerance to the euphoric and appetite-suppressant effects of the drugs, and avoidance of mental depression ("crashing") after drug use stops.

4. Cocaine is the most powerful CNS stimulant of natural origin and until recently enjoyed an unjustified reputation as a user-friendly drug.

5. Derived from coca plant leaves, cocaine has only limited medical uses at present.

6. Cocaine is snorted or sniffed, injected intravenously, smoked, freebased, and combined with CNS depressants ("speedballing"). The more serious health risks—toxic syndrome, drug dependency, lung damage, cocaine psychosis, formication, blood clots, infection, and burns—tend to be associated particularly with cocaine injection, freebasing, speedballing, and smoking crack. Crack, an intensified form of cocaine, is now considered one of the most addictive of all drug substances.

7. Using cocaine can result in death by sudden stimulation of the CNS, interference with normal heartbeat, and changes in heart action and blood pressure that can lead to heart attack and/or stroke.

8. Amphetamines (Benzedrine, Dexedrine, "meth" or "speed," and smokable "ice") are powerful, synthetic CNS stimulants with cocainelike effects. Although some of these stimulants have legitimate medical uses, amphetamines are often abused by those who want to extend themselves beyond their normal physiological limits.

9. Prolonged use of amphetamines sometimes leads to toxic conditions, mental confusion, assaultive behavior, amphetamine psychosis, and formication. Psychological dependence develops at low dose levels; tolerance to the euphoric and appetite-suppressant effects builds rapidly with repeated oral, injected, and smoked dosages; and serious withdrawal symptoms of mental depression and fatigue are evidence of a physical dependence.

10. Amphetamines are used medically as anorectics, as well as in treating narcolepsy and hyperkinetic disorders.

11. MAO inhibitors, tricyclics, and Prozac are antidepressant medications used to elevate mood and relieve mental depression. They are effective only with depressed people.

12. Caffeine is a widely used CNS stimulant present in coffee, tea, chocolate, and many nonprescribed medications.

13. The stimulating effects of caffeine are often perceived as beneficial, but some people experience unpleasant effects such as a toxic response, caffeinism with overindulgence, and caffeine dependence.

14. Two relatively new drugs of abuse that have surfaced in the United States are methcathinone (cat) and ephedrine, both of which have a stimulant effect.

Review Questions and Activities

1. What are the general drug actions or effects of the behavioral stimulants?

2. Why does intravenous injection of a CNS stimulant usually involve a greater potential health risk than taking the same drugs by mouth?

3. How does a CNS stimulant "flash" or "rush" differ from a CNS stimulant "crash"?

4. Explain why cocaine has often been perceived as a "safe" drug, despite its considerable potential for threatening health and life.

5. Read Bob Woodward's *Wired: The Short Life and Fast Times of John Belushi* (New York: Simon & Schuster, 1984) and identify several factors that you think contributed to Belushi's involvement with and death due to cocaine and other drugs.

6. What is the significance of the 800–COCAINE hotline? Contact local substance-abuse programs or clinics for information on this national service.

7. Explain the meanings of the following terms associated with cocaine use: *snorting, intravenous injection, speedballing, freebasing,* and *crack-smoking.*

8. Why is crack cocaine considered to be such a serious threat to the health of users?

9. Compare cocaine dependence with opioid dependence to reveal both similarities and differences.

10. Why do you think people try amphetamines and continue to use these cocainelike CNS stimulants?

11. How is "ice" similar to and different from "crack"?

12. What are the currently approved medical uses of amphetamine drugs?

13. Explain why antidepressants are not among the commonly abused drugs.

14. Identify ten common sources of caffeine that might be found in many American households.

15. In what ways does caffeine act as a CNS stimulant in the human body?

16. Survey several coffee drinkers. Determine if any of them have ever experienced caffeinism.

17. Do you think there is such a condition as caffeine dependence? What evidence have you observed or experienced that would support your answer?

18. What diseases are associated with consumption of coffee?

19. Under the brand names Zoom and Zing, tablets of guarana powder derived from seeds of a jungle shrub have begun appearing for sale in some health-food stores. What are the drug effects of Zoom and Zing? How are these products advertised?

References

1. Lester Grinspoon and James Bakalar, "Drug Abuse and Dependence," *Harvard Medical School Mental Health Review,* no. 1:7 (Boston: Harvard Medical School Mental Health Letter).

2. Drug Enforcement Administration, U.S. Department of Justice, *Drugs of Abuse* (Washington, D.C.: U.S. Government Printing Office, 1989), 37.

3. Basic descriptions of these stimulants are derived from the DEA, *Drugs of Abuse,* 37, 40.

4. Robert Julien, *A Primer of Drug Action* (New York: W. H. Freeman, 1992), 112.

5. DEA, *Drugs of Abuse,* 37.

6. J. Murdoch Ritchie and Nicholas Greene, "Local Anesthetics," chapter 15 in *Goodman and Gilman's The Pharmacological Basis of Therapeutics,* 8th ed., ed. A. G. Gilman, T. W. Rall, A. S. Nies, and P. Taylor (New York: McGraw-Hill, 1990), 319.

7. Elisabeth Kübler-Ross, *To Live until We Say Goodbye* (Englewood Cliffs, N.J.: Prentice-Hall, 1978), 22–23.

8. Nannette Stone, Marlene Fromme, and Daniel Kagan, *Cocaine: Seduction and Solution* (New York: Clarkson N. Potter, 1984), 6.

9. Patrick Macdonald, Dan Waldorf, Craig Reinarman, and Shigla Murphy, "Heavy Cocaine Use and Sexual Behavior," *Journal of Drug Issues* 18, no. 3 (summer 1988): 437–55.

10. Tibor Palfai and Henry Jankiewicz, *Drugs and Human Behavior* (Dubuque, Iowa: Brown & Benchmark, 1991), 305.

11. Lester Grinspoon and James Bakalar, *The Harvard Medical School Mental Health Review: Drug Abuse and Addiction* (Boston: Harvard Mental Health Letter, 1993), 17–18.

12. Ibid., 18.

13. Harold Doweiko, *Concepts of Chemical Dependency,* 2d ed. (Pacific Grove, Calif.: Brooks/Cole, 1993), 88–89.

14. Brian Hoffman and Robert Lefkowitz, "Catecholamines and Sympathomimetic Drugs," chapter 10 in *Goodman and Gilman's The Pharmacological Basis of Therapeutics,* 8th ed., ed. A. G. Gilman, T. W. Rall, A. S. Nies, and P. Taylor (New York: McGraw-Hill, 1990), 210–13.

15. Christina Dye, *Ice: Speed, Smoke and Fire* (Tempe, Ariz.: Do It Now, 1991), 2–3.

16. Bertram Katzung, ed., *Basic and Clinical Pharmacology,* 4th ed. (Norwalk, Conn.: Appleton & Lange, 1989), 387–88.

17. Edward M. Brecher and the Editors of Consumer Reports Books, "The Amphetamines," in *Licit and Illicit Drugs* (Mount Vernon, N.Y.: Consumers Union, 1972), 279.

18. "A New Look at Diet Pills," *University of California Wellness Letter* 9, no. 1 (October 1992): 1.

19. United States Pharmacopeia, *Complete Drug Reference* (Yonkers, N.Y.: Consumer Reports Books, 1991), 183–84.

20. Brecher and others, *Licit and Illicit Drugs,* 196.

21. Theodore Rall, "Drugs Used in the Treatment of Asthma," chapter 15 in *Goodman and Gilman's The Pharmacological Basis of Therapeutics,* 8th ed., ed. A. G. Gilman, T. W. Rall, A. S. Nies, and P. Taylor (New York: McGraw-Hill, 1990), 620–21.

22. Eric Strain and others, "Caffeine Dependence Syndrome," *Journal of the American Medical Association* 272, no. 13 (5 October 1994): 1043–48.

23. Laura Fenster, Brenda Eskenazi, Gayle Windham, and Shanna Swan, "Caffeine Consumption during Pregnancy and Fetal Growth," *American Journal of Public Health* 81, no. 4 (April 1991): 458–61.

24. Claire Infante-Rivard and others, "Fetal Loss Associated with Caffeine Intake before and during Pregnancy," *Journal of the American Medical Association* 270, no. 24 (22–29 December 1993): 2940–43.

25. Chuan Cheng Hsieh, Brian MacMahon, and others, "Coffee and Pancreatic Cancer," *New England Journal of Medicine* 315, no. 9 (28 August 1986): 587–89.

26. Diederick Grobbee and others, "Coffee, Caffeine, and Cardiovascular Disease in Men," *New England Journal of Medicine* 323, no. 15 (11 October 1990): 1026–32.

27. "Coffee and Health," *Consumer Reports* 59, no. 10 (October 1994): 650–51.

28. "Use of Cat, Potent New Stimulant, Called Epidemic in Michigan," *Substance Abuse Report* 24, no. 23 (1 December 1993): 8.

29. Avram Goldstein, *Addiction: From Biology to Drug Policy* (New York: W. H. Freeman, 1994), 157.

30. Gesina Longenecker, *How Drugs Work: Drug Abuse and the Human Body* (Emeryville, Calif.: Ziff-Davis Press, 1994).

31. Paul Glastris, "The New Drug in Town," *U.S. News and World Report,* (26 April 1993), 20–21.

32. Drug Enforcement Administration, *You Can't Trust Cat* (Washington, D.C.: U.S. Department of Justice, Drug Enforcement Administration, 1993), 2.

33. "New Law Attempts to Stop Spread of Cat," *Prevention Pipeline* 7, no. 2 (March–April 1994): 26.

34. "The Scoop on Ephedrine and Ma Huang," *University of California at Berkeley Wellness Letter* 10, no. 12 (September 1994): 6–7.

35. Julien, *A Primer of Drug Action,* 129.

36. Darryl Inaba and William Cohen, *Uppers, Downers, All Arounders,* 2d ed. (Ashland, Ore.: CNS Productions, 1993).

part

The Mind-Expanding Euphoriants

four

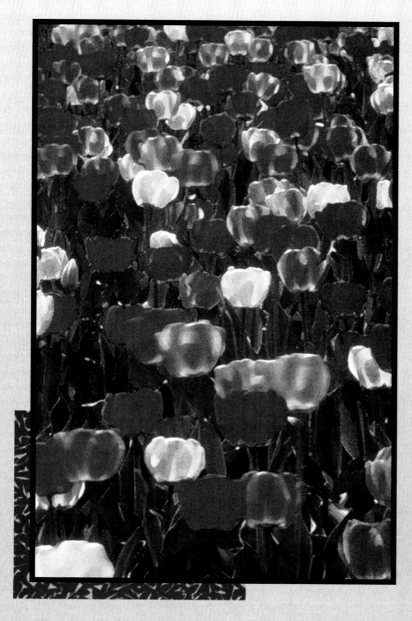

Questions of Concern

1. What would likely occur in our society if marijuana were legalized and sold for general consumption at relatively low cost and under strict government controls?

2. Why are the mind-expanding effects of the psychedelics so often feared by nonusers and many potential users?

3. How does the level of social acceptability of psychedelics, particularly LSD and peyote, compare with that of other mind-altering drugs, such as alcohol, tobacco cigarettes, and even marijuana?

Psychedelics

and

Phencyclidine

Psychedelics

and

Phencyclidine

chapter

9

psychedelics and phencyclidine

Cognitive Experience
Designer Drug
Ecstasy
Esthetic Experience
Flashback Reaction
Hallucination
Hallucinogen
Illusion
Lysergic Acid Diethylamide
Mescaline
Mind Expansion
Peyote
Phencyclidine
Psilocybin
Psychedelic
Psychodynamic Experience
Psychotic Experience
Synesthesia
Transcendental (Mystical) Experience
Trip

chapter objectives

After you have studied this chapter, you should be able to do the following:

1. Describe the major characteristics of the psychedelic state.
2. Define the following terms associated with use of the psychedelic drugs: *synesthesia, "high,"* and *flashback reaction.*
3. Distinguish among the following types of psychedelic experiences: psychotic, psychodynamic, cognitive, esthetic, and transcendental.
4. Identify several commonly experienced, physical side effects of psychedelic drugs.
5. Discuss the historical factors that were responsible for the beginning of the modern psychedelic era.
6. Explain the basis of the recent increase in the recreational use of LSD after several years of declining use.
7. Describe several mind-altering effects often experienced on an LSD "trip."
8. Identify three potential hazards associated with using LSD.
9. Compare the psychedelic effects of mescaline and psilocybin with those of LSD.
10. Name at least eight psychedelic substances in addition to LSD, mescaline, and psilocybin.
11. Explain why the designer drug MDMA is often called Ecstasy.
12. Describe the possible range of drug effects associated with use of PCP.
13. Discuss the continuing appeal of phencyclidine despite its notorious reputation as a dissociative anesthetic.

Introduction

Both an ancient and a contemporary undertaking, the expansion of consciousness continues to be a unique and persistent human endeavor. This search for the "beyond within" has led many to rely upon psychoactive drugs for personal insight and comprehension. Substances most often used for such elusive purposes have come to be identified popularly and legally as hallucinogens—generators of hallucinations.

Distinguished more by their ability to produce states of altered perception and thought than by hallucinations, the various psychedelic drugs—as they will be called in this chapter—include both natural and synthetic compounds. Though not the original psychedelic, LSD will be considered as the prototype and most powerful of these drugs. The abuse of these drugs is the major concern of this chapter.

Another psychoactive drug, phencyclidine (PCP), will also be examined. Quite distinct from the psychedelics, PCP resembles both the mind-expanders and the sedative-hypnotics. Yet PCP is in a class of its own, and it is quite possibly the most potentially dangerous of all "street" drugs.

The Psychedelic State: Mind Expansion

The major focus of this chapter is the psychedelics, which cause dose-related changes in perception, thinking, emotions, arousal, and self-image. Such altered states of consciousness cannot usually be achieved naturally except in dreams or during religious exaltation.

The terms currently used to describe the psychedelics include **hallucinogens** (inducers of **hallucinations**), *psychotomimetics*

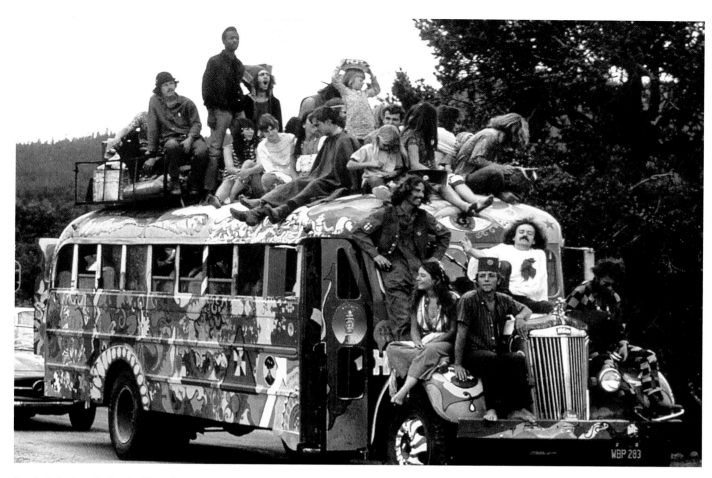

Psychedelic drugs had a significant impact on the counter culture of the 1960s as evidenced in clothing styles, hair lengths, music, language, and use of color. The school bus in the photo could be described as having a psychedelic paint job.

© Lisa Law/The Image Works

(drugs that mimic psychosis), *psychodysleptics* (substances that are mind-disrupting), and *psycholytics* (dissolvers of the psyche, or mind-looseners).[1]

Drugs such as lysergic acid diethylamide (LSD), mescaline, and psilocybin may indeed function in such bizarre ways. But each of these special labels, based upon a single pharmacological action, refers to only a very limited part of the wide range of psychological effects of the drugs.

A more inclusive term, **psychedelic** refers to **mind expansion** or *mind manifestation*—the ability of the mind to perceive more than it can tell and to experience more than it can explain. The major characteristics of the psychedelic state are these:[2]

Heightened awareness of sensory input, experienced as a flood of sensation

Especially vivid but unreal imagery, typical of one's childhood

An enhanced sense of clarity

Diminished control over what one experiences

A persistent feeling that one part of the self is a passive observer—the spectator ego phenomenon—while another part of the self participates and receives unusual sensory experiences

Replacement of the user's inward-focused attention by the seeming clarity and expansiveness of his or her thinking process

Assignment of profound meaning to the slightest of sensations

A lessened capacity to distinguish the boundaries of one object from another and of the self from the environment

The development of a sense of union with all humankind or the cosmos itself

As a group, psychedelics tend to distort the user's perception of objective reality, decrease logical thought, heighten sensation, and change or modify the user's state of consciousness. These drugs invariably bring about a central nervous system excitation that affects the senses—especially time sense—feelings, moods, experience, and mental processes. Stimulation of the sympathetic nervous system (described in chapter 3) also results in increased heart rate and blood pressure, sweating, loss of appetite, and sleeplessness.

In very large or toxic doses, psychedelic drugs also produce hallucinations (groundless or mistaken perceptions having no real external cause) and delusions (false beliefs that cannot be corrected by reason), although these are relatively rare. More commonly produced are **illusions** (erroneous perceptions of reality) and "pseudohallucinations" (misperceptions recognized as misperceptions). As a consequence, some people prefer to describe the psychedelics as illusionogenic rather than hallucinogenic in nature.

While mimicking some naturally occurring neurotransmitters of the brain and disrupting others, individual psychedelics have subtle, unique effects that are especially attractive to users. These may include speed of onset, duration of the psychedelic "high," and the particular sense that seems to be altered more than others, whether it is visual or auditory. Commonly shared properties are also part of the psychedelic allure. One of these is **synesthesia.** In this drug-related effect there is a mingling of the senses, in which one sensation may be translated into another. For example, sounds might be seen, smells might be felt, and colors might be heard.

Although the changes in perception, mood, and thinking usually are interpreted as euphoric, sometimes undesirable psychological effects do occur. Among these are acute anxiety and panic reactions, or *bad trips*—the most frequent adverse effect—characterized by terror, confusion, dissociation, and fear of losing control over oneself.[3] Such reactions last less than 24 hours in most instances, but occasionally they persist for days and eventually progress into a chronic, toxic psychosis. In some instances, depersonalization and depression become so severe that suicide is a distinct possibility.

Another psychological hazard is the **flashback reaction.** Long after psychedelics have been eliminated from the body, one might experience partial recurrences of psychedelic effects, such as the intensification of a perceived color, the apparent motion of a fixed object, or the mistaking of one object for another. In effect, the flashback is a free trip—a repetition of a drug's effects without using a drug. This sometimes alarming situation can be either spontaneous or triggered by physical or psychological stress, by medicines, or by use of marijuana. While the precise cause remains obscure, flashbacks are probably psychological in origin and might involve a "conditioned response" to a previous panic attack.

Psychological effects of the psychedelics, especially LSD, are influenced principally by the size of the dose taken, the basic emotional makeup of the user, the drug taker's mood at the time of use, and the setting or circumstances under which the drug is taken.[4] For instance, fearful individuals are likely to have a fear-filled psychedelic "trip"; those with repressed personalities and bottled-up desires or emotions might be confronted with a backlash of psychological problems that might or might not be solved. A darkened room is likely to promote gloomy thoughts. Loud music can increase tension. On the other hand, a nonthreatening environment and reassuring friends can be the difference between a "bad trip" and the euphoria of mind expansion.

Of course, dosage is a primary concern in relation to the effects of any particular drug. Since nearly all LSD comes from illegal domestic laboratories or is smuggled in from abroad, the quality of the drug will likely vary. Most street samples of LSD contain impurities and adulterants, and thus the actual amount of the drug per dose is often a surprise and a mystery.

Types of Psychedelic Experiences

Emotional responses to psychedelics can vary from a miserable, hopeless dysphoria (anxiety, restlessness, and depression) to an ecstatic, blissful sensation of well-being and pleasure. This latter response is referred to as euphoria. The expectation of this euphoria, or high, and the likely experience of chemical fantasies are the most common reasons for taking psychedelic drugs.

The Range of Responses

Researchers have identified at least five major kinds of potential psychedelic responses, described subjectively by those using mind-expanding drugs. Included are the following types.[5]

The **psychotic experience** is characterized by intense fear, panic, paranoid suspicion or delusions of grandeur, confusion, impairment of abstract reasoning, remorse, depression, and isolation or bodily discomfort or both. All of these experiences can be very powerful.

The **cognitive experience** is marked by astonishingly lucid thought. Various problems can be seen from a unique perspective in which inner relationships of many levels or dimensions can be viewed simultaneously.

The **esthetic experience** is defined by a change and intensification of all sensory input, including sight, sound, smell, taste, and touch. Fascinating changes in sensations and perceptions can occur, such as synesthesia, apparent lifelike movements in inanimate objects, the appearance of great beauty in ordinary things, an experience of powerful music, and extremely beautiful mental images.

The **psychodynamic experience** occurs when material that was previously unconscious or forgotten emerges in one's consciousness. A release of the tension or conflict from repressed emotions is sometimes reported subjectively as an actual reliving of incidents from the past or a symbolic portrayal of important struggles between hostile forces in the psyche.

The **transcendental,** or **mystical, experience** is often referred to as the "psychedelic peak" and involves the development of a sense of unity or oneness; transcendence of time and space; deeply felt moods of joy, peace, and love; a sense of awe, reverence, and wonder; meaningfulness of psychological or philosophical insight or both; and the inability to describe the experience of cosmic-type happenings in ordinary words.

It is important to note that a psychedelic experience rarely fits so neatly into

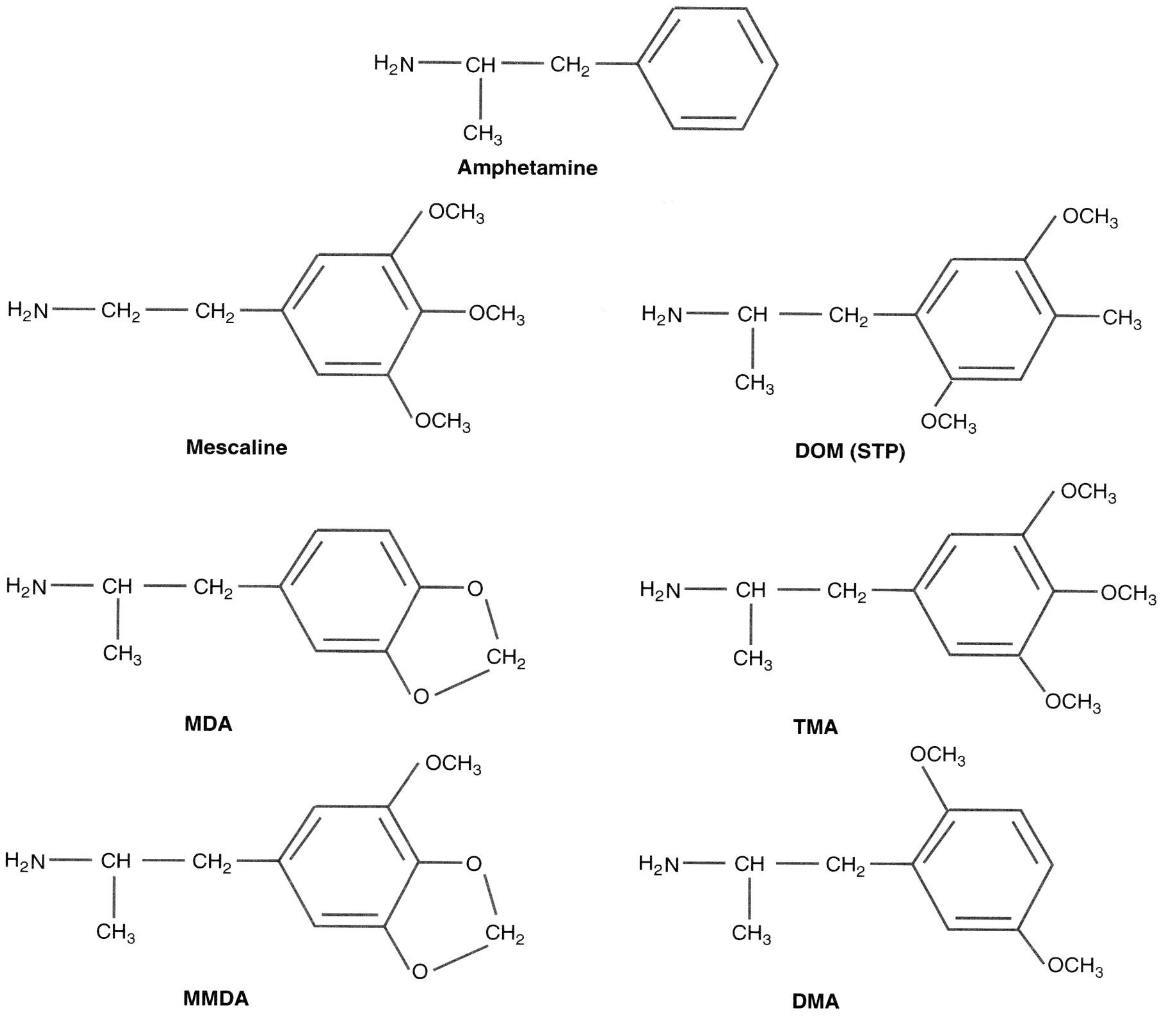

Amphetamine

Mescaline

DOM (STP)

MDA

TMA

MMDA

DMA

figure 9.1

Structural formulas of amphetamine and six phychedelic drugs. These drugs are related and produce simular effects.

any one particular category. Aspects of all five are likely to occur in each "trip." Nevertheless, the clear-cut types may be the result of biochemical actions that captivate the mind at any one time.

Psychedelic Side Effects

If the psychological effects of the psychedelics can be described as exciting, then the physical reactions are somewhat dull by comparison. The pupils of the eyes dilate, body temperature and blood pressure rise, heart rate increases, reflexes are increased above normal, and muscle weakness and tremors sometimes occur. Some "body trips," especially those induced by morning glory seeds and peyote, involve nausea, vomiting, diarrhea, and muscle tension.

Repeated use of the psychedelics leads to tolerance. For instance, after only three or four daily doses, the amount of LSD required to produce desirable psychological effects is increased markedly. However, sensitivity to lower doses returns after a comparable period of abstinence. There is a considerable degree of cross-tolerance among LSD, mescaline, and psilocybin, but none between LSD and such drugs as amphetamines and THC—the active ingredient in marijuana.

When the psychedelic drugs are withdrawn from a person, there is no detectable evidence of physical dependence. Whereas repeated use may result in psychological dependence in some instances, regular, compulsive daily use is somewhat rare. Episodic use of these substances tends to be the general pattern of abuse.

Historical Aspects

Many plants containing psychedelic drugs have been known and used for their mind-altering effects since prehistoric times. It is probable that the mushroom *Amanita muscaria*, which is neither deadly nor commonly eaten as food, was used both medically and recreationally by people in the early Aryan culture of present-day Afghanistan. Quite likely, this particular mushroom was the "Soma" described in 3,500-year-old Indian holy books.

Another variety of mushroom containing psilocybin, called "God's Flesh," was employed in the religious rituals of certain Mexican Indians. It is now presumed that the ancient Mayans of Mexico and Guatemala engaged in the worship of these mushrooms as long ago as 1000 B.C.

Meanwhile, other tribes of prehistoric Mexican Indians and the Aztecs utilized the peyote cactus as a religious sacrament. Peyote was still widely used centuries later at the time of the Spanish conquest. Eventually, its use spread northward into America, where several Indian tribes adopted the "peyote cult" with its mystical setting and religious rituals.[6] Presently, an estimated quarter million members of the Native American Church continue to use peyote legally as part of the church's ritual. This church has been exempted from specific provisions of the Controlled Substances Act of 1970. Nevertheless, a 1990 United States Supreme Court ruling declared that there is no constitutional right to take illicit drugs for religious reasons. Individual states are still free, however, to allow religious use of illegal substances, specifically peyote, although more than twenty states still forbid any use of peyote.

Sometimes the ancient Aztecs could not obtain or preferred not to use peyote. Then they considered sacred the seeds of the morning glory plant (*Rivea corymbosa*) which contain a relatively mild psychedelic substance chemically similar to LSD. More-modern Europeans employed *Atropa belladonna,* the deadly nightshade plant, as medicine as well as a poison. Later, the early white settlers in the New World accidentally discovered the psychedelic effects of *Datura stramonium,* the "Jamestown weed," soon shortened to "Jimsonweed" and also known as "loco weed."

It is fairly certain, then, that the use of plants with LSD-like effects was prevalent in both religious and therapeutic contexts long before Dr. Albert Hofmann and Dr. W. A. Stoll first synthesized lysergic acid

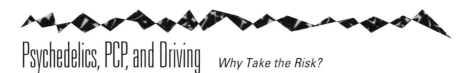

Psychedelics, PCP, and Driving — Why Take the Risk?

LSD, PCP, and other psychedelic or hallucinogenic drugs tend to distort judgment and reality and cause confusion and panic. They can also produce severe mental problems, resulting in strange and violent behavior. Clearly, individuals under the influence of these kinds of drugs should not drive.

Psychedelics are particularly hazardous because their effects are unpredictable. In addition, sensations and feelings are likely to change. Users may feel several different emotions at once or swing rapidly from one emotion to another. On occasion, an individual's sense of time and self changes, and the user may experience sensations that seem to "cross over," giving the perception of hearing colors and seeing sounds. All of these changes can be frightening, and they might cause panic.

PCP use, especially on a regular basis, can affect memory, perception, concentration, and judgment. Signs of paranoia, aggressive behavior, and a general disturbance of the user's thought processes may also appear. These distortions of normal mental functioning disqualify those who use PCP from attempting to drive an automobile.

Driving requires a combination of thought and motor skills, a great deal of common sense, and a concern for the safety of everyone on the road. Safe driving is based on observant eyes, steady hands, and a clear head. By mixing drugs with driving, you are only asking for trouble. Why take the risk?

Source: Modified from the National Institute on Drug Abuse.

diethylamide (LSD) in 1938. It was not until five years later, in 1943, that Dr. Hofmann took his very first "acid trip."

Working with the twenty-fifth compound in the lysergic acid series, Dr. Hofmann accidentally ingested a small amount of the untested LSD-25 substance in his Swiss laboratory. He experienced dramatic effects of restlessness, dizziness, and delirium, characterized by excited fantasies and fantastic visions of extraordinary realness, accompanied by an intense kaleidoscopic play of colors.[7] It was this single event that ushered in the modern Psychedelic Era. A few days later, Hofmann took another small dose of LSD and had his assistant record the psychedelic experience. This description was the very first account of the effects of uncontaminated LSD.

At first, psychiatrists and scientists felt that the new LSD-25 drug would assist the medical community in the study and treatment of mental illness. Some even thought that this strange compound would produce a temporary "model psychosis" that would help science better understand the mechanism of mental disease.

Many experiments were conducted with patients to determine if the psychedelic experience would help them overcome their mental conditions. In conjunction with psychotherapy, closely supervised research with LSD continued into the 1950s. At the same time, the use of this synthetic psychedelic spread from the medical community to the intellectual community, where the mystical potential and possible creative value of LSD were valued.

When the initial reports of LSD's therapeutic value were being questioned, the popularization of the drug was well under way. Students, writers, and philosophers became intrigued with LSD's mind-altering and nonaddicting qualities. Within a few years, nonmedical use of the drug spread to young people, who were being encouraged to join the "psychedelic revolution" of the 1960s. In some ways, LSD ushered in not only the psychedelic phenomenon but also the whole modern wave of nonmedical drug use. And the "psychedelic 1960s" also gave birth to new forms of popular music, art, and fashion styles. Many of these innovations are still

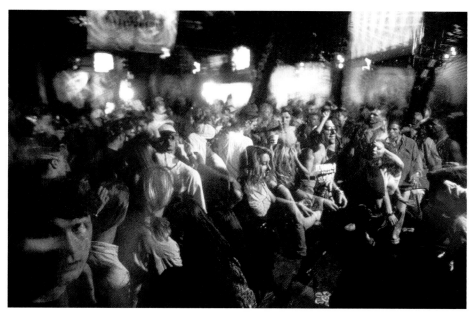

Psychedelics like LSD and Ecstasy are often taken at "rave parties."

© Mark Richards/PhotoEdit

with us today as "acid rock" music, special light shows at concerts, and brilliant neon or "day-glo" colors used in decorations as well as clothing.

Among the leaders of this "revolution" and chief advocates of LSD were Professors Timothy Leary and Richard Alpert of Harvard University. Although they made important contributions to "mainstream" psychology, these professors advised young people to "drop out, turn on, and tune in." "Dropping out" was any specific technique by which individuals detached themselves from the enslavement of habit, routine, convention, ambitions, and the symbolic rewards of society. Responding to abnormal states of consciousness produced by psychedelic drugs was the key to "turning on." Aware of one's own internal processes, a person could then "tune in" to a greater and more philosophical concern with beauty, peacefulness, and the fundamental questions of cosmic design.

After Leary and Alpert, joined by their students, began experimenting with LSD and other psychedelics, they were dismissed by the university in 1963. The resulting media coverage, however, served to increase national interest in LSD.

In reaction to the growing use of LSD and its association with the new permissiveness of the "hippie culture," new laws made the recreational use of the powerful psychedelic drug illegal. When new research was also restricted, the only drug company that had been making LSD stopped its production. As a consequence, practically no LSD-related research has been conducted since 1970.

Once legal production of LSD was stopped, illicit producers—"kitchen chemists"—supplied the demand of the street market. After several years of declining use, the early 1980s witnessed a significant upswing in LSD's popularity, which continues even today.

Using LSD today involves consuming powder pellets called "microdots," gelatin chips known as "windowpanes," or thin squares of absorbent paper soaked in liquid LSD—"blotter acid" or just plain "blotter." Supposedly, each square represents one dose. In contrast with bulky carriers (objects and substances containing LSD), such as sugar cubes, animal crackers, gelatin chips, and tiny pellets, "blotter acid" is practically undetectable. Moreover, the potency of today's LSD is not as strong as it was in the "acid" heyday of the early

1970s. Because of its weaker potency, LSD tends to produce more-manageable reactions today.

LSD's comeback is also related to one of the newest youth fads, "rave parties." These impromptu gatherings consist of hundreds or thousands of young people who meet at designated urban sites, such as abandoned warehouses or vacant racetracks, and party nonstop for several hours or even days. Alcohol is usually banned; the drugs of choice are LSD and another psychedelic, MDMA (Ecstasy), an amphetamine derivative.[8]

There is yet another factor contributing to LSD's resurgence: product packaging. Color-screening and printing on the surfaces of blotter paper, featuring cartoon figures of Mickey Mouse, Snoopy, dragons, stars, and flying saucers, make the "blotter acid" particularly appealing to the younger generation of users—packaging sells.

Lysergic Acid Diethylamide

LSD is derived from the ergot fungus that grows on rye or from lysergic acid amide, as found in morning glory seeds. The name *LSD* is an abbreviation of the German name for **lysergic acid diethylamide.** The best known and probably the most powerful of synthetic psychedelics, LSD has been estimated to be 100 times more potent than psilocybin and 4,000 times more potent than mescaline in producing altered states of consciousness.

Because it is so powerful, LSD doses are measured in extremely small quantities called micrograms, or "mikes" (millionths of a gram). Nearly all other drugs are measured in much larger units—milligrams, or thousandths of a gram. The average effective oral dose is about 30 micrograms (mcg); some "street" doses contain as much as 400 micrograms. Currently, the strength of LSD samples from illegal sources ranges from 20 to 80 micrograms LSD per dose.[9]

The amount per dosage unit varies considerably, as does the quality of the psychedelic itself, due mainly to the illegal sources of the drug: illicit domestic laboratories or smuggled imports from abroad.

Occasionally some samples of LSD are fairly pure, but they may also contain a variety of other psychedelic drugs, strychnine or other toxic stimulants, and even methamphetamine or speed.

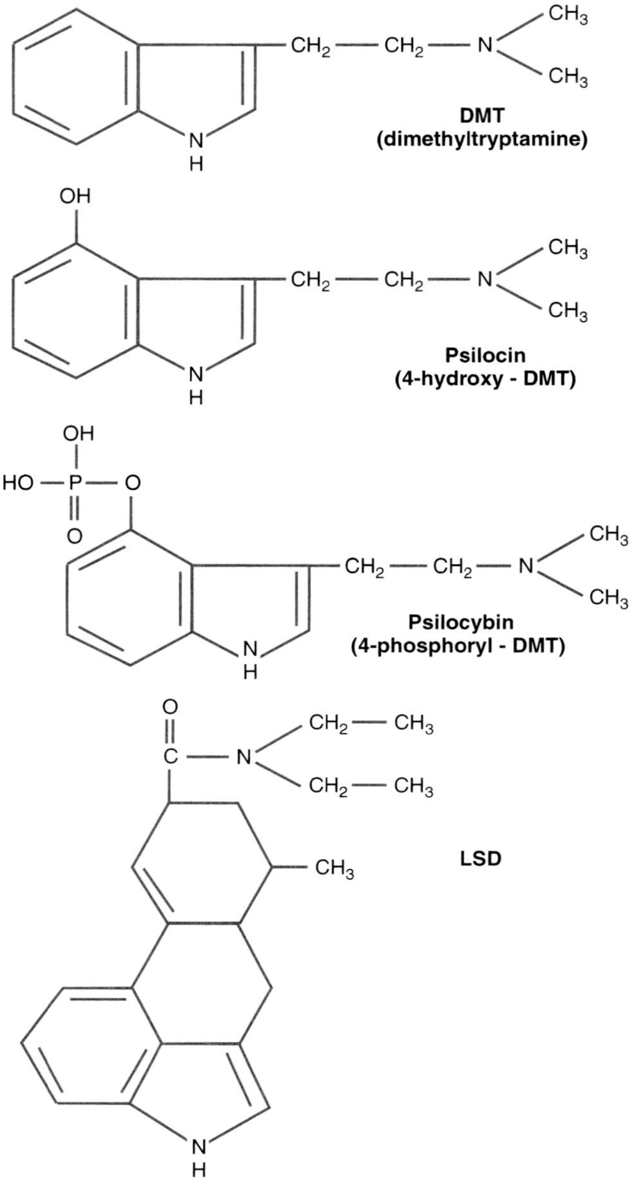

The LSD "Trip"

Sold on the street today in a variety of forms, LSD is generally taken by mouth. Only rarely is this drug injected. Sometimes LSD is mixed with tobacco and smoked, but the resultant high is typically unsatisfactory.

The mind-altering effects brought on by LSD and subjectively interpreted are often referred to as an "acid trip" or simply a **trip.** Whether a trip is new and exciting or frightening and unpredictable depends on several factors. Higher doses typically produce a more intense trip. However, the mind-set or mood, expectations, and existence of prior emotional disturbances can determine whether the trip will be pleasant or dangerous.

The anxious, unprepared, emotionally disturbed person is more likely to have a terror-filled "bad trip." However, a person need not be disturbed emotionally to have an adverse reaction. A bad trip can occur simply if a person is "uptight" about something. If the surroundings under which LSD is taken are comfortable, non-threatening, and provide for reassurance from concerned friends, then the chances for a pleasant trip are enhanced.

Although the effects of LSD are unpredictable and vary considerably from one person to another, and from one occasion to the next, several distinct, though somewhat subjective, phases with unique experiences may be anticipated.[10]

In the *first phase*, beginning shortly after taking LSD and lasting up to two hours, the user perceives a release of inner tension. Other characteristics of this phase include laughing or crying, a feeling of intense well-being (euphoria), restlessness, heightened awareness, and enhanced rapport with others.

About thirty to ninety minutes following use of the drug, the *second phase* begins and is usually marked by perceptual distortions, such as visual illusions and hallucinations. These changes in perception often involve the occurrence of

figure 9.2

Structural formulas of four psychedelic drugs. These drugs are structurally related to serotonin, and may act like serotonin at the synaptic level.

synesthesia—the mingling of senses in which one sensation is translated into another. Common physical effects include dizziness, weakness, drowsiness, nausea, rapid pulse, increased heartbeat and blood pressure, and loss of appetite.

Three to four hours after LSD is taken, the *third phase* begins. In this part of the trip, the drug user often reports a distorted sense of time—the psychedelic experience seems to move ever so slowly through the past, present, and future, all of which appear to fuse together. There might also be marked mood swings, and a feeling of ego disintegration—that is, a sense of being separate from one's body. LSD users mistakenly believe they possess magical powers of absolute control over

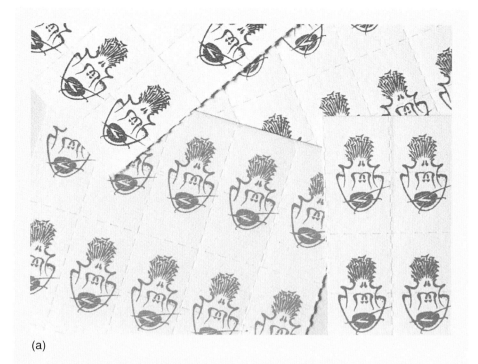

(a)

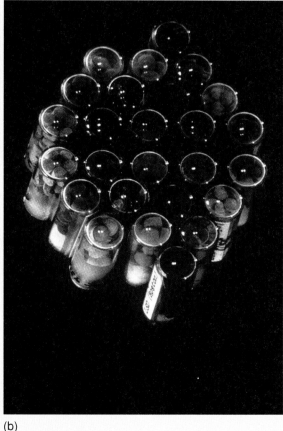

(b)

(a) Today LSD is often eaten in the form of drug-impregnated paper known as "blotter acid." Stamped with distinctive picture designs, blotter acid is printed in books of sheets of 1,000 unit doses. **(b)** LSD tablets or pellets called microdots were commonly "dropped" during the 1960s.

Drug Enforcement Agency.

their lives. Such false beliefs and loss of contact with reality have resulted in serious injury and even death.

Four to six hours after initial use, the effects of LSD begin to lessen. "Waves of normalcy" are experienced as the drug taker begins to recover and gradually returns to a nondrugged waking state.

LSD Hazards

A trip that begins in beautiful excitement can suddenly become frightening and take on the characteristics of a "bad trip," formerly known as a "bummer." Bad trips are the most common adverse effect of LSD and usually take the form of either a sudden, intense panic reaction or one or more psychotic reactions involving serious breaks with reality, persistent hallucinations, and delusions.[11] Sometimes there develops an intense oversuspiciousness leading to the false belief that one is being persecuted or harmed by others. In addition to such panic situations, depression and breaks with reality may develop.

If a person has suffered from emotional disorders before using LSD, the trip may trigger an emotional breakdown. However, bad trips can occur even among those who have had many earlier good trips. Bad trips usually end after eight to twelve hours, as the immediate effects of LSD wear off. In most instances, psychiatric help is not needed. The best treatment appears to be protection, companionship, and reassurance throughout the duration of the trip. On occasion, though, physician-prescribed tranquilizers may be required for some individual LSD users.

Whether LSD or any other psychedelic drug can cause permanent mental illness in otherwise normal, healthy individuals is still an open question. Some heavy users have developed impaired memory and attention span, mental confusion, and difficulty with abstract thinking. Reported periods of emotional imbalance and the experience of dreamlike states while awake may be evidence of structural damage to parts of the brain. But whether these abnormal occurrences are permanent or temporary has not been determined.

While LSD does not appear to cause genetic damage or cancer, street doses of the psychedelic are frequently cut or

box 9.2

Psychological First-Aid for Psychedelic Panic

Sometimes people who use psychedelic drugs experience a "bad trip" characterized by panic reactions—feelings of terror, confusion, depersonalization, and a fear of losing control over oneself. Rather than medical attention in a hospital emergency room, psychological first aid—"talking down" the person in such a panic situation—is often the best care that a friend can provide. The suggestions below are likely to help the person who has sustained such a panic reaction, whether it is drug-related or not, and focus on reassurance, reduction of stimuli, orientation to reality, and use of "alternative-focus" activities.

1. The first rule: Do no harm to those who are panicked. If you as a "guide" or first-aider become part of the problem by transmitting your fears and apprehension, then you cannot contribute to the solution. Stay calm yourself and smile. Do not yell or shout; do not cry or become hysterical. Do not tell the panicked individual how bad or serious his trip has been. In other words, don't make the situation worse!

2. Do not expect immediate or miraculous results. Remember that a bad trip might last several hours. Since trippers are often highly suggestible, you can help by turning a bad trip into a good trip.

3. Reassure individuals that the panic is temporary, that the drug's effects will not persist, and that they will return to normal. The best reassurance is your offer to stay with them as long as you are needed.

4. Help panicked individuals to relax. Encourage them to breathe calmly. Tell them to experience the trip as if they were watching a television program or a movie. Advise them to stop fighting the trip.

5. Calm the environment by dimming lights and reducing loud music or other noise. If the environmental setting cannot be altered favorably, then guide the "tripper" to a better one.

6. To orient people to reality, describe familiar objects to them: jewelry, photos, purse or wallet, chair, or toy. Ask them to describe such objects to you. Tell them where they are and, in very general terms, what is happening. Remind them that they are not crazy or psychotic, and that their psychic trip is drug-induced. Help them concentrate on controlling breathing and on the rising and falling movements of their stomachs. As their fears tend to subside, tell them about the longer periods of time between waves of fear.

7. When panicked individuals talk about specific problems or concerns, explain that the particular situation has been exaggerated or magnified by a drug, and the problem will appear less threatening after the trip.

8. If you cannot postpone consideration of a problem or divert the tripper's attention to another topic, such as art, music, or sports, then listen patiently in a friendly manner. If the tripper expresses fear or anger, do not be judgmental. Ask the person to explain why she or he is feeling those emotions; then you might provide alternative solutions for the tripper to consider.

9. Direct the tripper's attention to an external focus by suggesting alternative activities, such as taking a shower, going for a walk, eating, listening to music, or watching television.

10. Never give any medication to people experiencing a panic situation, even if you believe a particular drug might cure or reduce a bad trip.

11. If panic, fear, and anxiety do not appear to lessen, or if physical signs or symptoms of distress appear or become worse as time goes on, then take the tripper to a medical facility.

Source: Jim Parker, *Drug Crisis Response* (Tempe, Ariz.: Do It Now, 1990), 45–46.

---

adulterated with many unidentified drug substances, so that precise effects are uncertain and unpredictable. Consequently, pregnant women should not take this drug. Because LSD also causes uterine contractions, this psychedelic poses yet another threat to the pregnancy.

There are real dangers associated with the use of LSD. These can include a terrifying panic, a fear of losing one's mind that might lead to suicide, an unanticipated and terrifying flashback lasting up to ninety minutes, and accidents resulting in injury or death. Because persons on LSD are highly suggestible and often feel invulnerable, they sometimes step in front of moving automobiles or leap out of high windows in an attempt to fly. Such risks are reduced considerably when LSD is taken in a group situation. A nonuser might volunteer to serve as a guide, assisting those who are having bad trips and preventing users from harming themselves or others. The guide can give reassurance to the person on a bad trip and even change the surroundings favorably by reducing noise and light levels. Explaining the temporary nature of the psychedelic effects and that a bad trip will not last forever will tend to comfort the panic-stricken individual (see box 9.2).

The Other Psychedelics

While LSD is the primary example of a psychedelic drug, it is by no means the only one. Over one hundred other substances, both naturally occurring and synthetic, can induce mind-expanding and mind-manifesting effects. Some of these

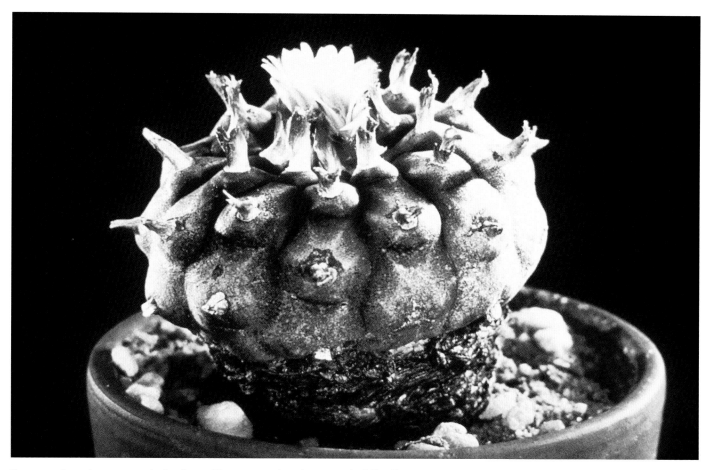

Peyote cacti may be eaten, smoked, or brewed into a tea, and produce a psychedelic effect.

Drug Enforcement Agency

are described in the following sections to highlight the differences as well as the similarities among these drugs.

Peyote and Mescaline

The peyote cactus, *Lophophora williamsii*, has been used in the religious rituals of Mexican Indians for thousands of years. Because of the visual and kaleidoscopic illusions produced by **peyote,** the ancients were convinced that they could communicate directly with their gods without the need for priests.

The fleshy green cactus tips—the mescal buttons—are dried in preparation for chewing and oral consumption. Rather than endure the bitter taste of the sliced mescal buttons as the Indians of the Native American Church do, some users prefer to smoke the ground-up material. Others brew a peyote tea or swallow capsules containing a powdery form of the cactus buttons. Regardless of the method of administration, peyote tends to cause stomach disorders, nausea, and vomiting. Afterward, psychedelic effects persist for six to ten hours and typically include feelings of weightlessness and depersonalization, perceptual distortions, and synesthesias.

Mescaline is the major psychoactive ingredient of the peyote cactus and is responsible for the mind-manifesting, LSD-like effects of the mescal buttons. In doses of 200 to 500 mg (the equivalent of twenty mescal buttons), mescaline causes increased heart rate, body temperature, blood pressure, and dilation of the pupils of the eyes, as well as a slowing down of both coordination and reflexes, and a diminished ability to concentrate.[12]

The chemical name for mescaline, which can now be synthesized in the laboratory, is 3, 4, 5-trimethoxyphenethylamine. Available as capsules, tablets, or in liquid form, synthetic mescaline usually produces less intense nausea and vomiting than does peyote, although the psychedelic effects are practically identical to those of LSD. Synthetic mescaline is rarely available on the street, and samples sold as mescaline frequently contain LSD, PCP, or amphetamine.

While mescaline induces altered perceptions, it tends to cause less mental or cognitive disorganization than is caused by LSD. Neither peyote nor its mescaline derivative produces physical dependence. Psychological dependence is rare, but tolerance develops rapidly, often within three days. Cross-tolerance with LSD and psilocybin exists. Along with LSD and other psychedelics, peyote and mescaline are Schedule I drugs under the provisions of the Controlled Substances Act. However, peyote is legal for members of the Native American Church who use mescal buttons sacramentally in their rituals.

It should be noted here that the mescaline derived from mescal buttons is not the source of tequila. A distilled spirit and popular alcoholic beverage, tequila is made from the fermented juice of the cactuslike agave plant, also known as mescal. However, unlike the mescal buttons of the peyote cactus, the mescal-based alcoholic beverage is intoxicating but not specifically psychedelic.

Psilocybin

When Psilocybe mushrooms (*Psilocybe caerulescens, Stropharia cubensis,* and several other members of the *Psilocybe* genus) are eaten, their effects on human perception and cognition are similar to those caused by mescaline and LSD. Before the onset of this drug's unique mental effects—visions perceived with eyes closed and altered states of consciousness—the intake of **psilocybin** may cause nausea, drowsiness, and feelings of numbness.[13]

The psychoactive ingredients of these sacred or "magic" mushrooms are psilocybin and psilocin, both chemically related to LSD. Both of these drugs can be made synthetically in the form of a white crystalline powder, but they may also be contained in mushroom preparations. Much of what is sold on the street, however, consists of LSD and other chemicals. Like mescaline, psilocybin is rarely available on the street, although some users have procured grow-your-own psychedelic mushrooms from special mail-order houses.

In order for psilocybin to produce psychedelic effects, it must first be changed (metabolized) to psilocyn in the body so that it can enter the brain.[14] After 1 to 5 grams of the appropriate dried mushrooms are eaten, or a dose of 20 to 60 mg of synthetic psilocybin is taken, effects begin within half an hour and last three to six hours. The duration of the psilocybin trip is considerably shorter than that of an LSD trip. Injection of psilocybin will initiate the trip somewhat earlier.

Generally, the effects are similar to but less intense than those of LSD. Psilocybin

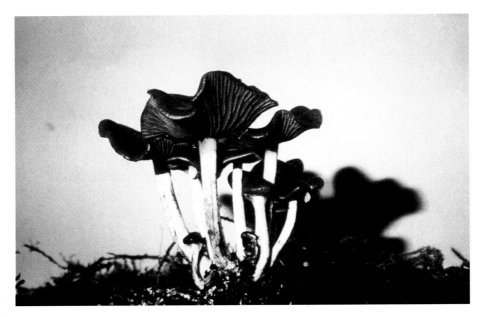

The psilocybe mushrooms pictured above produce effects similar to LSD.
Drug Enforcement Agency

has developed a reputation for producing very strong visual distortions, and it is believed to produce particularly vivid and colorful illusions. Tolerance to the effects of psilocybin builds rapidly with daily use, although physical dependence does not occur. Though psychological dependence is a possibility, it is thought to be rare.

DMT

A derivative of certain South American shrubs as well as a synthetic compound, DMT is a very powerful, fast-acting drug that produces psychedelic effects of an extremely short duration. Known chemically as dimethyltryptamine, DMT is produced in either liquid or powder forms. Usually DMT is combined with tobacco, parsley, or marijuana and smoked. Sometimes a finely ground powder of DMT is sniffed, eaten, or prepared in a solution for injection.

One of the surprising aspects of DMT is its almost instantaneous impact upon the user. Psychedelic effects often begin and reach their peak of intensity within 10 minutes after smoking. The trip lasts only 30 to 60 minutes, and then the visual and time-sense distortions subside

rapidly. In essence, a DMT trip is a compact version of an LSD trip, without the side effects of LSD.

As with most other psychedelics, use of DMT soon produces a tolerance, but there is no evidence of physical dependence. Despite its appeal as the "businessperson's trip"—allegedly a DMT trip can be taken during a lunch hour—there is little demand for this drug. Perhaps DMT's action as a MAO inhibitor is its greatest potential hazard. When taken in combination with various foods, liquids, and other drugs, DMT can cause life-threatening changes in blood pressure. (See chapter 8, box 8.4, on antidepressant drugs.)

Morning Glory Seeds

Pulverized seeds of the common morning glory plant (*Ipomoea purpurea* and various species of *Rivea* and *Argyreia*) contain a psychoactive substance, *d*-lysergic acid amide. This psychedelic drug is very similar to LSD but is much less potent. A dose of between 200 to 300 seeds will induce LSD-like effects within thirty minutes if taken as a powdery mixture or almost immediately if injected as a liquid preparation. Sometimes the seeds are chewed

Designer Drugs: Hallucinogens

box 9.3

Illegal drugs are defined in terms of their chemical formulas. To circumvent these legal restrictions, "underground chemists" modify the molecular structure of certain illegal drugs to produce analogues known as "designer drugs." (An analogue is a substance derived from a chemically similar compound.) These chemically engineered analogues can be several hundred times stronger than the drugs they are designed to imitate.

Analogues of amphetamines and methamphetamines cause nausea, blurred vision, chills or sweating, and faintness. Psychological effects include anxiety, depression, and paranoia. As little as one dose can cause brain damage. The analogues of phencyclidine cause illusions, hallucinations, and impaired perception.

Type	What Is It Called?	What Does It Look Like?	How Is It Used?
Analogues of amphetamines and methamphetamines (Hallucinogens)	MDMA (Ecstasy, XTC, Adam, Essence) MDM STP PMA 2, 5-DMA TMA DOM DOB MDEA (Eve) ET (Love Pills, Love Pearls) Nexus	White powder Tablets Capsules	Taken orally Injected Inhaled through nasal passages
Analogues of phencyclidine (PCP) (hallucinogens)	PCPy PCE TCP PHP TPCP	White powder	Taken orally Injected Smoked

Source: Modified from the U.S. Department of Education.

thoroughly before they are swallowed. The chewing process releases the psychoactive drug for absorption into the bloodstream.

After an initial period of apathy and irritability, the user typically experiences a pleasant state of elation and serenity, quite similar to the effects of a low dose of LSD. However, "pearly gates" and "heavenly blues," as the seeds are often called, are not ideal psychedelics unless a natural source can be located. Seed producers coat commercially available seeds with a poisonous substance to discourage their use as a recreational drug. Upon ingestion, the toxic substance of the coating induces dizziness, nausea, vomiting, chills, and diarrhea.

Nutmeg

A commercial spice derived from the tropical evergreen *Myristica fragrans*, nutmeg appears as either the whole, dried seed or as a preparation of coarsely ground powder. Both the seed and the powder can be eaten; the powder is occasionally sniffed.

Two to five hours after grated nutmeg is swallowed, a confusional state with mild euphoria and illusions develops. These effects are in response to a chemical identified originally as myristican. However, other psychoactive substances may also be involved. In most instances, nutmeg is used only when more powerful drugs are not available.

Mace, the orange, lacy covering of the nutmeg shell, also contains myristican. Sometimes the ground or whole mace is used as a kitchen spice. When swallowed in quantity, mace induces mild psychedelic effects. Although its use is infrequent, there have been occasional "mace parties" on various college campuses.

MDA

Nicknamed the "mellow drug of America" and "speed for lovers," MDA has the chemical name *3, 4-methylenedioxyamphetamine*. Derived from various plant oils, including sassafras, MDA can also be synthesized as a white powder. This product can be taken orally (in a capsule), sniffed, or injected as a solution.

Chemically similar to both mescaline and the amphetamines, MDA induces a euphoric, peaceful, dreamlike state beginning about an hour after a person first takes the drug. The average trip may last nearly eight hours. Although at very high doses MDA produces many physical reactions—some requiring emergency medical treatment—the most notable effect seems to be tranquility. The accompanying psychological warmth and tenderness permit the "tripper" to concentrate on interpersonal relationships. Communication with other people seems to be enhanced as a pervasive sensuousness overcomes the user.

MDMA

Known as **"Ecstasy,"** "Adam," "the Big E," and "XTC," MDMA is a chemical cousin of MDA. This psychoactive drug combines some of the hallucinogenic effects of mescaline with the stimulant effects of amphetamines.[15]

Originally synthesized in 1914, MDMA (methylenedioxyamphetamine) did not become a significant drug of abuse until the 1970s, when it enjoyed a sudden popularity among American college students. Although taking the drug by mouth is generally preferred, MDMA is inhaled on occasion, but only rarely injected. Derived by chemically engineering MDA, MDMA is considered a **"designer drug"**—an originally legal substance that acts similarly to its illegal cousin (see chapter 1).

Advocates of MDMA first labeled the drug "the LSD of the 1980s" and then the drug "fashion flash" of the 1990s, because it provides the euphoric rush of cocaine and some of the mind-expanding qualities of psychedelics.[16] As a consequence, MDMA has become a favorite attraction of "rave parties" in the United States, with their young partygoers dancing all night to heavily mixed, electronically generated sound, surrounded by computer-generated video and laser light shows.[17] In more practical terms, perhaps, MDMA is considered the successor to MDA and is often viewed as an aphrodisiac, despite its interference with erection and its inhibition of orgasm in both sexes.

Research indicates that MDMA is somewhat milder and shorter lasting than MDA and exerts amphetaminelike effects on the body (dilated pupils, dry mouth and throat, lower-jaw tension, grinding of the teeth, and overall stimulation). On the other hand, however, many users report a general relaxation effect, decreased use of psychological defense mechanisms, increased empathy for others, promotion of intimate communications, and enhanced sensual experiences, especially the pleasures of touching.

Some physicians and therapists have found MDMA to be a significant therapeutic aid in dissolving personal anxieties in certain patients. Research also suggests that MDMA tends to intensify feelings, facilitate personal insight, promote positive changes in attitudes and feelings, and facilitate close interpersonal relationships.

Although the claimed benefits sound very attractive, other investigations have revealed several undesirable effects of MDMA. Recreational users report that over time the desired effects of the drug become weaker, while the negative side effects become more likely.[18] Psychological difficulties reported by users include mental confusion, depression, anxiety, generalized panic, and even paranoia.

Common physical problems experienced are increased muscle tension, nausea, blurred vision, rapid eye movements, faintness, and increased heart rate and blood pressure. However, the greatest fears are associated with Ecstasy's potential for acting as a toxic substance within the brain and causing major changes in brain chemistry.

Because of its potential for abuse and its possible neurotoxic effect, MDMA was temporarily restricted as a Schedule I controlled substance in 1985 and permanently classified in Schedule I in 1988. Also that year, the Drug Enforcement Administration rejected arguments supporting its treatment value. As an analogue of MDA, MDMA is also illegal as a "designer-recreational" drug.

DOM (STP)

Another synthetic variation of mescaline and amphetamine, DOM (4-methyl-2, 5-dimethoxyamphetamine) was first introduced to the drug scene in 1967 as "STP." Named after a motor oil additive—scientifically treated petroleum—the original acronym was soon reinterpreted to stand for "Serenity, Tranquility, Peace."[19]

Usually taken orally, DOM at very low doses induces an amphetaminelike euphoria and feelings of enhanced self-awareness. At higher dose levels, LSD-like effects are experienced. Generally less potent than LSD, DOM is not metabolized rapidly, remains in the body much longer than most other psychedelics (from 12 to 24 hours), and produces a

table 9.1 Psychoactive Herbal Preparations

Recreational use of herbal intoxicants has increased in popularity as legal alternatives to illicit psychedelics. The herbal preparations are marketed as teas, cigarettes, capsules, and smoking mixtures. Such items are often available in health-food stores and by direct mail order from suppliers and importers.

Psychoactive Substances Used in Herbal Preparations*

Herbal Ingredient	Commonly Reported Use	Reported Effect
African Yohimbe Bark	Smoke or tea as a stimulant	Mild hallucinogen
California Poppy	Smoke as marijuana substitute	Mild euphoriant
Catnip	Smoke or tea as marijuana substitute	Mild hallucinogen
Juniper	Smoke as hallucinogen	Strong hallucinogen
Kavakava	Smoke or tea as marijuana substitute	Mild hallucinogen
Lobelia	Smoke or tea as marijuana substitute	Mild euphoriant
Mandrake	Tea as a hallucinogen	Hallucinogen
Periwinkle	Smoke or tea as euphoriant	Hallucinogen
Thorn Apple	Smoke or tea as tobacco substitute	Strong hallucinogen

*From Ronald K. Siegel, "Herbal intoxication: Psychoactive effects from herbal cigarettes, tea, and capsules." *Journal of the American Medical Association*, vol. 236, no. 5 (August 2, 1976): 473–476. Copyright 1976, American Medical Association. Reprinted by permission.

variety of physical problems, including nausea, sweating, tremors, and convulsions. The length and intensity of the DOM (STP) trip both contribute to an unusually high rate of bad trips produced by the drug.

Chemical Variations

An almost endless number of psychedelics have been synthesized by creative "kitchen chemists" for the illegal street market. Some of these, such as DOB (4-bromo-2, 5-dimethoxyamphetamine) and MMDA are mescaline-amphetamine variants similar to DOM and MDA, respectively. Other psychedelics with stimulant properties are PMA (paramethoxyamphetamine) and TMA (trimethoxyamphetamine). DET (diethyltryptamine) is similar in chemical structure to DMT.

All of these drugs differ from one another in terms of speed of onset, duration of action, potency, and capacity to modify mood. They are seldom pure, their capsule dosages are variable, and they are often misrepresented as other psychedelics.

Phencyclidine

Developed in the 1950s as a surgical anesthetic, **phencyclidine,** or PCP, was introduced into medical practice under the trade name Sernyl. In 1965, this drug was taken off the market for human use because it produced unpleasant side effects, including hallucinations, in many patients.

Originally designated a depressant by the federal government, and long considered a psychedelic or hallucinogen by many drug treatment professionals, phencyclidine is a unique drug. It has stimulant, depressant, psychedelic, hallucinogenic, psychotomimetic, analgesic, and anesthetic properties, all of which are dose dependent. Its precise pharmacological classification has not yet been agreed upon by the scientific community. Perhaps PCP will eventually be considered a "dissociative anesthetic," because during anesthesia this drug appears to make patients insensitive to pain by separating or dissociating their bodily functions from their minds without causing loss of consciousness.[20]

Contrary to popular belief, PCP, known chemically as 1-(1-phenylcyclohexyl) piperidine hydrochloride, is not a one-of-a-kind drug. Modifications of the basic PCP manufacturing process have yielded a number of chemically similar compounds referred to as *analogues*. These PCP variants, or analogues, including PCC, PCE, PHP, TCP, and an anesthetic, ketamine, produce similar psychic effects and have already been sold on the illicit street market as PCP. More commonly, PCP is sold under numerous other names that reflect its bizarre effects, such as "angel dust," "peep," "supergrass," "KJ," "killer weed," "ozone," "embalming fluid," and "rocket fuel." In the recent past, PCP was often misrepresented as more attractive drugs, such as THC or other marijuana components, mescaline, LSD, amphetamine, and even cocaine, because of phencyclidine's bad street reputation.

All PCP synthesized today for human use is illegal. Pure PCP is a white crystalline powder that has a very bitter taste. It can be mixed with dyes, dissolved in water, and cut with adulterants, and it can contain contaminants resulting from its makeshift manufacture. Additives that change its color and consistency give it the appearance of reliable drugs and increase the likelihood that it will be purchased and consumed. PCP is sold in powders of many colors and as gummy masses that are processed into tablets or capsules.

Phencyclidine can be inhaled or sniffed, taken by mouth, smoked, and injected intravenously. Today, however, PCP is most commonly smoked on "Sherman" or "More" cigarettes (known as "sherms" and "superkools"), which have thick brown wrappers that absorb liquid PCP and still allow the cigarettes to be smoked. Sometimes PCP powder is placed on parsley or other leaf mixtures and smoked as "angel dust" in cigarettes or joints. Less frequently, liquid PCP is drunk mixed with lemonade or some alcoholic beverage, or injected two to three times a day.

Effects of PCP

The pharmacological actions of PCP depend upon the route of administration and are dose-related.[21–23] Because PCP is so potent, however, the difference between a dose that produces a pleasant loss of sensation (sensory deprivation) and one that results in a very bad trip is quite small. Consequently, the effects of this drug differ widely from one PCP user to the next.

When PCP is eaten, it produces a high lasting five to eight hours; when smoked or snorted, the effects can last three to five hours. Small doses lead first to a mild depression, then to stimulation.

A common initial experience has been described as a drunken state, a floaty euphoria with numbness of the extremities—a result of PCP's anesthetic effect. Users often appear to be "stoned" and display a staggering gait and slurred speech. In addition, the PCP taker experiences a temporary state of depersonalization and detachment from his or her surroundings. Feelings of strength, power, and invulnerability may coexist with this dreamy sense of estrangement.

In moderate doses, both analgesia and anesthesia are produced, so that PCP users often do not know when they are being burned, when they have been cut, or when they have strained muscles or broken bones. A confusing psychic state resembling a form of sensory isolation is produced. As a result, the user dissociates, or disconnects from reality, and is no longer aware of what is happening. Changes in body image, disorganized thoughts, drowsiness, and hostile and even bizarre behavior also have been recorded.

While heart rate and blood pressure are elevated, the central nervous system undergoes a depression. Increased salivation, sweating, repetitive movements, and muscle rigidity may occur. With increasing dosage, analgesia and anesthesia are more pronounced, and stupor or coma may develop, but the eyes of the PCP taker remain open. In large doses, PCP may produce convulsions.

PCP Overdose

Research has revealed that some regular PCP users rarely appear in criminal justice or medical care statistics. These individuals often use phencyclidine along with alcohol and marijuana at parties or otherwise explore PCP's psychedelic properties without experiencing the undesirable reactions that often end in violent behavior, depression, and paranoia. Apparently such users have mastered the concept of dose control in order to maximize desired psychoactive effects and minimize undesired effects.

Because of the level of potency of any given dose, the effects of PCP are often unpredictable. Overdosing is a possibility. The victim of overdose is likely to experience muscular incoordination, oscillating movements of the eyeballs, inability to

Toads Hop into Current Drug Scene

One of the latest psychedelic fads involves the *Bufo alvarius* toad, whose venom contains bufotenine, a recognized hallucinogen. The toad secrets the venom, which is then dried and smoked in a pipe. Although bufotenine has been on both federal and state dangerous-drug lists for years and its possession is illegal, "toad smoking" is now a small but growing segment of America's drug culture.[a]

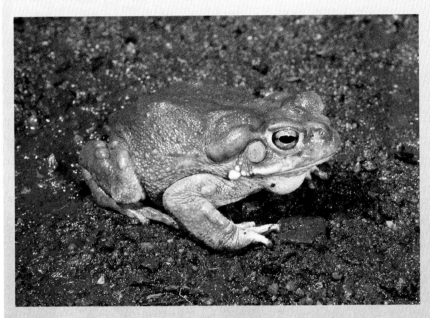

When smoked, the dried venom from this toad produces a psychedelic effect. Some people find that when "toad-smoking," one toke is enough!

© E. R. Degginger/Photo Researchers, Inc.

When smoked, the chemically active compounds in the venom produce an intense high that some claim eclipse the psychedelic properties of LSD. Feelings like being lifted up in an elevator, coupled with a sense of wonder and well-being, have been reported after just a single toke (inhalation). The experience of detachment from one's surroundings proves to be very intense and very strange.[b]

From all accounts, the practice of "toad smoking" is somewhat less dangerous than "toad licking," which involves the ingestion of venom that has been squeezed from live toads. The venom itself is poisonous. The heat of the smoking process in "toad smoking" largely detoxifies the venom, but its psychedelic effects persist.

a. "Toad Smoking Latest Threat in the War on Drugs," *Bottom Line on Alcohol in Society* 15, no. 2 (summer 1994): 90–92.
b. Andrew Weil and Winifred Rosen, *From Chocolate to Morphine*, rev. ed. (Boston: Houghton Mifflin, 1993), 201.

move from a fixed position, vomiting, skin flushing, noticeable perspiration, generalized anesthesia (loss of sensation), and psychotic episodes.

PCP-induced psychosis, which is most likely to occur in individuals who have already suffered severe mental disorders, may be characterized by violence, aggression, extreme anxiety, and tension.[24] The psychotic experience usually progresses through three stages, each lasting about five days.[25] The first stage is often the most severe and is marked by delusions, anorexia (lack of appetite), insomnia, and the possibility that the user will assault others. This is followed by an intermediate, second stage with continued paranoia, restlessness, and intermittent control over one's behavior. In the third stage, the PCP user undergoes a gradual recovery, but social withdrawal and severe depression often persist for months.

Of course, PCP can display the harmful properties of a CNS depressant, inducing cardiovascular instability, respiratory depression (stoppage of breathing), seizures, and coma. To prevent death, emergency medical treatment will include life-support measures, isolation of the victim to reduce sensory stimulation, and detoxification by gastric suctioning.

The number of deaths associated with combining PCP with alcohol or with heroin has been higher than expected, reflecting either a users' preference for taking these drugs in combination or some interaction in the effect of the drug combinations. Many of the reported PCP-related deaths, however, were not the result of overdose or drug interaction but rather resulted directly from external events, such as homicides, accidents, suicides, gunshot wounds, strangling, drownings, auto accidents, falls, and cuts.

Historical Aspects

Although the synthesis of PCP was originally described in 1926, it was not until the early 1950s that scientists first studied its potential use as a drug that could produce anesthesia without significant depression of heart and lung function. Clinical use of PCP soon raised serious doubts about its usefulness as an anesthetic, however. Humans sustained numerous postoperative difficulties, ranging from mild to profound disorientation, agitation, manic excitation, delirium, and even hallucinations. When subanesthetic doses of PCP were found to induce schizophrenia-like symptoms in normal subjects and to intensify primary symptoms of schizophrenic patients, PCP was restricted to its only legal use at that time, as a veterinary analgesic-anesthetic.

PCP first appeared on the illegal drug scene in 1965, but it did not attract much attention until it emerged as the "PeaCe Pill" during 1967, and as "hog" in New York City's "hippie" community in 1968.

As reports of increased adverse medical and psychiatric effects related to PCP were publicized, and as its recreational use spread throughout the United States, phencyclidine gained notoriety as a major drug menace. In 1977, the National Institute on Drug Abuse started a nationwide campaign to inform both professionals and the public of PCP-abuse hazards. Although today's use of PCP appears to be concentrated predominantly among former users and young adults, some preteens and adolescents are still being hospitalized for PCP-related emergencies in some large urban areas.

Phencyclidine: A Puzzle

Why PCP remains popular while it continues to have such a poor street reputation is a puzzle with seeming contradictions. With less misrepresentation of PCP as other drugs, perhaps the continuing demand is for what the drug really is—a risk to achieve subjective benefits, involving a challenge to manage the drug without being overwhelmed by the drug. In other words, difficulties in using the drug may have become part of the drug's attraction and appeal. "Doing a drug" that seems to melt away troubles or merely changes one's state of consciousness can also be a very pleasant happening in the company of good friends.

The popularity of phencyclidine may also be related to changes in the routes of administering the drug. Some users may be better able to avoid overdose when PCP is smoked or snorted rather than taken orally. When smoked, the doses are usually smaller and thus more manageable. This also applies to snorting PCP.

Nevertheless, phencyclidine does seem to produce a higher rate of unpredictably negative reactions with more frequent use than do most other psychoactive drugs. PCP has established a reputation for inducing frequent bad trips with severe mental confusion, total unresponsiveness to any sensory stimulation, muscle rigidity, bouts of depression, and even a chronic brain syndrome—in its most serious and rare form called the "Alzheimer's Disease of Adolescence" (an inability to function and periods of forgetfulness).[26]

Legal Prohibition

Responding to the national concern over the abuse of PCP and the severe behavioral toxicity of phencyclidine and its analogues, the federal government temporarily classified PCP as a Schedule II controlled substance and then, in 1979, permanently elevated it to Schedule I status. In 1978, the U.S. Congress enacted the Psychotropic Substance Act. This legislation imposed severe penalties for the manufacture of PCP and its analogues, as well as for possession with intent to distribute them. Legislation was also passed mandating that all sales of piperidine (a chemical intermediate in the synthesis of PCP) or its salts and derivatives be reported to the U.S. Attorney General and the Drug Enforcement Administration.

Whether such legal prohibition will indeed eliminate the abuse of PCP and prevent the "chemical wave of the future" remains to be seen.

Chapter Summary

1. Psychedelics are drug substances that change thinking and perception. Such mind expansion is characterized by heightened awareness of sensory input and sense of clarity, unusual sensory experiences and perceptions of the environment, assignment of profound meaning to the slightest sensation, lessened capacity to distinguish self from the environment, and a sense of cosmic union.

2. Synesthesia is a psychedelic drug-related effect in which there is a mingling of the senses. For example, sounds might be seen, smells might be felt, and colors might be heard.

3. Particular hazards of psychedelics are a "bad trip" (panic reaction) and a "flashback" (repetition of the drug's effects without using the drug again).

4. The types of psychedelic experiences are distinguished as psychotic, psychodynamic (surfacing of

subconscious ideas), cognitive (clearness of thought), esthetic (fascinating perceptions and sensations), and transcendental.

5. Physical side effects are dull compared to the psychological effects. They involve changes in temperature, blood pressure, heart rate, and reflexes; and include nausea, vomiting, and diarrhea. Repeated use often leads to tolerance and, in some instances, psychological dependence. Physical dependence has not been demonstrated.

6. Though plants with psychedelic effects had been used for many centuries, the synthesis and personal use of LSD by Albert Hofmann in 1943 ushered in the Psychedelic Era.

7. Initially used in the treatment of mental conditions, LSD was soon adopted by students, writers, and philosophers because of the drug's mind-expanding qualities. Eventually, LSD became associated with the "hippie culture," dropping out of conventional society, and antiestablishment social movements. Legal production of LSD was stopped in the mid 1960s.

8. Derived from ergot fungus or from lysergic acid amide, LSD is the most powerful synthetic psychedelic. It is 100 times more potent than psilocybin (derived from sacred mushrooms or synthesized) and 4,000 times more powerful than mescaline (derived from peyote cactus or synthesized).

9. Other psychedelics are DMT, morning glory seeds, and nutmeg (all naturally occurring), and MDA, MMDA, DOM, DOB, and DET (all synthesized).

10. MDMA, a designer drug derived chemically from MDA and often called Ecstasy, has become a popular recreational drug because it tends to combine the rush of cocaine with some of the mind-expanding qualities of psychedelics. MDMA's

potential therapeutic value has been rejected by the Drug Enforcement Administration.

11. In a drug class of its own, phencyclidine (PCP) has psychedelic, stimulant, depressant, hallucinogenic, psychotomimetic, analgesic, and anesthetic properties.

12. Introduced as a surgical anesthetic for humans, and then for use in veterinary medical practice, PCP was eventually classified as a Schedule I controlled substance due to its frightening and often violent side effects.

13. Though some users claim to maximize desired psychoactive effects of PCP by means of dose control, the drug's effects are unpredictable and subjectively experienced. A floaty euphoria, anesthesia, sensory deprivation, delusions, hallucinations, violent and assaultive behavior, paranoia, and a severe form of psychosis are all possible elements of a PCP trip.

Review Questions and Activities

1. In what specific ways do psychedelic drugs expand one's mind?

2. Some psychedelics produce psychotic experiences. What types of mind-expanding experiences might be interpreted as more desirable psychedelic effects?

3. How does the phenomenon of synesthesia differ from a flashback reaction?

4. Explain how people achieved psychedelic effects before the synthesis of LSD.

5. What roles did the following individuals play in the modern Psychedelic Era: Albert Hofmann, Timothy Leary, and Richard Alpert?

6. Describe the probable though variable experiences of an LSD "trip" in relation to dosage level, user

characteristics, drug-taking environment, and anticipated phases of effects.

7. Compare the following drugs in terms of their origin, their probable psychedelic effects, and their differences in use patterns and duration of action: peyote, psilocybin, DMT, and DOM.

8. Why is MDA sometimes referred to as "speed for lovers"?

9. What effects of MDMA make this drug, known as Ecstasy, so popular and yet so controversial?

10. Which classification of psychoactive drugs seems most appropriate and most accurate for phencyclidine?

11. Why is PCP often described as a drug menace?

12. Consult a reference text on herbs and herbal preparations and investigate the possible pharmacological effects of broom or Scotch broom, hops, maté, passion flower, prickly poppy, snakeroot, and wild lettuce.

References

1. Lester Grinspoon and James Bakalar, *The Harvard Medical School Mental Health Review: Drug Abuse and Addiction* (Boston: Harvard Mental Health Letter, 1993), 33.

2. Jerome Jaffe, "Drug Addiction and Drug Abuse," chapter 22 in *Goodman and Gilman's The Pharmacological Basis of Therapeutics*, 8th ed., ed. A. G. Gilman, T. W. Rall, A. S. Nies, and P. Taylor (New York: McGraw-Hill, 1990), 553.

3. Barry Stimmel and the Editors of Consumer Reports Books, *The Facts about Drug Use: Coping with Drugs and Alcohol in Your Family, at Work, in Your Community* (New York: Haworth Medical Press, 1993), 115.

4. Robert Julien, *A Primer of Drug Action* (New York: W. H. Freeman, 1992), 256.

5. Kenneth Blum, *Handbook of Abusable Drugs* (New York: Gardner Press, 1984), 558.

6. Edward M. Brecher and the Editors of Consumer Reports Books, *Licit and Illicit Drugs* (Mount Vernon, N.Y.: Consumers Union, 1972), 338.

7. Avram Goldstein, *Addiction: From Biology to Drug Policy* (New York: W. H. Freeman, 1994), 193.

8. H. Thomas Milhorn, *Drug and Alcohol Abuse* (New York: Plenum Press, 1994), 333.

9. National Institute on Drug Abuse, "LSD (Lysergic Acid Diethylamide)," *NIDA Capsules,* June 1992, 1.

10. Harold Doweiko, *Concepts of Chemical Dependency,* 2d ed. (Pacific Grove, Calif.: Brooks/Cole, 1993), 144.

11. Christina Dye, *Acid: LSD Today* (Tempe, Ariz.: Do It Now, 1992), 5–6.

12. Jennifer James, *Peyote and Mescaline: History and Use of the Sacred Cactus* (Tempe, Ariz.: Do It Now, 1990), 4.

13. Christina Dye, *Psilocybin: Demystifying the Magic Mushroom* (Tempe, Ariz.: Do It Now, 1991), 4.

14. Gesina Longenecker, *How Drugs Work: Drug Abuse and the Human Body* (Emeryville, Calif.: Ziff-Davis Press, 1994), 104.

15. Harvey Milkman and Stanley Sunderwirth, *Craving for Ecstasy: The Consciousness and Chemistry of Escape* (Lexington, Mass.: D. C. Heath, 1987), 53.

16. Christina Dye, *XTC: MDMA and the Chemical Pursuit of Ecstasy* (Tempe, Ariz.: Do It Now, 1991), 2.

17. Teri Randall, "Medical News and Perspectives: 'Rave' Scene, Ecstasy Use, Leap Atlantic," *Journal of the American Medical Association* 268, no. 12 (22–30 September 1992): 1506.

18. Doweiko, *Concepts of Chemical Dependency,* 150.

19. Tibor Palfai and Henry Jankeiwicz, *Drugs and Human Behavior* (Dubuque, Iowa: Brown & Benchmark, 1991), 315.

20. Leo Hollister, "Drugs of Abuse," in *Basic and Clinical Pharmacology,* ed. Bertram Katzung, 4th ed. (Norwalk, Conn.: Appleton & Lange, 1989), 389.

21. Robert C. Petersen and Richard C. Stillman, "Phencyclidine: An Overview," in *Phencyclidine (PCP) Abuse: An Appraisal,* ed. R. C. Petersen and R. C. Stillman (Washington, D.C.: U.S. Government Printing Office, 1978), 3.

22. Jaffe, "Drug Addiction and Drug Abuse," 557–58.

23. Grinspoon and Bakalar, *The Harvard Medical School Mental Health Review,* 36.

24. Ming Tsuang, Stephen Faraone, and Max Day, "Schizophrenic Disorders," in *The New Harvard Guide to Psychiatry,* ed. Armand Nicholi, Jr. (Cambridge: Belknap Press/Harvard University Press, 1988), 271.

25. Doweiko, *Concepts of Chemical Dependency,* 148.

26. Stimmel et al., *The Facts about Drug Use,* 119.

chapter

10 | marijuana

Unique and Controversial

KEY TERMS

Amotivational Syndrome
Antiparaphernalia Law
Anxiety/Panic Reaction
Cannabinoid
Cannabis
Cannabis sativa
Decriminalization
Flashback
Glaucoma
Hashish
Hashish Oil
Hemp Plant
Immunosuppressive Effect
Legalization
Marijuana
Marijuana High
Mutation
Paraquat
Sinsemilla
Teratogen
THC

chapter objectives

After you have studied this chapter, you should be able to do the following:

1. Identify the natural source of marijuana and name its principal psychoactive ingredient.

2. Name several different uses of cannabis products, other than as a recreational drug, in both ancient and modern times.

3. Explain the impact each of the following laws had on marijuana use, misuse, or abuse: Harrison Narcotics Act, Eighteenth Amendment to the U.S. Constitution, Marijuana Tax Act, and the Controlled Substances Act.

4. Distinguish between the concepts of decriminalization and legalization as they pertain to the possession of small amounts of marijuana for personal use.

5. Compare and contrast the major arguments offered for and against the legalization of marijuana and other illegal drugs of abuse.

6. Describe the probable psychological, emotional, and physiological aspects of the marijuana "high."

7. Identify the probable effects of marijuana on motor coordination, reaction time, tracking, cue detection, short-term memory, time sense, and oral communication.

8. Explain the probable effect of social levels of marijuana on driving ability.

9. Define each of the following terms as they relate to marijuana use: *anxiety/panic reaction, tolerance, dependence,* and *flashback.*

10. Discuss the amotivational syndrome and its controversial association with marijuana use.

11. Identify the major chronic effects of marijuana use on the respiratory, cardiovascular, and immune systems.

12. List three possible effects of marijuana on male reproduction and sexual function.

13. List three possible effects of marijuana on female reproduction and sexual function.

14. Distinguish between the following as they relate to use of marijuana: teratogen and mutation.

15. Discuss the therapeutic potential of marijuana in relation to specific diseases or abnormal conditions in humans.

Introduction

Marijuana has become a popular psychoactive drug—the most widely used illegal substance in the nation. It has frequently been described as relatively safe despite its illegal status, but it is now known to have significant health-threatening effects on users. This chapter examines the history of marijuana and the legal aspects of using it, along with the drug's pharmacology and potential health risks, thereby clarifying some of the uncertainties and myths surrounding this unique substance.

Of all the so-called recreational drugs, pot or grass—as marijuana is commonly called—is the most controversial. Since its use has become so widespread in the United States, those who favor marijuana and its legalization argue that its potential risks to health are no greater than those of alcohol or tobacco. Opponents

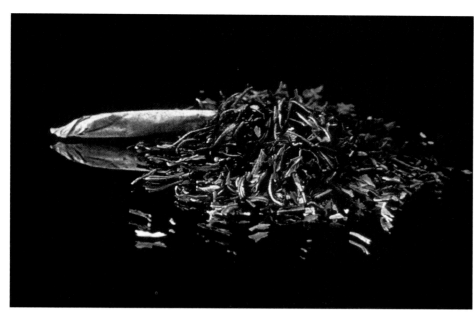

Shown in this photo is a marijuana plant, cannabis sativa, which is cultivated as well as grown wild throughout the world in temperate and tropical areas.

Drug Enforcement Agency

of marijuana insist that its proven and suspected hazards to personal and social health are so potentially harmful that any further legal approval would be unwise and undesirable.

Marijuana: A Brief Description

Marijuana is a prepared mixture of the dried, flowering tops, leaves, and stems of the **hemp plant**, *Cannabis sativa*.[1] Cultivated, as well as grown wild, throughout the world in temperate and tropical areas, the leafy cannabis plant grows for just one season, dies, and then reproduces through its seed.

Often incorrectly considered a narcotic, marijuana in low to moderate doses typically causes a sedative, dreamlike effect in the user, who is observed as relaxed, drowsy, and less socially interactive. However, at higher dose levels, marijuana produces effects quite similar to the mind-expanding psychedelics. As such, marijuana or cannabis shares the characteristics of two major drug classifications. But unlike the sedatives, marijuana's active ingredient does not produce anesthesia or death. And unlike the powerful psychedelics, there is little

cross-tolerance between marijuana and, for example, LSD. So marijuana is a unique psychoactive drug, best described in a class of its own.

Historical and Legal Aspects of Marijuana

Presumably first used by the Chinese as early as 2700 B.C., the hemp plant's fibers were valued highly and utilized in the manufacture of rope, cloth, and paper.[2] Before any intoxicating or drug effects were associated with the nonfood plant, a commercial application of cannabis was established. Since then, marijuana* seeds have been sterilized and processed for use in animal feed mixtures (the sterilization renders the seeds nonpsychoactive); cannabis fibers have been employed as raw materials in the production of canvas; oil extracts of the hemp plant have been combined with paint pigments.

*The preferred spelling of this word, *marijuana*, the Spanish variation, will be used throughout the chapter, except in direct quotations or publications containing the English variation, *marihuana*.

The ancient Chinese soon discovered the usefulness of cannabis in the medical treatment of a wide variety of ailments.[3] However, the Chinese eventually banned its use because of the plant's unpredictable intoxicating effects. The smooth, tranquil, and predictable sedation brought on by opium was preferred by the stable Chinese personality to the sometimes stimulative, sometimes sedative, psychological response to hemp.

Upon the introduction of cannabis into ancient India, its mind-altering effects were more generally appreciated. The cultivation of the hemp plant became an agricultural science, and its use eventually became widespread. The early Indian culture accepted the euphoria-producing ability of cannabis as both appropriate and as a blessing from the Almighty. In due time, the use of the hemp plant as an intoxicant and as a source of rope and cloth spread throughout Asia, Africa, Europe, and, more recently, the Americas.

By the time Europeans began exploring the New World, the cannabis plant was a commercial success. During the early seventeenth century, English settlers brought the plant to their colonies in America, where it was the first crop to be introduced in the Massachusetts Bay Colony.[4] Before long, hemp plants were abundant and the hemp fiber industry thrived.

Although the psychoactive properties of the cannabis plant were recognized, the general American public showed relatively little interest in marijuana as a nonmedical, recreational drug. In contrast, the medical uses of marijuana were expanded, and cannabis preparations were prescribed legally for numerous physical and mental ailments until 1940. When the Harrison Narcotics Act was passed by the U.S. Congress in 1914 in an attempt to control the distribution and use of medical narcotic drugs, cannabis products, including marijuana and hashish, were excluded from the provisions of the act.

In the view of the National Commission on Marihuana and Drug Abuse:

Marihuana smoking first became prominent on the American scene in the decade following the Harrison Act. Mexican immigrants and West Indian sailors introduced the practice in the border and Gulf state. As the Mexicans spread throughout the West and immigrated to the major cities, some of them carried the marihuana habit with them. The practice also became common among the same urban populations with whom opiate use was identified.[5]

It is also likely that marijuana use increased in popularity as a recreational intoxicant with the enactment of the Eighteenth Amendment to the U.S. Constitution. This prohibition amendment forbade the manufacture, distribution, and sale of alcoholic beverages. Inexpensive and easily available, marijuana became a substitute for ethyl alcohol. During the 1920s, marijuana "tea pads"—late-night smokeries similar to bars—operated in many large cities, including New York.

Allegations of abuse and an association with violence and crime came along with the increased use of marijuana among Mexican Americans, black cavalry soldiers, and the social elite. Exaggerated tales of the drug's bizarre effects, especially that it caused murder, rape, sexual excesses, and amnesia, were publicized widely. Marijuana horror stories were portrayed in the Hollywood film *Reefer Madness,* which is still shown occasionally on college campuses. By 1935, in reaction to the growing "epidemic" of marijuana puffing, most state governments enacted laws against the nonmedical use of cannabis. During this antimarijuana crusade, cannabis and its extracts were inaccurately classified as narcotics in scientific literature and in legal declarations.

The Marijuana Tax Act

In 1937, the U.S. Congress adopted the Marijuana Tax Act, which superimposed a federal prohibitory scheme on each of the state laws banning nonmedical use of marijuana. This federal statute mandated the registration and taxation of both buyers and sellers of marijuana and imposed criminal penalties for violations. In effect, the Marijuana Tax Act was a national ban on the nonmedicinal possession and use of cannabis preparations. Subsequent federal and state legislation prescribed even harsher penalties, including, in some states, life imprisonment for illegal possession.

box 10.1

Glossary of Terms for Marijuana-Related Products

1. *Bhang*—the dried leaves and flowering shoots of the cannabis plant, containing smaller amounts of THC; common name for a weak preparation of marijuana used in India and Jamaica.
2. **Cannabis**—a general term for any of the various preparations of the hemp plant, *Cannabis sativa,* and used interchangeably with the term *marijuana.*
3. *Ganja*—the resinous mass derived from the small leaves and brackets of the cannabis plant; common name for a slightly more potent form of marijuana used in India.
4. **Hashish**—the resinous secretions of the cannabis plant that are collected from the flowering tops, dried, and then compressed into various forms, such as balls, cakes, and cookielike sheets. This form of cannabis is generally more potent than marijuana, having a THC content ranging from trace amounts up to 20 percent, but averaging between 3 percent and 7 percent. Hashish is the major form of cannabis used in the Middle East and in North Africa. In the Far East, the dried resinous exudate is called *charas.*
5. **Hashish oil**—a dark viscous liquid produced by a process of repeated extraction of cannabis plant materials. A solvent, such as ether or chloroform, percolates through the marijuana mixture, thereby removing more of the existing THC. This extract contains a greater concentration of THC than does hashish, with some samples having a THC content of nearly 60 percent, but averaging about 20 percent.
6. **Marijuana**—a general term descriptive of any part of the cannabis plant, *Cannabis sativa,* or its extract that produces physical or psychic changes in the human. Marijuana is a tobaccolike substance produced by drying the leaves and flowering tops of the hemp plant.
7. **Sinsemilla**—a seedless variety of high-potency marijuana, originally grown in California and prepared from the unpollenated female cannabis plant.
8. *Thai sticks*—a cannabis preparation common in Southeast Asia, consisting of marijuana buds bound onto short sections of bamboo.

Source: Based on definitions and descriptions provided by the Drug Enforcement Administration and the Bureau of Justice Statistics, U.S. Department of Justice.

Until the early 1960s, the recreational use of marijuana was confined largely to underprivileged socioeconomic groups and certain insulated social groups, including jazz musicians and artists. Such use had little impact on the dominant social order. Nothing changed on the legal scene until millions of middle- and upper-class college youth—and their noncollege counterparts—adopted marijuana smoking as a common form of recreation. Marijuana became part of the youth and values revolution of the 1960s. Then, under the provisions of the Controlled Substances Act of 1970 (officially known as the Comprehensive Drug Abuse Prevention and Control Act), the U.S. Congress downgraded

possession and use of marijuana from a felony to a misdemeanor. Eventually, all fifty states relaxed their severe penalties for simple possession.

Decriminalization and Legalization of Marijuana

In 1973, Oregon became the first state to decriminalize marijuana; that is, the penalties for possession and use of this drug were reduced in severity. By 1980, another ten states had decriminalized the possession of this drug. However, antimarijuana initiatives—including the spraying of paraquat on marijuana crops and the adoption of zero tolerance

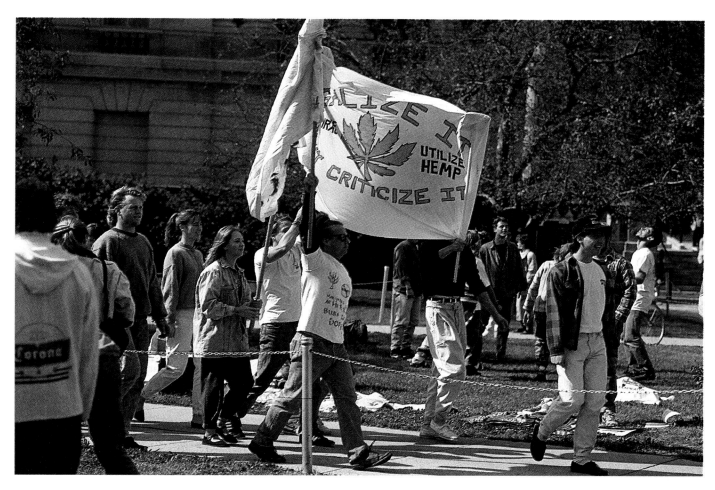

Efforts to legalize marijuana often take the form of peaceful demonstrations both on and off college campuses. Do you think marijuana will be decriminalized or legalized in the near future?

© James L. Shaffer

standards—were then undertaken by the federal government and the national mood of tolerance toward marijuana began to shift. In 1990, Alaska became the first state to recriminalize marijuana possession in a statewide referendum, although this antipot measure is now being challenged in a state superior court.

Decriminalization is the legal process of reducing the penalty for a particular behavior still restricted by law. In this instance, the behavior is the possession and use of small amounts of cannabis preparations. The former misdemeanor offense has been downgraded either to a minor misdemeanor—with no permanent criminal record—or to a mere civil offense requiring a civil fine and sometimes also mandating enrollment in a drug education program or involvement in public service

instead of a prison sentence. However, laws forbidding the sale of marijuana remain harsh. In many states, punishment for trafficking in marijuana has increased, while penalties for personal possession have decreased.

The decriminalization procedure is based on the philosophy that harsh criminal penalties are completely unjustified. Long prison terms and huge fines seem unreasonable and ineffective for punishing an individual who may be unaware of the consequences of taking marijuana. Moreover, noncriminal penalties appear to be more appropriate for such drug use that does not usually affect other people or society in general.

By contrast, when criminal penalties are applied, they have often resulted in otherwise law-abiding young people spending time in prison and incurring irreversible

damage to their careers and professional advancement. Such consequences apparently cause greater harm to human lives than any effects the drug would have had. As such, criminal penalties appear to be not only harsh and unjust, but counterproductive as well.

Legalization, on the other hand, is a legislative declaration approving or authorizing a particular action. In the legalization of marijuana, the state or federal government would not attempt to prohibit or penalize the use of marijuana. However, as in the legalization of alcohol after the period of national prohibition, laws could still regulate the place of use, minimum age of users, time of purchase, production, taxation, and consequences of combining drug use with driving or other public behaviors.

So far, neither the United States government nor any state has moved toward legalization of marijuana or any other presently illegal drug of abuse. However, support for both general and limited legalization has increased in recent years, due primarily to the perceived ineffectiveness of current, restrictive drug laws and the alleged failure of the continuing "war on illegal drugs" in America.

One vocal critic of the federal government's antidrug campaign is the National Organization for the Reform of Marijuana Laws (NORML), based in the nation's capital. NORML has been advocating both decriminalization and legalization of marijuana for more than twenty years, but it supports continued prohibition of cocaine. According to NORML, marijuana is a "softer" drug, with lower toxicity potential, than alcohol, cocaine, or heroin. So far, no one has ever died as a result of a marijuana overdose, and many fewer marijuana-related deaths occur each year in comparison with the huge toll of tobacco-related mortality. In addition, NORML has also spearheaded the challenge to the federal government's ban against the medical use of natural marijuana.

Today, an increasing number of individuals, including prominent politicians have indicated a willingness to consider legalization of drugs of abuse. This procedure is viewed as one viable alternative to what is perceived as unworkable antidrug measures now being applied without much success or effect. After spending billions of dollars to stop the spread of drugs, the nation is awash in illegal drugs, courts are jammed with drug-related cases, and drug arrests have more than tripled in some cities.

Those who support legalization of drugs, including marijuana, base their arguments on the following considerations.[6-8]

1. The current annual $10 billion cost associated with drug-abuse prevention efforts, mainly law enforcement and imprisonment, is far too high, and that sum could be better spent on drug-abuse education and treatment and rehabilitation of drug abusers.

2. Legalization would make drugs so cheap and available that organized

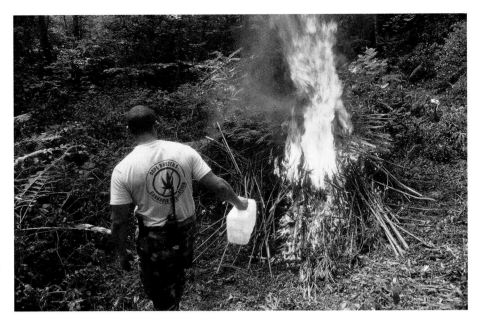

After a raid on a West Virginia marijuana plantation, a state police officer helps destroy thousands of plants as part of the Domestic Cannabis Eradication and Suppression Program, a coordinated effort between federal, state, and local agencies to eradicate domestically cultivated cannabis in the United States.
© William Campbell/Sygma

crime and "drug lords" would be deprived of at least $20 billion each year. Thus, the huge profits and violent crimes now related to the distribution and sale of illegal psychoactives would be reduced or even eliminated.

3. Revenues to finance drug treatment programs could be raised by placing "vice taxes" on drugs, similar to those now levied on alcoholic beverages and tobacco products.

4. Government at all levels should interfere as little as possible with individual rights—including drug taking. This argument is usually held by those who adopt a libertarian approach to human endeavors. Some libertarians would permit usage of drugs even if such action resulted in large numbers of drug users or proved to be life-threatening.

5. Legalization would not lead to an explosion of drug usage or drug users. Although there might be an initial

increase, as drugs become easier to use from a legal standpoint, they actually tend to become less popular.

6. Availability of legalized drugs would assure a higher standard of purity and controlled dosage levels—due to government regulation—and thus eliminate the uncertainty of potency and purity now associated with street drugs, especially marijuana and cocaine.

7. Because present antidrug laws are so frequently violated without consequence, many people have developed a disrespect for all laws. Legalization would allow law enforcement officials to concentrate on more serious crimes, where their efforts would likely be more effective, and thus generate renewed respect for laws in general.

8. Because some people have used, and always will use, mind-changing drugs, a society ought to adopt a drug-control policy that allows use but also promotes the reduction of harm in using psychoactive substances.

There are, of course, many valid counterarguments to the proposal for legalizing some or all psychoactive drugs. These are summarized in the following list:[9, 10]

1. The public does not want a change in the current antidrug laws. In fact, a majority of citizens want more, not fewer, restrictions placed on currently illegal drugs.

2. Greater availability of drugs would likely lead to more use, drug-use problems, and drug addiction. When prohibition of alcohol ended in 1933, the rate of drinking, alcohol-related diseases, and alcoholism soared. Today, alcohol-related problems plague not only individuals but the entire nation. With only 2 percent of the world's population, the United States now consumes an estimated 65 percent of the world's mind-changing chemicals. Making more drugs available will only contribute to more drug problems. The legal addictive drugs—alcohol and nicotine—already do enormous damage to both users and nonusers.

3. Legalization of drugs would likely increase the health costs of drug abuse, conservatively estimated at $60 billion annually. Hospitals would be filled with more drug-related emergencies, and more people would be involved in drug-related accidents. Job efficiency and productivity would decline still further, and unless some tax-supported government agency provides addicts with a free or low-cost supply of drugs, addicted individuals would still have to rob or steal to buy their psychoactives.

4. The right-to-privacy principle does not apply to using marijuana or any other illegal drug, because drug-taking behaviors are not completely private matters. Legalizing drugs will not save drug-abuse-related deaths, ease the pain of infants born addicted to drugs, or prevent drug-abusing parents from beating their children to death. And legalization will not reduce drug use in the workplace. Presently, drug-dependent individuals strain families, the

medical care system, and state and federal budgets in terms of treatment and rehabilitation services, and take their toll on the national economy by draining away productivity and shortening their own lives. In addition, the current crack cocaine epidemic has ruined entire neighborhoods and made violence common.

5. Although not formally proven, there is reasonable probability that marijuana smoking damages the bronchial passages in the same way that smoking tobacco cigarettes does. Moreover, there are other adverse health effects related to smoking marijuana, including disruption of short-term memory, distortion of perception, difficulty in learning, potential disruption of both the female and male reproductive functions, and the development of a drug dependence.

6. Legalization of marijuana and other drugs that alter perception or intoxicate would pose a major threat to nonusers through incapacitating operators of motor cars, planes, buses, and other types of machinery. One of the worst railroad tragedies in the United States occurred in January 1987 when two trains collided north of Washington, D.C. The accident, now attributed to marijuana-impaired engineers on one of the trains, resulted in the deaths of 16 passengers and injuries to another 175 people.

7. The alleged benefits of legalizing marijuana—the decrease in or disappearance of drug-related crime and the anticipated increased income for governments from taxes on cannabis products—are wishful thinking at best and desired outcomes that might never become reality. Once legalized, marijuana could lose its appeal, and illicit dealers would work harder to boost the market for cocaine and heroin. However, the illicit market for marijuana would persist for underage teenagers and children. And while

taxes collected on marijuana products might be significant, the economic gain must be weighed against the likely increase in compulsive drug use and drug-related problems.

8. Present law enforcement efforts have not been applied forcefully enough. Consequently, such efforts cannot be dismissed as ineffective or even counterproductive.

Antiparaphernalia Laws

Recent reaction to widespread marijuana use by young people has taken the form of **antiparaphernalia laws.** The term paraphernalia refers to items related to the use of illegal recreational drugs, such as pipes, bongs, roach clips, spoons, and roll-your-own cigarette papers. In many communities, local ordinances have been passed controlling or banning paraphernalia sales and the advertising of such accessories, usually sold at specialty shops ("head" shops) and some record stores.

Several states have also passed such antiparaphernalia laws. However, these statutes, along with local ordinances and proposed federal legislation against drug accessories, have been challenged as unjust or ineffective. Critics of such measures argue that these laws are akin to outlawing bottles and glasses to combat alcoholism.

The Current Scene

The marijuana of today is quite different from the cannabis available only a few years ago. Improved breeding techniques have resulted in American-grown marijuana that is many times stronger than the commonly used variety in the 1960s and 1970s. Average potency has increased from just 1 or 2 percent nearly twenty years ago to an average THC (tetrahydrocannabinol) concentration of 3 to 8 percent or even 10 percent. (THC is the main psychoactive ingredient in marijuana.) Marijuana cigarettes or "joints" that formerly contained 20 milligrams of THC now routinely contain 40 mg or more. And hashish samples typically are 100 times more potent than their earlier counterparts.

Because much of the research on the effects of marijuana has been based on users smoking less-powerful varieties of marijuana, many findings and conclusions may have little relevance to the use of stronger cannabis now prevalent in the domestic market.

The hazards of use are also somewhat controversial and ambiguous, because many of the adverse reactions were studied using an animal model, rather than a human one. Other factors complicating the interpretation of research studies are the youthfulness and generally healthy status of most marijuana users, and the common practice of many users of combining cannabis smoking with alcohol or tobacco use.[11]

Presently, marijuana is the number one illegal drug used in America. This psychoactive drug has become a common part of our social scene, with more than an estimated 67 million people having used either marijuana or hashish at least once in their lifetimes. Millions currently use marijuana on a monthly basis. Once again young people are increasing their use of marijuana, after nearly a decade of declining use rates. While alcohol remains the students' drug of choice, three times as many high school seniors report smoking marijuana on a daily basis than report daily beer drinking.[12] For young people, recreational use often begins as early as elementary school, and it has now spread to all age and socioeconomic groups, regardless of educational attainment and career preference.

In the past several years, large-scale production of marijuana in the United States has quadrupled the domestic pot crop. American-grown marijuana now accounts for at least 25 percent of all marijuana used in this country.[13] However, the bulk of marijuana used still comes from Mexico, Latin America, and countries in Southeast Asia, such as Thailand.

Domestically, marijuana is grown in small plots, and frequently in greenhouses by individual growers, or in large urban warehouses where plants are cultivated hydroponically (without soil). Outdoor plots are usually located in remote areas and have been found in some of our national parks and forests.[14] Marijuana is now one of this country's largest cash

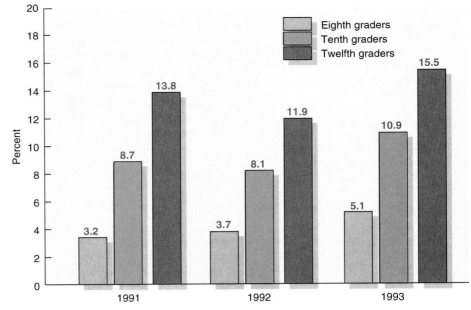

Past month use of marijuana by eighth, tenth, and twelfth graders, 1991–1993

Eighth graders
Tenth graders
Twelfth graders

figure **10.1**

Once again, marijuana use is increasing among young people after a decade of decline.

Sources: Data from National Survey Results on Drug Use from Monitoring the Future Study, 1975–1992, Volume I, Secondary School Students, *University of Michigan Institute for Social Research and National Institute on Drug Abuse, and U.S. Department of Health and Human Services, 1994; graph from* National Drug Control Strategy, *Office of National Drug Control Policy, 1994.*

crops and enriches the economies of several states, including California, Kentucky, and Hawaii.

New forms of marijuana use have also become evident. Alcohol and pot combinations are now common. Sometimes other illicit drugs, such as PCP, cocaine, hashish, and opium, are mixed with marijuana. In some communities, marijuana has also been laced with various insecticides and sold on the street as "Wac"—a preparation linked with psychiatric symptoms. Marijuana that has been soaked in formaldehyde and allowed to dry—a combination known as AMP—has effects common to both marijuana and PCP or phencyclidine intoxication. This toxic concoction has produced some very serious mental disturbances in users.

Once considered a "status" drug, a "cool" drug, and a relatively mild and harmless euphoriant, marijuana is now recognized as having a serious potential impact on social functioning and especially on physical health. Moreover, long-term heavy use has often been

related to the subsequent abuse of other illegal drugs. Consequently, marijuana is often called a "gateway" drug, because its frequent use has been the single best predictor of eventual cocaine use during adolescence. However, according to prominent drug-abuse experts, there is no convincing evidence for or against this "stepping-stone hypothesis"—that marijuana smoking leads to the use of other illicit psychoactive drugs.[15] Although almost everyone who uses any other illegal drug has smoked marijuana first, most marijuana smokers do not use cocaine or heroin, just as most alcohol drinkers do not use marijuana.

Marijuana and THC

Typically, cannabis products are smoked in pipes or in loosely rolled homemade cigarettes called "joints." Marijuana and its extracts might be used alone as well as in combination with other drugs. They might also be taken orally—eaten alone or as an ingredient in food preparations.

table 10.1 Marijuana: An Alphabet Soup of Chemicals

Listed below are some of the major types or classes of the known chemical constituents of cannabis preparations. When marijuana is burned, many additional chemicals are formed and are found in both the gas phase and the particulate phase of marijuana smoke.

Acids, simple and fatty	Ketones, simple
Alcohols, simple	Lactones, simple
Aldehydes, simple	Nitrogenous compounds
Amino acids	Phenols, noncannabinoid
Cannabinoids	Pigments
Esters, simple	Proteins
Enzymes	Sugars
Flavonoid glycosides	Steroids
Glycoproteins	Terpenes
Hydrocarbons	Vitamins

Source: Derived from the Institute of Medicine and the Marihuana Project, University of Mississippi.

The several plant parts of cannabis that make up the marijuana mixture are very complex chemically (see table 10.1). At least 426 individual compounds have been identified, more than 60 of which are specific to cannabis.[16] Chemical compounds found only in cannabis are referred to as **cannabinoids.** Several of these are routinely measured in identifying cannabis samples. When marijuana is smoked, some of the chemicals contained in the mixture of dried plant particles are further changed into many other compounds in the process of burning. One of these "new" chemicals, benzopyrene, is known to be cancer-causing and is 70 percent more abundant in marijuana smoke than in tobacco smoke.

At present, the most active and principal mind-altering ingredient of marijuana is identified as delta-9-tetrahydrocannabinol, or **THC** for short. The amount of this specific cannabinoid is an indicator of the psychoactivity of a drug sample, although other chemicals may eventually prove to be important for their drug effects upon the human body or their interaction with THC itself. Though the THC content determines the potency of marijuana, THC occurs in various concentrations in different parts of the plant. Thus the amount of THC in marijuana sold on the street is influenced by the source and selectivity of plant materials, and also by the plant strain, climate, soil conditions, harvesting process, and any added ingredients to the mixture.

Nonpsychoactive catnip and oregano have been substituted for or added to mixtures of marijuana, while some cannabis preparations may have been sprayed with **paraquat.** Used throughout the world as a powerful herbicide or weed killer, paraquat causes temporary damage to the heart, kidneys, central nervous system, liver, skeletal muscles, and spleen. However, lung damage, caused by continuous smoking of large quantities of paraquat-contaminated marijuana, has proved clinically to be permanent and in some cases severely injurious. The changes in lung tissue after smoking appear to be dose related. Paraquat has been banned on public land since 1983 because of environmental concerns, but it is still sprayed on private lands by the federal government and even in some foreign nations.

In the United States, the THC content of marijuana varies from 2 percent up to 8 percent, with a high of 15 percent in some strains of sinsemilla—a seedless variety of marijuana with increased resin content rich in psychoactive cannabinoids. Preparations of such marijuana, with relatively higher levels of THC, contribute to higher levels of intoxication and potentially to more severe and adverse consequences. Therefore marijuana can no longer be viewed as an innocuous drug, the "harmless little giggle" John Lennon referred to during the 1960s.

When smoked, the THC is rapidly absorbed by the blood in the lungs and transported to the brain in less than thirty seconds. Effects of cannabis also appear quickly, both psychologically and physically, and reach their peak about the time smoking is completed. By contrast, if the same amount of THC were eaten, absorption would take much longer, and effects would develop more slowly (over 2 to 3 hours), would last longer, but could not be controlled after the marijuana had been swallowed.

In a short period of time, the liver begins to change THC to many chemical byproducts, known as metabolites. However, approximately 25 to 30 percent of the original THC compound, together with various cannabinoid metabolites, remain in the human body one week after the initial dose is taken. Research further reveals that, in a frequent user, complete elimination of a single dose may require at least one month after the last use, during which time marijuana residuals can be detected in urine.[17] Because of the fat solubility of THC and other cannabinoids, these compounds accumulate in the fatty tissues and are eliminated slowly from the human body.

Laboratory tests of urine and other body fluids have been utilized increasingly by business and industry, drug treatment programs, the military services, and parole and probation officials to determine if individuals have been using marijuana. Current state-of-the-art marijuana detection procedures reveal the following:[18–20]

1. Urine screening and confirmatory testing can detect THC metabolites with a fair degree of accuracy and reliability.

2. The Enzyme Multiplied Immunoassay Technique (EMIT) is the primary method for detecting marijuana, and the Gas Chromatography/Mass Spectrometry (GC/MS) procedure is considered the method of choice for confirming positive urine samples.

3. After smoking a single marijuana cigarette, a positive test can be expected in about two to three hours, with the highest urinary concentration at five to six hours.

4. The detection period for a positive urine test ranges from 5 to 7 days for

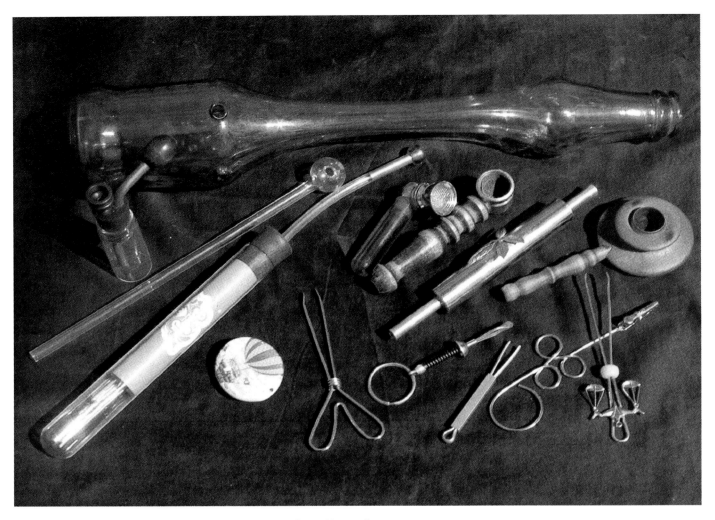

Cannabis paraphernalia, drug equipment or gadgets sold for use in smoking marijuana.

Drug Enforcement Agency.

casual use of up to four joints per week; 10 to 15 days for daily use; and one to two months for chronic heavy use.

5. A positive test has no relationship to marijuana intoxication (because THC metabolites do not usually appear in the urine until nearly two hours after smoking) and cannot distinguish between one time or regular use.

6. Urine tests cannot provide totally accurate results without confirmation.

7. An FDA-approved saliva test and a recently developed breath test can detect THC in persons for as long as three to five hours after they have smoked marijuana. Increasing use of hair analysis will now reveal a six-month history of drug use, including marijuana.

Although many problems have arisen with urine testing for marijuana—numerous false-positive test results and drug users who avoid detection by switching temporarily from pot to alcohol or cocaine—the effectiveness of preemployment drug screening for marijuana in predicting employment outcome has now been established.[21] Considerably less than previously estimated, those with marijuana-positive urine samples experienced 55 percent more accidents on the job, 85 percent more injuries, and a 78 percent increase in absenteeism. Moreover, for identified marijuana users, the relative risk for employment turnover was 56 percent. These rates are much less than earlier estimates, but it is quite evident that pre-employment drug screening that is positive for marijuana is associated with unfavorable employment outcome.

The Marijuana High

There is no doubt that the mind-altering effects of marijuana are the bases for its widespread popularity. Low to moderate doses tend to induce a sense of well-being and euphoria, and produce a feeling of relaxation, a dreamy state of sleepiness. This individually perceived, favorable response to marijuana intoxication is referred to as the **marijuana high**—peaking about thirty minutes after use and then disappearing altogether in two to four hours. Numerous behavioral and psychological effects have been reported, but they are often subjectively interpreted and influenced by several variables: (1) the *drug*—dose, type of preparation, route of administration, and grade or amount of THC present in any given dose; (2) the *marijuana user*—personality, psychological state, motivation, level of expectation or mind-set, and prior experience with the drug; and (3) the physical and psychosocial *setting* in which the use of the drug occurs. Nevertheless, when low social doses (one or two joints) are used, the effects of the high may go undetected by others, especially unknowing observers. As the THC concentration in marijuana increases, however, a low social dose may have some very observable effects.

Commonly reported reactions focus on changes in sensory perception, including sight, smell, taste, and hearing. The senses, in essence, seem to become more vivid. These experiences may be accompanied by alterations in thought formation and expression. Sometimes there may be shifting sensory imagery, rapid fluctuations of emotions, fragmentary thoughts with disturbed associations, and an altered sense of personal identity.[22] For some marijuana users, the body calms down to a quiet period of pleasurable introspection, while others develop a gregarious mood and engage in ridiculous conversation and laughter with friends.

Cannabis also tends to focus and intensify a person's concentration on the here and now. Regardless of its nature, the behavior or activity of the moment seems perfect to the user. Additionally, under the influence of marijuana, certain compulsions arise. Frequently reported are obsessive desires for food, especially sweets, and music—the louder and more rhythmic, the better.

While marijuana has not been clinically proven to be an aphrodisiac, there is a widely held belief that marijuana smoking enhances social effectiveness and heightens sexual pleasure. Marijuana use probably can reduce sexual inhibitions and enhance hearing, vision, and skin sensitivity—all of which are conducive to sexual enjoyment. However, it is fairly certain that cannabis preparations do not create sexual delights or passion. Like ethyl alcohol, too much marijuana can interfere with sexual performance and response, and might actually result in a loss of interest in sex.

Physical aspects of the high often include a temporary increase in heart and pulse rates, an increase in systolic blood pressure, and a marked reddening of the eyes.[23] Additional effects are a slight drop in body temperature, a decrease in intraocular pressure of the eye, and an increase in blood-plasma volume and in appetite.

Behavioral and Psychosocial Effects

In terms of immediate threat to one's life, marijuana is a relatively "safe" drug. There has never been a documented case of a lethal overdose due solely to marijuana. However, in some situations the pleasant effects of marijuana intoxication can be considered adverse and even dangerous. This is certainly true for the distorted perceptions that pose definite risks for driving motor vehicles or operating machinery. But there are other behavioral and psychological effects of using marijuana that pose additional risks for users.

Significantly more youth use alcohol than use marijuana. But unlike current drinkers, many more marijuana users report having bought and smoked this drug at or near school. This situation has raised a major, continuing concern about marijuana's effect on the learning process itself (see box 10.2).

Consider also those individuals who are receiving THC as therapy, but who are alarmed at the altered state of consciousness and perceived loss of control so frequently reported. As a consequence, for both practical and scientific interest, it is important to learn more about the effects of marijuana on the human brain and behavior.

Acute Effects

Changes in perceptual and psychomotor functions that can be seen after a single dose of marijuana are known as "acute effects." In general, these changes are related to THC's impact on the information-processing center of the brain, the limbic system, and the temporary disruption of the brain's neurotransmitters. Moreover, these effects are dose related; for example, low doses have small effects, whereas higher doses tend to have greater effects. Research has revealed numerous acute effects:[24–26]

1. *Motor coordination* is impaired; specifically, the drug affects hand steadiness, body sway, accuracy of carrying out body movements, and the ability to maintain postural stability. Although an individual under the influence of marijuana may feel graceful, he or she may become somewhat clumsy.

2. *Reaction time,* the time lag between a signal and a person's response to that signal, may be increased in some individuals, but not all. When intoxicated with marijuana, an individual is often less likely to pay attention to the reaction-time task of the moment.

3. *Tracking,* the act of following a moving stimulus, is significantly and consistently diminished. Tracking impairment often lasts for four to eight hours beyond the feeling of intoxication. Such a disability would interfere seriously with driving and flying skills.

4. *Signal or cue detection,* such as the ability to perceive a brief flash of light, is significantly impaired by low to moderate doses of smoked marijuana. This impairment of visual perception constitutes a major risk for users who operate machinery.

5. *Short-term memory* is diminished by a single moderate dose of marijuana. Remembering a sequence of numbers or memorizing and following a series of directions become most difficult to

accomplish. The memory deficit is particularly evident in acquiring and storing information, tasks that are dependent on attention.

6. *Time sense,* the ability to perceive accurately the passage of time, is adversely affected by moderate doses of marijuana. Users consistently overestimate the amount of time that has elapsed.

7. *State-dependent learning* occurs with marijuana. That is, material learned while under the influence of the drug is remembered best in the state of drug intoxication in which it was originally learned. It should be noted quickly that the quality of learning and recall is almost always impaired because the user's ability to acquire the information or skill will be impaired while the user is intoxicated.

8. *Oral communication,* even in low to moderate doses, is impaired. Users' ability to conduct a sequential dialogue with others is adversely affected. By impairing short-term memory, marijuana disrupts the continuity of speech. The introduction of irrelevant words and ideas into conversation further interferes with communication skills of speaking.

Automobile Accidents

Early studies comparing the relative effects of alcohol and marijuana on driving skills indicated that ethyl alcohol was by far the greater threat to highway safety. Of course, the marijuana used in those tests was considerably less potent than the marijuana commonly available today. Nonetheless, the potential effects of marijuana were minimized, and many people concluded that marijuana was somehow safe.

To complicate the marijuana/driving issue, the relationship between the drug's effects and driving skills has been less clearly established than for alcohol.[27] Moreover, there is no evidence today that marijuana use leads to increased aggressiveness. By

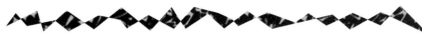

Developmental and Psychosocial Concerns Associated with Using Marijuana

box 10.2

1. Use of marijuana may impair or reduce
   - short-term memory,
   - comprehension,
   - concentration, and
   - attention span, with adverse effects on learning ability in both young people and adults.

2. While marijuana-intoxicated, users may display indicators of impaired psychological functioning, including
   - disjointed thinking and fragmented speaking,
   - reduced problem-solving ability, and
   - difficulty with concept formation.
   Most of these effects seem to share in common an impairment of short-term memory, which in turn can lead to a loss in one's train of thought.

3. Because marijuana use can contribute to
   - social withdrawal and
   - general lack of motivation,
   preteens and adolescents are disabled in forming their personal identities as they disengage from childhood attachments and parental controls to form new relationships and values.

4. As teenagers and young adults begin to experience heightened sexual awareness and develop their gender identities, use of marijuana can disrupt this important developmental process and cause severe sexual anxiety.

5. Many health care providers and medical organizations, including the American Academy of Pediatrics, now believe that marijuana, by providing a convenient chemical escape from normal "growing pains," can prevent young people from learning to become mature, independent, and responsible adults.

Source: Derived from the National Institute on Drug Abuse, and *Marijuana: Your Child and Drugs,* 2, American Academy of Pediatrics, 1986.

contrast, the aggressive tendencies of many who drive under the influence of alcohol are well publicized.

The issue of driving under the influence of marijuana is further complicated by the fact that numerous experienced marijuana users learn somehow to compensate for the drug's actions.[28] In some situations, these individuals appear not to be influenced by marijuana even when they are. This compensation phenomenon, which appears with other drugs, too, has perplexed researchers. However, the ability to override the effects of a drug does not confer any degree of safety on marijuana. Recent research proves otherwise.

Teenagers who are inexperienced drivers and who smoke marijuana as often as six times a month are more than twice as likely to be involved in traffic accidents.[29] In a study of accident victims admitted to a shock trauma unit in Baltimore, Maryland, one-third of all admitted patients had detectable levels of marijuana in their blood, indicating use of the drug within two to four hours prior to admission. Reported by the National Institute on Drug Abuse, this study also found that four of every ten persons 30 years of age or younger were under the influence of marijuana at the time of the accident.

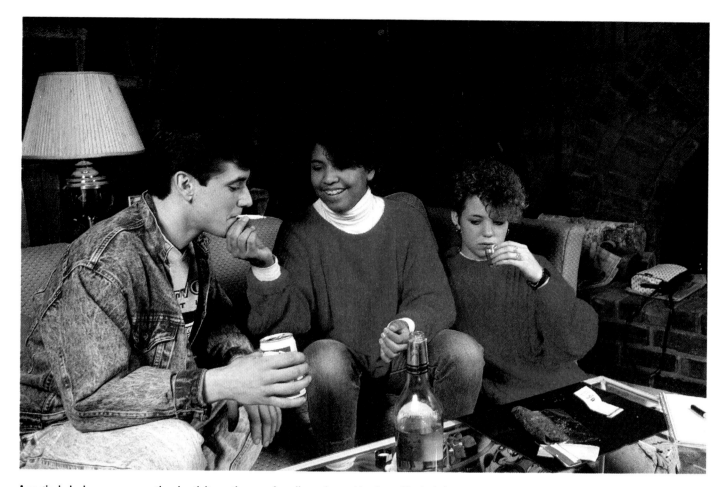

A particularly dangerous recreational activity—the use of marijuana in combination with alcohol—especially if such use occurs prior to driving.

© Mark M. Walker/The Picture Cube

In spite of the many variables associated with the impact of marijuana on human behavior, there is good evidence that the use of marijuana even at typical social levels definitely impairs driving ability and related skills. The marijuana user displays the common signs of what is now called "marijuana intoxication," a condition of euphoria accompanied by impaired motor coordination, anxiety, sensation of slowed time, impaired judgment, social withdrawal, memory and concentration impairment, psychological confusion, and feelings of fuzziness and dizziness.[30, 31]

Studies indicating such impairment were conducted with laboratory-based driving simulators, on "closed test" driving courses, in actual surveys of accidents, and in questioning marijuana users. In relation to operating a motor vehicle, the use of social levels of marijuana consistently

impaired motor coordination, i.e., specific car-handling skills of braking, steering, and tracking;

decreased consciousness of external stimuli, particularly flashing lights and other cues;

impaired judgment and concentration ability;

resulted in marijuana users' receiving higher-than-average numbers of tickets for driving violations and being involved in a higher-than-average number of auto accidents; and

caused the user to overestimate amounts of time that had elapsed.

The combination of these effects adds up to a severe reduction in driving abilities. Overconcentration and a shortened memory span will prevent detection of warning signals, and the adverse effects on time sense, and possibly depth perception and reaction time, can create confusion about traffic movement and appropriate drivers' responses. Just as alarming is the likelihood that the detrimental effects on driving skills may last several hours beyond the time when users experience either euphoria or sleepiness.

Another dangerous practice is the use of marijuana in combination with alcohol prior to or while driving. Such a combination will likely result in greater risks of accident than those posed by either substance alone.

Anxiety/Panic Reaction

Although the mind-altering effects of marijuana make its use attractive, some users report experiencing bad trips—anxiety/panic reactions perceived as unpleasant or undesirable. About one-third of regular users have reported that, while intoxicated, they experienced the most common disturbing reaction to marijuana—sudden panic, fears of dying or going insane, and paranoid thoughts (feelings of being ridiculed or persecuted). Sometimes, this anxiety/panic reaction is referred to as a delusional disorder, but it is not usually considered a cannabis psychosis. Hallucinations do not typically develop. While first-time users are more likely to have these adverse reactions, regular users also report that anxiety, fear of losing control, confusion, dependency feelings, and aggressive urges are common occurrences.

Such adverse reactions to marijuana are observed in subjects of laboratory experiments as well as reported by users themselves. Medical treatment is not usually needed, although thousands of people on marijuana seek assistance in hospital emergency rooms each year. People experiencing these anxiety/panic reactions need reassurance and calming support from friends or caregivers while waiting out this frightening period. The duration of these incidents ranges from only a few minutes to a few hours. Such undesirable reactions—milder versions of an LSD bad trip—generally decline after use of the drug is stopped.

While truly nightmarish experiences are rather rare, more-concentrated forms of marijuana have produced occasional psychedelic effects and even prolonged episodes that some describe as a "cannabis psychosis" with hallucinations, delusions, and acute schizophrenia in which thoughts and feelings do not relate to each other logically. More serious reactions have also been observed: (1) dysphoric reaction—severe anxiety, restlessness, and agitation—among the elderly on therapeutic doses of THC; and (2) acute brain syndrome—impaired attention span, memory, perception, and sleep pattern—in people who use cannabis products with extremely high levels of THC.

Tolerance and Dependence

Frequent, continuous use of most psychoactive drugs leads to the condition of *tolerance,* a diminished response to a repeated dose. A state of increased drug resistance, tolerance is related to (1) reduced sensitivity of target nerve cells to the drug's effects; and (2) probable increased rate of drug metabolism or elimination which lowers drug concentrations at sites of action. Tolerance to marijuana can occur under conditions of heavier, more regular use.[32] However, this condition does not appear to be a serious problem with most marijuana users, who appear to endure higher levels of marijuana without experiencing the severe mental and emotional effects often reported by first-time users.

Physical dependence, the likely result of temporary and compensatory changes in the human nervous system, is manifest by withdrawal signs and symptoms. The combination of these observable signs and individual complaints is known as the *withdrawal* or *abstinence syndrome* and appears following discontinuation of regular marijuana use. Marijuana's rather mild withdrawal syndrome includes restlessness, irritability, mild agitation, decreased appetite, sweating, insomnia, sleep disturbances, nausea, and occasional vomiting and diarrhea. Fortunately, most of these signs and symptoms disappear within two days, and the syndrome itself is not considered life threatening.

Although physical dependence can develop rapidly, the condition is usually associated with situations in which marijuana or THC doses were maintained at constant levels not typically seen in occasional social use. Notably, cannabis dependence does *not* necessarily equate with compulsive behavior to use more marijuana.

Nevertheless, there is now clinical evidence of a condition referred to as "primary marijuana addiction."[33] This disorder is occurring among people who have been smoking marijuana for more than fifteen years and have never perceived such behavior as dangerous, because of long periods of controlled use. Dosing themselves with progressively more-potent marijuana, these individuals report being sapped of their motivation, having undergone a deterioration of their sex life, and becoming chronically depressed mentally. This "addiction" is also characterized by loss of control over marijuana use, craving and obsession, continued use despite adverse consequences, and denial of problem usage. But unlike other drug addictions, marijuana does not present sudden and dramatic personality shifts, and withdrawal rarely requires hospitalization.

Passive Marijuana Smoking

Passive or involuntary smoking—inhaling secondhand, sidestream smoke from the burning tobacco products of others—is now associated with increased health risks, including lung cancer, as well as with indoor air pollution. Now research is being undertaken to learn if passive marijuana smoking also contributes to undesirable health and behavioral effects among nonusers of cannabis.

Since much of marijuana smoking occurs in closed and poorly ventilated environments, nonsmokers who are present sometimes experience mild forms of involuntary intoxication and discomfort in breathing. Some nonsmokers who associate with marijuana users might develop a sensitivity to secondhand marijuana smoke, experience a "contact high," and then become nauseated. It is likely that passive marijuana smoking is a potential threat to the safety and well-being of nonsmokers, as it is to smokers themselves.

Chronic Effects: Areas of Concern

Described in this section are various changes that can develop after prolonged marijuana use, as well as those that might continue even after use of cannabis preparations has stopped. Such persistent, lasting changes are termed "chronic," which means that they tend to be long-term in their duration.[34]

Amotivational Syndrome

There are few issues related to marijuana use that are more controversial than the so-called **amotivational syndrome,** a pattern of personality changes observed in some frequent users of marijuana. Generally characterized by apathy, lack of concern for the future, and loss of motivation, the syndrome tends to persist beyond the period of intoxication. Other aspects of the personality pattern include loss of ambition, loss of effectiveness, dullness, diminished ability to carry out long-term planning, difficulty in concentration, intermittent confusion, impaired memory, and a decline in work or school performance. When regular use stops, the syndrome usually disappears over a period of several weeks.

Clinical observations and self-reports by marijuana users support the common occurrence of this condition. However, interpretation of the evidence linking marijuana to amotivational syndrome is quite difficult. This constellation of symptoms is also observed in nonmarijuana users, and daily use of marijuana is not always associated with loss of motivation. Even if there is an association between the syndrome and use of marijuana, such a relationship does not prove that the drug causes the syndrome.

At present, there is no evidence that marijuana produces such an "amotivational syndrome." On the contrary, young people who are depressed, have low expectations for themselves, and whose parents expect little of them are more likely than others to resort to continuing marijuana use. In addition, heavy drug users are typically bored, depressed, listless, alienated, cynical, and rebellious. Quite possibly, drugs—including marijuana—might cause these mental states, but sometimes these states of mind are what lead to, rather than result from, drug abuse.[35] As such, marijuana abuse can be viewed as either an excuse for failure or a form of self-medication. Persistent concern about amotivation remains something of a chicken-or-egg question.[36] It has not been definitely shown whether marijuana causes lack of motivation through its drug effects, or whether unmotivated people use pot as a symptom of alienation.

Although it is likely that both personal qualities and certain drug effects contribute to motivational problems among some frequent marijuana users, the repeated use of any sedating drug, such as marijuana, alcohol, or barbiturates, can be hazardous to adolescents as well as to adults. It should be noted that adolescents are undergoing a period of rapid physical, mental, and emotional change. Their views of themselves and the world about them are also changing radically. Adolescents are engaged in processes of questioning, searching, and testing that eventually will determine their career and lifestyle choices. They are learning many cognitive, psychological, and social skills. Failure to acquire these skills can impair their maturation.

For the reasons cited above, and in light of the increasing daily use of marijuana by younger and younger adolescents and preadolescents, hundreds of parents' groups have banded together to form the National Federation of Parents for Drug-Free Youth. Organized and highly vocal, this group has been increasingly influential in the field of drug-abuse treatment and prevention. The major concerns of this group have been to prevent marijuana use among young people and to enact antiparaphernalia laws on the local level. Many parents view marijuana use as psychological escapism that interferes with growing up and becoming mature and responsible individuals.

Flashback

Self-reports indicate that some marijuana users experience an undesirable recurrence of the drug's intoxicating effects with no recent drug intake to explain the altered perceptions and disturbing emotions. This brief, spontaneous phenomenon is called a **flashback,** and it may range from mild puzzlement to full-blown panic. In some instances, marijuana reportedly has triggered LSD-type flashbacks in people with prior LSD experience. Although there is no pharmacological explanation of the flashbacks, reports of these somewhat frightening conditions tend to be consistent. It is probable that these bizarre effects have a

psychological origin. Such occurrences might be post-traumatic reactions when the drug user is fatigued or emotionally stressed.

Mental Illness

Available data indicate that marijuana use neither causes nor worsens mental illness. As with several other drugs, though, clinical reports show a temporary association between cannabis products and the return of mental symptoms. Marijuana appears to enhance the resurfacing of *preexisting* mental disorders. Patients with a history of schizophrenia, mood disorders, and depression may be especially sensitive to marijuana's effects. Sometimes the "renewed" emotional disturbances are quite severe.

The Brain

While the most clearly established effects of cannabis are upon behavior, there is considerable controversy about whether marijuana causes changes in brain structure or brain cells. Postmortem studies of rhesus monkeys trained to smoke marijuana daily for several months revealed dramatic changes in brain structures at the cellular level and even in synapses.

Animal research sponsored by the National Institute on Drug Abuse also suggests that long-term THC exposure damages and destroys nerve cells and causes other pathological changes in the brain. If this situation can be applied to humans, then mild functional losses due to aging might interact with the effects of marijuana and possibly place long-term users at risk for serious or premature memory disorders as they age.

Use of the electroencephalogram, or EEG, has demonstrated slight changes in the electrical activity of the brain as a result of marijuana use. Apparently, these functional changes do not persist when drug use is discontinued. Further brain studies suggest that marijuana does not appear to increase a person's susceptibility to epileptic seizure. The significance and clinical relevance of other chemical changes in the brain related to use of marijuana are unknown at this time. Nonetheless, the possibility of subtle and lasting alterations in brain function cannot be discounted with heavy and frequent marijuana use.

The Respiratory System

A major concern about marijuana smoking is its potential for harming the structure and function of the lungs. The unfiltered marijuana smoke is drawn into the lungs by way of the trachea, nasopharynx, bronchi, and alveoli—the "respiratory tree" of airway passages. Within the body, marijuana might be capable of assaulting not only the tissues of the lungs, but also specific self-cleansing and self-protective mechanisms that function in the lungs.

Unlike the tobacco cigarette, the marijuana cigarette often contains contaminants of unknown origin. Virtually the entire marijuana cigarette is smoked, and the smoke is held in the lungs for a much longer time than cigarette smoke is. Moreover, the marijuana smoke contains several chemicals similar to tobacco "tars" that contribute to lung cancer. Cigarette for cigarette, a marijuana "joint" contains about 50 percent more cancer-causing hydrocarbons than a tobacco cigarette.

Other than initial coughing, the short-term response to inhaled marijuana is *bronchodilation*, the opening of various airway passages of the lungs. With heavy, daily use of cannabis products, particularly hashish, long-term extensive inflammatory changes can be seen in lung tissue lining, and measurable airway obstruction occurs. Thus chronic exposure to marijuana smoke eventually leads to *bronchoconstriction*, the narrowing of the air passages. Such a condition impairs the lungs' ability to exhale air.

Scientists at the University of California, Los Angeles, have found that the daily use of just one to three marijuana cigarettes appears to produce approximately the same lung damage and potential cancer risk as smoking five times as many tobacco cigarettes. Biopsies of human lung tissues chronically exposed to marijuana smoke revealed abnormal cellular changes suggestive of precancerous and cancerous conditions. Results of this study also suggest that the way smokers inhale marijuana—more deeply, and holding it

At Issue

Shouldn't marijuana be legalized, since it really is safer than alcohol?

Point: Yes, indeed. Marijuana is relatively safer than alcohol in terms of its drug effects on the human individual and society. Marijuana is really a "tamed" drug, and does not cause a hundred thousand deaths each year—as does alcohol—and does not result in cirrhosis of the liver, "marijuanaism," or numerous other health problems now related to alcohol abuse. In addition, marijuana is not a contributing factor to half of all highway traffic deaths each year. Nor does pot contribute in any significant way to rape, spouse abuse, absenteeism, or any of the other social problems now associated with alcohol abuse in the United States. It is really strange that although marijuana is so much safer than alcohol, the former is illegal, while the latter is still legal.

Counterpoint: Wait just a minute! Such a description of marijuana sounds as if this mind-changing drug is practically harmless. Admittedly, alcohol is the "hardest" drug in terms of its total impact on both individuals and society in America. But marijuana is not without serious adverse consequences. And just because alcohol is legal does not mean that society needs or is ready for yet another legal psychoactive drug. Many people drink alcohol without getting "high," but getting "high" is generally the main purpose of smoking pot! Smoking marijuana presents a clear danger, especially since the potency of the THC content in the 1990s is several times greater than the THC content of samples available in the 1960s and 1970s. Because there are more cancer-causing agents in marijuana smoke than in tobacco cigarette smoke, some chronic marijuana users have now developed serious lung disease. We now know that marijuana can interfere with the body's immune response to various infections and diseases. And even small doses of pot can impair short-term memory function, distort perception, interfere with concentration, and degrade motor skills. Furthermore, long-term marijuana likely causes brain damage and changes in the brain similar to those that occur in aging. Such evidence of harmful consequences of use hardly justifies giving marijuana legal status. It may prove to be even more dangerous in the years ahead.

longer, than tobacco smoke—in addition to its chemical composition, increases the adverse physical effects. Experimental studies also indicate that the combination of tobacco and marijuana smoke is likely to have a greater cancer-causing potential than either substance used alone.

The Cardiovascular System

The term *cardiovascular* refers to the heart and blood vessels. Research indicates that during the marijuana high there are changes in the heart and circulation of the blood that are typical of stress. Marijuana increases the work of the human heart by increasing heart rate as much as 50 percent, and by moderately increasing blood pressure in some people. However, all research to date suggests that these changes are without permanently harmful effects on normal hearts and blood vessels. Marijuana's effects on the cardiovascular system are insignificant among healthy people, and even seem to become less severe following long-term exposure. Smoking marijuana while "shooting up" cocaine, however, has the potential to cause severe and rapid increases in both heart rate and blood pressure that could overload the cardiovascular system.

Another word of caution is in order. Any temporary increase in the workload of the heart poses a definite threat to patients with hypertension, cerebrovascular disease, and coronary atherosclerosis—serious disorders of the cardiovascular system. In individuals with heart disease, the use of marijuana may trigger chest pain (angina pectoris) more rapidly and following less effort than smoking tobacco does.

Reproduction and Sexual Function

The alleged effects of marijuana on human sexual function and reproduction have been reported widely in the media. Some of the research in these areas involved humans, but much of the scientific investigation has been conducted on animals. Thus the application of research findings to human physiology is somewhat uncertain and unclear.

Because of marijuana's effect on attention, some users proclaim the drug as an aphrodisiac that promotes sexual interest and improves sexual performance, whereas others admit to losing interest in sexual behavior. In contrast with these two extremes, other occasional users report no particular sexual effect whatsoever.

Various studies indicate that marijuana has a suppressive action upon the function of the testes in animals and men. A reduction in the weights of the prostate gland, seminal vesicle, and testis; reduced sperm production; and lowered levels of testosterone (the principal male sex hormone) have all been recorded following chronic use of cannabis or THC. Such effects are thought to be temporary and completely reversed one month after use of the drug is discontinued, because long-term reductions in male fertility and sexual performance have not been reported.

Additional research has not confirmed initial findings regarding lowered testosterone levels associated with marijuana use. In some experiments no change in blood levels of testosterone was recorded, whereas other research revealed an increase in hormone levels. Such conflicting and incomplete evidence prevents a definite statement on marijuana's effect upon testosterone. Still other studies have indicated that the sperm of chronic marijuana users are defective and nonfunctional. Decreased male fertility may be more closely related to abnormal sperm structure and impaired sperm movement than to reduced sperm count.

Few studies have been undertaken to determine the hormone profiles and menstrual patterns of women who use marijuana on a long-term and frequent basis. This situation is based on the several ethical issues surrounding research involving females of childbearing age. As a consequence, information on female reproductive and sexual functioning is particularly scarce.

The first controlled study in women on the acute effects of marijuana, reported by the National Institute on Drug Abuse, has shown that smoking marijuana after ovulation decreases the blood plasma level of luteinizing hormone (LH), essential for implantation of the fertilized egg in the uterus. A single dose of marijuana during the luteal phase of the menstrual cycle suppressed the level of luteinizing hormone and suggests the possibility that long-term use of marijuana may adversely affect reproductive functioning in women.

In studies of female animals, prolonged use of marijuana reduced the levels of FSH (follicle stimulating hormone) and suppressed the function of the ovaries, thereby stopping ovulation, production of estrogen and progesterone (the female sex hormones), and menstruation. The administration of THC also stopped the secretion of pituitary hormones affecting the ovaries.

Because it can cross the placenta of a pregnant female, THC is considered a potential **teratogen** (an agent that causes defects in a developing embryo). Initial reports indicate that low birth weight, prematurity, and a specific condition resembling fetal alcohol syndrome—the "fetal substance syndrome"—occur in some children of women who smoke marijuana heavily during pregnancy.

Earlier animal studies have revealed that crude marijuana extracts and THC are teratogenic at certain high-dose levels. Malformations of several body parts and organs of animals have been recorded, along with significant growth retardation. Because of the many unproven variables and the potential for harm, total abstention from marijuana seems most advisable for women during pregnancy. Smoking just one joint results in high-risk, prolonged fetal exposure to marijuana.

Widespread use of marijuana by young people in their reproductive years has generated real concern about the potential genetic effects of cannabis and its derivatives. When damaged or altered genes, known as **mutations,** occur in the reproductive cells, they can be transmitted to future generations by heredity. Animal studies have proven that marijuana smoke and tars can cause permanent changes in genes. Yet conflicting results of studies that link marijuana use with damaged chromosomes in white blood cells pose something of a genetic mystery for researchers. Chromosome breaks observed in earlier experiments could not be duplicated in later research.

Nevertheless, there is growing evidence that multiple-drug use, including marijuana, can induce mutations in genetic material and may adversely affect chromosome movement in cell division, resulting in abnormal numbers of chromosomes in daughter cells. Although this is worrisome, the clinical significance of these findings is not known at this time.

The Immune System

Various structural, cellular, and chemical defense mechanisms help protect the human body against assault. The mechanism that specifically protects an individual from disease-causing bacteria, viruses, molds, and toxins is the immune system. Animal studies indicate that THC has a mild, adverse, suppressant effect on the immune system, which would reduce the germ-fighting ability of the body. Human studies have produced contradictory results: Some marijuana users demonstrated a mild **immunosuppressive effect,** while other chronic marijuana smokers developed no significant differences in their immune systems in comparison with nonsmoking subjects.

Though a suppressant effect on the immune system has been produced in some experiments, there have been no human or animal studies indicating that marijuana smokers are more prone to infection or other diseases. If only a very weak suppression of the immune system were to exist, potential effects could be devastating, since so many people now use marijuana. Based on the likelihood that THC use can weaken the immune system, medical researchers are concerned that people who smoke marijuana may be predisposing themselves to more rapid development of end-phase acquired immune deficiency syndrome (AIDS) if they are infected with HIV. There is also an increased risk of bacterial pneumonia in marijuana smokers already infected with HIV.

In Conclusion

There is now sufficient evidence that marijuana has a broad range of physical, psychological, and behavioral effects, some of which can be harmful to human health. Available information does not yet indicate how serious the risk may be. Of growing concern is the realization that marijuana, its THC metabolites, and other cannabinoids remain in the human body up to thirty days or longer after smoking. How disruptive and health threatening these residual chemical compounds might be is still speculative.

According to the prestigious Institute of Medicine, what little is known for certain about the effects of marijuana on human health—and all that researchers have reason to suspect—justifies serious national concern. Although it does not appear to be as poisonous or lethal as ethyl alcohol, marijuana might eventually prove to be as life threatening as tobacco cigarettes.

By no means should marijuana be considered harmless or safe! In fact, some groups of individuals are at considerable risk of sustaining adverse effects of marijuana use. These include people who drive motor vehicles, fly airplanes, and operate machinery under the influence of marijuana; young people, particularly adolescents and preadolescents; those with a history of mental illness and depression; individuals who have sustained cardiovascular disease and/or lung disease, especially emphysema, lung cancer, and asthma; males with abnormal function of the testes; and pregnant females.

Medical Uses of Marijuana

For thousands of years, people have used marijuana for numerous medical purposes. It is probable that the ancient Chinese first employed the cannabis plant as a therapy; other cultures throughout history have followed. In the United States, until the Marijuana Tax Act of 1937 classified marijuana as an illegal narcotic and made the prescription of cannabis products difficult, marijuana was contained in nearly thirty medical products. As a pharmaceutical product, marijuana also fell into disfavor with the introduction of new, faster-acting, and dose-controlled synthetic drugs.

Modern scientific study of cannabis as a healing agent did not begin until the nineteenth century, but continued despite controversy until the early 1900s, when serious investigation of marijuana's therapeutic value was abandoned. Research was not resumed until cannabis and its derivatives emerged in the 1960s as popular, though illegal, "recreational" drugs.

In 1965, THC was totally synthesized and later proven to be the major psychoactive ingredient of marijuana. Then in 1985 the United States Food and Drug Administration (FDA) approved a version of this synthetic THC, called dronabinol. Marketed under the trade name Marinol, this synthetic THC was approved as a Schedule II controlled substance and prescription drug for relieving nausea accompanying cancer chemotherapy.[37] More recently, Marinol has also been designated an "orphan drug" by the FDA for use as a medication to stimulate appetite in AIDS patients, who often experience a severe loss of weight—evidence of the "wasting-away syndrome" or the "slim disease." (Orphan drug status is conferred on certain medicines to encourage pharmaceutical companies to develop drug treatments for rare diseases.)[38]

In reaction to both public and political pressure during the 1970s, the FDA and the Drug Enforcement Administration established a tightly controlled, experimental program to make not only THC capsules but also natural, cultivated marijuana cigarettes available to physicians who wanted to use marijuana as an antiemetic, a drug

that prevents nausea and vomiting. Although still classified as a Schedule I controlled substance, and therefore still illegal, marijuana is approved for medical use in thirty-four states.

Because the experimental federal program provided free cultivated marijuana to the seriously ill, legal efforts to give natural pot a legal status continue to the present time. In 1991, however, the U.S. Department of Health and Human Services began phasing out this approved medical use, because it undercut official administration policy against the use of illegal drugs. Although a very small number of patients already receiving marijuana will continue to do so, new applicants will be encouraged to try synthetic THC instead.

Marijuana allegedly has therapeutic effects for a number of disorders, including glaucoma, nausea and vomiting, asthma, epilepsy, muscle spasticity, anxiety, depression, pain, reduced appetite, and withdrawal from alcohol and narcotics. While marijuana's potential as a medical drug has been demonstrated in some of these areas, the dose needed to produce the desired therapeutic effect is often close to the amount that produces unacceptable and undesirable side effects.

However, cannabis has been found to exert its beneficial effects through mechanisms differing from those of other drugs. As a consequence, it is possible that some patients not helped by conventional therapies could be treated successfully with marijuana. Additionally, cannabis might be combined effectively and safely with other drugs to produce a treatment goal, but with each drug used at a much lower dose than would be required if either were used alone.

Glaucoma

The leading cause of blindness in the United States is glaucoma, a disease characterized by increased pressure within the eye. This pressure damages the optic nerve and leads eventually to loss of vision. When smoked, given intravenously, or taken orally, cannabis, THC, and other cannabinoid derivatives have been found to reduce the vision-threatening intraocular pressure of glaucoma. However, undesirable physical and psychological side effects have been demonstrated, especially among older patients. Recently, synthetic-THC eye drops have undergone testing with the hope that it can reduce unwanted side effects. Despite its beneficial effects for some patients, marijuana neither prevents glaucoma nor improves vision.

Chemotherapy-Caused Nausea and Vomiting

One of the more promising clinical uses of marijuana has been in the treatment of extreme nausea for patients undergoing cancer chemotherapy—the use of drugs to kill cancer cells. Because cancer chemotherapy can produce increased survival in patients with certain cancers, the nausea and vomiting that interfere with a person's willingness to continue therapy, in effect, become life-threatening side effects. THC and other cannabis derivatives have been proven effective in controlling these undesirable symptoms and are considered to be antiemetics—substances that tend to prevent nausea and vomiting. Some patients (especially older cancer patients), though, report having adverse anxiety/panic reactions, while others show little or no favorable antiemetic response.

However, marijuana may be losing ground as an antiemetic with the recent approval of a new, powerful, and effective antiemetic drug, odansetron, marketed as Zofran.[39] Odansetron produces no adverse side effects on functioning, no impairment of short-term memory, and no impairment of normal operation of a motor vehicle, as are sometimes experienced with medical marijuana.

Additional Medical Uses

Several actions of marijuana and its derivatives are presently being investigated for possible therapeutic applications. These are noted below:

Appetite stimulant—Social users often report that smoking marijuana increases the appetite. Research now suggests that there may well be a stimulating influence on food intake in advanced cancer patients who use marijuana as an antiemetic in conjunction with chemotherapy. Such an effect tends to overcome or reduce the severity of debilitating weight loss in such patients as well as in those with AIDS-related weight loss.

Anticonvulsant action—Limited human studies confirm results of animal research suggesting that specific components of marijuana—cannabinol and cannabidiol—protect against minimal and maximal seizures characteristic of epilepsy.

Antiasthmatic effect—As indicated earlier in this chapter, the long-term smoking of concentrated marijuana produces a constriction or obstruction of the airways. However, short-term smoking of cannabis and oral intake of THC have actually produced a bronchodilation effect in normal individuals and in patients with bronchial asthma. Cannabinoid compounds, such as cannabinol and cannabidiol, do not produce psychological effects or alterations in heart function commonly seen with marijuana itself. Therefore, these two compounds are potentially useful for their airway-expanding effect in the treatment of asthma.

Muscle-relaxant action—Limited studies suggest that THC is effective in relieving the muscle spasms or spasticity common in patients with multiple sclerosis.

Antianxiety effect—Although marijuana use often reduces anxiety, it sometimes produces undesirable psychological effects, including panic and anxiety. In addition, there is no indication that marijuana is any more effective or reliable than currently available antianxiety medicine.

Antidepressant effect—Presently, there is no controlled research indicating that marijuana reduces depression with any degree of consistency. Widespread use of marijuana for this reason would appear to be inappropriate.

Analgesic action—Test subjects demonstrating marijuana's analgesic (pain-relieving) effects also tended to experience "mental clouding" and other undesirable pharmacological effects. It is not likely that marijuana will be any more effective than currently available noncannabis analgesics.

Treatment for drug abuse—Research has failed to find marijuana useful in treating alcoholism. Moreover, there is no evidence at present that cannabis is likely to be more effective than currently available treatments for opiate withdrawal.

While marijuana has not been determined to be superior to any existing treatment for any of the conditions identified above, the therapeutic potential of cannabis and its derivatives merits continued research. The future could see "medical" marijuana approaching the popularity of "social" marijuana.

Chapter Summary

1. Marijuana is a derivative of the hemp plant, *Cannabis sativa*. Because at different dose levels it produces sedative, then psychedelic, effects, marijuana is a unique psychoactive drug.

2. Throughout history, the cannabis plant has had a variety of commercial and medical uses, in addition to its status as a recreational intoxicant.

3. The Marijuana Tax Act of 1937 effectively banned the nonmedical possession and use of cannabis preparations in America. Eventually, simple possession was reduced from a felony to a misdemeanor.

4. Several states decriminalized simple possession of small amounts of marijuana, thereby reducing the penalty to a minor misdemeanor or civil offense. However, the penalties

for trafficking remain harsh, and one state has already recriminalized possession.

5. Arguments in favor of legalizing marijuana and other illegal drugs of abuse are based on the high economic cost of prohibition and the war on drugs, the elimination of organized crime and violence linked with abused drugs, the desirability of taxing the legal drug trade for funding treatment programs, the reduced role of government in private lives of citizens, the reduced popularity of the legalized drug, an assurance of drug purity and dosage levels, and renewed respect for laws in general.

6. Arguments against legalizing marijuana and other illegal drugs of abuse are based on the opposition of most citizens to any changes in current antidrug law, the likelihood of creating more drug problems for both users and nonusers, increased health costs of legalized use, more drug-related accidents, limitations to the "right to privacy" principle, more anticipated health hazards for users, and the likely persistence of drug-related crime and black-market activities.

7. Antiparaphernalia laws control or prohibit the sale and/or advertising of marijuana-related items, such as pipes, bongs, roach clips, spoons, and roll-your-own cigarette papers.

8. Hundreds of chemicals have been identified in marijuana, but the principal psychoactive cannabinoid is THC. When marijuana is smoked, THC is readily absorbed by the blood in the lungs and transported rapidly to the brain. The THC content of today's marijuana is many times higher and more potent than that in marijuana samples during the 1960s and 1970s.

9. The marijuana "high" from low to moderate doses is a sense of well-being, euphoria, relaxation, and a dreamlike state. Common reactions include changes in sensory perception; alterations in thought formation, emotions, and personal identity; and pleasurable introspection or gregariousness.

10. Adverse "acute effects" relate to motor coordination, reaction time, tracking ability, cue detection, short-term memory, time sense, and oral communication.

11. The use of marijuana at typical social levels definitely impairs driving ability and related skills.

12. Some users report having bad trips, whereas frequent continuous use develops tolerance and non-life-threatening withdrawal, sometimes involving compulsive drug-seeking behavior.

13. Areas of concern related to long-term effects of using marijuana include the amotivational syndrome; flashback; resurfacing of preexisting mental disorders; potential for harming lung structure and function; temporary increase in workload of the heart; possible suppressant effect on testes, the male sex hormone, female reproductive function, and the human immune system; and potential for causing mutations.

14. Because THC is also a potential teratogen (an agent that causes defects in embryonic life), pregnant women are advised to abstain completely from marijuana.

15. Possible medical uses of marijuana include treating glaucoma, chemotherapy-caused nausea and vomiting, and AIDS-related weight loss.

Review Questions and Activities

1. What is marijuana, and how does it differ from cannabis, hashish, and sinsemilla?

2. In what ways was marijuana used among the ancient Chinese, ancient Indians, Americans up to 1940, and Americans after 1965?

3. Do you believe the Marijuana Tax Act of 1937 has been effective in restricting the nonmedical possession and use of cannabis preparations? Support your response.

4. If you could vote to prohibit, decriminalize, or legalize the possession of small amounts of marijuana for personal use, how would you vote? What factors might influence your vote?

5. If you were debating the desirability of legalizing all presently illicit drugs of abuse, what three arguments do you think would be most effective? Why? What three counterarguments to legalization or decriminalization would likely be most effective? Why?

6. What are the penalties in your state for possessing small amounts of marijuana for personal use?

7. Define the nature and purpose of antiparaphernalia laws. Are there any such laws in your community or state?

8. Why is the nonmedical use of marijuana so often regarded as a major drug problem and a threat to American society?

9. What is THC and what effect does it have on the marijuana user?

10. What factors influence the nature and intensity of the marijuana high?

11. Do you believe that using marijuana could have an adverse effect upon driving an automobile? Be specific in your response.

12. Explain what is meant by "state-dependent learning." Relate this phenomenon to using marijuana.

13. What evidence exists in support of the amotivational syndrome resulting from use of marijuana?

14. Compare the effects of smoking marijuana on the human respiratory system with the effects of smoking tobacco on the same body system.

15. Discuss the possible adverse effects that use of marijuana might have on human reproduction and sexual function.

16. What specific properties of marijuana make it useful as a therapeutic drug?

17. Based upon your own knowledge of your community or school/college, do you believe that the use of marijuana constitutes a major drug problem? What evidence might be offered in support of your response?

18. Can you identify any popular entertainment figures who promote or encourage the use of marijuana or other drugs? Do you think they are successful? What might their motives be?

19. Explain why so many people use marijuana despite its illegal status and controversial reputation.

References

1. H. Thomas Milhorn, *Drug and Alcohol Abuse* (New York: Plenum Press, 1994), 301.

2. Ernest L. Abel, *Marihuana: The First Twelve Thousand Years* (New York: Plenum Press, 1980).

3. Edward R. Bloomquist, *Marijuana: The Second Trip,* rev. ed. (Beverly Hills, Calif.: Glencoe Press, 1971), 14–15.

4. J. Terry Parker, ". . . And the Grass Keeps Growing: A Brief History of Marijuana Use through the 1600s," *Eta Sigma Gamman* 20, no. 2 (Spring 1989): 17–19.

5. National Commission on Marihuana and Drug Abuse, *Marihuana: A Signal of Misunderstanding* (Washington, D.C.: U.S. Government Printing Office, 1972), 29.

6. ABC News, *This Week with David Brinkley* [transcript of a telecast on 17 December 1989] (New York: Journal Graphics, 1989).

7. Barry Stimmel and the Editors of Consumer Reports Books, *The Facts about Drug Use: Coping with Drugs and Alcohol in Your Family, at Work, in Your Community* (New York: Haworth Medical Press, 1993), 312.

8. Ethan Nadelmann, "America's Drug Problems: A Case for Decriminalization," in *Taking Sides: Clashing Views on Controversial Issues in Drugs and Society,* ed. Raymond Goldberg (Guilford, Conn.: Dushkin, 1993), 4–14.

9. Eliot Marshall, *Legalization: A Debate* (New York: Chelsea House, 1988), 95–107.

10. James Wilson, "Against the Legalization of Drugs," in *Taking Sides,* ed. Goldberg, 15–25.

11. Leo Hollister, "Drugs of Abuse," in *Basic and Clinical Pharmacology,* ed. Bertram Katzung, 4th ed. (Norwalk, Conn.: Appleton & Lange, 1989), 392.

12. "Kids Say They Use Pot More Frequently than Alcohol," *Alcoholism and Drug Abuse Weekly* 5, no. 19 (10 May 1993): 4.

13. Drug Enforcement Administration, *Domestic Cannabis Eradication/Suppression Program* (Washington, D.C.: U.S. Department of Justice, 1992), 1.

14. Office of Justice Programs, Bureau of Justice Statistics, U.S. Department of Justice, *Drugs, Crime, and the Justice System* (Washington, D.C.: U.S. Government Printing Office, 1992), 50.

15. Lester Grinspoon and James Bakalar, *The Harvard Medical School Mental Health Review: Drug Abuse and Addiction* (Boston: Harvard Mental Health Letter, 1993), 32.

16. Tibor Palfai and Henry Jankiewicz, *Drugs and Human Behavior* (Dubuque, Iowa: Brown & Benchmark, 1991), 452.

17. Stimmel and others, *The Facts about Drug Abuse,* 126.

18. Sidney Cohen, "Marijuana Use Detection: The State of the Art," in *The Substance Abuse Problem.* Vol. 2: *New Issues for the 1980s* (New York: Haworth Press, 1985), 35–39.

19. Datafax Information Series, *Urine Testing* (Tempe, Ariz.: Do It Now Foundation, 1990), 2.

20. Darryl Inaba and William Cohen, *Uppers, Downers, All Arounders,* 2d ed. (Ashland, Ore.: CNS Productions, 1993), 222–28.

21. Craig Zwerling, James Ryan, and Endel Orav, "The Efficacy of Preemployment Drug Screening for Marijuana and Cocaine in Predicting Employment Outcome," *Journal of the American Medical Association* 264, no. 20 (28 November 1990): 2639–43.

22. Drug Enforcement Administration, U.S. Department of Justice, *Drugs of Abuse* (Washington, D.C.: U.S. Government Printing Office, 1989), 45.

23. Jerome Jaffe, "Drug Addiction and Drug Abuse," chapter 22 in *Goodman and Gilman's The Pharmacological Basis of Therapeutics,* 8th ed., ed. A. G. Gilman, T. W. Rall, A. S. Nies, and P. Taylor (New York: McGraw-Hill, 1990), 550.

24. Council on Scientific Affairs, American Medical Association, "Marijuana: Its Health Hazards and Therapeutic Potentials," *Journal of the American Medical Association* 246, no. 16 (16 October 1981): 1823–27.

25. Committee to Study the Health-Related Effects of Cannabis and Its Derivatives, Institute of Medicine, *Marijuana and Health* (Washington, D.C.: National Academy Press, 1982), 26–27, 112–28.

26. National Institute on Drug Abuse, "Marijuana Update," *NIDA Capsules,* May 1989, 1–3.

27. Gail Winger, Frederick Hofmann, and James Woods, *A Handbook on Drug and Alcohol Abuse: The Biomedical Aspects,* 3d ed. (New York: Oxford University Press, 1992), 125.

28. Andrew Weil and Winifred Rosen, *From Chocolate to Morphine,* rev. ed. (Boston: Houghton Mifflin, 1993), 121.

29. Harold Doweiko, *Concepts of Chemical Dependency,* 2d ed. (Pacific Grove, Calif.: Brooks/Cole, 1993), 101.

30. American Psychiatric Association, *Diagnostic and Statistical Manual of Mental Disorders,* 4th ed. (Washington, D.C.: American Psychiatric Association, 1994), 218.

31. Norman Miller, *The Pharmacology of Alcohol and Drugs of Abuse and Addiction* (New York: Springer-Verlag, 1991), 200.

32. Robert Julien, *A Primer of Drug Action* (New York: W. H. Freeman, 1992), 283.

33. "Marijuana Addiction: The Legacy of the '60s?" *Substance Abuse Report* 22, no. 5 (1 March 1989): 1–2.

34. Committee to Study the Health-Related Effects of Cannabis and Its Derivatives, *Marijuana and Health,* 57–106, 124–26.

35. Grinspoon and Bakalar, *The Harvard Medical School Mental Health Review: Drug Abuse and Addiction,* 31–32.

36. Christina Dye, *Marijuana: Personality and Behavior* (Tempe, Ariz.: Do It Now, 1994), 3.

37. Jim Parker, *Marijuana: Medical Uses* (Tempe, Ariz.: Do It Now, 1994), 3–4.

38. "Synthetic THC Approved for Treatment of AIDS-Related Weight Loss, *Substance Abuse Report* 22, no. 6 (15 March 1991): 5.

39. "Survey: Other Drugs Better Than Marijuana and Marinol for Nausea," *Substance Abuse Report* 25, no. 11 (1 June 1994): 7.

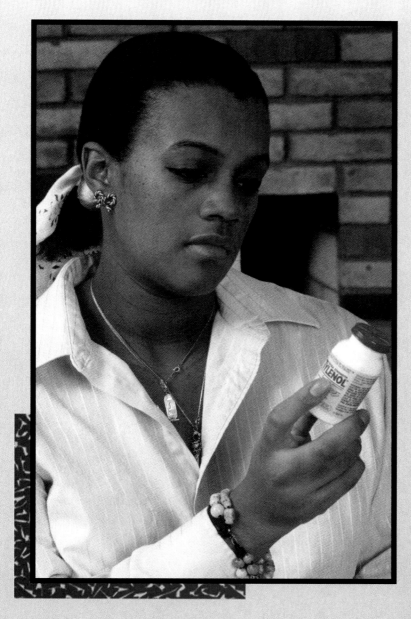

Questions of Concern

1. Why do so many people believe so firmly in the concept of fail-safe medication?

2. What factors really influence the selection and purchase of specific over-the-counter drugs?

3. How much government control is needed to assure drug-consuming patients that medicines are safe and effective?

counte
drugs
over-th
counte

chapter

11 over-the-counter drugs

Acetaminophen
Adverse Drug Reaction
Analgesic
Antihistamine
Appetite Suppressant
Aspirin
Brand-Name Drug
Caffeinism
Drug Misuse
Fixed-Ratio Combination Product
Food and Drug Administration (FDA)
Generic Drug
Ibuprofen
Naproxen Sodium
Nonsalicylates
NSAID
Over-the-Counter (OTC) Drug
Prescription Drug
Reye's Syndrome
Salicylates
Salicylism
Self-Limiting Condition
Self-Medication
Side Effect
Sleep Aid
Stimulant

chapter objectives

After you have studied this chapter, you should be able to do the following:

1. Explain how the use of medications can present a significant potential hazard to a drug taker's health.

2. Define the term *drug misuse*, and list several examples of such a drug-taking practice.

3. Distinguish between over-the-counter and prescription drugs in terms of their procurement, conditions of use, powerfulness, and potential for meeting individual needs of patients.

4. Compare and contrast the general drug actions or uses of the following drug classes: anorectal products, antibacterials, dermatologicals, diarrhea preparations, emetics, and nausea medications.

5. List the major anticipated effects of the following types of OTC drugs: analgesics, antipyretics, sleeping aids, stimulants, decongestants, and antihistamines.

6. Describe the similarities and differences between salicylate and nonsalicylate analgesics.

7. Define the following terms as they relate to OTC drugs: *salicylism, caffeinism, fixed-ratio combination product*, and *starch blockers*.

8. List at least eight guidelines for wise and relatively safe use of OTC drugs in the process of self-medication.

9. Distinguish between a drug "side effect" and an "adverse reaction" to a drug.

10. Identify at least eight different items of information that must be listed on the labels of OTC medications.

11. Explain why some drugs might remain on the market despite the conclusion of the FDA OTC drug-review process that their effectiveness is doubtful.

Introduction

This chapter provides a consumer's guide to the use of over-the-counter (OTC) drugs in America. In our country the practice of self-medication is common and often beneficial, but because OTC drugs are used so widely, there is also considerable drug misuse in the general population.

Early in the chapter a distinction is made between over-the-counter drugs and those prescribed by a physician. Then a classification of OTC drugs is presented with a description of various drug classes or types, based upon the primary function of drug products in relieving minor symptoms of illness.

Several major OTC drug classes frequently used by adults are examined in detail: analgesics, appetite suppressants, cold preparations, sleep aids, and stimulants. To promote the safe and beneficial use of OTC drugs, several guidelines for sensible use are also provided. A final section on the safety and effectiveness of nonprescribed drug products offers a special message to all people who engage in self-medication and are concerned about their health.

Our Fascination with Drugs

Influenced by advertising on television and radio and in the print media, many individuals firmly believe that some miracle

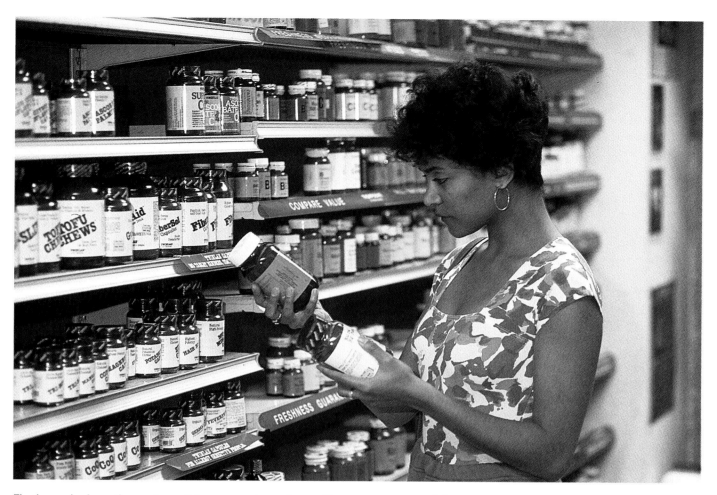

The thousands of over-the-counter medicines present the purchaser with numerous consumer choices in selecting nonprescribed drugs. What factors influence your purchase of OTC medicines?

© David Young-Wolff/PhotoEdit

drug is available for almost every human ailment. Many also feel that if a physician's treatment is to be effective, the therapy must include the use of some drug. These beliefs have achieved the status of national expectations and are reflected in the continuing demand for medicines. And legitimate, reputable drug manufacturers have responded in kind to this persistent demand with hundreds of thousands of drug products designed to relieve, cure, and prevent illness.

In addition to the large quantities of illegally produced and marketed drugs, billions of doses of physician-prescribed medicines and those purchased for self-treatment are used each year. Recent estimates of prescription drug sales exceed $49.2 billion annually, and Americans spend another $28 billion on nonprescription drugs each year.[1] The price tag for our national "pill-popping" is considerable indeed, and it is even higher when we take into account the human cost of the millions of drug-induced adverse reactions that occur each year in the United States.

Drugs, nevertheless, remain popular because they can have wonderful effects upon the human body and mind. The drugs in medicines can aid in the diagnosis of illness; they can also be used to relieve symptoms of disease, including pain and fever. Some drugs are used to kill or inactivate disease-causing microorganisms; others—vaccines and toxoids—are employed to prevent disease. Drugs in some medications can slow down or speed up body functions, as well as suppress them entirely, as seen in the effect of oral contraceptives on the process of ovulation. While some diseases can be cured by drugs, others, including epilepsy and diabetes, can only be controlled.

However, healing and disease-preventing drugs, especially those taken by mouth, also involve potential risks. Sometimes drugs taken with the intention of restoring or improving health can harm the body and endanger life itself, as described in earlier chapters. Depending upon their use, certain drugs can act as poisons and intoxicants, alter the effects of other medications, and cause some very undesirable and unanticipated side effects, including adverse drug reactions and drug dependencies.

People have continued to spend billions of dollars for nonprescription drugs despite the fact that the U.S. Food and Drug Administration recently identified—and then banned—over two hundred ingredients as ineffective.[2] In addition, evidence of improper labeling, listing of ineffective drugs as active ingredients, and inadequate warnings about proper use and possible adverse reactions all suggest that safety and effectiveness are not guaranteed absolutely.[3] Although a drug may be "generally recognized as safe" (GRAS), it isn't necessarily safe for everyone. And a drug "generally recognized as effective" (GRAE) is not guaranteed to be completely effective for everyone. Those most at risk are the very young, the elderly, pregnant women, and patients being treated for long-term diseases.

In part, the continuing demand for OTC drugs reflects a national ethic of impatience with any frustration and of insistence on an instant "fix" for every possible discomfort. Frequent victims of advertising tactics, American consumers also continue to buy drugs for imagined illnesses or to calm basic insecurities or fear of pain. But after the purchase is made, at least one in five individuals takes nonprescription medicines without ever reading the product label! Thus, many people buy drugs that not only do them little good but could actually cause them harm. Thus, the very use of medicines constitutes one of the greatest potential hazards to drug takers' health, as well as to their pocketbooks.

Equally alarming and life-threatening is the occurrence of **drug misuse,** the widespread inappropriate use of medicines resulting in impaired physical, mental, emotional, or social well-being. Drug misuse involves taking medications in excess of recommended doses, not following directions regarding time intervals between doses or other conditions of use specified on the drug label, and providing personally prescribed medicines to other individuals. (Other examples of drug misuse have been identified in chapter 1.) Sometimes the drug misuser is lucky and no adverse reactions occur. On occasion, though, such drug-misuse practices can have tragic consequences.

Over-the-Counter Versus Prescribed Drugs

As determined by the federal **Food and Drug Administration (FDA),** drugs are classified into two basic groups: (1) *over-the-counter medicines*, and (2) *prescription medicines* (see box 11.1).

Over-the-counter, or **OTC, drugs** include that vast assortment of medications that can be purchased without a physician's prescription. Sometimes these drugs are also known as patent medicines. Nonprescription medicines are regarded as safe if consumers follow the directions and heed the required warnings on the label. In general, OTC drugs have a relatively low risk of causing toxicity (a poisonous condition) and a high margin of safety.

More than 300,000 OTC drugs are now on the market, and almost everybody has used them at one time or another. Typically these drugs are taken or applied on a temporary basis for conditions that do not warrant a visit to a physician.

OTC drugs are sold widely at pharmacies, supermarkets, and department stores. Such drugs include everything from a bar of antibacterial soap to a nighttime sleep aid, headache remedy, or antacid preparation. When directions and warnings on OTC drug labels are followed, most people can use the medicines with relative safety and with beneficial results.

However, OTC drugs rarely, if ever, cure any illness or disease. The major effect of these nonprescription drugs is to relieve minor symptoms of illness, such as headache or menstrual cramping. For example, a cold remedy might make a person feel more comfortable by reducing sniffles and sneezes, but the cold itself will last as long as it would with no medicine at all. In effect, many OTC medicines mask or cover up the signals from the body—the symptoms that usually alert people to take some corrective action. Therefore, OTC drugs should never be used on a regular basis over an extended period of time. If symptoms persist, an appointment should be made with one's family physician, who can identify and treat the basic problem underlying the symptoms.

Prescription drugs can be obtained only by the direction of a physician. Bearing the *Rx* symbol on their labels, these prescribed drugs can be sold only by a registered pharmacist. Defined primarily as unsafe for use except under professional medical supervision, prescription drugs include certain habit-forming substances and any other drug that is unsafe due to its toxicity or potential for causing a harmful effect, its method of use, or related measures necessary to its proper use.[4]

By comparison with OTC drugs, prescription medicines have a relatively high risk of causing toxicity and a low margin of safety. Because prescription drugs generally are more powerful than OTC medicines, they are also more likely to cause unanticipated and adverse side effects. Consequently, to assure the safety and effectiveness of these medicines, prescription drugs are to be used under a physician's supervision. Each prescription is individualized for a patient in terms of dosage and frequency of use, according to the nature of the illness, the patient's age, weight, sex, general health status, and potential for allergic reaction.

Classification of OTC Drugs

The following classification of basic OTC drugs has been established by the OTC drug review process of the U.S. Food and Drug Administration. Unless otherwise indicated, examples of specific drug classes were derived from the *Physicians' Desk Reference for Nonprescription Drugs*. Brand names of drugs appear within parentheses, as capitalized, or are referred to specifically as OTC drug preparations.

Allergy relief products—These relieve symptoms of sneezing; watery nose and eyes; itching of the nose, mouth, and throat; headache; irritability; insomnia; and lack of appetite associated with an allergy (a special sensitivity to some ordinary harmless substance). Symptoms of allergies are often treated by OTC antihistamines (drugs that block histamine secretion responsible for excess mucus production, tissue swelling, sneezing, and itchy nose

box 11.1

The Switch Is On: From Prescription to OTC Drugs

An ever-increasing number of drugs, formerly available by prescription only, are now OTC preparations. These newly designated OTC medications represent a trend on the part of the U.S. Food and Drug Administration and drug manufacturers to convert all appropriate drugs from prescription to OTC classification.[a] These new OTC drugs are now more effective and powerful than ever. Will they be used safely and correctly by consumers?

Listed below are the generic or product names of formerly prescription-only drugs, followed by one or more brand names of the OTC counterparts—enclosed within parentheses—and a definition or drug-class identification to suggest the major function of the medicine.

Brompheniramine maleate (Dimetane, Dimetapp)—antihistamine

Chlorpheniramine (Chlor-Trimeton, Coricidin Nasal Mist)—antihistamine used to relieve hay fever and other allergic reactions

Cimetidine (Tagamet HB)—an acid reducer used to relieve and prevent heartburn and acid indigestion

Clemastine fumarate (Tavist–1 and Tavist–D)—antihistamine, antihistamine/decongestant

Clotrimazole (Gyne-Lotrimin)—an antifungal drug used to treat vaginal yeast infections

Diphenhydramine (Benadryl)—relieves allergy symptoms; and also contained in certain OTC sleep aids (Compoz, Sleep-Eze 3, Sominex)

Doxylamine succinate (Unisom)—a sleep aid; also to be marketed soon as an OTC antihistamine

Famotidine (Pepcid AC)—an acid controller used to relieve and prevent heartburn and acid indigestion

Fluoride dental rinse containing sodium fluoride in solution (Act, Fluorigard)—helps prevent dental cavities

Hydrocortisone creams (Cortaid, Lanacort)—relieve minor itchy skin irritations, inflammation, and rashes

Ibuprofen (Advil, Motrin-IB, Nuprin)—analgesic

Loperaminde (Imodium A-D)—relieves common diarrhea

Miconazole (Micatin)—an antifungal agent used in treating athlete's foot and "jock itch"

Naproxen sodium (Aleve)—analgesic

Oxymetazoline hydrochloride (Afrin, Neo-Synephrine)—nasal decongestant; and (OcuClear, Visine L.R. Eye Drops)—decongestant solution designed to relieve redness of the eyes due to minor irritations

Tolnaftate (Tinactin)—an antifungal agent used in treating athlete's foot, "jock itch," and other fungal infections

Triprolidine and pseudoephedrine (Actifed)—an antihistamine and decongestant combination used to relieve cold and allergy symptoms

Probable "Switches" in the Near Future:

For use as antacids, the following drugs now prescribed as treatment for peptic ulcer disease:
Ranitidine (Zantac)—preliminary approval for OTC sale already granted

Sucralfate (Carafate)

For use as cold/allergy medications, the following drugs now prescribed as antihistamines for the relief of allergies:
Astemizole (Hismanal)

Terfenadine (Seldane)[b]

For use as nonsteroidal anti-inflammatory medicines, the following drugs now prescribed for relief of mild to moderate pain and inflammation:
Piroxicam (Feldene)

Sulindac (Clinoril)

[a] Marian Segal, 1991. Rx to OTC: The Switch Is On. *FDA Consumer*, Vol. 25, No. 2 (March): 9–11.
[b] Recently identified adverse reactions when taken with certain other medications may postpone indefinitely Seldane's conversion to OTC status.
Source: U.S. Food and Drug Administration.

and throat), and decongestants (drugs that open up stuffed noses). These are among the same drug preparations used in relieving symptoms of the common cold (Actifed, Allerest, Benadryl, Chlor-Trimeton, Contac, Coricidin, Dimetapp, Dristan, Drixoral, Sudafed, Teldrin).

Analgesics—These provide relief of minor aches and pain, and tend to bring down a fever. The most popular of these nonprescription pain relievers are aspirin, acetaminophen, ibuprofen, and naproxen sodium. (This drug class will be examined more fully later in this chapter.)

Anorectal products—These are OTC ointments, creams, foams, and suppositories that provide temporary relief of symptoms associated with hemorrhoids (enlarged, swollen, knotted veins of the lower portion of the rectum and the tissues about the anus) and other anorectal disorders. Drugs containing a local anesthetic, benzocaine, may relieve pain, irritation, itching, or burning; protectant drugs (calamine and mineral oil) provide a coating over inflamed tissues and relieve itching; counterirritants (menthol in aqueous solution) detract from the sensation of pain; astringent drugs, zinc oxide and witch hazel lotion, relieve irritation and burning; and keratolytics, such as alcloxa, tend to relieve itching. These OTC products are primarily for the relief of symptoms and not the treatment of disease (Anusol, Medicone, Nupercainal ointment, and Preparation H suppositories).

Antacids—These relieve symptoms of heartburn, sour stomach, and/or acid indigestion by neutralizing stomach acid or stopping the production of irritating digestive chemical enzymes. These products are available in tablets, liquids, powders, and capsules as well as in combinations with pain relievers and antiflatulents (drugs that relieve or prevent the formation of gas or flatulence in the stomach or intestine). Most of the OTC antacids contain one or more of the following active ingredients: sodium bicarbonate, calcium carbonate, aluminum hydroxide, magnesium hydroxide, and H_2 antagonistic drugs.

Antibacterials and antiseptics—These are used generally to treat infections caused by bacteria and include antimicrobial skin cleansers, topical antiseptics applied to the skin to destroy bacteria (Campho-Phenique, Bactine), and topical antibiotics, also applied to the skin as first aid to help prevent bacterial infection in minor cuts, scrapes, and burns (Mycitracin, Neosporin, Polysporin).

Appetite suppressants—These are weight-control preparations, such as diet pills, that reduce an individual's desire to eat food (see pages 277–278).

Arthritis medications—These are used in the treatment of arthritic conditions to reduce both the pain and the inflammation associated with these illnesses. Many physicians still consider OTC aspirin (acetylsalicylic acid) the drug of first choice for arthritic diseases. Aspirin not only reduces arthritic pain but also reduces inflammation in joint

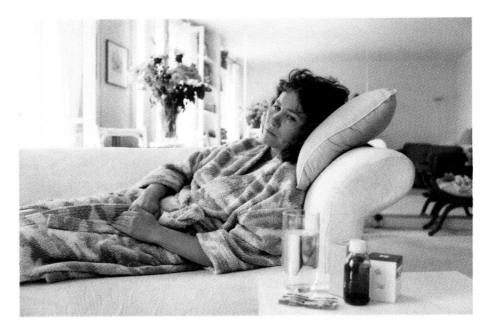

Over-the-counter cold relief medications do not cure the common cold; they merely suppress some of the symptoms.

© Didier Ermakoff/The Image Works

tissues and surrounding structures. The anti-inflammatory action counteracts the cause of pain. In addition to plain aspirin, acetylsalicylic acid also comes in buffered formulas to reduce gastritis (Ascriptin, Arthritis Pain Formula, Bufferin). By contrast, acetaminophen products relieve pain and reduce fever, but they do not produce the anti-inflammatory effects sought in antirheumatic medications. The anti-inflammatory effects of OTC ibuprofen and naproxen sodium drugs are generally equivalent to those of aspirin.

Asthma preparations—These are drugs that increase or widen the caliber (diameter) of the air passages within the lungs. OTC medications containing bronchodilators, such as ephedrine, epinephrine, methoxyphenamine, and theophylline, cause tightened air passageways in the lungs to expand, thus relieving shortness of breath and an acute sense of suffocation symptomatic of asthma (Bronkaid tablets, Primatene Mist).

Cold preparations—These provide relief for symptoms of the common cold. Typical OTC remedies include antihistamines, decongestants, and combinations of these medications with analgesics, cough suppressants, and expectorants. However, none of these drugs or combinations can actually cure a cold. (This drug classification will be examined more fully later in this chapter.)

Contraceptives—These include OTC gels, foams, suppositories, jellies, and vaginal inserts. A related product category includes OTC pregnancy tests (Advance, Clearblue Easy, Daisy 2, e.p.t. Stick Test, First Response).

Cough preparations—These are drugs that suppress coughing; they are referred to as antitussives (Benylin cough syrup, Halls Mentho-Lyptus cough tablets, Robitussin, Sudafed cough syrup, TheraFlu, Vicks Formula 44M multisymptom cough medicine). Some of these remedies for coughing also contain an expectorant that tends to loosen and liquefy mucus in the bronchial airways and thus makes the phlegm easier to cough up (Benylin expectorant, Fedahist, Naldecon, Novahistine, Triaminic expectorant). Some OTC cough preparations are combinations of antitussives, expectorants, antihistamines, and decongestants.

Dental preparations—These include anticavity and antitartar agents, such as toothpastes, gels, fluoride rinses, antiseptic and anesthetic gels, and denture preparations.

Dermatologicals—These are products applied to the skin for relief of various skin disorders, and include facial scrubs, acne preparations (Acnomel, Clearasil), topical analgesics (Americaine, Aspercreme, Icy Hot Cream, Therapeutic Mineral Ice), topical anesthetics (Bactine, Dermoplast, Solarcaine), antiperspirants, bath oils, burn relief medications (A and D Ointment, Nupercainal Pain Relief, Polysporin Spray), dandruff medications and shampoos, dermatitis relief drugs (Aqua Care lotion, Aveeno lotion, CaldeCORT cream, Cortaid lotion, Desitin ointment), fungicides (Cruex, Desenex, Micatin, Tinactin), sunburn preparations, sunscreens, and wound cleansers.

Diarrhea medications—These control or relieve the abnormally frequent passage of watery stools (feces). Diarrhea is usually a self-limiting condition, often without an identifiable cause. Commonly used OTC preparations, such as kaolin and pectin mixtures, are generally less effective than prescribed opioids, including opium powder, tincture of opium, paregoric, codeine tablets, diphenoxylate, and loperamide.[5] All of these prescription drugs are narcotics or closely related synthetic derivatives. However, liquid and tablet forms of loperamide (Imodium) are now available OTC. Although the FDA has not favored

the use of bismuth subsalicylate as an antidiarrheal drug, it has been proven somewhat effective in conferring a degree of protection from "traveler's diarrhea"—diarrhea that often occurs when people travel in other countries.[6] Bismuth subsalicylate is the major active ingredient in Pepto-Bismol, an OTC preparation.

Laxatives—These promote or induce defecation or bowel movements, and are used generally to relieve the condition of constipation. Most medical authorities, however, recommend nondrug remedies or preventives, including the addition of fiber or roughage to one's diet, increasing liquid consumption, and getting more physical exercise. Laxatives are usually classified according to their method of action in causing stool evacuation, and are marketed as bulkformers, stimulants, salts, hyperosmotics (water attracters), lubricants, stool softeners, and carbon-dioxide-releasing agents.

Mouthwashes—These are oral hygiene aids consisting of antimicrobial or antiseptic mouthwashes or anesthetic sprays, drops, or lozenges that may temporarily reduce bacteria in the mouth, freshen the breath, or relieve mouth and gum discomfort or pain associated with minor sore throat (Chloraseptic Spray, Listerine Antiseptic, Listermint Mouthwash).

Nausea medications—Known as antiemetics, these tend to prevent unpleasant gastric sensations resulting in vomiting, as well as reduce motion sickness (Dramamine, Emetrol, Pepto-Bismol).

Sleep aids—Originally these were promoted as drugs that would reduce nervousness during daytime as well as relieve sleeplessness. Presently, these nonprescription medications are used only to help people fall asleep, and they contain

antihistamine ingredients that cause drowsiness. (This drug class will be examined more fully later in this chapter.)

Stimulants—These tend to increase physical activity (motor performance) and mental alertness. Most OTC stimulant drugs are composed primarily of caffeine. (This drug class will be examined more fully later in this chapter.)

Vitamins and minerals—These are substances that regulate various normal biochemical reactions within the body. Vitamin supplements (organic substances) might contain one or more of the following nutrients: vitamins A, C, D, E, K, B_1, B_2, B_6, B_{12}, niacin, pantothenic acid, biotin, folic acid, choline, inositol, para-aminobenzoic acid, and rutin. Mineral supplements might contain one or more of the following inorganic substances: calcium, phosphate, magnesium, iron, zinc, copper, iodine, manganese, molybdenum, chromium, selenium, and cobalt. Also included are various dietary supplements (brewer's yeast, tonics, and liquid diet preparations).

Analgesics

Drugs taken internally to relieve pain without the loss of consciousness are referred to as **analgesics** or *painkillers*. Some OTC analgesics also act as *antipyretics* (agents that reduce fever), and as *anti-inflammatory drugs*, useful in relieving symptoms associated with arthritic diseases—pains, aches, and swelling of joints.

There are two different ways of classifying OTC internal analgesics. The first is based on ingredients (the presence or absence of salicylic acid), while the second is determined by a major effect of the drugs (relief or nonrelief of inflammation). In the first classification, OTC pain relievers are identified as either **salicylate** painkillers (such as Bayer Aspirin, St. Joseph Aspirin, and generic aspirin) or **nonsalicylates,** including acetaminophen (marketed as Tylenol, Excedrin, and other brand-name products), ibuprofen (sold OTC as Advil, Motrin IB, and Nuprin), and now naproxen sodium (available OTC as Aleve).

Both the salicylates and the nonsalicylates have been combined with other ingredients, resulting in a variety of cold remedies, antacids, decongestants, antihistamines, buffered analgesics, and medicated gums—all containing a painkiller.

The other major classification distinguishes among the several analgesics according to whether or not they reduce inflammation—the localized heat, redness, swelling, and pain in a body part that occurs usually in response to some injury or illness. Because certain of these internal analgesics also act as anti-inflammatory drugs, but not as cortisone-like medications, they are referred to as nonsteroidal anti-inflammatory drugs, or **NSAIDs.** Aspirin, ibuprofen, and naproxen sodium are all NSAIDs that produce their desirable effects by suppressing or blocking the action of specific prostaglandin chemicals. Such chemicals, produced naturally by the human body, contribute to the perception of pain.

Acetaminophen, in contrast, is not a nonsteroidal anti-inflammatory drug and likely relieves pain by acting on particular nerve endings or pain centers in the brain. While acetaminophen-based analgesics are as effective as aspirin in relieving mild to moderate pain, as well as fever, they do not reduce inflammation.

Salicylates

Until very recently, **aspirin** had been the most widely known and used OTC painkiller. Belonging to a family of drugs containing *salicylic acid*, aspirin is so easily available that many people hardly consider it a drug. Others have no idea that aspirin (acetylsalicylic acid) is an active ingredient in such products as Anacin, Bufferin, Alka-Seltzer, Empirin, Ecotrin, and Vanquish. Despite the increasing use of nonsalicylate analgesics, Americans consume nearly 80 billion aspirin-containing tablets each year.

Another salicylate, magnesium salicylate, is the active ingredient in Doan's Caplets and Mobigesic Tablets, also marketed as analgesics. Both salicylates are

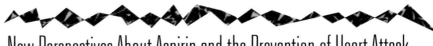

New Perspectives About Aspirin and the Prevention of Heart Attack

box 11.2

1. Aspirin appears to prevent heart attacks by interfering with the clotting mechanism in which blood platelets clump together to form clots. Consequently, aspirin inhibits the formation of blood clots in the arteries. However, aspirin does not reverse atherosclerosis in the coronary arteries.

2. Nonaspirin analgesics, such as acetaminophen and ibuprofen, do not share aspirin's clot-preventing action.

3. Some people should not take aspirin under any circumstances, especially those who have an aspirin allergy, hypertension, asthma, or problems with wound healing, including bleeding ulcers.

4. The recommended dose for heart attack prevention might prove to be much less than one regular-strength

aspirin every other day. Some researchers believe that the "ideal" daily dose may be as little as one-eighth of an aspirin. Doses larger than currently recommended may actually have the opposite effect—the formation of blood clots.

5. After considering age, gender, and other heart attack risks, the prime candidates for using aspirin as a preventive measure appear to be the following:
   a. Any male or female with a family history of heart attack and high cholesterol levels, inactive lifestyle, diabetes, and smoking cigarettes.
   b. Postmenopausal women with one or more risk factors for heart disease.
   c. Males over 35 with one or more risk factors besides gender, and those over 45 with no risk factors except for gender.

relatively safe and effective as painkillers, fever reducers, and anti-inflammatory drugs. However, the FDA has expressed concern about the prolonged use of these OTC drugs for treating symptoms of arthritic diseases without medical supervision. The recommended dosage of these analgesics may relieve the pain and swelling of arthritic conditions but may be insufficient to treat the disease that causes the inflammation. Improperly diagnosed and treated arthritis can lead to crippling and permanent disability.

Versatility of Aspirin

A remarkably useful drug, aspirin is valuable in the treatment of many conditions. As a painkiller, fever reducer, and anti-inflammatory drug, aspirin is present in hundreds of different OTC products on the market. When taken properly, aspirin works best on pain of mild to moderate severity, such as muscular aches, backaches, toothaches, and headaches. Using aspirin as an analgesic does not lead to

physical dependency, and it is less toxic than more-powerful analgesics, and much less expensive, too. Aspirin works well for arthritis pain because it reduces swelling in joint tissues and surrounding structures. This salicylate is also helpful in treating rheumatic fever.

Although the precise mechanisms by which aspirin achieves its wide range of effects is not completely known, newly discovered powers of this analgesic extend far beyond reducing pain, fever, and inflammation.

1. Less than one tablet per day is often used to treat and prevent heart attacks and to prevent strokes. In fact, men over 50 years of age can cut the risk of having their first heart attack by nearly half, if they take just 325 mg (one ordinary tablet) every other day.[7–9] And among both men and women who survive an initial heart attack, low-dose aspirin therapy appears to reduce the risk of subsequent heart attacks.

2. The "antiprostaglandin action" of aspirin might help reduce undesirable blood clotting that in turn contributes to reduced blood supply to specific, localized tissues—a condition known as transient ischemic attacks (TIA). A TIA is considered a "mini-stroke" and a strong predictor of having a future stroke.

3. In the same study that found aspirin effective in preventing a first heart attack, it was also discovered that taking an aspirin every other day resulted in a 20 percent reduction rate of migraine headaches. Though further research is needed to confirm this finding, combining low-dose aspirin with other drugs could become the standard therapy for the control of migraines.[10,11]

4. Aspirin has also proved useful in slowing the development of cataracts (clouding of the eye's lens), limiting periodontal disease, strengthening the human immune system, and preventing deaths due to colon cancer.

As popular and versatile as aspirin is, it does have its limitations. Aspirin may no longer be used in topical analgesic products that are applied to the skin. Gargles containing aspirin have no therapeutic effect on a sore throat. Aspirin also has no effect on bacteria or viruses, so it will not cure a cold or the flu, or shorten the duration of either condition. By reducing fever and relieving the pain of headache and muscle aches, aspirin might allow the cold sufferer to become more active prematurely, before the self-limiting disease has run its course in a body that is resting. In this respect, aspirin can do more harm than good.

Side Effects of Aspirin

Despite their history of therapeutic usefulness, aspirin and the other salicylates are not harmless. These analgesics can produce a variety of undesirable side effects, often affecting the gastrointestinal tract. Commonly reported problems include heartburn, stomach discomfort, nausea, and vomiting. In addition, aspirin may injure the stomach by causing an erosion of and bleeding from the stomach's lining.

Such a condition is evidence of a stomach ulcer, which often occurs in those who repeatedly take high doses of aspirin. To lessen the chances of such side effects, individuals are often urged to take aspirin shortly after meals.

Buffered aspirin, or aspirin coated with or combined with an antacid, may prevent some of the common side effects. The chemical "buffer" makes aspirin dissolve more quickly, thus speeding its absorption into the bloodstream. This buffering effect reduces but does not eliminate the irritating effects of aspirin on the stomach. A recently introduced form of aspirin has a microfilm coating that protects the tablets from dissolving in the stomach and is less likely to cause stomach irritation. While this "enteric-coated" aspirin is dissolved in the small intestine, pain relief is somewhat delayed. However, less stomach irritation associated with taking enteric-coated aspirin is a special benefit to those on high daily doses.

Pregnant women are cautioned about taking aspirin, especially during the last three months of pregnancy. There is a remote possibility that aspirin taken in excessive amounts might cause birth defects in the fetus. Since aspirin also interferes with blood clotting, it can prolong pregnancy and labor, and cause bleeding both before and after delivery. Excessive bleeding tendencies also occur in babies whose mothers use aspirin during their pregnancies.

Unfortunately, the unsupervised taking of aspirin continues to be a major cause of childhood poisoning, although it is no longer the leading cause of accidental poisoning and poisoning deaths in children since "childproof" containers were introduced. However, another life-threatening aspect of aspirin use among children and teenagers has been identified recently. Because the use of salicylates (aspirin) by young people who have influenza and chicken pox has been associated with **Reye's syndrome,** the surgeon general has advised against the use of salicylate preparations for children and teenagers with these diseases.[12]

Reye's syndrome is a rare, acute, brain-damaging, and sometimes fatal condition. It is characterized by vomiting and lethargy that may progress to delirium and coma. The syndrome occurs commonly in young children and teenagers who are recovering from viral infections. To emphasize the seriousness of the link between Reye's syndrome and drug products containing aspirin, the following warning must occur on the labels of nonprescription aspirin and products containing aspirin: "Warning—Children and teenagers should not use this medicine for chickenpox or flu symptoms before a doctor is consulted about Reye's syndrome, a rare but serious illness reported to be associated with aspirin."[13]

Salicylism, another undesirable side effect of using aspirin, is poisoning due to acetylsalicylic acid taken in excess. Overdosing with aspirin can result in a condition with symptoms such as nausea, vomiting, ringing in the ear (tinnitus), deafness, or even severe headaches. These are warning signals that a person has taken too much aspirin. Sometimes, hyperventilation, difficulty in hearing, and even diarrhea may occur. Such symptoms should be sufficient reminders to stop taking the painkiller or to reduce the dosage.

Even small doses may be too much for the significant number of individuals who are aspirin-sensitive or allergic to aspirin. These people cannot tolerate aspirin; if they ingest it, they may develop minor skin itching, abdominal pain, facial swelling, swelling of the larynx or voice box, and falling blood pressure. Some may develop physiological shock and eventually die.

Nonsalicylates

Drugs that do not contain salicylic acid are known as **nonsalicylates.** At present, **acetaminophen** is the most popular nonsalicylate drug determined to be safe and effective for the relief of minor pain and as a fever reducer. However, acetaminophen does not reduce inflammation and should not be used in the treatment of arthritic symptoms except under the supervision of a physician. Consequently, its status as the top-selling ingredient of OTC painkillers is being challenged by Advil and other ibuprofen-based analgesics.

Derived from coal tar, acetaminophen was developed in 1893 but was not promoted widely as an aspirin substitute until the 1970s. Since then, acetaminophen sales have soared under the brand names Tylenol, Datril, Anacin-3, and Panadol. Some analgesics, such as Vanquish caplets, now contain combinations of acetaminophen and aspirin.

Until the 1982 poisoning epidemic involving cyanide-laced Tylenol, this one medication was the leading brand of nonprescribed analgesic, accounting for one-third of all OTC analgesic sales. Although its capsule form was recalled, Tylenol was not reformulated or renamed. It was reintroduced to the market in triple-sealed, tamper-resistant packages, and it is once again the leading nonprescription painkiller in terms of market share. In response to the Tylenol tampering, the U.S. Food and Drug Administration required nonprescription drug manufacturers to package their products in sealed, tamper-resistant containers to protect consumers from contaminated medicines.

Milligram for milligram, acetaminophen has no advantage over aspirin either as a painkiller or as an antipyretic. The standard tablet for each has 325 milligrams of medication. Yet many people have switched from aspirin to acetaminophen because aspirin has acquired a rather nasty reputation. To be certain, acetaminophen is less irritating to the stomach than aspirin. The aspirin substitute can be used safely by those who are allergic to aspirin. Moreover, acetaminophen does not cause stomach bleeding or affect blood clotting and is stable in liquid preparations.

Although acetaminophen is free of most of the side effects of the salicylates, an overdose can result in permanent liver damage. This is especially true in people who combine acetaminophen with alcohol use. Severe and possibly fatal liver disease may occur within two to four days of an acetaminophen overdose, without any warning symptoms of toxicity. Unfortunately, an overdose of this aspirin substitute does not cause a ringing in the ears or any other abnormal condition or easily recognized symptom as experienced in salicylism.

Ibuprofen, a prescription-only painkiller until 1984, is now a widely available and effective OTC analgesic. Its popularity is linked to its convenience, inasmuch as just one or two OTC ibuprofen tablets can reduce inflammation as well as a dozen aspirin tablets. Because of this particular effect, ibuprofen is designated as a nonsteroidal anti-inflammatory drug (NSAID). As a prescribed drug, ibuprofen has been one of the best-selling medications in America.

Consisting of 2–(p-isobutylphenyl) propionic acid, ibuprofen has been used extensively in the treatment of rheumatoid arthritis and osteoarthritis, as well as for the relief of mild to moderate pain and for treatment of painful menstruation.

Since the FDA approved lower-dose ibuprofen for nonprescription sale, it has been available under the brand names of Advil, Nuprin, Ibuprin, Motrin IB, and Medipren. These OTC analgesics are promoted as both pain relievers and fever reducers. In addition, these new, nonacetaminophen nonsalicylates have anti-inflammatory effects and are useful in relieving muscular aches, menstrual cramps, backaches, and the minor pain of arthritis. Despite the fact that it has only recently been introduced to the OTC market, ibuprofen has become a major competitor to both aspirin and acetaminophen.

Compared to aspirin, ibuprofen generally causes fewer side effects and tends to be more gentle to the stomach, although daily use can result in heartburn, indigestion, and gastrointestinal bleeding, even peptic ulcers and perforated ulcers. Consequently, doctors often advise individuals aged 60 and older not to use ibuprofen, because of their increased risk of sustaining such serious and sometimes life-threatening events.[14] Other adverse reactions may include skin rashes, digestive upsets, or dizziness. People with gout, ulcers, or aspirin allergies should not take ibuprofen products without first consulting a physician. The warning to aspirin-sensitive people applies even though ibuprofen drugs contain no aspirin or salicylates. Cross-reactions may occur in those individuals who are allergic to aspirin (see box 11.3).

Perhaps the most frightening adverse reaction to the use of ibuprofen, including OTC preparations, is the drug's potential for causing damage to the kidney.[15] Even a brief course of ibuprofen may result in acute renal or kidney failure in those individuals who already have mild, asymptomatic (without symptoms) chronic renal failure.

Such a serious condition could result in about 1 percent of the people who use ibuprofen, because early kidney failure does not often produce noticeable symptoms.

Naproxen sodium, the most recently approved OTC analgesic, is now marketed under the brand name Aleve. Like aspirin and ibuprofen, naproxen sodium is a nonsteroidal anti-inflammatory drug. It is only the second prescription analgesic ever approved for sale over the counter.[16] The last such nonprescription pain reliever based on a new analgesic ingredient was ibuprofen, approved for over-the-counter sales in 1984.

For many years, naproxen (Naprosyn) and naproxen sodium (Anaprox) have been sold exclusively by prescription as arthritis medications. However, in 1994, because of naproxen's established record as a relatively safe and effective analgesic, the FDA approved naproxen sodium—which works more rapidly than plain naproxen—as a nonprescription pain reliever.[17] In its approval process, the FDA required the drug's manufacturer to change dosage instructions to reflect its new OTC status.

Nonprescription naproxen sodium is sold in tablets containing 200 milligrams of naproxen and 20 milligrams of sodium. For the temporary relief of minor aches and pain associated with the common cold, headache, toothache, muscular aches, backaches, arthritis, or menstrual cramps, and for the relief of fever, adults and children 12 years of age or older are advised to take one tablet (220 mg) every eight to twelve hours as needed. Some people, however, may get even better relief by taking two tablets for the first dose, then one tablet twelve hours later on the first day only.[18]

Naproxen sodium provides longer-lasting relief in comparison with other OTC analgesics. Consequently, this analgesic is ideal for use at bedtime. It is also especially effective for menstrual cramps and pain occurring in females after childbirth. However, children under the age of 2 ought not take naproxen sodium, and those under 12 years old, as well as pregnant or breast-feeding women, should use this medication only on medical advice.

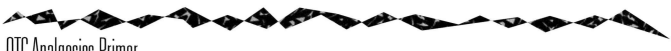

OTC Analgesics Primer
Aspirin, Acetaminophen, Ibuprofen, and Naproxen Sodium

box 11.3

	Aspirin Products	Acetaminophen Products	Ibuprofen Products	Naproxen Sodium Products
Analgesic effect	Reduces pain.	Reduces pain.	Reduces pain.	Reduces pain.
Antipyretic effect	Reduces fever.	Reduces fever.	Reduces fever.	Reduces fever.
Anti-inflammatory effect	Reduces inflammation.	None.	Reduces inflammation.	Reduces inflammation.
Dosage	325 mg.	325 mg.	200 mg.	200 mg.
Common brands	Anacin, Ascriptin, Bayer, Bayer Plus, Bufferin, Ecotrin.	Anacin-3, Excedrin, Pamprin, Midol, Tylenol.	Advil, Motrin-IB, Nuprin, Pamprin-IB.	Aleve.
Special uses	Often used in treating arthritis and preventing heart attacks, strokes, and cataracts.	Fewer side effects than aspirin; used by those with ulcers or aspirin allergies. Gentler on the stomach than aspirin; reduces fever without risk of Reye's syndrome.	Fewer side effects than aspirin; very effective in relief of menstrual cramps. Less toxic in large doses than other pain relievers. May be better for fever and muscle aches associated with a cold.	Often proves effective when other OTC analgesics have not helped. Provides longer-lasting relief.
Possible side effects	Nausea, vomiting, stomach irritation, dizziness, diarrhea. Accidental overdose, allergic reactions, salicylism, Reye's syndrome. Prolonged use may cause gastrointestinal bleeding, especially in heavy drinkers; may increase risk of maternal and fetal bleeding and cause complications during delivery if taken in the last trimester.	Upset stomach, nausea, and vomiting. Accidental overdose or long-term use may cause liver damage, hepatitis, reduced white blood cell and platelet count. May cause liver damage in drinkers and those taking excessive amounts (more than 4,000 mg daily) for several weeks.	Similar to those of aspirin; skin rash, sensitivity to sunlight. Accidental overdose, allergic reactions, including anaphylaxis, gastrointestinal bleeding, kidney damage. Gastrointestinal bleeding, especially in heavy drinkers; stomach ulcers; kidney damage in the elderly, people who have cirrhosis of the liver, and those taking diuretics.	Accidental overdose may cause stomach upset and stomach bleeding in some people; not recommended for pregnant women or those with ulcers, asthma, or kidney disease, or for heavy users of alcohol. Gastrointestinal bleeding; stomach ulcers; kidney damage in the elderly, in people who have cirrhosis of the liver, and in those taking diuretics.

Source: Modified from the U.S. Food and Drug Administration.

Weight-Control Products

The OTC products that help individuals curb their appetites are known variously as *diet aids,* **appetite suppressants,** and *anorectics* or *anorexics.* Although many drugs have been included in diet aids in the past, the U.S. Food and Drug Administration has now limited the active ingredients in these products to phenylpropanolamine hydrochloride and benzocaine.[19] Other nonprescription products used in the control of weight, as well as the regular appetite suppressants, are available in a variety of preparations (see box 11.4).

Phenylpropanolamine (PPA) is a mild stimulant as well as a decongestant often used in shrinking swollen nasal passages. Related to amphetamine, PPA has been considered useful as an appetite suppressant. As the result of an FDA OTC drug review panel's findings, PPA was identified initially as a safe and effective OTC drug for curbing appetite. Consequently, nearly all of the diet aids at one time or another contained this drug, varying only in dosage form (capsules, tablets, or drops), and dosage schedule (25 mg three times a day vs. 75 mg in one time-release capsule).

Some drug authorities, however, disagree about the safety and effectiveness of PPA. Side effects of PPA can include nervousness, restlessness, insomnia, headache, nausea, elevated blood-sugar level, and dangerous increases in blood pressure. Individuals who are at risk of heart disease, stroke, hypertension, kidney disease, or diabetes have been cautioned to avoid PPA. Increasingly, this drug is being recognized as potentially dangerous to at least 20 percent of the population.[20]

While PPA diet aids might suppress appetite for short periods of time in some individuals by stimulating the central nervous system, their effect is modest at best.

Benzocaine, a topical anesthetic often used to relieve sore throats and the pain associated with minor cuts, scrapes, burns, and hemorrhoids, is the only other active ingredient now approved by the FDA for weight-control products. Contained in lozenges, candies, and gums, the benzocaine supposedly numbs the tongue and taste buds mildly and temporarily. This numbing effect supposedly reduces one's ability to taste and results in a decreased appetite. However, the anesthetic effect of benzocaine-based candies and gums may interfere with the swallowing process. If these products are sucked or chewed on a continuous basis, hypersensitivity reactions can occur.

Other so-called diet aids are *bulk-formers, laxatives, diuretics, and food supplements* containing methyl-cellulose compounds and fiber from grains and fruits. Sometimes, in combination with PPA, the bulk-producers actually absorb liquid in the stomach, produce a feeling of fullness, and thus reduce the desire to eat. Bulk-forming laxatives are also used inappropriately to control weight by "purging" the body (see box 11.5). Such laxatives relieve constipation and promote elimination by providing

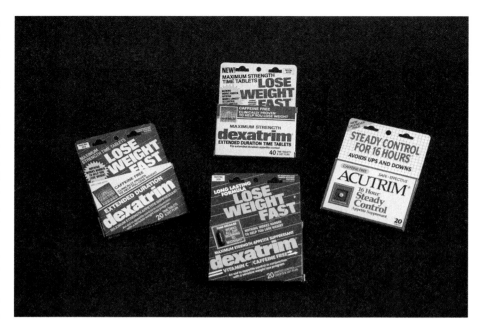

Of limited value in controlling weight, many over-the-counter diet pills contain the same active ingredient. Notice how these products feature their caffeine-free content, since caffeine was banned from weight-control products by the U.S. Food and Drug Administration.

© *James L. Shaffer*

box 11.4

Selected OTC Products Used in Controlling Weight

Phenylpropanolamine-Based Drugs

Acutrim
Appedrine
Dex-A-Diet
Dexatrim
Permathene-12
Prolamine

Benzocaine-Based Drugs

Diet Ayds

Diuretic-Based Drugs

Aqua-Ban
DeWitt's Pills
Diurex Water Capsules
Natural Herbal Diuretic Water Tablets

Meal Replacement and Food or Fiber Supplements

Fiber Full
Slim Fast
Spicer's Diet Shakes
Ultra Rich & Slim
Ultra Slim Fast

Bulk-Forming Laxatives

Citrucel
Effer-Syllium
Fiberall
Fibercon
Metamucil
Perdiem Fiber
Serutan
Syllact Powder

Eating Disorders and Weight-Control Products

box 11.5

Anorexia nervosa and *bulimia* are two serious eating disorders about which dieters and users of OTC weight-control products should be concerned. Basically, both are food obsessions in which the core symptom is the unending pursuit of thinness.

The anorexic individual finds food to be repulsive and strives to avoid it; the bulimic, by contrast, craves food and indulges in periodic episodes of binge eating that are followed by self-purging. Use of certain weight-control products and diet plans can contribute to both disorders, which often begin in adolescence or young adulthood and affect females almost exclusively.

The person suffering from *anorexia nervosa* has a distorted view of personal body image and body weight. The anorexic rejects food, engaging in a persistent self-starvation process in order to achieve a desired thinness. After being detected and forced to eat, the anorexic will often induce vomiting in secret and redouble efforts to lose more weight. Frequently, the person becomes so emaciated that hospitalization is necessary.

Bulimia is characterized by a fear of fatness and by "binge-purge" behavior. The bulimic first binges on high-calorie food, then seeks to prevent its absorption by inducing vomiting (for example, by taking an emetic drug such as syrup of ipecac), or by using laxatives or other cathartic drugs to cause bowel movements. Sometimes diuretics are also used compulsively to help remove body water. Such purging endeavors can result in severe dehydration, chemical imbalances within the body, and other physical problems.

Both of these eating disorders are serious and potentially life threatening, and they usually require a combination of therapies in order to change the patient's self-perception and basic belief system. Psychiatric care is often required.

---

fiber (bulk) to the diet. Diuretics, or "water pills," aid in the relief of simple water retention or bloating. These diuretic drugs cause a temporary weight loss by reducing body fluid, evidenced by increased urination. None of these products is considered safe and effective in promoting a permanent loss of weight.

Many *diet foods, meal replacements,* and *food supplements* are available to help people maintain or slowly lose body weight. Most such products are accompanied by detailed plans for dieting, which can help some individuals lose weight. Basic ingredients typically include proteins (peanuts, whey, calcium caseinate, egg whites, and soy), and vitamins and minerals. Other products may contain artificial sweeteners to provide a sweet taste without sugar's calories, while glucose preparations raise blood-sugar levels and make individuals feel as if they do not need as much to eat.

Although there is no magic wand or "no-work" way to lose weight, many consumers have gladly accepted numerous spurious concoctions that, according to the Consumers Union, are both worthless and even dangerous fat-melting pills and potions.[21] Among these allegedly fraudulent products are the following:

1. *Starch blockers,* popular in the early 1980s and derived from legumes, effectively prevented the digestion of starch, but resulted in nausea, vomiting, and stomach pains that often required hospitalization. These products were eventually banned by the FDA, but stayed on the market for a number of years due to the ineffectiveness of enforcement procedures.

2. *Growth-hormone releasers* containing various amino acids were supposed to cause overnight weight loss. Taking these products on an empty stomach supposedly caused the pituitary gland to secrete growth hormone, which in turn would burn fat and cause weight loss during sleep. As a result of government enforcement actions, most of the growth-hormone-releasing preparations have been removed from the marketplace.

3. *Sugar blockers,* derived from an Indian plant, were sold to help prevent the body from absorbing the sugar in various foods. Such an action could never be proved.

4. *Calories-ban,* made from guar gum, was advertised as a product that prevented the absorption of a major portion of calories, thus assuring automatic weight loss. Guar gum, a soluble fiber that thickens foods, has only minimal value as a bulk laxative, and the substance has never been proven effective. It has remained available in several states because the FDA is conducting a lengthy OTC drug review process on the product.

Despite the current popularity and appeal of weight-control products and the often sensational advertising claims for such items, it should be noted that no OTC drug can cause a weight loss itself. At most, even PPA and benzocaine can only help reduce a dieter's appetite. Ideally, drugs ought to be considered only as temporary, short-term measures in conjunction with a well-planned weight reduction program.

In addition, all reducing diets should be undertaken only with the supervision of a physician. In the final analysis, only a reduction in calories consumed or an increase in exercise to burn off excess calories can cause a loss of weight. This effort will likely involve significant, long-term changes in lifestyle.

Contrary to what many consumers believe, popping a diet pill will not result in the magical disappearance of fat. And those individuals who engage in "yo-yo" dieting—swinging through repeated cycles of losing weight followed by gaining back weight—can be endangering their own lives. Such "off-again on-again" dieters run a 70 percent higher risk of dying from heart disease than people whose body weight stays fairly steady, even if they are overweight.[22] In general, being moderately overweight is less dangerous than yo-yo dieting.

Cold Remedies

One of the most common causes of human misery and disability is the "common cold," a viral infection of the upper respiratory tract. The infection usually localizes in the head, throat, or chest. Fortunately, colds tend to be a **self-limiting condition;** that is, they run their course to recovery without treatment.

However, the various signs and symptoms of a cold can be most discomforting: sneezing, watery eyes, chills, fever, sore throat, stopped up nose, runny nose, postnasal drip, sore chest, coughing, and the tired, ache-all-over feeling. Although none of these symptoms in itself indicates a cold, together this group of complaints forms the "cold syndrome."

Because antibiotics such as penicillin have no effect against viruses, the treatment of a common cold is aimed at the relief of symptoms. The drug companies have responded to this human desire for relief with thousands of cold remedies. While some of these drugs will relieve several of the cold symptoms, none of these products will prevent, cure, or even shorten the course of the common cold.

Certain single-ingredient cold products can provide symptomatic relief of a cold's discomforts; nearly all cold and cough remedies contain a combination of two or more drug ingredients intended to relieve a number of different symptoms. Ordinarily, these combination drug preparations appear to be logical drug mixtures for treating multiple symptoms. However, these OTC **fixed-ratio combination products** are considered generally undesirable, for the following reasons:[23,24]

1. Combination remedies treat a cold with a "shotgun" approach; that is, the multidrug often contains ingredients that are not really needed by the cold sufferer. Those who undertake self-medication, therefore, expose themselves to unnecessary drugs.

2. It is not possible to formulate multidrugs for individual needs, body weight, and metabolism. Certain fixed-ratio combinations might not be appropriate for some individuals.

3. Cold remedies might contain effective ingredients in less-than-therapeutic doses. Consequently, these drugs often have little or no effect.

4. Consumers expose themselves to more risks and side effects of drugs, often due to the interaction of various ingredients in the multidrug preparation. In addition, the combination remedy might interfere with the healing process. For instance, many cold preparations contain an analgesic. Whether the cold sufferer has a headache or not, the individual is dosed with the drug. Moreover, the analgesic also tends to lower fever that in most instances runs its course without harm. While high body temperatures can be extremely dangerous, a lower fever may actually stimulate the body's immune system into operation. Therefore, drugs taken to lower temperature might also interfere with the body's own healing strategy. Fever reducers might also reduce the effectiveness of *interferon,* a natural antiviral agent within the body.

5. These combination products invariably cost more money than the single-ingredient medications that are recommended generally and preferred by medical authorities in treating symptoms of the "common cold."

Some precautions should be observed when using any combination- or single-ingredient cold remedy. Cold medications are intended for temporary use only. They should never be taken on a persistent or continuous basis, even if the drugs produce a beneficial effect. People with asthma, emphysema, or smoker's cough should only use these OTC medicines with their physicians' approval. In addition, individuals with diabetes, high blood pressure, heart disease, and thyroid problems should carefully read all package labels and inserts that may indicate special warnings pertaining to those ailments.

Lacing oral cold remedies with alcohol is a widespread practice, although there is little evidence that ethyl alcohol relieves the symptoms of either colds or coughs. When the combination medication contains an antihistamine, the alcohol heightens the antihistamine's effect and often produces drowsiness. Such an effect presents a real danger when persons must drive an automobile or operate machinery.

The numerous cold remedies, such as Actifed, Benadryl, Comtrex, Contac, Coricidin, Dimetapp, Sudafed, and Triaminic, might be marketed as combinations of the following major drug ingredients:

Antihistamines block the effects of the allergy chemical (histamine) in the body and relieve sneezing, watery eyes, runny nose, and itching of the nose or throat. While effective in controlling allergic reactions, antihistamines do not relieve sinus or nasal congestion and have no direct action on colds. They continue to be one of the most common ingredients of cold preparations, primarily because of antihistamine's side effects—drowsiness and a slight drying of nasal secretions. Still considered as "blank ammunition" in the "shotgun therapy" approach of most cold remedies, commonly occurring antihistamines include brompheniramine maleate, chlorpheniramine maleate, doxylamine succinate, and triprolidine hydrochloride.

Decongestants, such as pseudoephedrine, phenylpropanolamine, oxymetazoline, and xylometazoline, unclog blocked nasal passages and sinuses, and prevent postnasal drip into the throat. Marketed as either oral (taken by mouth) or topical (applied in the form of nose drops or sprays) preparations, these decongestants generally cause a *vasoconstriction* (narrowing) of the blood vessels in the nasal passages and thus help clear up stuffy noses.

Although the decongestants are quite effective, those applied in the form of

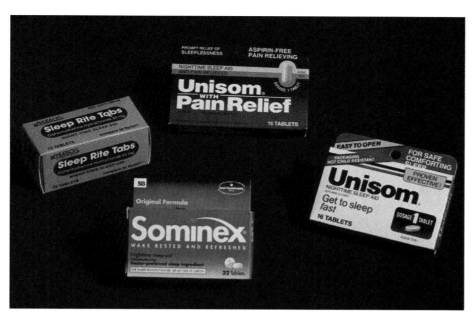

Virtually all OTC sleep aids contain an antihistamine that produces a degree of drowsiness or mild sedation in many users.

© James L. Shaffer

nose drops and nasal sprays present a potential problem. Initially, the active ingredient causes the swollen blood vessels in the nose to shrink. When the nose drops or sprays are used too long or too frequently, a phenomenon known as the "rebound effect" is likely to occur. After excessive use of the decongestant, the blood vessels become fatigued and undergo a swelling or dilation when the effect of the drug wears off. The swollen blood vessels contribute to greater congestion and nasal stuffiness. In response to this rebound swelling or vasodilation, the cold sufferer uses more and more of the nasal decongestant, resulting in a vicious cycle of drug dependency.[25]

Analgesics and antipyretics are drugs that relieve pain and reduce fever, respectively. As indicated earlier in this chapter, the major analgesics and antipyretics present in most OTC cold remedies are aspirin, acetaminophen, and ibuprofen. Acetaminophen is a common ingredient because it does not irritate the stomach lining and cause bleeding.

Antitussives or *cough suppressants*, such as dextromethorphan, diphenhydramine hydrochloride, and codeine (a prescription-only drug in some states), are useful in controlling coughs that cause

chest pain or interfere with sleep or breathing. (A cough that brings up phlegm—a "productive cough"—should not be suppressed. Such a cough helps clear the respiratory passages.)

Expectorants are drugs that tend to thin and loosen the thick mucus that often accumulates in the respiratory airways of a cold sufferer. Although this drug action may be desirable, an FDA OTC drug review panel concluded that expectorants, including *guaifenesin* (the most widely used), are of limited therapeutic effectiveness. Perhaps in a somewhat irrational combination, some cold preparations contain both an expectorant and a cough suppressant. Such a mixture has both a drug intended to make phlegm easier to cough up and another drug intended to suppress coughing.

Sleep Aids

At present, several OTC preparations are marketed exclusively as **sleep aids.** Some popular ones are Compoz, Nervine, Nytol, Sominex, Sleepeze-3, and Sleepinal—all of which contain the same active ingredient, diphenhydramine hydrochloride, a common antihistamine. Other sleep aids, such as Doxysom, Ultra Sleep,

and Unisom, contain another antihistamine, doxylamine succinate, while Excedrin PM contains both an antihistamine and an analgesic.

The antihistamine drugs reverse the action of a naturally occurring substance, histamine, which causes allergic reactions like runny nose, itching, tearing of the eyes, and sneezing. In addition to relieving allergy symptoms, antihistamines tend to act on the central nervous system and produce a mild form of drowsiness or sedation in some individuals. However, many physicians and pharmacologists oppose the use of antihistamines as sleep aids because they expose users to several other possible side effects. Frequently reported problems include dizziness, incoordination, fatigue, nervousness, blurred vision, double vision, loss of appetite, dryness of the mouth, throat and respiratory passages, nausea, vomiting, increased urination, constipation, and even diarrhea.

For those considering the use of OTC sleep aids, the following advice is offered.

1. Sleeping pills are for short-term use only. If insomnia persists for more than two weeks, even after taking sleeping pills, consult a physician without delay. Persistent insomnia may be a symptom of some serious underlying medical problem.

2. Take sleep aids with extreme caution if alcohol is also being consumed. Drinking an alcoholic beverage while taking an antihistamine, another CNS depressant, can lead to excessive drowsiness and confusion, and, in extreme cases, coma and death.

3. Unless discomfort from minor pain is causing sleeplessness, avoid those sleep aids that also contain a pain and fever reducer.

4. Never give OTC sleep aids to children under 12 years of age. Such medication is for adults only.

5. Do not use these products if you are presently taking another prescribed or OTC medicine without medical consultation, or if you are pregnant or nursing an infant, or if you are suffering from asthma, glaucoma, or enlargement of the prostate gland.

6. Be careful not to exceed the recommended dosage. When the standard dose does not seem to be effective, there is the temptation to take more pills. Overdose then becomes a danger.

Today, millions of people rely on OTC sleeping pills to purchase elusive sleep. Insomnia and the fear of sleeplessness are considered among the worst of human miseries. Sleep aids remain popular and convenient remedies, although a variety of nondrug alternatives exist that can promote sleep, including these: modification of eating, drinking, exercise, and relaxation habits; establishing regular times for retiring at night; elimination of caffeine or other stimulants; resolution of personal crises; synchronization of lifestyle with natural body rhythm; biofeedback; and relaxation techniques. Specific recommendations for relieving insomnia are detailed in chapter 6.

Stimulants

When improved mental alertness or motor performance is desired, OTC **stimulants** are used to mask or cover up conditions of fatigue, and thus permit the successful completion of a required task. Common nonprescription stimulants include Caffedrine, Dexitac, NoDoz, Quick Pep, Tirend, and Vivarin. While these drugs might help individuals stay awake, they might not be sufficient to promote the alertness or efficiency needed to drive an automobile skillfully and safely.

The only approved effective ingredient of OTC stimulants is caffeine. This drug can help restore mental alertness or wakefulness in people experiencing fatigue or drowsiness. Each stimulant tablet or capsule contains from 100 to 325 milligrams of caffeine. Generally, the recommended dosage ranges from 100 to 200 mg of caffeine every three to four hours. Some products, until restricted by the FDA, also contained phenylpropanolamine hydrochloride and ephedrine sulfate, both mild stimulants. A variety of vitamins and small amounts of sugar have also been added

to some OTC stimulants. Since vitamins have no stimulating effect, they do not help people stay awake.

Use of an OTC stimulant may be considered reasonable on an occasional basis, especially when used to reduce fatigue or tedium associated with long, boring, and repetitive tasks. However, self-treatment with a stimulant should not last more than a week. It is also very important to remember that there is no drug substitute for adequate sleep. Although an OTC stimulant may relieve the feeling of tiredness, the body is still fatigued.

Caffeine is a natural component of various plants that are sources of coffee, tea, kola nut extracts, cocoa, and chocolate. Present in many prescription drugs, caffeine is also an ingredient in nearly two thousand OTC medicines, such as analgesics and cold remedies. Because it is used typically in very dilute forms, caffeine is a relatively safe drug. However, excessive intake—whether in coffee, tea, cola drinks, OTC stimulants, or OTC analgesics—can contribute to sleep disturbances, nervousness, and irritability.

Caffeine overdoses can result in mood changes, anxiety, insomnia, headache, and restlessness; these are all characteristics of **caffeinism,** which is described in chapter 8. When caffeine doses exceed 5 to 10 grams, convulsions may occur and, on rare occasions, even death.

Since OTC stimulants are concentrated doses of caffeine, enough coffee, tea, or caffeine-containing cola drinks should be as effective and probably much less expensive.

Self-Medication

Many human ailments are distressing only temporarily and produce no lasting changes in the human body. When used with care and discrimination on a temporary basis, over-the-counter drugs can provide a significant degree of relief from various minor discomforts.

The OTC drugs serve yet another function in overall health care. In programs of **self-medication,** nonprescription drug use allows medical doctors to concentrate their efforts on more serious health problems of treatment, rehabilitation, and prevention.

Without the wise and responsible use of nonprescription medications, and the application of home remedies (rest, sleep, hot water bottles, and ice caps), physicians would be so overwhelmed with patients complaining of minor illnesses that their services would be severely limited. The practice of treating oneself with nonprescription medications has some very important advantages, which will likely increase as the cost of health care continues to rise.

Guidelines for Self-Medication[26]

Before purchasing any OTC drug for self-medication, *read the label* carefully to make sure the drug is the right one for your own symptoms. Federal law requires that OTC drug labels provide sufficient directions for use needed by the average person, as noted in box 11.6. Then, *follow the directions for use.* If symptoms persist, stop taking the OTC drug and seek professional advice from a physician. Additional guidelines for self-medication follow.

1. *Do not expect a "miracle cure."* At best, OTC drugs can only relieve symptoms of illness. Though regulated by the Federal Trade Commission, advertising for OTC drugs tends to exaggerate the need for a particular drug, creates health problems that do not exist in reality, or promises more results than one can reasonably expect. In all likelihood, the analgesic promoted as the one remedy to end all headaches will not prevent the next one from occurring.

2. *Never use old medicines.* Leftover drugs often become stale, harmful, or ineffective over long periods of time. At regular intervals, clear your medicine cabinet of both OTC and prescription drugs that have been on hand for a long time. Since many OTC medications either lose or increase their strength as time goes by, the large economy size may not be economical if it will remain unused for several months. Check the medicine's expiration date, which is often listed on the label or elsewhere on the container itself.

box 11.6

Labeling of Over-the-Counter Drugs

Federal law requires that labels of OTC drugs provide adequate information on safe and effective use and on the conditions under which the drugs should not be taken. Look for the following items on OTC drug labels.

1. Name and address of manufacturer, packer, or distributor.
2. The lot, control, or batch number—any distinctive combination of letters, symbols, or numbers from which the complete manufacturing history of the drug can be determined.
3. Name of the product and what type of drug it is, such as an antacid, nasal decongestant, analgesic, or antiseptic.
4. Statement of the active ingredient or ingredients in the medication.
5. Declaration of the presence of the dye Yellow No. 5. People who are allergic to aspirin will also be allergic to this dye and should be careful to look for it on product labels. Other than Yellow No. 5 and certain other inactive ingredients, such as alcohol, most such ingredients do not have to be declared on OTC labels. However, due to a voluntary program established by the Proprietary Association (a trade organization) in 1987, virtually all OTC products on retail shelves or in distribution list all inactive ingredients on their outer packages. In the case of very small packages, inactive ingredients are listed on counter or shelf displays.
6. The amount of the product in the container, that is, the number of tablets or ounces of liquid, cream, or ointment.
7. Indications for use—the symptoms or conditions for which the product should be used.

8. Directions for use—sometimes designated as dosage—explain how much of the drug to take (per dose, time between doses, and maximum number of doses) and when to take it. The directions may also indicate how to take or use the product.
9. Warnings or cautions—who should not take the drug, when the drug should not be taken, what adverse reactions might develop, and what symptoms signal the need for professional help. The label might also warn that the product should not be taken for more than a specific number of days or that it should be discontinued and a doctor consulted if symptoms persist. Labeling of all OTC drug products to be taken internally must include this warning: "As with any drug, if you are pregnant or nursing a baby, seek the advice of a health professional before using this product." Other warnings advise about the habit-forming tendency of certain drugs and the recommendation that all medicines be kept out of the reach of children.
10. Drug interaction precautions—some ingredients in OTC drugs can counteract or interfere with the effectiveness of other drugs. Mixing drugs and alcohol is discouraged, especially when the drug tends to cause drowsiness.
11. Expiration date—the month and year beyond which the drug should not be used. However, not all OTC drug products will carry such a date.

Source: Modified from the U.S. Food and Drug Administration.

Old, outdated drugs should be discarded, preferably by flushing them down a toilet. When no expiration date is listed, one year from the date of purchase should be the maximum time to keep any medication.

3. *Store medicines properly to prolong their effectiveness.* OTC and prescription drugs should be stored away from bright lights in a cool, dry place that cannot be reached by children. Kitchen cabinets and bedrooms are preferred to bathrooms as storage places, because bathrooms tend to be too warm and humid. Unless directed to do so, do not store medicines in the refrigerator. In addition, keep all drugs in their original containers, capped tightly when not being used.

4. *Consult your physician and/or pharmacist for information on OTC drug effectiveness and selection of appropriate medications.* While a pharmacist may be more readily available, both professionals can assist consumers in selecting OTC products that suit their needs. In particular, a pharmacist may help consumers make informed choices on drug purchases by providing information on comparative drug effectiveness and by advising individuals on the appropriate use of drugs and proper storage of various medicines.

5. *Avoid identical medicines.* Many OTC drugs contain exactly the same ingredients and differ from one another only in brand name, container, and the amount of each ingredient. The major difference is often in the advertised claims, especially for the multidrug combinations. Unknowingly, consumers often purchase these "identical" medications and take them concurrently, and consequently become victims of drug overdose and adverse reactions. By comparing drug labels for lists of ingredients and their specific amounts, you may be able to guard against both overdose and adverse reactions, and save money as well.

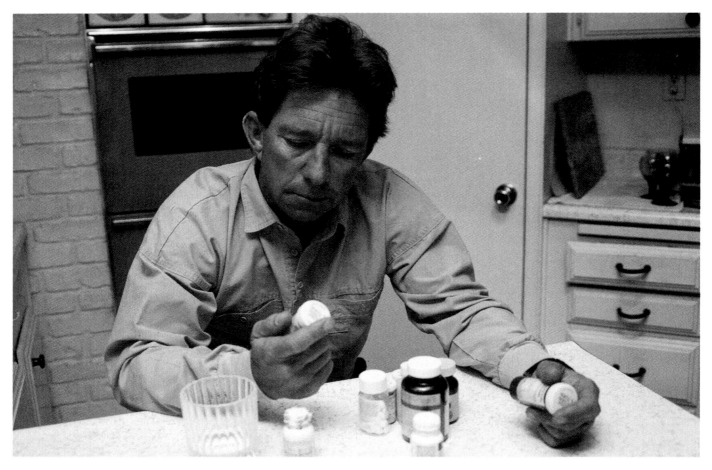

Always check medicine's expiration date, and discard outdated drugs.

© *Felicia Martinez/PhotoEdit*

6. *Save money on the purchase of OTC drugs.* Shop around at discount drugstores and take advantage of special sales and bargains. Undertake a price comparison survey to determine where specific medicines can be bought more economically. Be sure to check the expiration date on the drug container or label before you make your purchase. If a large quantity of drugs must be procured for long-term use, buying the large or king-size container of drugs may result in significant savings, if it has a sufficiently distant expiration date.

If you have reservations about low-priced drugs, look for the abbreviation *N.F.* or *U.S.P.* on certain OTC drug labels. These symbols stand for the *National Formulary* and the *United States Pharmacopeia,* reference books containing standards for identity, strength, and purity of various drugs and for the inactive ingredients in drug dosage forms. When a drug label lists one of these abbreviations, the drug itself was made according to official standards and can therefore be purchased with confidence and assurance of the highest quality.

7. *Consider generic OTC drug substitution.* As a potential money-saving technique, the substitution of **generic drugs** for **brand-name drugs** has received much publicity regarding prescription medicine purchases. However, this practice can also apply to buying OTC drugs. Generics (chemical equivalents of brand-name drugs) or store brands provide identical medications found in their brand-name counterparts. For instance, *aspirin* is the generic name for a leading analgesic. *Bayer* and *St. Joseph* are brand names for different manufacturers' aspirin. Whether you purchase the house or store brand, a generic aspirin, or one of the nationally advertised brands, there should be no differences in the painkilling quality of the aspirin products.

Nearly fifteen years ago, tests of Bayer, Norwich, Squibb, and several store (house) brands of aspirin revealed that no one brand performed significantly better than any of the other brands.[27] The tests, conducted by Consumers Union, evaluated the aspirin and salicylic acid content, and the dissolution speed of nine competing brands. Such tests are often used to indicate therapeutic effectiveness and superiority. Despite the various advertising claims of the 400-plus brands of aspirin in the United States, all aspirin is essentially the same according to these tests. As Consumers Union advises, buy the cheapest! Such advice is still valid today.

8. *If an adverse reaction occurs, stop taking the OTC drug.* On occasion, any drug will produce some effect other than the intended or anticipated one—the so-called drug **side effect.** When this side effect is unusual, undesirable, discomforting, or life threatening, the side effect is described as an **adverse drug reaction.** If you experience an adverse reaction, stop taking the OTC drug immediately and consult with a physician or pharmacist. These individuals know what actions a drug should have and what adverse effects may be expected. Follow their advice before using the drug again.

9. *Beware of the drug overdose danger.* Although OTC drugs are relatively safe when used in recommended doses, large overdoses and persistent overuse of such products can prove to be very dangerous. This is especially true with large doses of aspirin, which can result in accidental poisoning. Overuse of certain analgesics can cause kidney damage, and antacids can produce an imbalance in the body's secretion of enzymes. Prolonged use of laxatives to relieve constipation can actually lead to constipation. In order to avoid such dangers, never use any OTC drug on a regular, continuous basis or in large quantities, except on the advice of a physician. Additionally, never mix different medicines in one container. Such a practice may be confusing and lead to taking the wrong medication. To avoid another drug-taking error, never take any medicine in the dark.

10. *Exercise extreme caution and consult your physician or pharmacist when using several medications at the same time.* Each drug acts on the body in a characteristic way. However, each drug is also capable of altering the effect of any other drug a person may be taking. On occasion, the combination of drugs can be harmful and even fatal. For instance, aspirin increases the blood-thinning effect of some medicines prescribed for heart attack patients. Individuals taking such medicines risk hemorrhage if they use aspirin to relieve headaches. Some combination nasal decongestant-antihistamine cold and allergy remedies should not ordinarily be used with prescription antihypertensive or antidepressant drugs containing a monoamine oxidase inhibitor. Therefore, before using any combination of drugs (prescription with OTC drugs or several OTC drugs taken at the same time), consult your physician or pharmacist.

11. *Never combine OTC sleeping pills or antihistamines with alcohol.* Since ethyl alcohol can increase the CNS depressant effect of such drugs, the combination can produce extreme drowsiness, accident, or injury. Whenever taking either prescription or OTC drugs, ask your physician whether drinking beverage alcohol could be hazardous in combination with the medication.

Safety and Effectiveness of OTC Drugs

Each day millions of Americans engage in self-medication. They rely on the purity, safety, and effectiveness of various OTC remedies they purchase, and the adequacy of label information to get the benefits they expect. Such reliance and expectations were not always justified, because neither purity and accurate or truthful labeling nor safety and effectiveness of OTC medications had to be assured before enactment of the first national Food and Drug Act. Passed by the U.S. Congress in 1906, the law forbade interstate commerce in *misbranded* and *adulterated* (impure) drugs.

It was not until 1938, when the federal Food, Drug, and Cosmetic Act (FDC Act) was approved, that new drugs were required to be proven *safe* before their distribution. However, drug manufacturers were not required to prove the *effectiveness* of their products until passage of the Kefauver-Harris drug amendments to the FDC Act in 1962. Since then, drugs used as medicines must be proven both safe and effective to the Food and Drug Administration (FDA) before being sold in the United States. New drug products were affected immediately, but the monumental problem was the thousands of OTC and prescription drugs already on the market that had never been demonstrated to be effective.

In 1972, the FDA began a long-range regulatory program to apply the "drug efficacy" amendments to drugs sold over the counter. The ambitious program was designed to assure consumers that every OTC drug is safe, adequately and truthfully labeled, and that it will do what the manufacturer claims it will do.

To carry out the project, sixteen advisory drug review panels composed of nongovernment experts were formed to evaluate eighty basic OTC "drug classes"—antacids, laxatives, cold remedies, analgesics, etc.—for safety and effectiveness. These advisory review panels attempted to place the active ingredients in each OTC drug in one of three categories, namely:

Category I—drugs determined to be safe, effective, and not mislabeled.

Category II—drugs not generally recognized as safe and effective, or mislabeled. Such drugs must be removed from medications within six months after the FDA issues its final regulations.

Category III—drugs for which there are insufficient data to determine general recognition of safety and effectiveness.

After reviewing the advisory panels' findings—which were not binding on the FDA itself—the FDA then began establishing standards for various OTC drugs. These standards are first published in the Federal Register (an official document of the U.S. government) to elicit both consumer and industry comments and reactions to the proposals. Then a tentative monograph or report is followed several months later by a final monograph. Both are published in the Federal Register. The final monograph then has the effect of law.

Until 1981, the FDA permitted continued marketing of Category III drugs while manufacturers sought to substantiate claims for their products through further study. Because of legal pressures by a variety of consumer advocacy groups, the FDA eventually dropped the use of Category III from its final drug monographs.

Now, when the final monographs are published, only drugs found to be both safe and effective may remain on the market. Those evaluated as ineffective, unsafe, or needing further study must be removed. Such a policy reversed an old procedure that permitted drug makers to continue marketing those drugs thought to be probably safe and effective on the basis of long use, so long as the manufacturers were conducting additional tests.

Nevertheless, some drugs of doubtful effectiveness remain on the market, since a drug manufacturer can request a hearing on whether its drug should be ruled ineffective. If such a formal hearing is denied or results in an unfavorable ruling, the drug maker may initiate a legal challenge against the FDA. The drug product in question remains on the open market pending the outcome of the court proceedings—a lengthy process often lasting several months or even years.

Sometimes budgetary limitations prevent the FDA from acting as rapidly as possible. For instance, several months after "starch blockers" had been banned by the FDA, numerous stores continued to sell the controversial diet aids. Without sufficient personnel and lacking enforcement resources, neither the FDA nor its counterparts at the state level could visit each retail outlet and confiscate the illegal pills. It is interesting to note, however,

that during the entire OTC drug review process (1972–88), the FDA did not initiate any enforcement actions against those drugs that its own panels of experts had found to be unsafe.

Despite the best intentions of the U.S. Congress, the FDA, and the state agencies dealing with drug products and claims, American consumers have been subject to unreasonable and unnecessary risks to their health by purchasing OTC drugs lacking evidence of safety and effectiveness. It is estimated that the FDA's multi-year evaluation of OTC drugs and the issuance of final monographs will not be completed until the late 1990s, although the various advisory panels completed the review process in 1988.

Initial results of the OTC drug-review process indicated that only about 31 percent of the ingredients in the 300,000 brands of nonprescription drug products were both safe and effective for their intended uses. By contrast, the effectiveness review process of prescription drugs, completed in September 1984, some 22 years after the project was begun, found that, of the 3,300 prescribed drugs that were reviewed, 2,208 (66 percent) were effective for their indicated use.

Chapter Summary

1. There is a widespread belief in the effectiveness of drugs to heal discomfort and prevent disease. In some instances, however, drugs can act as poisons, cause undesirable side effects including adverse drug reactions, alter the effects of other medicines, and produce drug dependency.

2. Common usage of over-the-counter drugs—those purchased without a physician's prescription—has been accompanied by widespread drug misuse and by the inappropriate use of medicines, resulting in impaired physical, mental, emotional, or social well-being.

3. Used on a temporary basis for illnesses not requiring a physician's

supervision, OTC drugs typically do not cure diseases but do relieve symptoms.

4. The hundreds of thousands of OTC drugs are classified generally according to their primary or intended effect, such as relieving acid indigestion, controlling diarrhea, providing vitamin supplements, stopping growth of bacteria, and relieving symptoms of sneezing, watery nose, and itching of the throat.

5. There are two major types of internal analgesics: the salicylate painkillers containing aspirin, and the nonsalicylate painkillers containing acetaminophen, ibuprofen, or naproxen sodium. Aspirin, ibuprofen, and naproxen sodium also reduce fever and act to reduce inflammation, and are known as nonsteroidal anti-inflammatory drugs (NSAIDs). Acetaminophen does not reduce inflammation.

6. OTC preparations sold as sleeping aids tend to produce drowsiness. This effect is due to an antihistamine, the major ingredient of nonprescribed sleeping pills and many cold remedies.

7. OTC stimulants typically contain caffeine and help some individuals to stay awake. Usually these drugs do not improve mental alertness or motor performance to the level needed to safely operate an automobile.

8. Fixed-ratio combination products (drugs containing two or more ingredients intended to relieve a number of different symptoms), are often sold as OTC cold remedies. Frequently such multidrug mixtures contain ingredients not really needed by cold sufferers.

9. Most diet aids or appetite suppressants contain a mild stimulant (PPA) or a topical anesthetic such as benzocaine. Other weight-control products contain bulk-formers that reduce the desire to eat.

10. Self-medication is often advantageous when guidelines for responsible use are followed. Such guides pertain to reading labels; following directions; discarding old medicines; properly storing drugs; consulting with one's physician or pharmacist on the appropriateness of medications or when using more than one OTC drug at the same time; avoiding identical medicines; stopping drug usage when an adverse reaction occurs; guarding against drug overdose; and not combining OTC sleeping pills or antihistamines with alcohol.

11. Due to congressional actions, misbranded and adulterated drugs have been outlawed, and since 1962 all new drugs have been required to be proven both safe and effective.

12. Despite the regulations of the federal Food and Drug Administration and its state-level counterparts, many OTC drugs are of doubtful effectiveness and safety. Final monographs from the multiyear OTC drug review process will not likely be published until the late 1990s.

Review Questions and Activities

1. In what ways can drugs taken to restore or improve health actually harm the body and endanger life?

2. How does drug misuse differ from drug abuse?

3. List all of the OTC drugs you have taken in the past year. Which of these do you feel were beneficial? Do you think that any of the OTC drugs you have taken were a waste of money? Why? Could you have done anything else to remedy the health problem other than take a nonprescribed drug?

4. What sources are available at your college or in your local community to help you evaluate the effectiveness of OTC drugs?

5. Explain the major function or anticipated effect of each of the following OTC drug types: antiemetic, antihistamine, antiseptic, analgesic, antitussive, and dermatological.

6. Survey a variety of liquid cold remedies and allergy-relief medications at a local drugstore, and determine the relative alcohol content of each item surveyed.

7. In what ways do salicylates and nonsalicylates differ as analgesics? Investigate the names of fifteen oral analgesics available at local drugstores and classify them as either salicylate or nonsalicylate painkillers.

8. How do the NSAID analgesics differ from pain relievers that contain acetaminophen?

9. In what ways might the use of aspirin products cause harm to the body or threaten health status?

10. Why is the use of OTC fixed-ratio combination cold remedies considered to be undesirable?

11. List the anticipated effect of each of the following OTC drug ingredients: appetite suppressant, asthma preparation, expectorant, decongestant, and topical antibiotic.

12. What precautions should be observed when using OTC sleep aids and stimulants?

13. Discuss the practice of self-medication in terms of general guidelines to assure reasonable safety and effectiveness in using OTC drugs.

14. Describe the various activities of the U.S. Food and Drug Administration to assure the safety and effectiveness of OTC drugs sold in the United States.

References

1. United States Pharmacopeia, *Complete Drug Reference (1995 Edition)* (Yonkers, N.Y.: Consumer Reports Books, 1994), iv.
2. "Drug Ingredients Banned," *FDA Consumer* 25, no. 2 (March 1991): 3.
3. "FDA Bans Ineffective OTC Drug Ingredients and Adds a Warning," *Health Letter* 7, no. 1 (January 1991): 3–4.
4. Marian Segal, "Rx to OTC: The Switch Is On," *FDA Consumer* 25, no. 2 (March 1991): 9–11.
5. Editors of Consumer Reports Books, *The New Medicine Show*, rev. ed. (Mount Vernon, N.Y.: Consumers Union, 1989), 60.
6. Joe Graedon and Teresa Graedon, *Graedons' Best Medicine: From Herbal Remedies to High-Tech Rx Breakthroughs* (New York: Bantam Books, 1991), 40.
7. Steering Committee of the Physicians' Health Study Research Group, "Preliminary Report: Findings from the Aspirin Component of the Ongoing Physicians' Health Study" *New England Journal of Medicine* 318, no. 4 (28 January 1988): 262–64.
8. Gerald Weissmann, "Aspirin," *Scientific American* 264, no. 1 (January 1991): 84–90.
9. Ken Flieger, "Aspirin: A New Look at an Old Drug," *FDA Consumer* 28, no. 1 (January–February 1994): 19–21.
10. Julie Buring, Richard Peto, and Charles Hennekens, "Low-Dose Aspirin for Migraine Prophylaxis," *Journal of the American Medical Association* 264, no. 13 (3 October 1990): 1711–21.
11. "The Health Beat: Migraine and Aspirin," *Harvard Health Letter* 16, no. 3 (January 1991): 7.
12. Public Health Service and the Food and Drug Administration, *A Message from the Surgeon General about Reye Syndrome*, U.S. DHHS Pub. No. (FDA) 86–3154.
13. Evelyn Zamula, "Reye Syndrome: The Decline of a Disease," *FDA Consumer* 24, no. 9 (November 1990): 21–23.
14. "Over-the-Counter Ibuprofen May Be Hazardous to Your Health, Too," *Public Citizen Health Research Group Health Letter* 5, no. 6 (June 1989): 8.
15. Andrew Whelton, Robert Stout, Patricia Spilman, and David Klassen, "Renal Effects of Ibuprofen, Proxicam, and Sulindac in Patients with Asymptomatic Renal Failure," *Annals of Internal Medicine* 112, no. 8 (15 April 1990): 568–76.
16. "Another OTC Pain Reliever," *FDA Consumer* 18, no. 3 (April 1994): 4.
17. "Over-the-Counter Pain Relief," *University of California at Berkeley Wellness Letter* 10, no. 10 (July 1994): 3.
18. United States Pharmacopeia, *Complete Drug Reference*, 1237.

19. "FDA Bans Ineffective OTC Drug Ingredients and Adds a Warning," *Public Citizen Health Research Group Health Letter* 7, no. 1 (January 1991): 3–4.

20. "Do Not Use Phenylpropanolamine-Containing Products," *Public Citizen Health Research Group Health Letter* 7, no. 1 (January 1991): 3.

21. "Tales from the Bazaar: Automatic Weight Loss with Cal-Ban? Send for Your Refund Now!" *Consumer Reports Health Letter* 2, no. 6 (June 1990): 46–47.

22. Lauren Lissner and others, "Variability of Body Weight and Health Outcomes in the Framingham Population," *New England Journal of Medicine* 324, no. 26 (27 June 1991): 1839–44.

23. Neshama Franklin, "Dubious Drugs for Coughs and Colds," *Medical Self-Care* no. 17 (Summer 1982): 38.

24. S. M. Wolfe, M. Coley, and the Health Research Groups, *Pills That Don't Work* (New York: Farrar, Straus & Giroux, 1981), 12.

25. "Decongestants," *Consumer Reports Health Letter* 1, no. 3 (November 1989): 21.

26. United States Pharmacopeia, *Complete Drug Reference*, 1713–20.

27. "Is Bayer Better?" *Consumer Reports* 47, no. 7 (July 1982): 347–49.

chapter

12 | prescription drugs

Additive Drug Reaction
Adverse Drug Reaction
Analgesic
Anorexic (anorectic)
Antagonistic Drug Reaction
Antihypertensive Drug
Anti-infective Drug
Benefit-Risk Equation
Bioavailability
Bioequivalence
Cardiovascular Drug
Chemically Equivalent Drug
Combination Oral Contraceptive Drug
Controlled Drug
Depo-Provera
Diuretic
Drug Classes or Families
Fail-Safe Medicine
Food-Drug Interaction
Generic Drug
Insulin
Major Tranquilizer
Minipill
Minor Tranquilizer
Norplant
Patient Medication Instructions (PMIs)
Physicians' Desk Reference
Polypharmacy
Potentiation Drug Reaction
Prescription
Prescription Drug
Sedative-Hypnotic Drug
Side Effect
Stimulant
Subdermal Implants
Therapeutic Index

chapter objectives

After you have studied this chapter, you should be able to do the following:

1. Explain why so-called prescription drugs, unlike OTC drugs, can be obtained only by the direction of a physician.

2. Discuss the concepts of fail-safe medicine and the benefit-risk equation as they apply to the use of prescription drugs.

3. Identify the common elements appearing on (a) a typical prescription and (b) a typical Rx drug label.

4. Compare and contrast the restrictions placed on the prescribing of drugs under the provisions of the Controlled Substances Act.

5. List at least eight questions to be answered or guidelines to be followed in order to assure the wise use of prescription drugs.

6. Identify the major anticipated effects of the following drug classes or families: anorexics, antiasthmatics, antidepressants, antihypertensives, antispasmodics, and diuretics.

7. Describe the differences between the major and the minor tranquilizers in terms of their psychotherapeutic uses.

8. Explain the similarities and differences between the combination oral contraceptive pill and the minipill.

9. Identify five of the most serious and life-threatening side effects associated with using oral contraceptives.

10. Name several noncontraceptive benefits associated with the use of oral contraceptives.

11. Define the following related to drug-based contraception or birth control: estrogen hormone agents, progestin hormone agents, Depo-Provera, Norplant, and RU 486.

12. Describe several relatively mild side effects and several adverse reactions associated with the use of prescription drugs.

13. Explain the significance of the therapeutic index.

14. List at least five guidelines for preventing or minimizing adverse drug reactions.

15. Discuss the relationship between polypharmacy and drug interactions in terms of drug absorption, distribution, metabolism, excretion, and drug reactions.

16. Distinguish between additive and potentiating drug interactions.

17. Describe the potential usefulness of the *Physicians' Desk Reference* to the consumer.

18. Define the following in relation to the "generic" versus "brand-name" drug controversy: chemical drug name, generic drug name, brand drug name, chemical equivalence, bioavailability, and bioequivalence.

several guidelines are offered for the wise use of prescription drugs. Next, there is an investigation of the most frequently prescribed drugs, including psychoactives. Separate drug classes are described briefly.

Since many patients apparently fail to comply with directions for using drugs, because they lack information on what can happen if they deviate from instructions, an extensive section explores the potential for side effects and adverse reactions accompanying drug use. A concluding investigation focuses on the issue of generic versus brand-name drugs.

Prescribed Drugs: Potent Chemotherapeutic Agents

According to the Food, Drug, and Cosmetic Act, drugs are substances intended for use in the diagnosis, cure, mitigation, treatment, or prevention of disease. Many of these drug substances or medicines are used beneficially in programs of self-medication that relieve minor symptoms. Such drugs that can be purchased over the counter (OTC) and taken without a physician's supervision have been identified and described in chapter 11.

There are many other drugs that also have a legally recognized therapeutic value, such as Amoxil, Zantac, Premarin, Seldane, and Xanax. Unlike OTC drugs, these medicines can be obtained only by the direction of a physician and are referred to as **prescription** or *Rx* **drugs.** Sold only by licensed pharmacists, prescribed drugs are used in treating specific disease conditions of a more serious nature, are generally more powerful than OTC drugs, and are more likely to cause unexpected and adverse side effects. In comparison with OTC drugs, prescribed medicines have a relatively higher risk of causing toxicity and a lower margin of safety.[1]

Potent chemotherapeutic agents, prescription drugs require professional supervision in their use because of the complex and powerful actions they can have on human structure and body function. Presently, several nonphysician specialists, such as dentists, podiatrists, and some pharmacists, optometrists, physician assistants, and nurse practitioners—all of

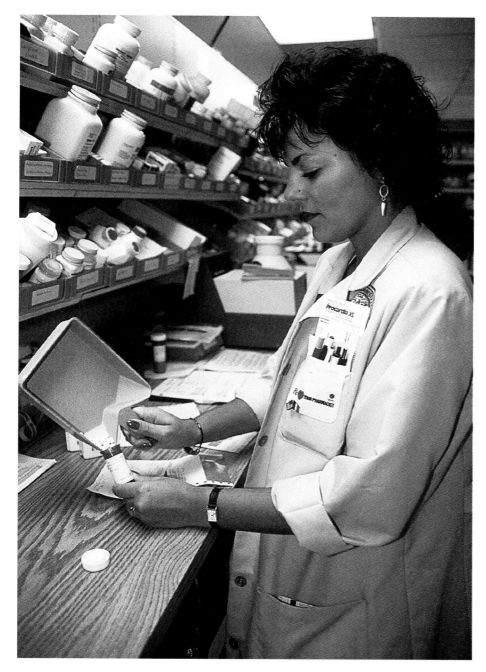

Prescription drugs may be sold only by licensed pharmacists in a variety of drug stores, as well as through pharmacist-supervised mail-order programs.

© Jeff Greenberg/PhotoEdit

Introduction

Although the major concern of this text is psychoactive drugs and their abuse potential, a related American drug problem is the widespread misuse of all prescribed drugs—not just those having their primary impact on the human mind. Therefore, a chapter on physician-prescribed medications seems most appropriate.

To counter the widespread belief in "fail-safe" medicines, the "benefit-risk" equation is described, portraying all medications as having the potential for harm as well as for health and cure. After prescriptions and drug labels are examined,

whom have been granted limited prescribing privileges in specific states—are qualified to determine the nature of a particular health problem and recommend an appropriate medication.[2] Nevertheless, only physicians are trained professionally to use a broad range of therapeutic drugs safely. Only these professionals can determine how long a specific drug can be taken—and in what amounts—without harm.

The Benefit-Risk Equation

Many people believe in the myth of **fail-safe medicine,** that is, the expectation that all drugs work safely on all people at all times. However, there is a common and not well-publicized reality that exists in all medical practice as well as in many aspects of human endeavor—the so-called **benefit-risk equation.** According to this equation, there is a high probability that absolute safety does not exist. This is particularly true with regard to drugs.

Whether at the conscious or subconscious level, nearly all regulatory judgments are based on a compromise between benefits and risks. This benefit-to-risk judgment applies to crossing a busy street, driving a car, chewing a piece of meat that could cause choking, and undergoing surgery, as well as to taking a prescribed medicine. The probability of the good outweighs the possibility of the bad. If a medication poses an unusual or serious risk to the user, then, to justify prescribing it for that person, its benefits must be proportionately high and urgently required.

Indeed, every drug has the potential for causing unanticipated and unintended drug reactions or **side effects.** These side effects may range from relatively minor complaints that are undesirable and discomforting to the more serious effects that can be life threatening, even fatal. The more serious side effects are usually described as **adverse drug reactions.**

It is the competent physician then, together with an informed patient, who must decide if the health-giving or medicinal characteristics of an Rx drug are greater than the drug's potential hazards. Consequently, pharmacists can dispense these powerful drugs only to individuals who have a physician's prescription.

 table 12.1 Some Common Prescription Symbols

Latin Origin	Abbreviation	Meaning
ad libitum	ad lib.	Freely, as needed
ante cibos	a.c.	Before meals
auris dextra	A.D.	Right ear
auris laeva	A.L.	Left ear
auris	a.u.	Both ears
bis in die	b.i.d.	Twice a day
—	C	100
capsula	caps.	Capsule
cum	c̄	With
—	cc	Cubic centimeter
—	disp.	Dispense
dentur tales doses	dtd #	Give this number
—	ext.	For external use
guttae	gtt.	Drops
hora	h.	Hour
hora somni	h.s.	At bedtime
mitte	mitt. #	Give this number
—	ml	Milliliter
oculus dexter	O.D.	Right eye
oculus laevus	O.L.	Left eye
oculus uterque	O.U.	Each eye
per os	p.o.	Orally, by mouth
post cibum	p.c.	After meals
pro re nata	prn.	As needed
quaqua	q.	Every
quaqua die	q.d.	Once a day
quaqua 4 hora	q. 4h.	Every 4 hours
quater in die	q.i.d.	4 times a day
semis	ss.	Half or half unit
sine	s̄	Without
signa	sig.	Label as follows
statim	stat.	Immediately, at once
sub lingua	sl.	Under the tongue
—	sol.	Solution
—	tab.	Tablet
—	top.	Apply topically
ter in die	t.i.d.	3 times a day
unguentum	ung. or ungt.	Ointment
ut dictum	ut dict, UD	As directed

Prescriptions and Drug Labels

A **prescription** is a physician's order to a pharmacist to dispense a specific drug product to a patient.[3] The prescription itself may be written or given orally to a pharmacist or nurse, in person or by telephone. According to the Pharmaceutical Manufacturers Association, nearly 70 percent of all Rx drugs are dispensed through prescriptions; the remainder are administered directly to patients or provided in hospitals or by physicians themselves.

Reading a Prescription

Although a prescription may appear to be a foreign, garbled handwritten message to a pharmacist, there is no mystery about reading a physician's order if the pharmacists know the special shorthand and can decipher the physician's handwriting. The prescription actually follows a uniform procedure and includes the following elements on a preprinted form:[4]

The *physician's name, address, phone number, and DEA* (Drug Enforcement

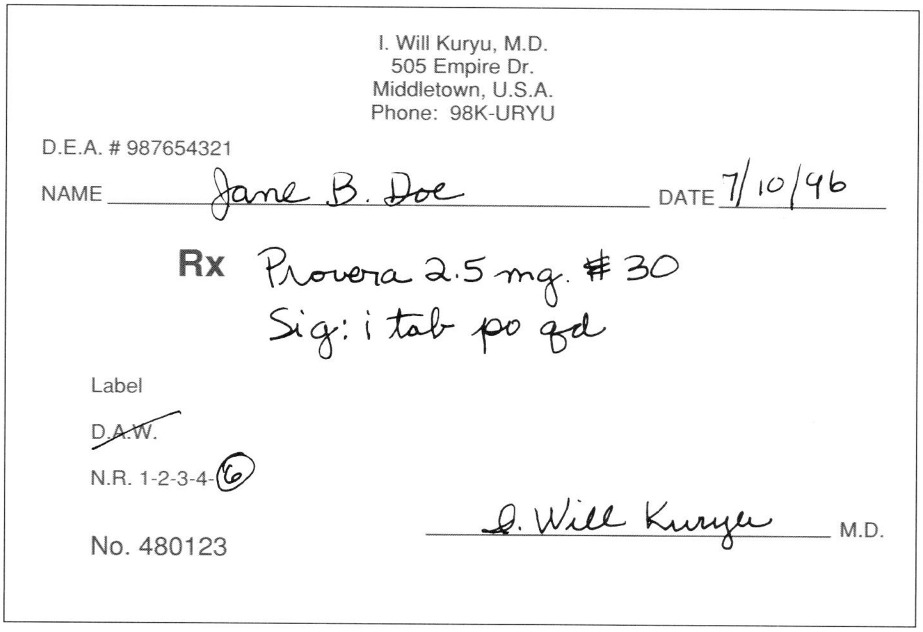
I. Will Kuryu, M.D.
505 Empire Dr.
Middletown, U.S.A.
Phone: 98K-URYU

D.E.A. # 987654321

NAME Jane B. Doe DATE 7/10/96

Rx Provera 2.5 mg. # 30
Sig: i tab po qd

Label

~~D.A.W.~~

N.R. 1-2-3-4-(6)

No. 480123

I. Will Kuryu M.D.

figure 12.1

The sample prescription above is for a medication named Provera, a synthetic female hormone used to treat abnormal menstrual bleeding, difficult menstruation, lack of menstruation, and several other conditions as determined by one's physician. According to the prescription, the pharmacist is directed to provide the patient with 30 tablets (#30) of Provera, 2.5 mg. dosage level. One tablet (i tab) is to be taken by mouth (po) once every day (qd). The prescription also states that the label on the container should list the name of the drug (Label is not crossed out), that the pharmacist may substitute a less expensive generic drug (D.A.W. or dispense as written is crossed out), and that the patient may receive 6 refills (N.R. with 6 encircled).

Administration) *number,* which is required if the prescription is for a controlled substance.

The *patient's name.*

Date of the prescription.

Name of the drug being prescribed.

Dosage form. If there is a choice of the form in which the medication is to be dispensed, it will be indicated by an abbreviation, such as *caps* for capsule, *tab* for tablet, *el* for elixir, *sy* for syrup, or *sol* for solution.

Strength of the dose. Usually this information is stated in a metric measure, such as *50 mg,* which means 50 milligrams.

Amount to be dispensed. This is the number of units of the drug to be given. If four capsules are to be taken every day for four days, the amount to be dispensed would be sixteen.

Directions for use. Sometimes beginning with the abbreviation *Sig,* the last line of the prescription tells the pharmacist the instructions for the patient that should appear on the container label. These instructions are written in a Latin form of medical shorthand, as noted in table 12.1, which must be interpreted by the pharmacist.

The *number of times the prescription can be refilled,* if at all.

Labeling instructions. The prescribing physician may indicate whether the drug container should state the name of the drug to be dispensed.

Generic drug substitution. When **generic** equivalent **drugs** may be substituted for prescribed brand-name medicines, a physician may allow such a practice by signing the substitute line or crossing out the dispense as written (D.A.W.) designation. On the other hand, if a physician wants a patient to receive the specific brand drug noted on the prescription form, then the signature is placed on the "dispense as written" line or the D.A.W. designation is not crossed out.

The physician's signature. In some states, controlled substances (drugs having an abuse potential that are regulated by state and federal laws) must be prescribed on triple-copy pads. One copy is sent to state public safety officials, while the other copies are kept by the prescribing physician and the dispensing pharmacist.

Labels on Prescribed Medicines

Though prescription drugs are more powerful and more likely to produce serious side effects than OTC drugs, the labels on prescribed medicine containers have somewhat limited information in comparison with their OTC counterparts. Prescription drug labels generally carry the following information:

Name, address, and *phone number* of the dispensing pharmacy.

Prescription number, which is sometimes followed by the initials of the dispensing pharmacist.

Prescribing *physician's name.*

Date when prescription was filled.

Patient's name.

Drug name. In some instances, state laws may require the listing of the originally prescribed drug name and the product's manufacturer, if a generic drug has been substituted.

Directions for use, such as *dosage, frequency of use, when to take the medicine, how to take the medicine, and specific instructions for storage or preparation for use.* (See figures 12.1 and 12.2.)

On controlled substances (psychoactive therapeutic drugs having an abuse potential) as well as noncontrolled medicines, a *special legend* regarding *federal prohibition of the transfer of the drug* to any person other than the patient for whom the medication was prescribed.

Expiration date indicates the month, day, and year after which the medicine's potency is not likely to be maintained and/or the date beyond which the prescription cannot be refilled.

Number of allowable refills, if any.

Labels on prescribed medicines are not required to indicate precisely what the drug will likely do or why the medicine is being prescribed. Common side effects or precautions are not routinely listed. Only a general warning may be provided by the pharmacist, who may attach a small adhesive tag to the drug container or provide a small sheet detailing various precautions to observe, as a service by the dispensing pharmacy. Even the required directions for use might be inadequately stated. For instance, the direction to take a medication "before meals" is not specific enough for most individuals. Adequate instructions would indicate exactly how long before meals the medication should be taken.

All of this detailed information should come from one's own physician. It will not likely be printed on the drug container's label.

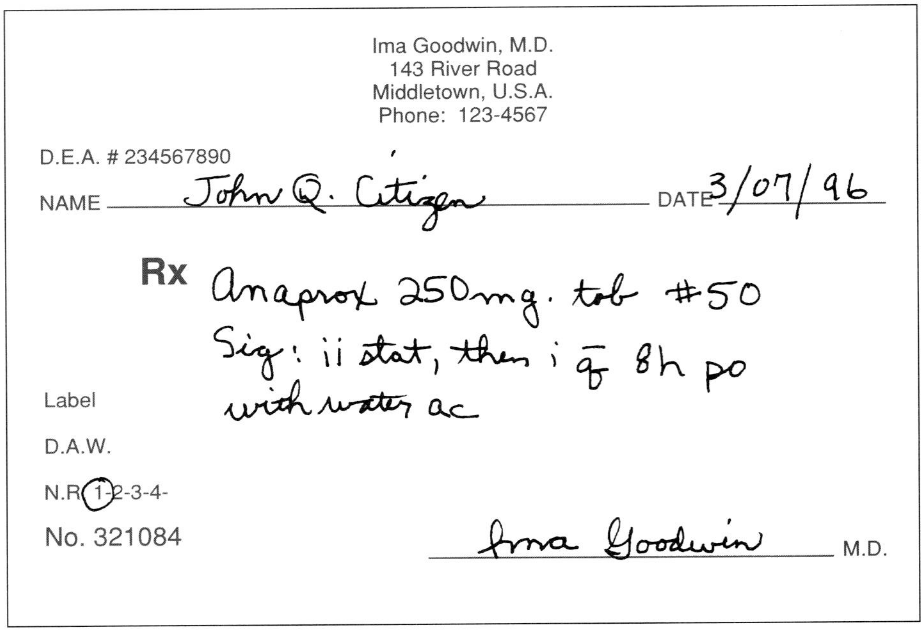

Ima Goodwin, M.D.
143 River Road
Middletown, U.S.A.
Phone: 123-4567

D.E.A. # 234567890

NAME ___John Q. Citizen___ DATE 3/07/96

Rx Anaprox 250mg. tab #50
Sig: ii stat, then i q̄ 8h po
with water ac

Label

D.A.W.

N.R (1)-2-3-4-

No. 321084

___Ima Goodwin___ M.D.

figure 12.2

The sample prescription above is for Anaprox, a brand name for a specific nonsteroidal anti-inflammatory analgesic often used to control pain, swelling, and stiffness accompanying certain types of arthritis. As indicated on the prescription, the pharmacist is directed to give the patient 50 tablets (#50) of Anaprox, 250 mg. dosage level. The label also states that two tablets should be taken at once as the first dose (ii stat), then the dose should be decreased to one tablet every 8 hours (i q̄ 8h) by mouth (po) with water before meals (ac). The label on the drug container should list the name of the medication (Label is not crossed out); the pharmacist must fill the prescription as written and no generic is allowed (D.A.W. is not crossed out); and the patient may receive just one refill.

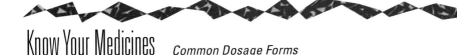

Know Your Medicines *Common Dosage Forms*

Caplet—a round or elongated tablet with a coated or smooth surface.

Capsule—a thin gelatin case or shell that encloses a medicine.

Inhalant—a breathable mist or fine powder that is introduced into the body through the lungs.

Injectable—typically, a liquid medication that enters the body by way of a syringe and needle.

Liquid—a solution in which a drug is completely dissolved. A *suspension* is a liquid in which the active drug is only partially dissolved, while an *elixir* or tincture is a solution of a medicinal substance in alcohol. By contrast, a *syrup* is a concentrated solution of sugar that contains the active drug ingredient along with flavoring and stabilizing agents. *Drops* are solutions or suspensions containing a drug that is

introduced behind the eyelid or into the ear. *Nasal sprays* or drops are solutions of a drug in water intended to produce a localized effect in the nostrils.

Suppository—a solid medication that is inserted into the rectum or vagina, where the drug dissolves.

Tablet—a solid form of medicine made by compressing the powder form of the same drug. Frequently, the term *tablet* is used interchangeably with "pill," although a pill is more generally described as a solid form of medicine in a globular or oval mass.

Topical—a drug form such as an ointment, cream, lotion, or liquid that is applied to an external surface of the body.

Transdermal—a medication that is absorbed into the body through the skin.

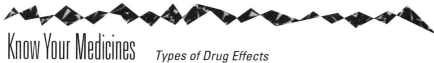

Know Your Medicines
Types of Drug Effects

box 12.2

Buccal—general or whole-body effects resulting from the slow absorption of a medicine through the cheek.

Dental—localized effect when a drug is applied to the teeth or gums.

Inhalation—local or even systemic (general) effects when a drug is inhaled into the lungs in breathing.

Mucosal—local drug effect when a medication is applied to mucous membranes, such as the inside of the mouth.

Nasal—local drug effect when a medicine is used in the nose or nostrils.

Ophthalmic—local drug effect when a medication is applied directly to the eyes.

Otic—local drug effect when a medication is introduced into the ear.

Parenteral-local—localized effects in a specific body area, when the drug is injected.

Rectal—local or systemic (general) effect when a drug is used in the rectum.

Sublingual—general or whole-body effects resulting from the slow absorption of a medicine placed under the tongue.

Systemic—general or whole-body effect; descriptive of medicine taken by mouth or by injection.

Topical—local drug effect when a medication is applied directly to the skin.

Vaginal—local or systemic (general) effect when a drug is used in the vagina.

The label on an Rx drug will indicate the number of times the medicine can be refilled. Under the provisions of the Controlled Substances Act (see chapters 1 and 13), those therapeutic drugs having a significant potential for producing psychological or physical dependence are restricted according to the following schedule.[5]

1. *Schedule I* drugs, such as heroin, marijuana, and LSD, are used for closely supervised research purposes only, and are not legally available at present for medicinal use by prescription.

2. Prescriptions for currently used *Schedule II* drugs (those having the highest abuse potential and dependence liability), such as morphine, methadone, Demerol, certain short-acting barbiturates, and specific amphetamines, must be written, not telephoned, to a pharmacy, and they may not be refilled. In order to obtain more drugs, the patient must return to a physician to obtain another written prescription.

3. Prescriptions for *Schedule III* drugs (codeine, hydrocodone, some hypnotics, such as Doriden and Noludar, and some appetite suppressants, such as Didrex, Tenuate, and Sanorex) and *Schedule IV* drugs (pentazocine [Talwin], propoxyphene [Darvon], all benzodiazepines, and certain hypnotics, such as Placidyl, Noctec, and Valmid) may be either written or telephoned to a pharmacy and may be refilled on the patient's own decision up to five times, and at any time within six months from the date of the initial dispensing. Until 1987, if no renewals had been authorized on the prescription as originally written, a physician would have needed to authorize a new prescription if the patient required more medication. Now, physicians may later authorize a pharmacist to dispense additional medication based on the original prescription.

4. *Schedule V* drugs include both prescribed and several OTC narcotic preparations of antitussives and antidiarrheals that contain codeine. Schedule V drugs requiring a prescription are processed as any other nonscheduled prescription drug. Some OTC drug preparations can be sold only upon approval by a pharmacist. In addition, the buyer must be at least 18 years old and is required to sign his or her name in a special record maintained by the pharmacist.

Using Prescribed Drugs Wisely

Because labels provide relatively little information about prescribed medicines, and due to the widespread public ignorance regarding drugs and their effects, numerous consumer action groups, along with the Food and Drug Administration, suggest that patients obtain such detailed information from their physicians. But getting the facts, the precautions, the early-warning signs of adverse reactions, and related information on drug effects may involve developing a degree of assertiveness with one's own physician. By all means, do not be intimidated by your health care consultant. Remember, your health is at stake!

Ask plenty of questions. Refuse complicated explanations offered in "medical jargon." If you do not understand certain instructions, ask—even demand—that the physician repeat them slowly so you can write them down. The wise patient is one who has answers to the following questions *before* taking prescribed drugs.[6]

1. *What is the name of the medicine?* Write it down or have your physician write it legibly for you, even if the drug's name will occur on the label. It is advisable that you keep a record of all medications that you take.

2. *When and how often should the drug be taken?* If your physician tells you to take the drug three times a day, be

sure to notice whether it should be taken before or after meals. If "every six hours" is specified, does that mean when you are awake, or should you get up during the night to take the medicine every six hours? (See fig 12.3.)

3. *What is the medicine supposed to do?* Will it reduce the pain or get to the cause of the pain, reduce fever, lower blood pressure, or cure infection? Does the drug merely relieve symptoms or eliminate or control an underlying condition?

4. *Can the new medicine be taken along with others?* If you are taking other medications, tell your physician. On occasion, drugs may interact to cause either a decrease or an increase in the desired effect.

5. *What unwanted side effects might occur?* In some individuals, medicines might cause drowsiness, nausea, vomiting, dizziness, nervousness, or other reactions. Should an unexpected reaction occur, inform your physician as soon as possible. He or she may want to change your medication.

6. *What precautions should you take?* For example, if the expected reaction to a medicine is drowsiness, dizziness, or unsteadiness, you should not drive or operate machinery.

7. *Are there any particular foods you should avoid while taking the medicine?* Some antibiotics, for example, will not work if you drink milk or eat milk products. Alcoholic beverages should not be used when some drugs are being taken.

8. *Should you take the medicine until it is all gone or just until you feel better?* Some medicines must be taken for long periods of time to cure the disease. If you stop taking the medicine too early, even when you feel better, the symptoms and disease may recur.

Supplied with the answers to the foregoing questions, the consumer-patient may wish to consider several additional guidelines in using prescription medicines.

All of the following suggestions are designed to safely enhance the effectiveness of a drug.[7]

- *Follow the directions for using a drug* as specified on the label.

- *Inform your physician and pharmacist about any medication problems you may have and all medications you are now taking* or have taken during the past few weeks.

- *If you are pregnant, planning to become pregnant, or breast-feeding, consult with your physician* before taking any medicines, including OTC drugs.

- *Before surgery of any kind,* including dental surgery or emergency treatment, *inform your physician, surgeon, or dentist of any medication you are taking.*

- After completing your course of medication, *discard the remaining prescribed drugs.*

- To avoid medication errors, *never take a medicine in the dark or from an unlabeled container.*

- *Store your medication properly* in its original container, away from bright lights, and in a cool, dry place, out of the reach of children.

- *Do not use outdated medications,* because certain drugs lose their effectiveness or potency with age.

- *Never give your prescribed medications to another person,* and never take medicine prescribed for anyone else.

Frequently Used Prescription Drugs

Each year, a nationwide survey, the National Prescription Audit (NPA), indicates which drugs are most often dispensed in chain, independent, and food store pharmacies in the United States (see table 12.2).[8] The NPA, a continuing study of the movement of prescription drugs from retail pharmacies to patients, is based on

prescriptions dispensed by pharmacists, not on prescriptions written by physicians. Such a procedure reflects the growing importance of retail pharmacists' decision-making authority regarding multiple-source drugs, when generic products may be substituted for brand-name drugs.

An analysis of the National Prescription Audit reveals that the total number of prescriptions filled each year in the United States is 1.96 billion. This number includes both refills (0.83 billion) and new prescriptions (1.13 billion), and both brand-name and generic drugs. By the mid 1990s, the average cost of a prescribed drug had risen to nearly $27. Furthermore, the audit confirmed once again the growing trend of physicians to prescribe generic drugs when writing new prescriptions. At least 15 percent of all new prescription drugs are now generic.

Of all prescribed drugs, other than those administered to hospitalized patients, only a small proportion (5 percent or less) are **controlled drugs,** scheduled medications that have a significant potential for abuse and addiction. These psychoactive drugs are under the regulatory control of the Drug Enforcement Administration (DEA), an agency of the U.S. Department of Justice. Most of these controlled medicines are anti-anxiety drugs, the so-called minor tranquilizers, narcotic analgesics, sedatives, and hypnotics.

Prescription Drug Classes

The huge numbers of prescription medications are often subdivided into major groups. These **drug classes or families** share important characteristics in terms of their chemical composition or in their actions within the human body. Typically, the several drugs within a class or family all behave in particular and somewhat similar ways. There are, to be sure, some important exceptions.

Careful analysis of the various drug classes reveals that within each class or category there may be several medications containing the same or very similar basic drug ingredients that are marketed under different brand names. Identified below

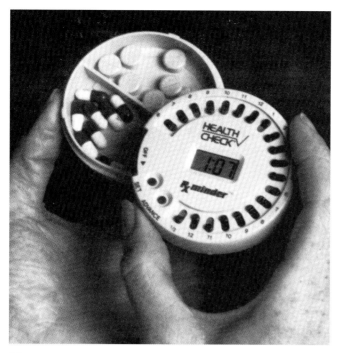

(a)

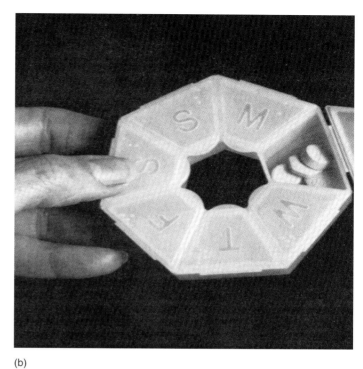

(b)

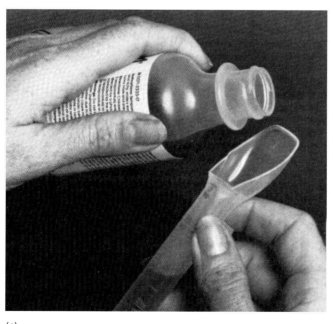

(c)

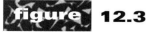

(d)

figure 12.3

Taking the right dose. (a) Several types of aids are available to help people take the right dose of medicine at the right time, like this pill container with a quiet, wristwatch-like alarm that can be set for specific times of day or specific intervals. (b) A pill container with Braille markings that holds a week's worth of pills, divided into days of the week. (c) A spoon marked with the appropriate dosages for liquid medications. (d) An oral medication syringe, similarly marked.

Source: U.S. Food and Drug Administration.

table **12.2** The Top 30 Drugs of All New and Refill Prescriptions in the United States, 1993

Rank	Drug Name	Generic Name	Therapeutic Use
1	Premarin Oral	conjugate estrogen	Replacement female hormone therapy
2	Amoxil	amoxicillin	Antibiotic
3	Zantac	ranitidine	Antiulcer drug
4	Procardia XL	nifedipine	Antianginal, antihypertensive, calcium channel blocker
5	Synthroid	levothyroxine	Thyroid hormone
6	Lanoxin	digoxin	Improves contraction force of heart muscle
7	Trimox	amoxicillin	Antibiotic; anti-infective, penicillin
8	Vasotec	enalapril	Antihypertensive
9	Xanax	alprozolam	Anti-anxiety drug; minor tranquilizer
10	Ceclor	cefaclor	Antibiotic
11	Augmentin	amoxicillin	Antibiotic
12	Proventil Aerosol	albuterol	Bronchodilator
13	Prozac	fluoxetine	Treatment of mental depression
14	Cardizem CD	diltiazem	Relieves and controls angina (chest pain) with heart disorder, calcium channel blocker
15	Naprosyn	naproxen	Analgesic, anti-inflammatory drug
16	Provera	medroxyprogesterone	Female sex hormone
17	Mevacor	HMG-CoH reductase inhibitor	Lowers blood cholesterol levels
18	Ventolin Aerosol	albuterol	Bronchodilator
19	Tagamet	cimetidine	Relieves duodenal ulcer pain, speeds ulcer healing
20	Seldane	terfenadine	Antihistamine
21	Capoten	captopril	Antihypertensive
22	Ortho-Novum	norethindrone and mestranol or ethinyl estradiol	Oral contraceptive
23	Cipro	ciprofloxacin	Anti-infective; antibacterial
24	Coumadin Sodium	warfarin	Anticoagulant
25	Lopressor	metaprolol	Antihypertensive, beta blocker
26	Micronase	glyburide	Antidiabetic
27	Dilantin	phenytoin	Anticonvulsant
28	Calan	verapimil	Relieves and controls angina; calcium channel blocker
29	Amoxicillin Trihydrate	amoxicillin	Anti-infective; systemic penicillin; antibiotic
30	Propoxyphene N/APAP	propoxyphene napsylate	Narcotic analgesic with acetaminophen

Source: Data from the National Prescription Audit.

are several of the major drug classes or drug families, together with representative brand-name medications.

Analgesics relieve pain and produce insensibility to pain without loss of consciousness. Mild analgesics include Darvon, Darvocet, Percodan, Talwin, and Valadol. Some stronger analgesics are Demerol, Dolophine (methadone), and Leritine.

Anorexics, many of which are amphetaminelike central nervous system stimulants, are occasionally prescribed for weight loss because they tend to reduce one's appetite. Commonly prescribed diet pills are Desoxyn, Didrex, Fastin, Ionamin, Preludin, and Tenuate.

Antialcohol preparations produce a sensitivity to ethyl alcohol resulting in an unpleasant reaction when the patient takes even small amounts of alcohol. Antabuse is a brand name of disulfiram frequently used to deter drinking of ethanol in the management of alcoholism.

Antiarthritics are used to treat joint diseases, specifically rheumatoid arthritis, osteoarthritis, and related arthritic conditions. The anti-inflammatory action of these drugs reduces joint swelling, pain, and duration of morning stiffness and improves functional ability of arthritic patients. Both nonsteroidal (Ansaid, Feldene, Indocin, Motrin, Naprosyn, and Voltaren) and corticosteroidal (Decadron and Prednisone) medications are examples of antiarthritic drugs.

Antihistamines block the action of a specific chemical, histamine, and are used in the treatment as well as prevention of various allergic reactions, especially the prevention of allergic rhinitis. This condition is the inflammation of the nose and upper airways, resulting from a reaction to an allergen, such as pollen, dust, or animal fur. These antihistamine drugs are used to relieve itching, swelling, and redness characteristic of allergic reaction involving the skin. Among the frequently prescribed antihistamines are Actidil, Atarax, Hismanal, Polaramine, and Seldane.

Antiasthmatics, or bronchodilators, by dilating bronchial tubes (airways) that are in sustained constriction, relieve difficult breathing associated with acute attacks of bronchial asthma and with other disorders characterized by spasm of the bronchial tubes. Bronkodyl, Bronkosol, Choledyl, Intal, Isuprel, Neothylline, Theo-Dur, and Theolair are antiasthmatics.

Anti-infective drugs, or antimicrobials, such as antibiotics, sulfonamides (sulfa drugs), antifungal preparations, and antiseptics are pharmaceutical agents that inactivate and eliminate invading, disease-causing microbes. Drugs in this family destroy bacteria or inhibit the growth and multiplication of infecting microorganisms. Among the most frequently prescribed drugs are the antibiotics, represented by cephalosporins (Ceclor), erythromycins (E.E.S.), penicillins (Amoxil, Augmentin), and tetracyclines (Achromycin). Gantrisin is a commonly used sulfa drug.

Antidepressants are prescribed for the relief of emotional depression, dejection, and withdrawal. Sometimes these drugs also reduce feelings of anxiety and produce a sedative effect. The foremost antidepressant is Prozac, a relatively new and somewhat controversial psychopharmacological medication. The tricyclic antidepressants include Aventyl, Elavil, Surmontil, and Tofranil. Another group of antidepressants, the monoamine oxidase (MAO) inhibitors, are represented by Parnate, Marplan, and Nardil. These drugs have amphetaminelike actions, inhibit a particular brain enzyme, and produce neurotransmitters that tend to maintain normal mood and emotional stability.

Antidiabetic agents, taken by mouth as well as by injected forms of **insulin,** help to maintain the diabetic patient's blood sugar at a nearly normal level and keep the urine as free of sugar as possible. Prescribed oral antidiabetics help the body to release its own insulin and are represented by Diabinese, Dymelor, Micronase, and Orinase. Injected insulin, for which a prescription is not required, is used to restore the body's ability to utilize sugar normally in the condition of diabetes. Examples of injected insulin preparations are Iletin, Lente Insulin, Regular Insulin, and Ultralente Insulin.

Antidiarrheals are used in the management and control of diarrhea (increased frequency and fluid content of fecal discharge). Antidiarrheals containing narcotics or narcotic derivatives tend to reduce intestinal movements. Other drugs in this family relax the smooth musculature of the intestinal tract or destroy specific bacteria causing the diarrhea. Donnagel-PG, Lomotil, Paregoric, and Parepectolin are frequently prescribed to control diarrhea.

Antihypertensive drugs are special types of cardiovascular (heart and blood vessel) drugs used to reduce high blood pressure. Some of these drugs act directly on the heart to lower heart rate and blood pressure (the alpha- and beta-blockers), while others—the diuretics—help rid the body of excess water and salt and thus produce an antihypertensive effect. Aldomet, Capoten, Inderal, Loniten, Lopressor, Minipress, Tenormin, and Vasotec are common antihypertensive drugs.

Antineoplastics are used in treating specific cancerous conditions. These drugs are often prescribed to reduce the pain and other symptoms of cancer and include various pharmaceutical agents, such as antibiotic derivatives, antimetabolites, hormones, steroids, and derivatives of nitrogen mustard. Among prescribed antineoplastics are Adrucil, Fluorouracil, Mexate, Cytoxan, Megace, and Leukeran.

Antispasmodics and antiulcer agents are prescribed for the control of various disorders of the stomach and intestinal tract. These drugs tend to reduce the muscular contractions or spasms of the gastrointestinal tract or reduce acid secretion in the stomach. Examples of these drug families are Anaspaz, Bentyl, Darbid, Robinul, Donnatal containing phenobarbital, Tagamet, and Zantac.

However, recent medical research has revealed that almost all duodenal ulcers are due to a spiral-shaped bacterium, *Helicobacter pylori,* as are nearly 80 percent of gastric ulcers.[9] As a consequence, treatment of ulcers—the open sores in the lining of the stomach or the upper part of the small intestine—will likely involve more use of the antibiotic tetracycline or amoxicillin.

Cardiovascular drugs affect the function of the heart and blood vessels of the body. In addition to the widely used antihypertensives that control high blood pressure, cardiovascular drugs include (1) calcium channel-blocking *antianginal*

preparations (Calan, Cardizem, and Procardia), which dilate blood vessels supplying the heart and thus relieve pain; (2) *antiarrhythmics* (Inderal, Norpace, Tonocard), which help restore normal rhythm to one's heartbeat—Inderal also has other positive effects on heart function; (3) *digitalis* (Digoxin, Lanoxin), which increases the strength of the heart's contraction; (4) *coronary vasodilators,* such as nitroglycerin (Arlidin, Nitro-Bid, Vasodilan), which increase the blood flow to heart muscle; and (5) *vasopressors* (Aramine), which increase both systolic and diastolic blood pressure and are thus used in treating low blood pressure.

Cholesterol-lowering drugs tend to reduce the amount of damaging blood fats that contribute to the build-up of fatty deposits in the arteries of the body. Some of these (Colestid, Questran) block the reabsorption of cholesterol-carrying bile salts, while others (Atromid-S, Lorelco, and Lopid) prevent the conversion of fatty acids to lipids in the liver.

Diuretics help the body to pass excess water and salt and cause a sudden and copious flow of urine. Drugs such as Aldactone, Dyazide, Diuril, Lozol, and Lasix are frequently prescribed to lower blood pressure and to manage symptoms of liver and kidney diseases and congestive heart failure.

Sedative-hypnotic drugs are prescribed to induce sleep or to produce a reduction in tension and anxiety. Noludar and Placidyl are hypnotics used to counter insomnia on a short-term basis. Another nonbarbiturate sedative is Phenergan, an antihistamine with sedative action. Halcion, Dalmane, and Restoril (representing the benzodiazepine anti-anxiety drug family) are used frequently as bedtime sedatives to induce sleep. The barbiturates, Amytal, Nembutal, Phenobarbital, Seconal, and Tuinal, may be prescribed as sleeping drugs due to their depressant effect on the central nervous system.

Stimulants are drugs that speed up the function of the central nervous system. Biphetamine and Dexedrine may be used to treat children with attention deficit disorders as well as the condition of narcolepsy (uncontrollable desire for sleep or sudden attacks of deep sleep). Cylert, another CNS stimulant that is structurally

The Drug Approval Process

Before any new over-the-counter or prescription drug can be marketed in the United States, an enormous amount of research and testing must be accomplished. Such an extensive undertaking involves many people and a great deal of money and can often span many years. The drug approval process consists of two major stages, as indicated below:

Preclinical stage. During this part of the approval process, researchers test a newly discovered drug to determine its effects as well as unanticipated side effects. They use laboratory tests, usually involving animals, to demonstrate both safety and effectiveness. This phase often takes two years or more, during which time researchers conduct other tests to establish the most effective method of administering the drug, *i.e.*, by injection or by capsule, tablet, or liquid. After the manufacturer notifies the United States Food and Drug Administration (FDA) that the drug company wants to investigate a new drug, then the formal approval process begins. In its notification to the FDA on an Investigational New Drug (IND) application, the manufacturer must explain how and why human tests will be conducted.

Clinical stage. After the FDA approves the drug company's IND application, human testing is conducted in three distinct phases. Phase 1 begins when the drug is given first to a small number of healthy adults. This initial phase of clinical testing establishes the safety of the drug, records side effects experienced in the test population, and sets maximum dosage levels.

In phase 2, researchers administer the drug to a small number of patients with the disease the new drug is supposed to help. Assuming that the drug proves to be both safe and effective in a small test population, phase 3 involves administration of the drug to many more patients—ranging from several hundred to several thousand. All of these people also have the particular disease the new drug is intended to relieve or cure. This stage of clinical testing may take from two to seven years or even longer. During this extended trial period, additional evidence of effectiveness is established. Studies of adverse drug reactions are also undertaken.

Test data compiled in the earlier portion of the clinical phase are then submitted to the FDA on a New Drug Application (NDA). These data must prove that the new drug is both safe and effective. The FDA review of the NDA may require two or more years. Once the FDA grants its approval for marketing the new drug, the manufacturer then begins a period of postmarketing surveillance to collect information about side effects, including adverse reactions, as well as other possible uses of the drug other than the one for which it was originally developed and approved. According to the FDA, only one in five drugs tested is eventually approved, and some FDA-approved drugs have been removed from the market due to the occurrence of adverse reactions that did not surface in either preclinical or clinical testing.

Recently, the FDA implemented new procedures to speed up access to new drugs and improve the drug review process as described above. Under the accelerated approval initiative, so-called breakthrough drugs will be approved at the earliest time at which safety and effectiveness can reasonably be established. In making such decisions, the FDA will use physical signs that indirectly indicate patients are improving, rather than wait for the final evaluation of clinical studies. This faster approval process will likely be applied to anti-obesity drugs, which will undergo only one year of human testing, instead of two, prior to FDA review.

In applying a parallel track initiative, patients with AIDS and other HIV-related conditions who are unable to participate in clinical trials will be able to receive investigational therapies for which there are no satisfactory alternatives. Safety-testing harmonization based on animal testing in just one of the nations of the European Community, Japan, or the United States will be accepted by each of the other participating countries, thus eliminating duplicative animal testing. Lastly, in an effort to reduce the backlog of new drug applications, the FDA will utilize qualified experts from outside the federal government to review certain routine types of applications. However, the FDA will retain final approval authority.

Sources: Modified from "Updates: Initiatives Speed Access to Drugs," in *FDA Consumer*, vol. 26, no. 6, pages 2–3, July–August 1992; and Ken Flieger, "Testing Drugs in People" in *FDA Consumer*, vol. 28, no. 6, pages 16–19, July–August 1994.

---

different from the amphetamines, is used as part of a management program for children with attention deficit disorders and hyperkinetic syndrome.

Tranquilizers include two different types of psychotherapeutic drugs used in the management of various physical or psychological disorders.

Major tranquilizers, such as Haldol, Mellaril, Prolixin, and Thorazine, are prescribed to relieve symptoms of a psychotic nature. And one new drug, Clozapine, has been most effective in relieving chronic schizophrenia.

By contrast, the **minor tranquilizers** are used in treating anxiety and reducing tension. These anti-anxiety drugs function somewhat like the sedative-hypnotics in restoring emotional calm. Minor tranquilizers include Atarax, Ativan, Librium, Serax, Tranxene, Valium, and Xanax. When these drugs are used in large doses for an extended period of time, they often produce a psychological or physical dependence, or both, along with tolerance and withdrawal symptoms when the drug is discontinued (see chapter 6). Some of these anti-anxiety agents also control vomiting in stressful situations, relieve muscle or skeletal disorders, prevent convulsions, and prevent withdrawal reactions in drug-dependent individuals.

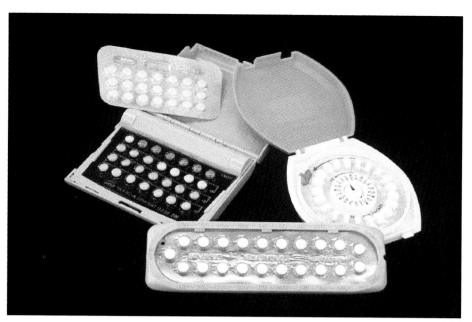

Oral contraceptive pills are frequently prescribed birth control drugs, because they are very effective despite their potential for adverse and harmful effects.
© *James L. Shaffer*

There are, of course, many other drug classes or families, including *anticoagulants* (which reduce blood clotting), *anesthetics* (which produce a loss of sensation), *eye and ear preparations, hormones* (which regulate various body processes), *muscle relaxants, narcotic antagonists,* and *narcotic detoxification agents.* However, from the consumer-patient's viewpoint, knowing what drug has been prescribed, to which drug class or family the prescribed medicine belongs, and the other members of the same drug class, may prove useful in

1. preventing any interactions that could reduce the effectiveness of drug actions, and

2. lessening the chance of experiencing unanticipated and sometimes hazardous, adverse drug effects.[10]

Oral Contraceptives

Prescription drugs that prevent pregnancy by keeping the ovaries from developing and releasing mature ova or eggs are referred to as oral contraceptives. Formulated in the late 1950s by Dr. John Rock

and his associates, oral contraceptives are among the most effective ways of preventing conception. (The only known method that is more effective is sterilization.) Although these drugs are convenient and relatively free of major side effects for most women, they are still available only by prescription. Moreover, the use of these drugs cannot guarantee absolute safety or effectiveness. And when used alone, birth control pills offer no protection against the transmission of HIV (the AIDS-causing virus) or other sexually transmitted diseases.

Two major types of oral contraceptives (OCs) are currently on the market.[11] By far, the most widely used is the **combination oral contraceptive drug**—a combination of two synthetic female hormones, estrogen and progestin. It is this combination OC that is generally referred to as "birth control pills" or simply "the Pill." It is also this same, combined oral contraceptive, but in much higher doses, that is occasionally prescribed as a "morning-after pill," an emergency form of postcoital contraception that prevents the implantation of a fertilized egg into the wall of the uterus.

Nearly forty different formulations of oral contraceptives are listed in the

Physicians' Desk Reference, reflecting numerous brand names with varying dosage levels of hormonal ingredients. Therefore, any reference to the oral contraceptive must consider the many different pills and their unique characteristics.

The combination drug or pill has proven to be more effective (approaching 99 percent) than the minipill, although the combined OC is associated with the more serious side effects and health risks. The estrogen component appears to be responsible for both the greater effectiveness and the greater potential dangers of the Pill. All of the present brands of OCs, it should be noted, contain far less estrogen and progestin than the combined products first available almost 35 years ago. Because of extensive research, doctors and their patients can now choose from "highest dose" combined pills (more frequently related to serious complications), "lowest dose" pills (associated with "spotting" and "missed menses"), and the "intermediate dose" variety. Most physicians now prescribe the lowest dose type for new patients.

By contrast, the progestin-only minipill is somewhat less effective (only about 97 percent) than the combination OC. However, the minipill apparently has fewer undesirable side effects, particularly headaches, high blood pressure, and leg pain. Because certain physical conditions, such as irregular genital bleeding, indicate a potentially dangerous consequence of using minipills, the absolute contraindications to the use of estrogen-containing combination pills also apply to the minipill.

Estrogen Hormone Agents

From a contraceptive point of view, estrogen has several major actions.[12] The first action is the blocking or inhibition of the process of ovulation, the release of an egg from the ovary. This blocking action is the result of estrogen's effect on the hypothalamus, a tiny portion of the brain that regulates several body functions and influences the pituitary, the so-called master gland located at the base of the brain. With the presence of relatively high levels of estrogen in the blood, the hypothalamus does not stimulate the pituitary to produce follicle-stimulating hormone (FSH) and luteinizing hormone (LH). Without these two chemical messengers, the ovaries cannot produce mature ova.

Second, the implantation or "nesting" of the fertilized egg in the uterine lining is inhibited by the presence of relatively high blood levels of estrogen. This action is especially effective when the estrogen is given after an unprotected act of intercourse during the middle of the menstrual cycle. Estrogen brings about certain changes in the lining of the uterus and makes the lining inhospitable so that the attachment of a fertilized egg is not likely to occur. High-dose oral estrogens have been given in emergency situations as a "morning-after pill," consisting of a substance known as diethylstilbestrol (DES).

Other actions of estrogen include changing the rate of passage of the ovum within the oviduct, and the degeneration of the corpus luteum. This latter effect results in a decline in blood levels of progestin and thereby prevents normal implantation of a fertilized egg or placental attachment.

Progestin Hormone Agents

Whether occurring in the combination pill or in the minipill, progestins also have major contraceptive effects. The progestin changes the cervical mucus so that it becomes thicker and forms a plug that makes sperm movement through the cervix more difficult. Progestin also inhibits ovulation by disturbing the hypothalamus/pituitary gland/ovary interaction, resulting in a reduction of FSH and LH hormones. As in the case of the estrogenic effect, there is no ovulation without these two pituitary hormones.

Implantation of the fertilized egg may also be blocked when progestins are given before ovulation. It is probable that progestins interfere with the process of capacitation, a complex action occurring in the uterus and oviducts that enhances the sperm's ability to penetrate the egg. Normal transport of the ovum may also be slowed when progestins are taken before fertilization.

Side Effects of Oral Contraceptives

Although oral contraceptives are highly effective in preventing pregnancy, many women do not use the Pill because of their concerns about safety and side effects. The following are among the most serious side effects associated with oral contraceptives.

1. *Cardiovascular* (heart and blood vessel) *disorders,* specifically, abnormal blood clotting in the veins or lungs in women using "intermediate" and "highest" dose OCs, stroke due to hemorrhage, heart attack, and pulmonary embolus—a blood clot that forms in the leg or pelvis, then breaks off and travels to the lungs. Any of these conditions can be fatal. For oral contraceptive users in general, it has been estimated that in females aged 15 to 34 years, the risk of death due to a circulatory disorder is about 1 in 12,000 per year. For nonusers, the rate is approximately 1 in 50,000 per year.

   The actual risk of a heart attack among Pill users is increased with age and cigarette smoking. The highest risk of all is among women over the age of 35 years who smoke cigarettes heavily. Other factors such as hypertension, diabetes, or a history of heart or blood-vessel disorders also increase the risk of cardiovascular disease.

2. *Benign* (nonmalignant) *tumors of the liver.* While such unwanted tumors or growths do not spread, they may result in the rupture of the liver's outer capsule, with extensive bleeding that could be fatal.

3. *Primary liver cancer.* Although an exceptionally rare disease in most developed countries, hepatocellular carcinoma (malignant tumors of liver cells that may infiltrate surrounding tissues and give rise to metastases) in noncirrhotic livers has now been attributed to long-term oral contraceptive use.

4. *Dangers to a developing fetus.* If oral contraceptives are used during or immediately preceding a pregnancy, there may be an increased risk of birth defects in the fetus, including defects of the heart and limbs.

5. *Gallbladder disease.* Associated with the liver, the gallbladder is a small saclike organ that stores and concentrates bile. Oral contraceptive use is not an important risk factor for development of gallbladder disease, but may speed up the development and appearance of gallbladder problems in women who are susceptible to such conditions.

6. *Hypertension.* Although hypertension (high blood pressure) resulting from the use of oral contraceptives is usually reversible, it can lead to permanent complications unless closely monitored by a physician. Fewer than 5 out of 100 women develop elevated blood pressure associated with using OCs.

Other side effects that are sometimes experienced by users of the Pill, but are not likely to be life threatening, include nausea, vomiting, breast tenderness, weight gain or loss, swelling of the ankles, spotty darkening of the skin (especially on the face), and unexpected vaginal bleeding (spotting) between periods. More serious side effects observed are worsening of migraine headaches, asthma, epilepsy, kidney or heart disease due to edema (retention of water in the body), and mental depression. Though only 50 to 75 percent of females who start using oral contraceptives still use them after one year, most of those who discontinue their pills "do so for nonmedical reasons, that is, they have not developed a complication or major side effect."[13] The vast majority of pill users have only minor difficulties.

Noncontraceptive Benefits

Although the scientific literature details many potential side effects of oral contraceptives, millions of women in the United States and throughout the world

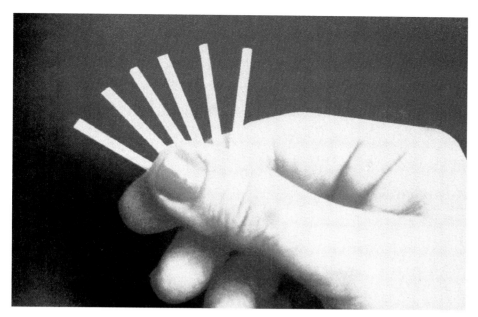

Norplant, the subdermal contraceptive, consists of six small capsules that are surgically implanted just beneath the skin on a woman's upper arm. Each capsule contains a progestin-only substance that is released slowly and provides a long-acting contraceptive effect.

Courtesy Wyeth-Ayers Laboratories.

have continued to use these pregnancy-prevention drugs with relative safety and a minimum of adverse reactions. In comparison with all the possible risks and discomforts associated with conception, pregnancy, and childbirth, the risks from oral contraceptive side effects are virtually negligible. Effectiveness, convenience of use, and the lack of interference with the act of intercourse have all combined to make the Pill so very popular.

There are, in addition, a number of noncontraceptive benefits associated with oral contraceptive use. The Pill appears to provide a "protective effect" against pelvic inflammatory disease. Oral contraceptives tend to relieve a variety of unwanted menstrual symptoms, particularly menstrual cramping. The number of days of bleeding is shortened and the amount of blood loss is reduced. Premenstrual tension is often milder.

Most studies in the past have demonstrated no increased risk of breast cancer in users of OCs. Research now suggests that OCs might have a breast-cancer-promoting effect on a specific subgroup of women. Some studies have also shown an increased risk for cervical cancer

among Pill users. Nevertheless, use of oral contraceptives lowers the risk of ovarian cysts, ovarian and endometrial cancers, and benign breast disease.[14] Use of oral contraceptives may also improve acne conditions as well as enhance the enjoyment of sexual relations for both females and males, presumably by reducing the fear of pregnancy.

The Future of Drug-Based Contraception

It is quite likely there will never be an absolutely safe and perfectly effective oral contraceptive for either the female or the male. However, new techniques now being researched and developed may enable many people to select what is appropriate and reasonably safe.

Long-acting injectable progestin, commonly known as **Depo-Provera** (depomedroxyprogesterone acetate, or DMPA) is now approved for use in the United States. A single intramuscular injection of DMPA, given every three months, blocks ovulation by suppressing FSH and LH blood levels. The development of an "inhospitable endometrium"—one that does

not allow implantation of a fertilized egg—and a thickening of cervical mucus that decreases sperm penetration, are additional contraceptive actions.

Subdermal implants consisting of Silastic capsules are inserted beneath the surface of the skin, where a slow-release, progestin-only chemical, levonorgestrel, exerts a contraceptive effect for as long as five years. The FDA approved this **Norplant** subdermal implant as an implantable contraceptive in 1990. The implant itself is a fanlike arrangement of six match-size, silicon rubber rods, each containing a progestin-only hormone. Surgically inserted just beneath the skin at the inner arm just above the elbow, the rods slowly release the hormone into the bloodstream. While not visible, the rods can be felt under the skin.

According to the FDA, Norplant is more than 99 percent effective in women weighing less than 150 pounds, but its effectiveness may decrease in heavier women.[15] If a woman wants to become pregnant or experiences undesirable effects, including irregular menstrual bleeding, headaches, and mood changes, the patient can have the implants removed by outpatient surgery.

One entirely new drug product now being tested makes use of a chemical substance, LHRH, originating in the hypothalamus of the brain. This chemical influences the pituitary gland and thus affects the ovulatory cycle. It is hoped that this new drug will not have the potentially serious side effects associated with present-day oral contraceptives.

The future of drug-based contraception may include an antipregnancy vaccine for women, an antifertility vaccine for men, and a recently tested injectable hormone preparation of testosterone that suppresses sperm production. Presently, an extract from cotton plants, known as *Gossypol,* is being used experimentally on a limited basis in the People's Republic of China to suppress sperm production and to change the structure and transport of sperm cells. Such a contraceptive would help males assume more responsibility for birth control. However, this will not likely be available in America for many years, if ever.

Chemical Induction of Menses with RU 486

Extensive studies in France have determined that the drug *mifepristone (RU 486)* is highly successful in causing menstruation in a woman whose menstrual period is up to six weeks late.[16,17] A single dose of RU 486 is given by mouth and is then followed 36 to 48 hours later by the administration of prostaglandin (another chemical) in the form of a suppository or an intramuscular injection.

RU 486 is an antiprogesterone chemical that was first used to terminate human pregnancies in 1982. The drug causes menses, when given late in the menstrual cycle, and prevents implantation or causes sloughing (casting off or rejection) of a fertilized egg, when administered within several days after ovulation.

Available in several nations now, but only in limited clinical studies in the United States, RU 486 is considered variously as a form of postcoital contraception, menses induction, voluntary pregnancy termination, and abortifacient—a substance or device that causes an abortion. As such, its approval by the FDA is somewhat controversial and is subject to legal and political forces, as well as ethical concerns.

Side Effects and Adverse Reactions of Prescribed Drugs

Earlier in this chapter it was emphasized that all medicines ought to be considered as having the potential for both helping and harming an individual. Indeed, all medicines are double-edged swords. Most people are surprised, however, to learn that nearly 7 percent of all hospitalizations in the United States are due to drug-induced illnesses.[18]

Drugs can reduce symptoms and cure disease—the primary, intended, and expected functions of medicine. Nevertheless, the same medicine can also produce secondary side effects that are sometimes unintended, unexpected, and often undesirable or fatal (adverse drug reactions). Such side effects can result from the use of both Rx and OTC medicines, and they are related to variations in individual responses to drugs, such as sensitivities, allergies, and changes in body chemistry. Every person reacts somewhat differently to medicine; some will sustain undesired effects, while most will have beneficial results.

Relatively minor side effects of certain medicines may include skin rash, mild headache, nausea, and drowsiness. More severe adverse reactions appear as prolonged vomiting, bleeding, extreme weakness, or impaired vision or hearing. Such symptoms are the body's own way of telling an individual that the medicine is acting in an unfavorable, adverse way. Prolonged usage of some drugs may even result in a variety of nutritional deficiencies. For instance, aspirin can decrease the body's ability to absorb and use vitamin C, folic acid, and vitamin K; tetracycline antibiotics can reduce the body's uptake of vitamin C; and anticonvulsants used in treating epilepsy can lower the level of folic acid and vitamin D, and thus contribute to anemia and rickets (or bone-softening disease). Unless appropriate nutrient supplements are prescribed, these side effects can lead to drug-caused malnutrition.

Because of the potential for side effects and adverse reactions, pharmacologists have established an index for assessing the relative safety of drugs for use in large populations. This index is known as the *therapeutic ratio,* or **therapeutic index.** The therapeutic index is a measure that relates the dose of a drug required to produce a desired effect to that which produces an undesired effect.[19]

The therapeutic index is expressed as the ratio between the median lethal dose (LD_{50}) and the median effective dose (ED_{50}) of a particular drug used for a specific effect (see chapter 3). Those drugs with a low ratio have a relatively small margin of safety between an effective (therapeutic) dose and an overdose effect, whereas drugs having a high therapeutic ratio possess a relatively greater margin of safety. For instance, a therapeutic index of 3 indicates that the 50 percent lethal dose is only three times the 50 percent effective dose. Accordingly, 1 milligram of a drug will produce the desired effect in half of the test population, but just 3 milligrams of the same drug will kill half of the test population.[20] Evidently, the higher the ratio, the safer is the drug; that is, the drug can be taken safely by most individuals, and even if the recommended dose were slightly exceeded, adverse effects would not likely occur. Nevertheless, for thousands of individuals, even the therapeutic dose causes harm.

While the incidence of drug-related illness and death is alarming, serious adverse reactions are relatively uncommon considering the huge national use of prescribed medications. Nevertheless, renewed emphasis should be placed on safeguarding one's health from adverse drug reactions, many of which are predictable and preventable.[21]

Preventive measures involve the prescribing physician, the dispensing pharmacist, and the consumer-patient, and focus on

informing one's physician of previous adverse reactions to a drug;

reporting of general and specific allergic conditions to one's physician, dentist, and pharmacist;

respecting known contraindications (situations that would prohibit the use of a drug) regarding any particular drug;

exercising precautions in using drugs, such as intermingling of two or more drugs without consulting a physician, and avoiding alcoholic beverages when using depressant drugs;

following prescribed dose recommendations;

recognizing and reporting early warning signals of adverse reactions to one's physician;

having your physician monitor the drug's effects through periodic exams, if necessary; and

having your physician submit to the U.S. FDA an "Adverse Reaction Report" or file one yourself (see fig. 12.4).

There are two special areas of concern in preventing adverse drug reactions. One deals with polypharmacy; the other

DEPARTMENT OF HEALTH AND HUMAN SERVICES
PUBLIC HEALTH SERVICE
FOOD AND DRUG ADMINISTRATION (HFN-730)
ROCKVILLE, MD 20857

ADVERSE REACTION REPORT
(Drugs and Biologics)

Form Approved OMB No. 0910-0230

FDA CONTROL NO

ACCESSION NO

REACTION INFORMATION

1. PATIENT IDENTITALS (In Confidence)   2. AGE YRS   3. SEX   4-6. REACTION ONSET MO DA YR

8-12. CHECK ALL APPROPRIATE:
- [ ] PATIENT DIED
- [ ] REACTION TREATED WITH Rx DRUG
- [ ] RESULTED IN, OR PROLONGED, INPATIENT HOSPITALIZATION
- [ ] RESULTED IN PERMANENT DISABILITY
- [ ] NONE OF THE ABOVE

7. DESCRIBE REACTION(S)

13. RELEVANT TESTS/LABORATORY DATA

II. **SUSPECT DRUG(S) INFORMATION**

14. SUSPECT DRUG(S) (Give manufacturer and lot no. for vaccines/biologics)

20. DID REACTION ABATE AFTER STOPPING DRUG?   [ ] YES [ ] NO [ ] NA

15. DAILY DOSE   16. ROUTE OF ADMINISTRATION

17. INDICATION(S) FOR USE

21. DID REACTION REAPPEAR AFTER REINTRODUCTION?   [ ] YES [ ] NO [ ] NA

18. DATES OF ADMINISTRATION (From/To)   19. DURATION OF ADMINISTRATION

III. **CONCOMITANT DRUGS AND HISTORY**

22. CONCOMITANT DRUGS AND DATES OF ADMINISTRATION (Exclude those used to treat reaction)

23. OTHER RELEVANT HISTORY (e.g. diagnoses, allergies, pregnancy with LMP, etc.)

IV. ONLY FOR REPORTS SUBMITTED BY MANUFACTURER
24. NAME AND ADDRESS OF MANUFACTURER (Include Zip Code)

V. INITIAL REPORTER (In confidence)
26-26a. NAME AND ADDRESS OF REPORTER (Include Zip Code)

24a. IND/NDA NO FOR SUSPECT DRUG   24b. MFR CONTROL NO   26b. TELEPHONE NO (Include area code)

24c. DATE RECEIVED BY MANUFACTURER   24d. REPORT SOURCE (Check all that apply) [ ] FOREIGN [ ] STUDY [ ] LITERATURE [ ] HEALTH PROFESSIONAL [ ] CONSUMER

26c. HAVE YOU ALSO REPORTED THIS REACTION TO THE MANUFACTURER?   [ ] YES [ ] NO

25. 15 DAY REPORT? [ ] YES [ ] NO   25a. REPORT TYPE [ ] INITIAL [ ] FOLLOW-UP

26d. ARE YOU A HEALTH PROFESSIONAL? [ ] YES [ ] NO

Submission of a report does not necessarily constitute an admission that the drug caused the adverse reaction.

NOTE Required of manufacturers by 21 CFR 314.80

FORM FDA 1639 (7/86)   PREVIOUS EDITION MAY BE USED

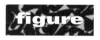 **12.4**

Adverse reaction report.

Source: U.S. Food and Drug Administration (HFN-730).

involves food and drug interactions. Both areas require the active involvement and cooperation of the consumer-patient.

Polypharmacy: Drug-Drug Interactions

The use of two or more drugs at the same time during the course of treatment for a particular illness is known as **polypharmacy.** Mixing two different medications can result in unexpected and sometimes dangerous chemical interactions within the body. Such a practice requires your physician's close supervision and knowledge of other drugs you may be taking, including those prescribed by another physician.

In general, the occurrence of adverse reactions increases in proportion to the number of drugs being taken. Sometimes the drug interactions influence the treatment outcome. Consequently, the best policy is to use the fewest drugs possible at any one time. The common practice of patients demanding "overtreatment" by their physicians is therefore unwise and often an invitation to experience an adverse drug reaction.

Drugs interact in a variety of ways. One medication may make another act faster or slower, or more powerfully or less powerfully than it normally would act. As a consequence, one drug may change the effect another has on the body. Some of these interactions are described below.

Changes in drug absorption, distribution, and metabolism may take place when one drug interacts with another. For example, if a person having a circulatory problem due to clotting of blood in an artery or vein is prescribed an anticoagulant drug, the prescribed medicine would tend to thin the blood and help dissolve a clot. However, if this individual were to take an antacid, even an OTC drug, the anticoagulant may be absorbed at a much slower rate than required to do its job properly.

Alteration of a drug's excretion can also occur with polypharmacy. One drug can either inhibit or hasten the excretion of another drug from the body, thus exaggerating or reducing its effect. Such is the case in which an individual takes an OTC drug that changes the acid level of the urine. Rx drugs are formulated on the basis of a normal level of acid in the urine. However, certain nonprescription drugs containing ammonium chloride, sodium bicarbonate, or citrate change the acid level and thus interfere with the beneficial impact of the prescribed medicine.

As indicated in chapter 3, when drugs are taken in combination, the drug effects can usually be classified as either *independent, antagonistic, additive, or potentiating.* Drugs taken together may work independently of each other; that is, neither one affects the drug action of the other. However, when drugs taken together interact so that the effect of either or both agents is blocked or reduced, the action is described as an **antagonistic drug reaction.** For example, certain antibiotics, barbiturates, and tranquilizers tend to reduce the effectiveness of oral contraceptives.

An **additive drug reaction** may occur when two or more drugs that are similar in their general effects interact in the body. The impact of adding one drug's action to that of another so that a doubling of the drug effect takes place is described as a "cumulative" reaction. The end result (effect) is the sum of the parts.

Potentiation or synergistic **drug reactions** describe the interactions of two or more drugs that produce an exaggerated effect—one that goes beyond what might be expected from adding the effect of one to another. With such drugs, the end result is greater than the sum of the parts. Such a drug reaction, in which the effects of the two drugs are multiplied, can speed up the beneficial effect of a particular medicine, as when the antibiotic trimethoprim may be used to enhance the activity of another drug, sulfamethoxazole, in combating certain infections.

But potentiation can also pose dangers, especially when alcoholic beverages are mixed with sleeping aids, pain relievers, or tranquilizers. Even OTC drugs can have potentiating effects. Aspirin greatly increases the blood-thinning action of oral anticoagulants. People taking such medication may risk hemorrhage if they use aspirin to alleviate a headache. OTC cold remedies containing antihistamines can produce potentiating effects when combined with CNS depressants, including anesthetics, barbiturates, hypnotics, sedatives, and analgesics.

Food-Drug Interactions

When a person is taking a drug, the food that he or she has eaten could make the drug work faster or slower or even prevent it from having any effect at all. More alarming is the possibility of severe adverse reactions to drugs that can be caused by specific foods or alcoholic beverages. Some of the reactions, if left unchecked, can be life threatening. As indicated in box 12.4, there are several potentially harmful **food-drug interactions.**

To prevent such undesirable food-drug interactions, be certain to follow your physician's directions about when to take drugs and what foods and beverages to avoid while taking medications. Read any patient information materials distributed by your physician or pharmacist. Never be afraid to ask how drugs might interfere with your favorite edibles. While taking medicines, always report to your physician about any unusual complaints or experiences that occur when you consume specific foods and beverages.

Drug Information for Patients

Nearly twenty years ago, because of increasing public concern about the lack of adequate information on prescription drugs, the U.S. Food and Drug Administration proposed the adoption of *Patient Package Inserts* (PPIs) for virtually every Rx drug. A PPI is a brief informational pamphlet provided by a pharmacist along with each new prescription. The pamphlets, similar to the printed inserts accompanying oral contraceptives, would

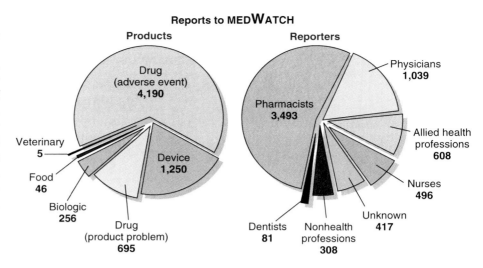

Reports to MEDWATCH

figure 12.5

In one recent 8-month period, MedWatch, the U.S. Food and Drug Administration's medical product reporting program, received reports of 6,442 events or other problems. The chart on the left shows reports according to type of product; the chart on the right depicts reports by profession of the reporters.

As a partner in the MedWatch program, the independent, nonprofit organization of medical and pharmaceutical professionals and consumers, known as the United States Pharmacopeia, has established a Practitioners' Reporting Network (PRN) that consolidates concerns and suggestions involving drugs, radiopharmaceuticals, medical devices, animal drugs, actual or potential medication errors, and adverse events so that product manufacturers and regulatory agencies are kept informed of the problems observed. The reporting network and consequent actions of the Food and Drug Administration (FDA) have resulted in product improvements, corrections, and recalls in support of federal and state government efforts to protect the public health by helping to identify serious adverse effects.

Source: U.S. Food and Drug Administration.

have provided basic knowledge regarding the drug's effects, dosage form, possible side effects, and precautions in using the drug.

However, in 1983, the FDA abandoned its proposed mandatory PPI program and backed instead the American Medical Association's voluntary program that makes **Patient Medication Instructions (PMIs)** available to practicing physicians for distribution to their patients. Use of PMIs now promotes improved effectiveness of drug therapy, reduces the risk of improper drug use, decreases the occurrence of preventable and serious drug reactions, and helps patients comply with instructions about taking their medication properly.

Due to a perceived reluctance on the part of many physicians to share basic information on Rx drugs with patients, a growing number of laypersons have

sought pertinent facts about drugs from a variety of sources. One of the more popular and authoritative sources of such information on prescription drugs is the *Physicians' Desk Reference* (PDR), compiled by representatives of pharmaceutical companies. An annual publication, the PDR has nearly 2,700 pages and includes detailed information on thousands of drug products, accounting for practically all of the leading prescription drugs.[22]

The *Physicians' Desk Reference* provides "full disclosure" of how a specific drug product works, what it is used for, possible side effects and adverse reactions, contraindications, and other precautions and warnings about potential hazards. In the front of the massive volume there are several convenient indexes and sections, the more useful of which are described as follows:

Potentially Harmful Food-Drug Interactions

box 12.4

Tetracycline (a commonly prescribed antibiotic) and *dairy products*—calcium in milk, cheese, and yogurt impairs absorption of this drug, thus interfering with its effectiveness in the body.

Drugs in combinations with soda pop or acid fruit or vegetable juices—these beverages can result in excess acidity that may cause some drugs to dissolve quickly in the stomach instead of in the intestine, where they can be more readily absorbed into the bloodstream.

High blood pressure medications in combination with *natural licorice products*—the natural licorice extract, still used in imported products, counteracts the effect of the medicine.

Anticoagulants (drugs that prevent blood clotting) and *liver* and *green leafy vegetables*—excess consumption of foods rich in vitamin K, as are liver and spinach, hinders the effectiveness of anticoagulants.

Monoamine oxidase (MAO) *inhibitors*—drugs used to counter depression and high blood pressure—and *foods containing tyramine*—tyramine is found in foods such as aged cheese, chicken livers, pickled herring, fermented sausages, yogurt, sour cream, beef liver, canned figs, bananas, soy sauce, active yeast, and specific alcoholic beverages, including Chianti wine, sherry, and other wines in large amounts. MAO inhibitors react with tyramine to force the blood pressure to dangerously high levels, thus causing severe headaches, brain hemorrhage, and possibly even death. MAO inhibitors also are suspected of reacting adversely with cola beverages, coffee, chocolate, and raisins.

Colchicine (a prescription drug for gout) and *mineral oil* (an ingredient in some OTC laxatives) block the proper absorption of nutrients by the intestines.

Diuretics, or "water pills," used over a long period of time can lead to severe potassium depletion in the body. Potassium is an important mineral needed for proper body function.

Oral contraceptives tend to deplete the blood's content of folic acid and vitamin B$_6$. Such vitamin loss is not usually serious among healthy women with good diets, but it can present serious problems in women with poor nutrition, such as impoverished women.

OTC antacids, used persistently without a physician's supervision, can cause phosphate depletion—a body condition producing muscle weakness and vitamin D deficiency.

Source: Modified from the U.S. Food and Drug Administration.

---

1. *Manufacturers' Index*—a listing of all drug manufacturers who have provided information to the PDR. Addresses and emergency phone numbers of manufacturers are also listed.

2. *Product Name Index*—an alphabetical listing of drug products by their brand names available from participating manufacturers.

3. *Product Category Index*—a listing of products according to their appropriate category (classification or drug type), such as analgesics, diuretics, antihistamines, etc.

4. *Product Identification Section*— approximately 30 pages of full-color photographs that depict tablets and capsules in actual size under company headings. Pictures of tubes and syringes are reduced in their dimensions.

5. *Product Information Section*—a list, in alphabetical order according to the name of the manufacturer, of more than 2,500 pharmaceuticals that are fully described as to brand name, generic or chemical name, indications for usage, dosage, administration, description, clinical pharmacology, supply, warnings, contraindications, adverse reactions, overdosage, and precautions in usage.

The PDR also contains diagnostic product information, a listing of poison-control centers throughout the United States, and a guide to the management of drug overdose. Once the exclusive domain of physicians, the PDR is now purchased by drug companies, health care professionals, pharmacists, dentists, nurses, hospitals, nursing homes, and a growing number of laypersons. Some libraries also have copies of recent PDRs. The publisher of this reference on prescription drugs has recently issued a companion pharmaceutical directory, the *PDR for Non-Prescription Drugs.* This latter volume is also proving to be a best-seller in the wake of the consumer movement.

Generic Drugs

One of the more complex issues pertaining to prescription drugs is the "generic vs. brand name controversy." With the increasing cost of health care, some consumers as well as physicians, pharmacists, the Food and Drug Administration, and the pharmaceutical companies that make drugs have become concerned about the quality and cost of comparative drugs. The controversy includes the naming of drugs, possible differences in quality between brand-name drug products and their generic counterparts, the cost differential between the two name types of medication, and the substitution of the generics for brand-name drugs.

Drug Names

To better appreciate the nature of this controversy, it should be noted that drugs prescribed for therapy are named in three different ways.

1. The *chemical name* describes the chemical structure of the drug molecule. Typically, such a name is rather long, unwieldy, and written in a complex chemical jargon seldom used by either physicians or pharmacists. For instance, a common antibiotic drug has the following chemical name: *D-(-)α-amino-p-hydroxybenzyl penicillin trihydrate.*

2. The *generic name* refers to a drug's official or nonproprietary name, that is, a name that is *not* patented, trademarked, or owned by a private individual or company. Assigned to a drug after it has demonstrated some therapeutic usefulness, the generic name is usually a contraction of the more complex chemical name. The antibiotic drug identified in #1 above has the generic name *amoxicillin.* Drugs are frequently referred to by their generic names in academic and scientific situations.

3. The *brand name* or trademark (registered with the U.S. Patent Office) is assigned to a generic-name drug by a particular pharmaceutical company. Generally, the brand name is shorter than the generic name, easier to remember, and often devised to suggest the pharmacological action of the drug. For instance, SmithKline Beecham Laboratories' brand name of amoxicillin is Amoxil; Wyeth-Ayerst's is Wymox; and Squibb's is Trimox. There are several other brand names and generic versions of amoxicillin marketed in the United States by different drug manufacturers. It is the brand name of a drug, however, that is advertised to the medical profession, although the generic name must also appear in both advertising and labeling in letters at least half as big as that of the brand name.

Chemical Equivalence Versus Bioavailability

According to the Food and Drug Administration, all drugs, whether sold under their brand names or their generic names,

must meet the same FDA standards for safety, strength, purity, and effectiveness. Even after a recent scandal involving certain generic drug manufacturers and three former FDA employees, who accepted illegal gratuities, was investigated, an extensive sampling and analysis of frequently prescribed generics revealed no significant differences in the quality of the generics compared to the brand-name products.[23] None of the samples tested posed a health hazard to patients when the drugs were examined for potency, dissolution rate, and content uniformity.[24] Consequently, the FDA believes there is no significant difference in quality between generic and brand-name drugs. Supposedly, generic drugs are equivalent to those sold under their brand names.

While generics contain the same amounts of active ingredients in the same dosages—and are, therefore, **chemically equivalent drugs**—many physicians, pharmacists, and drug manufacturers contend that the quality of the generics varies considerably. This variation is expressed usually as **bioavailability,** a measure of a drug's activity within the body, determined by the quantified levels of that particular drug in the blood. Considered as trade secrets, various fillers, binders, coloring agents, lubricants, preservatives, drying agents, flavors, disintegrants, coatings, and wetting agents—the inactive ingredients used in formulating and manufacturing a drug product—are actually what determine how available the active ingredient will be in the body. Sometimes these inactive substances affect the drug's absorption, how much of the active ingredient gets to its desired destination, and how fast it gets there.

This variation can make an important difference between apparently similar drugs. When the bioavailability of brand-name drugs and generics are the same, the drug products are described as having the same **bioequivalence.** This means that the medications produce the same therapeutic effect in the body. But any difference in bioavailability between brand names and generics may alter the clinical or therapeutic effects of the medications. In such a situation, then, the drugs would not share the characteristic of bioequivalence because they might not function similarly at the site of action within the human body.

To be regarded as therapeutically equivalent to an already FDA-approved, brand-name drug, a generic product may differ only in such characteristics as color, taste, tablet shape, packaging, and inert or inactive ingredients. In comparison with their brand-name counterparts, generics must contain the same active ingredients; be identical in strength, dosage form, and route of administration; be used generally for the same illnesses (with the same precautions, warnings, and instructions); and be bioequivalent, meaning that they must release the same amount of drugs into the body at the same rate and must affect the body in the same way.

Despite the antigeneric position of the pharmaceutical manufacturing industry, a majority of all generics are made by the major drug firms in the United States. These drug companies are often the very same ones that also research, develop, and market the brand-name drugs. Some of the large firms even distribute, under their own brand names, drug products that have been manufactured, packaged, and labeled by firms that make only generic drugs.

Generic Drug Prescription

The consumer-patient will likely find that generic drugs cost less. The savings can be as much as 50 percent. Such a difference can translate into a significant dollar amount, especially if the drug must be taken over a long period of time.

To benefit from such savings, the consumer needs the cooperation of both physician and pharmacist. Ask your physician to write a prescription so that it permits a generic version to be dispensed, and tell your pharmacist you want the least expensive version of the medicine that has been prescribed for you. In addition, the consumer should compare prices both at chain stores and independent pharmacies because some generics have cost even more than brand-name drugs, on occasion. Although pharmacists generally pay less at wholesale for generics, they often have a higher markup than their brand-name counterparts. Sometimes, a pharmacy might feature a bargain price on a brand-name drug—lower than the generic price—due to a special order or deal from a pharmaceutical manufacturer.

Consumer-patients can also save money by purchasing OTC generics. For instance, aspirin is the generic name for one of the most frequently used nonprescription painkillers. Bayer and St. Joseph are brand names for different manufacturers' aspirin. Whether the "house brand" aspirin or a nationally advertised brand name of aspirin is purchased, there should be no difference in the painkilling quality of the analgesic products.

During the past several years, generic prescription has increased rapidly, surpassing the smaller annual increase in brand-name perscription. As more patents expire on brand-name drugs, it is anticipated that not less than 80 percent of the top-selling prescribed medications will soon be open to generic competition.

The trend to generic prescription has been promoted now that all fifty states have laws allowing, and in some instances requiring, pharmacists to substitute a generic drug for a brand-name medication, unless the prescribing physician mandates the use of a specific brand-name product. Additional factors advancing the trend to generics are the many hospitals, military installations, and other government health care facilities that routinely dispense generics whenever possible. Today, even cost-conscious employers and health insurance companies encourage members to urge their physicians to write prescriptions that can be filled with generic drugs.

The upswing in generic prescribing indicates that more and more physicians are convinced that generic drugs are good drugs, despite the deluge of pro-brand-name propaganda by the major drug-developing companies. But the trend to generics may also represent the effort by consumer-patients to take some control of their own health care costs.

Chapter Summary

1. Prescription medicines are chemotherapeutic agents, more powerful than OTC drugs, that require a physician's supervision in their use. They are also more likely to cause unexpected side effects and adverse drug reactions.

2. Although many people believe that all drugs work safely on all people at all times (the fail-safe concept), there is no absolute safety regarding the use of prescription drugs. The benefit-risk equation applies in the use of such medications.

3. A prescription typically lists the physician's name, address, phone number, and DEA number; patient's name and address; date; name of drug prescribed; dosage form; strength of dose; amount to be dispensed; directions for use; number of refills allowed; and the physician's signature.

4. By contrast, the label on an Rx drug container typically lists name, address, and phone number of the dispensing pharmacy; prescription number; prescribing physician's name; date of dispensing; patient's name; drug name; directions for use; federal restriction; expiration date; and number of allowable refills.

5. Dispensing of controlled drug substances is restricted according to major drug schedules, under the provisions of the Controlled Substances Act.

6. Guidelines for the wise use of Rx drugs pertain to knowing medication's name, directions for use, expected drug effects, possible side effects, precautions in use, avoiding use of other drugs and particular foods, and duration of recommended use.

7. Additional guidelines for responsible use of Rx drugs relate to informing one's physician about medication problems, possibility of pregnancy, and multiple-drug use; discarding old drugs; proper storing of medicines; and avoiding medication errors.

8. According to the National Prescription Audit, new and refill prescriptions total nearly 2 billion per year. Nearly 15 percent of all new prescriptions are for generic drugs. Psychotropic drugs (minor tranquilizers, sedatives, hypnotics, antidepressants, major tranquilizers, and antimanics) account for just 5 percent of prescriptions.

9. Rx drug classes or families are composed of drugs that share important chemical characteristics and tend to produce similar effects in the human body. Major drug classes include anti-infectives, antihypertensives, antineoplastics, cardiovascular drugs, diuretics, sedative-hypnotics, and stimulants.

10. Both the combination pill and the minipill are types of oral contraceptives that prevent pregnancy by keeping the ovaries from developing and releasing mature ova.

11. Highly effective and relatively safe to use, oral contraceptives can produce serious but rare adverse reactions, such as cardiovascular disorders, benign liver tumors, increased risk of birth defects, primary liver cancer, and gallbladder disease.

12. Rx drugs that reduce symptoms of illness and cure disease can also produce unexpected side effects as well as life-threatening adverse drug reactions.

13. Mixing two or more different medications can result in changes in drug absorption, distribution, and metabolism; alteration of a drug's excretion; and either additive or potentiation drug interactions.

14. Patient Medication Instructions and the *Physicians' Desk Reference* are two important sources of information on Rx drugs.

15. There has been an increase in the prescription of generic drugs that have an official, nonpatented, nontrademarked name. Although generics tend to be chemically equivalent to brand-name Rx drugs, some physicians believe the generics produce variable levels of drug activity in the body. As such, generics may alter the therapeutic effectiveness of a brand-name drug.

Review Questions and Activities

1. In what ways do Rx drugs differ from OTC drugs?

2. How does the benefit-risk equation apply to the use of prescribed drugs?

3. Can you think of any reason why directions for use on a prescription often include a Latin form of medical shorthand?

4. Examine a prescription drug container and determine if the recommended information elements are included on the label.

5. Do you believe the federal government should continue to restrict the prescription of controlled drug substances, under the provisions of the Controlled Substances Act?

6. Develop a "plan of action" to enhance your chances of using a prescription drug safely and responsibly.

7. Investigate how you as a patient might improve your communication skills with a physician, especially regarding the use of prescribed medications.

8. Identify some of the major Rx drug classes or families that are prescribed frequently in America.

9. What are some of the more frequently prescribed psychoactive drugs?

10. How do major tranquilizers differ from the so-called minor tranquilizers?

11. From both a female and male viewpoint, discuss the "pros" and "cons" of using oral contraceptives.

12. Explain in detail precisely how oral contraceptives prevent pregnancy. Distinguish between the effects of estrogen hormone and those of progestin hormone.

13. What are some of the common side effects of using oral contraceptives? What are some adverse reactions associated with these Rx drugs?

14. In what ways can the practice of polypharmacy affect drug actions within the human body?

15. What foods can sometimes cause adverse drug reactions?

16. Interview local pharmacists to determine the level of generic drug prescriptions in your community.

17. Survey several pharmacies and compare the prices of various brand-name drugs with their generic counterparts. What conclusions might be reached as a result of your comparative study?

18. Contact a regional or district official of the Federal Food and Drug Administration for information on testing of new drugs, actions taken recently concerning Rx drugs already in use, and related matters concerning drug safety and effectiveness.

References

1. Marian Segal, "Rx to OTC: The Switch Is On," *FDA Consumer* 25, no. 2 (March 1991): 9–11.
2. Andrew Purvis, "Unlocking the Pill Bottles," *Time,* 17 December 1990, 95.
3. Pharmaceutical Manufacturers Association, *Key Facts about the U.S. Prescription and*

Medical Device Industries (Washington, D.C.: Pharmaceutical Manufacturers Association, n.d.), 2.

4. Editors of Consumer Guide, *Prescription Drugs* (Lincolnwood, Ill.: Publications International/Signet Reference, 1995), 6–11.

5. James Long and James Rybacki, *The Essential Guide to Prescription Drugs* (New York: HarperPerennial, 1994), 1162.

6. Ibid., 14–16.

7. United States Pharmacopeia, *Complete Drug Reference* (Yonkers, N.Y.: Consumer Reports Books, 1994), 1713–20.

8. Laura Simonsen, "Top 200 Drugs of 1993: Price of Average Rx Up Only 2.9%," *Pharmacy Times* (April 1994): 18–32.

9. Ricki Lewis, "Surprise Cause of Gastritis Revolutionizes Ulcer Treatment," *FDA Consumer* 28, no. 10 (December 1994): 15–18.

10. Long and Rybacki, *Essential Guide to Prescription Drugs,* 1060.

11. Robert Hatcher and others, *Contraceptive Technology,* 16th rev. ed. (New York: Irvington, 1994), 285–86.

12. Ibid., 224.

13. Ibid., 227.

14. Ibid., 231.

15. "Implantable Contraceptive Approved," *FDA Consumer* 25, no. 2 (March 1991): 2–3.

16. Louise Silvestre and others, "Voluntary Interruption of Pregnancy with Mifepristone (RU 486) and a Prostaglandin Analogue," *New England Journal of Medicine* 322, no. 10 (8 March 1990): 645–48.

17. Hatcher and others, *Contraceptive Technology,* 418.

18. S. Kerr, quoted in Paul Spannbauer, "Prescription Drug Database," *American Clinical Laboratory* 10, no. 5 (June 1991): 16, 18.

19. Henry Boune and James Roberts, "Drug Receptors and Pharmacodynamics," chapter 2 in *Basic and Clinical Pharmacology,* 4th ed., ed. Bertram Katsung (Norwalk, Conn.: Appleton & Lange, 1989), 24.

20. Tibor Palfai and Henry Jankiewicz, *Drugs and Human Behavior* (Dubuque, Iowa: Brown & Benchmark, 1991), 76.

21. Long and Rybacki, *Essential Guide to Prescription Drugs,* 16–18.

22. *Physicians' Desk Reference,* 48th ed. (Montvale, N.J.: Medical Economics Data Production, 1994).

23. Frank Young, "Ensuring the Safety of Generic Drugs," *FDA Consumer* 23, no. 10 (December/January 1989/1990): 5–7.

24. "Generic Drugs: Still Safe and Effective According to New Study," *Public Citizen Health Research Group Health Letter* 6, no. 10 (October 1990): 8–10.

Prevention of Alcohol, Tobacco, and Other Drug Problems

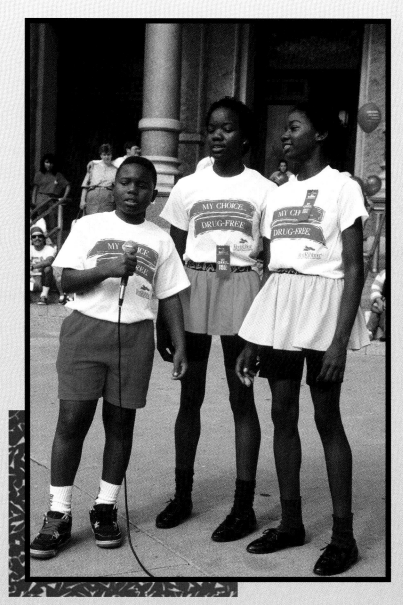

Questions of Concern

1. What strategies should communities and schools use to prevent the use of alcohol, tobacco, and other drugs by youth, and to prevent drug and alcohol abuse among adults?

2. Some drug-abuse prevention programs promote only abstinence from illegal drugs. Does this adequately prepare young people for their probable interactions with legal drugs after they leave the school setting?

3. Why are so many prevention programs directed at the illegal drugs, when alcohol and tobacco appear to cause more personal and social problems than the illegal psychoactives?

4. Although legalizing drugs might increase the number of deaths due to drug use and abuse, would it not eliminate the enormous profits of drug dealers, spare users the high costs of drugs, and reduce the cost of crime to society?

of alcohol,

tobacco,

and other

drug

chapter

13

drug-abuse prevention

chapter objectives

After you have studied this chapter, you should be able to do the following:

1. Describe a potentially effective program of drug-abuse prevention.

2. Distinguish among the following general strategies of drug-abuse prevention: supply reduction, demand reduction, and inoculation.

3. List two examples that reflect the application of each general strategy in a drug-abuse prevention program.

4. Identify the three interrelated factors of the public health model of abuse prevention.

5. Explain the public health model of abuse prevention as it might be applied in a program preventing drug abuse.

6. Discuss the significance of the macro approach to preventing drug abuse.

7. Differentiate among the following intervention levels of drug-abuse prevention: primary, secondary, and tertiary.

8. List two examples of each intervention level (primary, secondary, and tertiary) that might be applied in a drug-abuse prevention program.

9. Identify at least five routine law-enforcement techniques used by law-enforcement agents in their drug-abuse prevention activities.

10. Describe the nature and objectives of the federal government's strategy in combating drug abuse.

11. Name at least four federal law-enforcement agencies concerned directly with drug-abuse prevention activities.

12. Explain how the Comprehensive Drug Abuse Prevention and Control Act of 1970 attempts to control the manufacture, purchase, and distribution of controlled substances.

13. Compare the advantages and disadvantages of using a "summons" rather than making an "arrest" of an underaged person caught using alcoholic beverages.

14. Describe the general purpose and activities of the antiparaphernalia movement.

15. Compare, in general terms, the drug laws of other nations with those of the United States.

16. Explain the meaning of the "alternative behaviors" approach as a drug-abuse prevention measure.

17. Identify at least ten alternative behaviors appropriate to the various levels of experience or types of satisfaction sought.

18. Discuss in detail the concept of "responsible drug use" as a drug-abuse prevention measure.

19. Describe "responsible drug use" in terms of situational responsibilities, health responsibilities, and safety responsibilities.

20. Explain why drug abuse is often seen as a family affair.

21. Identify several common signals or indicators of drug use among young people and adults.

22. List at least five guidelines parents could use to help their children overcome a drug problem.

23. Describe the major stages frequently seen in adolescent chemical use.

24. Explain how the family can function in the primary prevention of drug abuse.

Introduction

Prevention activities are undertaken to avoid, reduce, or eliminate altogether the adverse consequences of using, misusing, and abusing psychoactive drugs. Various prevention strategies of reducing the drug supply, lessening the demand for drugs, and protecting users from the more negative consequences of drug abuse are explained. In addition, alcohol, tobacco, and other drug-abuse prevention is described within the framework of the public health model, with its related components of host, agent, and environment.

Primary, secondary, and tertiary prevention efforts are identified as levels of program intervention or application. Because various therapies for drug dependencies have already been described in earlier chapters, the major emphasis here is on substance-abuse prevention in the workplace, drug law enforcement, the promotion of alternative behaviors as a substitute for taking drugs, and the consideration of responsible drug use, a somewhat controversial proposal.

Although prevention activities take place at school, in the workplace, and in the community at large, the final section of this chapter focuses on the role of the family in preventing drug problems. It is within the family unit that both primary and secondary interventions are likely to have their greatest potential effect.

Prevention: The War on Drugs

What can be done to prevent alcohol, tobacco, and other drug problems? From time to time, a coordinated national effort—a so-called war on drugs—is declared or renewed by the president. Such a "war" has many dimensions. For instance, officials at the federal, state, and local levels pledge their best efforts to reduce, if not entirely eliminate, the many personal and social difficulties related to the use and abuse of mind-changing substances. Often reflecting the political and economic expediency of the federal government's legislative branch, the U.S. Congress enacts tougher antidrug laws, threatens or suspends foreign aid to drug-producing countries, and slashes prevention programs considered too expensive, ineffective, or not punitive enough. Meanwhile, the U.S. military services, as well as businesses and industries, continue programs of drug testing to deter drug use and chemical dependency in the interest of national security and worker productivity, respectively.

All of the foregoing activities demonstrate this nation's ongoing anxiety and frustration about a serious and potentially life-threatening issue. Because of the widespread use of both legal and illegal psychoactives (fig. 13.1), there is a persistent concern about stopping or reducing the tragic consequences and mounting expenses associated with the use, misuse, and abuse of these drugs. The need for countermeasures seems obvious, because we pay a staggering price for our own national drug problem. A huge part of the cost of national health care is related directly to alcohol, tobacco, and other drug-related medical expenses, and amounts to over $5 million every single hour—money some believe could be better used in reducing the national debt or funding health care reform.

However, our continuing preoccupation with drug-related problems is also due to increasing interest in health promotion and the growing awareness that alcohol, tobacco, and other drug abuse often results in serious problems for family life, school performance, and worker efficiency. Of course, there is another factor responsible for the need to act against these drugs—the growing awareness that using alcohol, tobacco, and other drugs often contributes to crime, violence, homelessness, urban decay, and preventable illnesses and injuries. Presently, at least half a million Americans die each

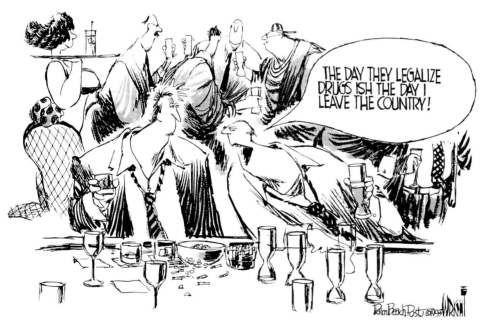

figure 13.1

Although the debate over legalizing certain psychoactive drugs continues, prevention of alcohol, tobacco, and other drug-related problems is often hampered by commonly held misconceptions, as noted in this cartoon. Does the "war on drugs" overlook certain mind-changing chemicals by focusing so narrowly on illegal psychoactives?

Reprinted by permission: Tribune Media Services.

year from alcohol, tobacco, and illicit drugs, thus making substance abuse the single largest preventable cause of death in this country.[1] (See fig. 13.2.)

Health, social welfare, educational, and law enforcement agencies, among others, have placed greater emphasis on efforts to block, avert, forestall, or eliminate those unfavorable results of using, misusing, and abusing psychoactive chemicals. Such efforts are particularly evident in the rapid growth of parent groups alarmed by their children's drug usage. Parents are more than concerned. They are furious and feel frustrated in their attempts to halt the increasing acceptance of a drug culture where one "gets by" by being "high."

Realistically, can the war on drugs be won? Or has the nation already lost such a war? Despite billions of dollars spent and more than a million arrests each year, the war on drugs has turned into a war on drug users, and drug-related violence, crime, ill health, social tension, and compromised civil liberties have all increased.[2] Reasonable answers to such questions can be given only when and if the "enemy" in this war is better understood and recognized for what it is. Because of the country's continuing demand for psychoactive drugs—both legal and illegal—the war will not likely be won soon. There can be no significant victory until there is a basic change in the national acceptance of and reliance upon mind-altering substances. People have yet to learn that taking pills is not the best way to handle indigestion, stress, or emotional conflict, and that drinking alcoholic beverages is not necessary for a successful party or essential for gracious living.

As long as the demand for drugs is great, the supply will be there, despite the antidrug wars on the local and even national levels. It is a basic fact that illegal drugs, and the legal ones too, are "big business," and a profitable one at that! The inhabitants of the earth are estimated to spend more on illegal drugs than on food, housing, clothes, education, medical care, or any other product or service. In the United States, consumers of illegal drugs spend an estimated $140 billion annually on illicit drugs alone.[3] In this instance, the enemy in the war against drugs is a formidable international narcotics industry described as ruthless, rich, and largely unseen. This menacing operation consists

of criminals in an underground empire in which crime and governments embrace in the promotion of drug trafficking.

But the enemy is also a nation in which the annual advertising budget for just one brand name of "light beer" is more than twenty times greater than the annual prevention budget for the National Institute of Alcohol Abuse and Alcoholism. And while urging other nations to destroy their major cash crops of cocaine, heroin, and marijuana, we Americans continue to subsidize the number one drug killer in our country today—tobacco. In these ways, we ourselves are the enemy too!

The war on drugs will not likely be won for a long, long time, if ever. But we cannot afford to stop fighting; we cannot retreat; we cannot lose. The stakes are too high, and defeat would be too costly in terms of human lives. In theory, the battle plan in this war consists of various countermeasures, referred to generally as *prevention activities,* to combat alcohol, tobacco, and other drug abuse. These activities are aimed at ensuring healthy, safe, and productive lives for all Americans. In general, prevention includes

those efforts that keep alcohol, tobacco, and other drug (ATOD) problems from occurring by reducing risk factors, and by making certain that "at risk" populations do not use such substances.[4] Prevention also occurs when people do not use certain substances in conjunction with other behaviors, such as drinking alcoholic beverages and then driving, and when those who have already developed an ATOD problem stop using these substances.

Prevention activities are usually based on general strategies or plans in terms of desired outcome, and they are applied at three different yet related levels of intervention, described in the following sections.

General Strategies of Preventing Drug Abuse

Although alcohol and other drug abuse is hardly a new phenomenon, it was not considered a major problem in the United States until the "youth rebellion" of the 1960s. When middle-class teenagers and young adults suddenly adopted a wide range of unconventional behaviors, including the

Over 20,000 deaths related to *illegal drug abuse* and drug-related AIDS deaths.

1.6 million deaths related to all other *causes.*

At least 400,000 deaths related to *tobacco.*

100,000 deaths related to *alcohol abuse.*

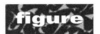 **13.2**

Of the nearly 2.1 million deaths per year in the United States, about one in four—approximately 520,000—is now related to alcohol, tobacco, and other illegal drugs.

The Role of Colleges and Universities in Preventing Alcohol, Tobacco, and Other Drug (ATOD) Problems

- Increase student awareness about alcohol and the use of other drugs in relation to academic and social problems on campus, particularly vandalism, date rape, poor academic performance, dropping out, injuries, disease, death, and disturbance of nondrinkers and nondrug users.

- Make certain that students with ATOD problems know where they can go for help with their abuse of mind-changing drugs.

- Provide alternatives to drinking by keeping campus facilities open, expanding recreational activities at nights and on weekends, and responding to needs for "on-the-spot" alternatives.

- For students who are under 21 years of age, prevent drinking, limit alcohol advertising in the college newspaper, and ban alcohol industry sponsorship of college activities.

- For students who are over 21 years of age, limit times and places for drinking, prohibit drunkenness, regulate conditions of alcohol use, and refuse sponsorship of a bar on campus.

- Develop and encourage designated driver programs among the student body.

- Train faculty and administrators on how to recognize substance-abuse problems and how to refer students to sources of assistance.

- Encourage faculty to incorporate substance-abuse education into their curricula.

- Educate students about the connection between alcohol and other drug abuse and unprotected sexual behaviors, which can lead to transmission of HIV and other sexually transmitted diseases.

- Provide smoke-free environments in student living areas, such as cafeterias and residence halls.

- Encourage art students, student athletes, and campus media to disseminate substance-abuse prevention messages.

- Involve both students and faculty in the development of policies regarding ATOD abuse.

- Enforce campus rules and regulations consistently and fairly.

- Develop aggressive media campaigns to counterbalance the alcohol industry's advertising and promotions, which are often aimed at young people.

- Encourage students and faculty to direct their studies in their special disciplines toward college drinking problems in particular.

Source: Modified from the Center for Substance Abuse Prevention.

---

recreational use of illicit psychoactive chemicals, the nation realized that something had to be done.

Initial efforts at combating drug abuse were aimed at scaring youths into nonuse through information-only school programs and at finding and treating drug abusers for their illness or penalizing them for their criminal behavior. Evaluation of early school-based drug education programs revealed that such efforts had little or no effect on drug-using behavior. In some instances, students seemed to increase their recreational drug usage after exposure to drug education programs.[5] It was also recognized that there would never be sufficient treatment facilities or caregivers to "cure" the mounting numbers of "addicts," and the jails were not big enough to accommodate a whole generation. Countermeasures were eventually devised that focused on preventing the problem before it developed. Today, effective programs of alcohol, tobacco, and other drug abuse prevention combine a variety of activities—as noted in Box 13.1—that reflect the following general plans or strategies.

Supply Reduction Strategy

This concept of drug-abuse prevention is not new. Both the Harrison Narcotic Act of 1914 and the Eighteenth (Prohibition) Amendment to the U.S. Constitution—later to be repealed by the Twenty-First Amendment—represented early attempts at drug-abuse prevention (see fig. 13.3). Both were based on the idea that enforcement of laws controlling the manufacture and distribution of certain drugs would stop people from using those drugs. These and similar laws reflect a plan of **supply reduction**—one that intends to lower, restrict, or eliminate the availability of a drug. With less and less use, eventually there will be no use at all. Without use, there can be no misuse or abuse.

Reducing the supply of illegal drugs and limiting the availability of therapeutic drugs with abuse potential are important parts of the current abuse prevention policy in the United States.[6,7] Other aspects of supply reduction include disrupting major drug-trafficking organizations, eradicating American and foreign marijuana crops, driving drug prices higher by limiting availability and discouraging use, interdicting foreign-manufactured drugs at the nation's borders and ports of entry, heavy taxation of ethyl alcohol, criminal penalties for trafficking in drugs, and limiting the number of retail beverage alcohol outlets and their hours of operation. The implementation of supply reduction techniques has not always produced the desired effect, however. In fact, some people believe that laws curtailing the supply of drugs have virtually no impact whatsoever on drug-taking behavior.

Recently, the relationship between the average level of consumption in a population and the percentage of heavy consumers has been debated and extended to the phenomenon of alcohol and drug abuse. According to this **distribution of consumption theory,** there is a relationship between the per capita consumption of all drugs used in a society and the prevalence of heavy drug use and abuse. Therefore, highly restrictive controls on accessibility to drugs will lead to lower consumption which in turn, will result in fewer drug abuse problems. Although the theory supporting supply reduction has some validity, the social, economic, and political costs of implementation are often perceived as outweighing their potential benefits. Moreover, the severity of restrictions—often known in the alcohol-abuse prevention field as "neoprohibition" tactics—would likely be found unconstitutional.

Demand Reduction Strategy

Another major plan for preventing drug abuse is to reduce the actual demand for drugs. Techniques based on **demand reduction** include a wide range of activities that help individuals (primarily youth) create positive mental attitudes, values, behaviors, skills, and life-styles that will enable them to mature as adjusted and competent citizens who will not need to resort to the use of drugs. Demand reduction also involves medical or other therapy for current drug abusers and drug dependent individuals who will no longer be in the drug-using population.

Information programs conducted via various media can provide accurate and objective information about all types of drugs and their effects on the body. This effort is often referred to as information dissemination and aims at increasing awareness of the effects of drugs on families, communities, and individuals. Such a program also attempts to increase perceptions of the risks associated with alcohol, tobacco, and other drug use.

Educational experiences can be designed to help individuals develop skills in decision making, coping with stress, problem solving, and interpersonal communication. These activities can prove valuable for young people who are not using drugs or for those having only initial or experimental contact with psychoactives.

Although drugs may be available "on the street," the demand, desire, or need for their use and anticipated benefits are hopefully reduced or eliminated altogether by this strategy. The outcome of such demand reduction is the lessening, delay, or absence of drug-abuse behavior that is not within the bounds of medical therapy and that disrupts normal human development and functioning.

Too often, substance-abuse specialists view supply reduction and demand reduction strategies as conflicting approaches to the prevention of alcohol and other drug problems. However, reciprocal relationships that exist between these strategies should not be overlooked. For instance, while overseas crop eradication and border interdiction activities work primarily to reduce the supply of drugs, they often make the purchase of certain imported drugs more difficult, and therefore, less likely. Similarly, drug education and treatment work primarily to reduce demand, but in doing so they may force suppliers to cut back on production and distribution in an effort to sustain consistent profits in the illegal drug marketplace.

Inoculation Strategy

Abuse prevention based on the **inoculation strategy** attempts to immunize or protect drug users against unhealthy, irresponsible drug-taking behavior and thus reduce the harmful and negative consequences so often associated with drug abuse. Rather than reduce either

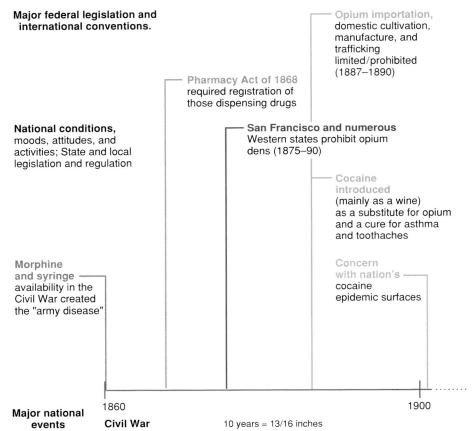

 13.3

Some historic milestones in early drug control efforts in the United States.

Source: Office of Justice Programs, Bureau of Justice Statistics, U.S. Department of Justice.

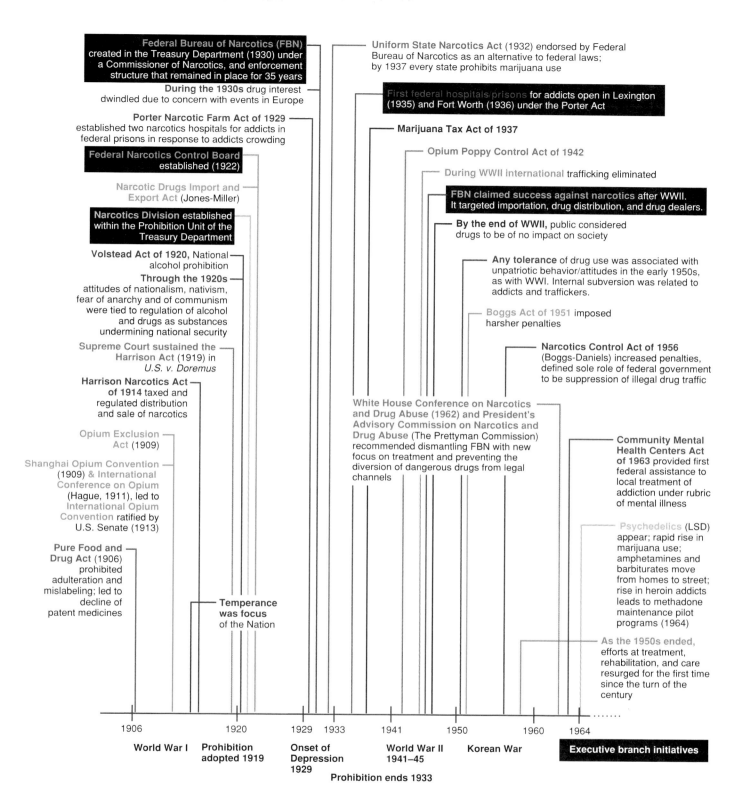

Federal Bureau of Narcotics (FBN) created in the Treasury Department (1930) under a Commissioner of Narcotics, and enforcement structure that remained in place for 35 years

During the 1930s drug interest dwindled due to concern with events in Europe

Porter Narcotic Farm Act of 1929 established two narcotics hospitals for addicts in federal prisons in response to addicts crowding

Federal Narcotics Control Board established (1922)

Narcotic Drugs Import and Export Act (Jones-Miller)

Narcotics Division established within the Prohibition Unit of the Treasury Department

Volstead Act of 1920, National alcohol prohibition

Through the 1920s attitudes of nationalism, nativism, fear of anarchy and of communism were tied to regulation of alcohol and drugs as substances undermining national security

Supreme Court sustained the Harrison Act (1919) in *U.S. v. Doremus*

Harrison Narcotics Act of 1914 taxed and regulated distribution and sale of narcotics

Opium Exclusion Act (1909)

Shanghai Opium Convention (1909) & International Conference on Opium (Hague, 1911), led to International Opium Convention ratified by U.S. Senate (1913)

Pure Food and Drug Act (1906) prohibited adulteration and mislabeling; led to decline of patent medicines

Uniform State Narcotics Act (1932) endorsed by Federal Bureau of Narcotics as an alternative to federal laws; by 1937 every state prohibits marijuana use

First federal hospitals/prisons for addicts open in Lexington (1935) and Fort Worth (1936) under the Porter Act

Marijuana Tax Act of 1937

Opium Poppy Control Act of 1942

During WWII international trafficking eliminated

FBN claimed success against narcotics after WWII. It targeted importation, drug distribution, and drug dealers.

By the end of WWII, public considered drugs to be of no impact on society

Any tolerance of drug use was associated with unpatriotic behavior/attitudes in the early 1950s, as with WWI. Internal subversion was related to addicts and traffickers.

Boggs Act of 1951 imposed harsher penalties

Narcotics Control Act of 1956 (Boggs-Daniels) increased penalties, defined sole role of federal government to be suppression of illegal drug traffic

White House Conference on Narcotics and Drug Abuse (1962) and President's Advisory Commission on Narcotics and Drug Abuse (The Prettyman Commission) recommended dismantling FBN with new focus on treatment and preventing the diversion of dangerous drugs from legal channels

Community Mental Health Centers Act of 1963 provided first federal assistance to local treatment of addiction under rubric of mental illness

Psychedelics (LSD) appear; rapid rise in marijuana use; amphetamines and barbiturates move from homes to street; rise in heroin addicts leads to methadone maintenance pilot programs (1964)

As the 1950s ended, efforts at treatment, rehabilitation, and care resurged for the first time since the turn of the century

Temperance was focus of the Nation

| 1906 | 1920 | 1929 | 1933 | 1941 | 1950 | 1960 | 1964 |

World War I | Prohibition adopted 1919 | Onset of Depression 1929 | World War II 1941–45 | Korean War | **Executive branch initiatives**

Prohibition ends 1933

 13.3

continued

the supply of or demand for psychoactive drugs, inoculation activities seek to increase the proportion of individuals practicing certain styles of moderate and responsible drug use. Emphasis is placed on responsible decision making, that is, decisions involving obligations, accountability, rational limits on use, and the exercise of various precautions as individuals interact with specific drugs.

An example of the inoculation strategy is the development of a drinking etiquette for those who use alcoholic beverages. Such an etiquette refers to manners and behaviors that meet standards generally accepted by a particular social group of drinkers. When practiced, the basic rules of etiquette tend to lessen the number and severity of adverse consequences resulting from drug use or abuse. It is important to note that while inoculation activities may make the drug user resistant to harm, they can never guarantee absolute protection from negative effects. There is some risk associated with use of all drugs, including alcohol.

Public Health Model of Abuse Prevention

What may be a comprehensive abuse prevention strategy involving elements of the three preceding plans is the so-called **public health prevention model.** Rather than focus on just one major outcome, this model identifies points or targets of intervention within a conceptual framework.

The public health model assumes that a *host-agent-environment relationship* exists, through which diseases are transmitted and into which various interventions can be made in order to prevent illness or promote wellness. Prevention activities might occur appropriately in any or all of the three sectors of the model at levels that range from the individual to the community. Although critics doubt whether the public health field is capable of preventing drug problems that may be more social than medical in nature, the model has provided many innovative opportunities for prevention activities.

Applied to the prevention of drug abuse, the term **host** refers to individuals and their knowledge about psychoactive

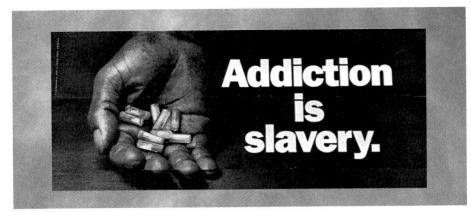

Public awareness campaigns that communicate the adverse effects of psychoactive drugs are important parts of any overall effort to promote a drug-free environment.

© Toni Michaels/The Image Works

drugs, the personal attitudes that influence drug use and patterns of abuse, and drug-taking behavior itself. Host-targeted prevention activities include

- helping children to resist peer pressure to use drugs;

- mandating product-warning labels that can assist drug users in avoiding harmful effects of drugs;

- providing alternative experiences to drug-taking behavior;

- enhancing coping skills to reduce individual stress factors that might lead to drug use;

- encouraging people to stop pushing drugs at social gatherings; and

- helping children of alcoholics to reduce their chances of developing drinking problems.

The term **agent** pertains to the various drug substances—their content, formulation, distribution, prescription, and availability. Agent-targeted prevention activities are often intended to reduce the supply of drugs and are represented by

- enforcing laws that prohibit the growing of marijuana and the entry of cocaine into the nation;

- eradicating overseas drug crops;

- forbidding the placement of cigarette dispensing machines in areas accessible to young people under the age of 18 years;

- increasing the taxes on alcohol and tobacco products and increasing the penalties for dealing in or possessing illegal drugs;

- lowering the tar and nicotine content of cigarettes;

- banning the manufacture of look-alike drugs;

- limiting so-called "happy hours" and other practices that encourage beverage alcohol consumption; and

- encouraging physicians to exercise more caution in prescribing psychoactive drugs and pharmacists to check with physicians when in doubt about prescriptions for psychoactive drugs.

The **environment** is the setting or context in which drug use occurs, and the group or community customs, mores, or folkways that influence drug takers. This element allows for a sociocultural interpretation of drug abuse that originates in social stress factors of ambivalent and conflicting values assigned to drug taking, unemployment, racial discrimination, sexist employment and educational policies, and harshness of ghetto living. Environmental change would involve

- altering the social climate that accepts and approves of widespread drug use, especially that which reduces tension;

- deemphasizing the portrayal of smoking and drinking in television programs;

box 13.2

A Community-Based Approach to Preventing Alcohol, Tobacco, and Other Drug (ATOD) Problems

The Washington, D.C., Community Prevention Partnership uses a macro-approach that emphasizes a total community-based prevention effort against ATOD disorders and dysfunctions. Twenty-seven public and private agencies formed separate teams in each of the District of Columbia's eight wards. Each team consists of volunteers of all ages and backgrounds who meet monthly to discuss ATOD issues and problems in their neighborhoods.

The Asian American Drug Abuse Program of South Central Los Angeles is a federally sponsored High Risk Youth Project that is a model collaborative effort between the Korean Youth Center and the Search to Involve Philippine Americans. These three agencies provide ATOD programs and services to high-risk Asian Pacific Islander youth in the area. This project was especially visible during the 1992 south-central Los Angeles riots, working closely with other local organizations to stop violence and restabilize the community. A related prevention effort, the Communications and Community Partnership, attempts to shift social norms away from illicit drug use and excessive alcohol consumption, and to halt the rebuilding of liquor stores destroyed in the recent riots.

Another communications program seeks to change the norm of excessive alcohol consumption by Native Americans in Oklahoma by focusing on the strengths of Native American tradition and the strengths of the current culture.

Source: Center for Substance Abuse Prevention.

---

developing and adopting a standard of acceptable alcohol use;

rejecting intoxication as funny, and therefore tolerable, behavior;

holding "party hosts" liable for guests' drunken driving and its life-threatening consequences; and

reducing various social stress factors through government programs, economic policies, and planned group practices.

Among drug-abuse prevention specialists, focusing prevention efforts on the entire environment in which any individual lives is called the **macro-approach.** (The word *macro* means large, great, or all-inclusive.) Such a prevention approach involves a number of coordinated activities designed to create a total community climate of nondrug use. Acceptance or even tolerance of recreational drug usage, including the legal social drugs, would not be among the objectives of a macro-prevention program.

The promotion of a drug-free environment would be focused on helping various components of a community provide effective prevention and treatment services for ATOD disorders.[8] Specific activities identified by the federal government's Center for Substance Abuse Prevention include organizing, planning, and enhancing the efficiency and effectiveness of services, implementation assistance, interagency collaboration, and coalition building among public and private agencies (see box 13.2).

In addition, such an approach would also attempt to establish or change written and unwritten community standards, codes, and even attitudes that influence the occurrence of ATOD problems in the general population. Particularly important are laws and regulations that restrict availability of and access to ATOD substances, thereby increasing the price of ATOD products, and area-wide prevention actions initiated by citizen advocacy groups and reinforced by governmental policy. Such a total, community-wide effort to reduce or prevent ATOD problems might include an integrated undertaking of community activities, parent and family actions, school-based programs, and workplace initiatives (see box 13.3).[9]

Developing comprehensive *community-wide projects* to prevent or reduce drug and alcohol abuse involves many segments of the community, including civic, youth, and voluntary organizations as well as professional and medical associations, industry, law enforcement and other government agencies, and the mass media. A community-based task force might consider the following.

1. Establishing youth programs that emphasize drug- and alcohol-free behavior and provide positive peer influence to prevent drinking/drug-taking and driving fatalities.

2. Developing social policies, norms, laws, and regulations that provide consistent messages about drugs and alcohol. Restricting "happy hours," banning drug paraphernalia sales, and not allowing youths to leave school during the day can all help prevent chemical abuse problems.

3. Providing community-based counseling that would refer clients to other programs, and providing resources that might better prevent or reduce problems of substance abuse.

4. Assessing community needs and involving youth in constructive community service projects.

5. Highlighting and supporting health promotion techniques that advocate healthy life-styles and alternatives to drug-taking activities.

6. Encouraging local newspapers and radio and television stations to deglamorize drug and alcohol use, and to provide current and accurate information regarding drug use and abuse.

7. Promoting "networking" (working together through developing interrelationships) among public and private groups to assure consistent and comprehensive solutions to drug-related problems.

8. Forming coalitions of concerned people to provide a public forum for the sharing of ideas and perceptions about issues related to alcohol and other drugs in the local community.

Parents and families are often affected the most by drug and alcohol problems in the community. However, they are often the most dedicated antidrug abuse activists on the local level. Some actions to consider include

1. forming parent support groups through which parents help one another as they cope with drug and alcohol problems in their homes and neighborhoods;

2. establishing parent action groups that work with state and local governments, schools, law enforcement agencies, and businesses to influence social policies regarding alcohol and drug use;

3. enabling parents and children to communicate more effectively and learn personal and interpersonal skills through family life skills development programs;

4. encouraging parent drug and alcohol education programs emphasizing pharmacology of abusable substances and the impact of such drugs on personal health status; and

5. training service providers and informing the elderly about the proper use of medicines and effective communication skills with physicians and pharmacists.

Today's *school-based programs* to prevent alcohol and drug abuse consist of more than information sessions to discourage the use of psychoactive drugs. Working together, students, teachers, parents, school administrators, school counselors and nursing personnel, community officials, local professionals, and other concerned citizens have made a significant impact on young people's use of mind-altering chemicals. Some effective school strategies include the following.

1. Adopting and enforcing fair and clear school policies regarding use and possession of drugs and alcohol both on and off school property.

---

box 13.3

What Communities Can Do about Drug and Alcohol Abuse

Community Projects

Youth Organizations

Social Policies, Laws, and Regulations

Community-based Counseling

Assessment of Community Needs

Health Promotion

Media Impact

Networking Resources

Community Coalitions

School Programs

School Policies

Positive Peer Programs

Peer Resistance to "Gateway Drugs"

Drug and Alcohol Information Programs

Comprehensive Health Education Curriculum

Student Assistance Programs

Alternative Programs

Parent/Family Activities

Parent Support Groups

Parent Action Groups

Family Life Skills Development

Parent Drug and Alcohol Education

Training for Service Providers and the Elderly

Workplace Initiatives

Drug and Alcohol Policies

Employee Assistance Programs

Family Assistance Programs

Health Promotion

Drug and Alcohol Information Programs

Encouragement of Social Responsibility

Source: National Institute on Drug Abuse and Center for Substance Abuse Prevention.

---

2. Establishing positive peer programs that use student peers as role models, facilitators, helpers, and leaders for other school-age children. Such programs can help young people who are having problems, undergoing normal adolescent stresses, wanting to confide in someone, and who want to take part in school and community service activities.

3. Developing peer resistance programs relating to use of cigarettes, marijuana, cocaine, and alcohol. These programs generally help students learn that the use of such drugs is not as common as they perceive, that not "everybody" is doing it, and that there are clear ways to say no to the use of drugs.

4. Offering school team training for teachers, administrators, support staff, and other interested community people who can then implement action plans in schools that will improve the school's

emotional climate and address alcohol and other drug-related issues.

5. Introducing comprehensive health education and other curricula that increase students' knowledge about their own health and help them assess their feelings and values. Sometimes these curricular offerings focus on specific chemicals of abuse, whereas others seek to enhance healthy, constructive lifestyles.

6. Initiating student assistance programs for those who may be at high risk for developing drug, alcohol, and other problems. Such programs, modeled after the Employee Assistance Programs in business and industry, can also serve as an intervention tool with students who have already developed problems.

7. Offering alternative programs that provide specific activities and involvements that are healthy,

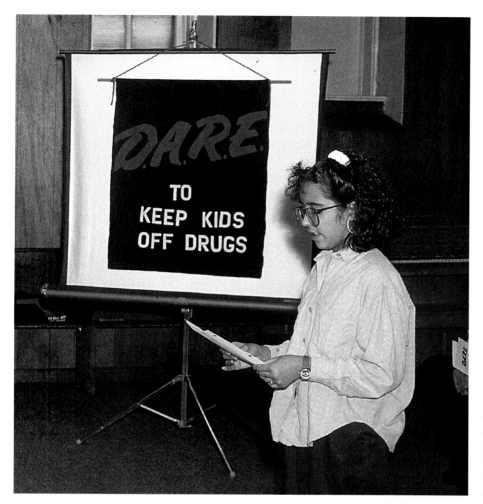

Learning to say no to drugs is the major goal of Project D.A.R.E. Now focused on fifth and sixth graders, Drug Abuse Resistance Education (D.A.R.E.) is a school curriculum involving specially trained police officers who teach young students to resist drug usage, build self-esteem, manage stress, and withstand pro-drug media messages.

© James L. Shaffer

positive options to drug use (see table 13.4). Some alternatives already being promoted for youths include helping the elderly, preventing crime and vandalism, finding jobs and learning job skills, restoring historic sites, and building community parks and playgrounds.

Substance abuse continues to pose a major problem to *business and industry* in terms of worker health and productivity. Listed below are some of the strategies now being used to prevent alcohol and drug abuse in the workplace.

1. Adopting appropriate, clear, and fair policies relating to drug and alcohol use and abuse, and their consistent enforcement.

2. Implementing employee assistance programs (EAPs) that help troubled employees, including those with drug and alcohol problems, through referral to counseling, treatment, and rehabilitation agencies.

3. Establishing family programs that provide counseling and referral services to workers' family members when employee problems originate from nonwork issues. Flexible work schedules and maternity leaves have been used to help families in periods of stress.

4. Developing health-promotion endeavors that inform employees about general health issues and provide them with opportunities to improve their fitness, nutrition, and other health-related behaviors.

5. Offering drug and alcohol education programs that provide information about the negative health effects of drug and alcohol use as well as positive reinforcement for nonuse of drugs and alcohol.

6. Encouraging social responsibility by offering training programs about use of safety belts and the hazards of drinking and driving. A corporation may also exercise crowd control procedures and offer nonalcoholic alternatives to consumption of alcoholic beverages at holiday parties and company picnics, in the interest of promoting more responsible behavior of its employees.

Another version of the macro-approach interprets alcohol, tobacco, and other drug use as a major health problem influenced by various risk factors in five life areas of young people—individual, family, school, peer group, and community. In each of these five risk areas, specific risk factors are identified and then appropriate intervention strategies are proposed (see box 13.4).[10] While no single initiative can ever address all such risk factors, various "high-risk" youth demonstration programs have been implemented to develop and field test innovative approaches aimed at preventing ATOD use and helping young people make healthy, productive, and self-affirming life decisions.

This rather detailed description of two macro-approaches to drug abuse prevention reveals the many interrelated efforts that can be used to influence the host, agent, and environment in solving a community-wide problem. It is essential that all parts of the community work together to address the various factors and causes underlying alcohol, tobacco, and other drug use and abuse. Slowly, many communities are discovering the great power they have to solve their own drug-related predicaments.

Risk factors for alcohol, tobacco, and other drug problems and examples of promising countermeasures for addressing these risk factors.

Individual-Based Risk Factors

Individual life skills
Lack of self-control, assertiveness, peer-refusal skills
Low self-esteem and self-confidence
Emotional and psychological problems
Favorable attitudes toward ATOD use
Rejection of commonly held values and religion
School failure
Lack of school bonding (commitment)
Early antisocial behavior (lying, stealing, aggression)

Promising Countermeasures

Social and life skills training in problem solving, decision
  making, controlling anger and aggression
Alternative activities to build self-esteem and self-confidence

Individual and group counseling

Tutoring and homework support
Mentoring (intergenerational) and surrogate nurturers

Family-Based Risk Factors

Family conflict and domestic violence
Family disorganization and lack of family rituals
Lack of family cohesion
Social isolation of family
Heightened family stress
Family attitudes favorable to drug use
Ambiguous or inconsistent rules regarding ATOD use
Poor child supervision and discipline
Unrealistic expectations for development

Promising Countermeasures

Family therapy
Family skills training in effective parenting

Play therapy, especially for young children of ATOD-abusing parents
Parent training

Parent involvement in youth activities

School-Based Risk Factors

Ambiguous or inconsistent rules regarding drug use and
  student conduct
Favorable staff and student attitudes toward ATOD use
Poor student management practices
Availability of ATOD on the school premises
Lack of school bonding (commitment, lack of motivation)

Promising Countermeasures

Teaching reform that involves youths as active learners;
  educational planning
School alcohol and drug policy that is clear and consistently
  enforced
Availability of ombudsperson or advocate for both parents and
  students
Availability of prevention services to youths and professionals
  in contact with the youths

Peer-Based Risk Factors

Association with delinquent, ATOD-using peers
Association with peers having favorable attitudes toward ATOD use

Susceptibility to peer pressure
Strong sense of external focus (locus) of control, that is, the
  belief that oneself is controlled by outside pressures, family,
  friends, chance, or even luck

Promising Countermeasures

Membership in positive peer clubs or groups
Correcting perceptions of norms concerning ATOD use in peer
  and general population
Peer resistance training to develop skills of saying no
Positive peer/youth models who do not use ATOD

Peer leadership and counseling interventions

Community-Based Risk Factors

Community disorganization with few potential leaders
Lack of community bonding (no identification)
Lack of cultural pride
Lack of bicultural competence
Community attitudes favorable to ATOD use
Ready availability of alcohol, tobacco, and other drugs

Inadequate youth services and opportunities for prosocial
  involvement

Promising Countermeasures

Cultural enhancement via learning of group's history,
  traditions, values, identity, and pride
Orientation to community services
Rites of passage to become responsible, mature members of society

Positive drug-free youth groups
Community service and media education activities
Provision of "safe havens" that provide secure areas for those
  wishing to avoid gangs and drug dealers
Community advocacy for changes in social policy that
  glamorize ATOD use
Involvement of the faith community that links ATOD use with
  the moral authority of a church institution

Source: Modified from the Center for Substance Abuse Prevention.

Ten Steps to Help Young People Say No to Alcohol and Other Drugs

1. *Talk with your child about alcohol and other drugs.* Parents can intervene to help change mistaken ideas their children may have obtained from peers and the media, such as "everybody drinks."

   Challenge the common myths; clearly explain why young people should not drink or take drugs.

2. *Learn to really listen to your child.* Children are more likely to communicate when they receive positive verbal and nonverbal cues that show their parents are listening.

   Rephrase your child's comments to show you understand; watch your child's face and body language; give nonverbal support and encouragement; use the right tone of voice for the answer you are giving; use encouraging phrases to show your interest and to keep the conversation going.

3. *Help your child feel good about himself or herself.* Self-regard is enhanced when parents praise efforts, as well as accomplishments, and when they correct by criticizing the action rather than the child. Give lots of praise; help children set realistic goals; don't compare your child's efforts with others; use "I messages" to take responsibility for your own negative feelings; give your children real responsibility.

4. *Help your child develop strong values.* A strong value system can give children the courage to make decisions based on facts rather than pressure from friends.

5. *Be a good role model or example.* Parental drinking and drug-taking habits may strongly influence children's perceptions about alcohol and other drugs, including medicines.

6. *Help your preteen deal with peer pressure.* Children who have been taught to be gentle and loving may need parental "permission" to assertively say no to negative peer pressure. Teach your child to value individuality; explore the meaning of friendship with your child; encourage your child to practice saying no.

7. *Make family policies that help your child say no.* It's helpful when parents verbalize specific family rules against alcohol and other drug use by minors, and the consequences of breaking those rules.

8. *Encourage healthy, creative activities.* Hobbies, school events, and other activities may prevent children from experimenting with alcohol, tobacco, or other drugs out of boredom.

9. *Team up with other parents.* When parents join together in support groups, they can take steps that will reinforce the guidance they provide at home.

10. *Know what to do if you suspect a problem.* Parents can learn to recognize the telltale signs of alcohol and drug abuse and even experimentation.

Source: Modified from the National Institute on Alcohol Abuse and Alcoholism.

Intervention Levels of Abuse Prevention

Activities undertaken to prevent the occurrence of some disease or disabling condition are often described on three different levels of intervention or application. Each intervention level is intended to reduce the total number of individuals who suffer from a disease or are afflicted by some impairment. According to public health practices, these levels refer to the timing when intervention (prevention) activities are first begun. Identified as **primary, secondary,** and **tertiary prevention,** the three levels are described below.

Primary Prevention Level

The first level of intervention pertains to activities that are begun before drug abuse occurs. Primary prevention takes place "before the fact" and prevents an individual from becoming diseased or impaired in the first place. As a consequence, no new cases of drug abuse develop. Common primary prevention techniques include legislation and law enforcement, information programs, education for responsible decision making, knowledge of risk factors, and the development of non-drug-related alternative behaviors.

One example of primary prevention aimed at the host is helping young people say no to alcohol and drugs. Also a demand reduction procedure, the task has been formalized into a ten-step program to be used by parents and others who work with preteens—those in the 9- to 12-year-old age group (see box 13.5). During these "in-between" years, young people are old enough to understand various adult subjects but still young enough to accept guidance from parents and other family members.

The ten-step program is based on proven communication techniques that can lead to strengthened parent-child relationships. Furthermore, each of the specific steps can be implemented independently. Whether one or all of the steps are used, they can provide young people with the solid foundation needed for the confusing adolescent years just ahead.

Secondary Prevention Level

On the second level of intervention are those prevention activities applied during the early stages of drug abuse. Through crisis intervention, early diagnosis, crisis monitoring, and referral for treatment, efforts are made to detect the problem as soon as possible and to get it treated effectively so that the condition does not progress. Secondary prevention attempts to restore to health those who have been drug abusers, and thus reduces the number of existing drug-problem cases.

Many initial activities of the war on drugs have been secondary prevention endeavors. Two of these—early **detection** and *referral* and *family intervention*—are

Indications of Possible Chemical Abuse

Common Signs

Changes in attendance patterns at work or school.

Change from typical capabilities, such as work habits, efficiency, self-discipline, mood or attitude expression.

Poor physical appearance, including lack of attention to dress and personal hygiene.

Unusual effort to cover arms in order to hide needle marks.

Association with known drug users.

Increased borrowing of money from friends or family members; stealing from employer, home, or school.

Heightened secrecy about actions and possessions.

Specific Indications

Narcotics:

Appearance of scars ("tracks") on the arms or back of hands, caused by injecting drugs.

Constricted pupils.

Frequent scratching of various parts of the body.

Loss of normal appetite.

Immediately after a "fix," user may be lethargic, drowsy, i.e., "on the nod," an alternating cycle of dozing and awakening.

Restlessness, sniffles, and red, watery eyes and yawning, which disappear soon after drug is administered.

Users often have syringes or medicine droppers, bent spoons or metal bottle caps, small glassine bags or tinfoil packets.

Depressants:

Behavior like that of alcohol intoxication, with or without the odor of alcohol on the breath.

Sluggishness, difficulty in thinking and concentrating.

Slurred speech.

Faulty judgment, moody.

Impaired motor skills.

Falls asleep while at work.

Anxiety, weakness, tremors, sweating, insomnia relieved by another dose.

Stimulants:

Excessively active, irritable, nervous ("wired") or impulsive.

Abnormally long periods without eating or sleeping, with the likelihood of being or becoming emaciated.

Repetitive, nonpurposeful behavior.

Dilated pupils.

Chronically runny nose, respiratory problems related to snorting cocaine.

Users may have straws, small spoons, mirrors, and razor blades.

Psychedelics (Hallucinogens):

Behavior and mood vary widely. The user may sit or recline quietly in a trancelike state or may appear fearful or even terrified.

Difficulty in communicating.

Profound changes in perception, mood, and thinking.

May experience nausea, chills, flushing, irregular breathing, sweating and trembling of hands after consuming the drug.

Phencyclidine (PCP) and Related Drugs:

User is likely to be noncommunicative and exhibit a blank, staring appearance with eyes repeatedly flicking from side to side.

High-stepping, exaggerated gait.

Increased insensitivity to pain.

Amnesia.

Profound changes in perception, mood, and thinking, which can include self-destructive behavior and mimic an acute schizophrenic disorder.

Marijuana:

Shreds of plant material in pockets, bobby pins or other small clips used to hold end of cigarette (joint), cigarette papers, pipes.

Intoxicated behavior.

Lethargy, inability to concentrate.

Impaired motor skills.

Distorted sense of time and distance that would make driving hazardous.

Source: Modified from the U. S. Drug Enforcement Administration.

---

described here in some detail because of their potential for success and their widespread application in the general population.

Early Detection and Referral

Most people interested in alcohol and drug problems probably begin their informal education by reading newspaper articles, magazine stories, and pamphlets distributed by various local organizations and by both state and federal government agencies. This type of self-learning is absolutely essential for those who want preparation in detecting drug abuse problems in their family members and loved ones.

More formalized drug education programs may be offered by such community groups as drug rehabilitation programs, mental health agencies, churches, and civic organizations. Parents' groups, including the National Federation of Parents for Drug Free Youth, Parents' Resource Institute for Drug Education (PRIDE), and Families in Action, sometimes have local chapters that provide organized programs on drug prevention and education.

Fortified with a better understanding of the nature of chemical abuse and drug dependence, individuals are more prepared to observe others' behaviors and interpret such signs as possible indicators of drug abuse in its early stages (see box 13.6). It is important to recognize the outward indicators of chemical abuse because many drug abusers tend to conceal their drug-taking behavior. Though one should be alert to both general and specific signs of possible drug abuse, it is necessary to realize that even drug experts themselves have difficulty on occasion in early identification of chemical abuse.

Therefore, it is recommended that concerned individuals not act solely on their own, because such an undertaking could lead to falsely accusing an innocent person. After identifying an indicator of possible drug abuse, seek professional advice and help from the "experts"—physicians and the agencies specializing in drug problems.[11]

Those who attempt to detect early signs of chemical abuse ought to remember that a diabetic, for example, has a legitimate reason for having a syringe and needle and is not necessarily a "junkie." Possession of tablets and capsules may reflect that an individual is on prescribed medication rather than an abuser of illegal drugs. And having the sniffles and runny eyes may be due to a head cold or an allergic condition and not to narcotics addiction. Such unusual or even odd behavior may not be related in any way to substance abuse.

After early detection and the willingness to break the silence of denial, the next task involves getting the drug abuser into some form of treatment so that chemical dependence does not progress to its more serious and devastating phases. This sometimes frustrating and complex procedure is the **referral process**—directing, convincing, and encouraging the drug abuser to contact some drug and alcohol treatment program for assistance. Typically, some form of intervention (described in the next section of this chapter) may be needed in order to get the early-phase drug abuser evaluated by professional personnel and involved with a treatment program leading to recovery.

Just as difficult may be the location of appropriate information and treatment centers, as well as other agencies that support either the drug abuser or members of the drug abuser's family. Consulting the local telephone directory for such valuable knowledge is a recommended first step. Look on the inside front cover, and in both the white and yellow pages, for numerous listings of information and referral centers, treatment and rehabilitation programs, and self-help groups. Examining just one telephone directory from a medium-size city revealed the multiple

sources of assistance listed in box 13.7. Self-help organizations for family members of a drug abuser may also be available, including Al-Anon Family Groups, Nar-Anon Family Groups, Families Anonymous, and TOUGHLOVE.

The Intervention Process

One example of secondary prevention that focuses on the host or drug abuser is the **intervention process.** Sometimes this process or procedure is referred to as a form of crisis intervention because the family and friends of the drug-dependent individual attempt to create a crisis that will motivate or persuade the drug abuser to seek help.[12] In practice, the process of intervention is a technique used in helping drug abusers overcome their psychological denial and accept the fact that a problem exists.

Planned and implemented under the supervision of a trained counselor or family therapist, the intervention process is structured to help drug-dependent individuals become aware of and desire recovery from their dependency. Such intervention can assist drug abusers to achieve the first steps in recovery—identification of the need to make significant lifestyle changes and recognition of the need for help in the recovery process itself.

Until recently, many therapists as well as the general public were convinced that drug abusers had to "hit bottom" before they were ready for help. To "hit bottom" involves the drug abusers' recognition of the seriousness of their dependency, admitting their need for help, and eventually asking for help. Often such recognition occurred only after the breakdown of psychological defense mechanisms that allowed addicts and alcoholics to deny their need for assistance. And the recognition, level of awareness, and the eventual "cry for help" were reached only after loss of physical and mental health, family and friends, job, and self-respect in many cases.

The unique aspect of intervention is that drug abusers do not always have to "hit bottom" before they can be helped. Through compassionate communication, family members and friends of the drug-dependent individual explain the adverse consequences of continued drug abuse as

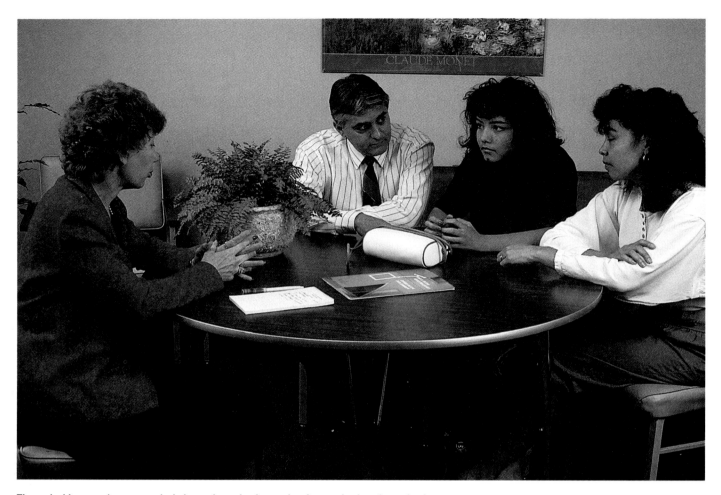

The typical intervention process includes a planned, rehearsed and supervised confrontation between family members and the drug dependent individual. This effort is an attempt to motivate or persuade the drug abuser to seek help for his or her drug problem.

© Bob Daemmrich/The Image Works

they experience them. Using planned and rehearsed nonjudgmental confrontation, directed self-evaluation of the drug abuser, identification of various treatment options, and a statement of expectation on the part of family members, the intervention process can interrupt drug abuse and drug dependence before they progress to their most serious, advanced, and devastating phase.

Typically, family members and friends require several weeks of training prior to the intervention. The following tasks must be accomplished by the interventionists.[13]

1. *Realization that drug dependency (e.g., alcoholism) is the family's primary problem,* not just one of several problems. Regardless of why the abuser started drinking or drugging,

the continuing use of drugs is the cause of problems and no longer a symptom of problems.

2. *Recognition of how drug dependency affects its victims at its various stages.* Eventually, the family members must accept the idea that the drug abuser cannot seek help alone; therefore, they must initiate the intervention.

3. *Admission that worrying about the drug abuser and playing the roles of "enablers" are basically useless endeavors.* The only helpful thing is to get the addict to accept treatment through their combined influence.

4. *Determination of how drug dependence has affected each member of the family.* Enabling, denial, hurt,

and powerlessness resulting from disturbed family relationships must be replaced by love, courage, and the readiness to risk intervention.

5. *Preparation of a written list detailing how each family member and friend has been adversely affected by the drug abuser over a period of time.* Sharing the specifics of exact time and setting reveals the different pain, danger, embarrassment, and guilt experienced within the family.

6. *Phrasing of all statements on individual lists in a straightforward and objective way and without any hostility or blame.* Effective intervention relies upon the emotional impact of presenting

numerous documented facts that do not allow room for denial. Love and concern must be the basis for identifying the harm to relationships, responsibilities, job, school, church, health, personality, and self-esteem—all created by drug use.

7. *Rehearsal of the directed self-evaluation by practicing the presentation of lists in a calm and courageous way.* Each family member should read aloud from his or her list and receive coaching from the supervising therapist.

8. *Determination of exactly what action the drug abuser will be asked to take.* In preparation for the actual intervention, the therapist and the interventionists must determine what sources of help are available, what treatment options and support groups will be utilized, how hospitalization will be arranged, and how the drug abuser's employer will be notified or involved.

9. *Establishing the time and place for the actual confrontation.* Depending upon circumstances, the best time for confrontation is when the drug dependent's psychological defenses are at a low ebb, for example, shortly after a threatened divorce or loss of job, a drunk-driving arrest, or a warning from a physician.

After thorough preparation, the intervention is held usually in the therapist's office and under the therapist's direction. The confrontation begins with the presentation of the evidence so that the drug abuser perceives the relationship between continued use of drugs and important relationships and responsibilities. Then, the chief interventionist presents the drug abuser with a program of treatment and aftercare that he or she is expected to undertake. At this point in the intervention, the family members announce their intention to enter treatment also, part of the total treatment approach found in family therapy. Their willingness to admit their need for help and their resolve to seek help make the drug abuser's response easier and more favorable.

Provided the planning is thorough and the preparation is adequate, the person being addressed agrees to get help in the vast majority of cases.[14] However, the interventionists should also consider the possibility of failure or noncompliance on the part of the drug abuser. Sometimes, an alternative treatment plan may have to be proposed. On occasion, a final ultimatum can be used as leverage to convince the drug abuser to enter treatment. Because drug-dependent individuals rarely seek help on their own until faced with a crisis, an ultimatum might create the crisis that will cause them to enter treatment.

Tertiary Prevention Level

As the third level of prevention, tertiary intervention is initiated during the later or advanced stages of drug abuse. To avoid the relapse of recovering drug abusers and to maintain their health status after therapy, the following techniques are used: various physical, mental, social, and even spiritual treatment procedures; detoxification of chemically dependent individuals; and institutionalization or drug-maintenance programs (see box 13.8). Tertiary efforts are intended to prevent the reactivation of the drug abuse phenomenon. In this text, tertiary prevention techniques are described more fully in chapters pertaining to specific psychoactive drugs.

Although treatment is the major feature of tertiary prevention, it is essential that common barriers to treatment be removed or reduced. Emotional support must be available for continuing recovery and rehabilitation of the drug-dependent individual. Financial support, often inadequate, must be assured through job counseling, job training, and eventual employment. Special treatment needs of recovering addicts and drug abusers may require support groups, child care, and various medical therapies. If these treatment enhancers are not present, tertiary prevention often fails.

Substance Abuse in the Workplace

Although there is no precise measure of the extent of drug use in American businesses and industries, there is a general consensus that illegal drugs have become pervasive in the workplace among both blue- and white-collar workers. Indeed, people who use drugs regularly are likely to use them at work on occasion, and sometimes arrive at work already "high" or intoxicated. Consequently, one of the major battlefields in the war on drugs is the workplace, where both new and old procedures are being used to assure a drug-free place of employment for both labor and management.

While cocaine often replaces marijuana as the most common workplace drug, the misuse of prescription and OTC drugs has also become an extensive problem for both industry and business. And alcohol, America's number one drug problem, continues to contribute to absenteeism, expensive medical bills, and reduced employee productivity.

Available statistics suggest that substance abuse in the workplace and drug usage affecting the workplace present a truly staggering problem.[15,16]

- Approximately 70 percent of all users of illegal drugs are currently employed.

- An estimated 1 out of 5 workers 18 to 25 years of age, and 1 out of 8 workers 26 to 34 years of age, abuse drugs on the job.

- Workplace ATOD problems cost U.S. companies over $100 billion each year. The costs to individual companies usually exceeds 2.5 percent of payroll.

- Drug-abusing employees acquire 300 percent higher medical costs and benefits, which consequently increases health insurance rates.

- Illicit-drug users are five times more likely to file a workers' compensation claim.

- Employees using drugs are 3 times more likely to be late for work and 2.5 times more likely to have absences of eight or more days. Absenteeism among problem drinkers or alcoholics is 3.8 to 8.3 times greater than normal. Statistics also show that drug users ask for early dismissal or additional time off 2.2 times more often than nonusers do.

- Drug use in the workplace breeds drug dealers in the workplace. Of workers surveyed, nearly one-third know of drug use by fellow employees on the job, and 10 percent have been offered drugs while at work.

- Drug users in the workforce are 3.6 times more likely to have workplace accidents. They also are 9 times more likely to have a domestic altercation or accident away from work. And according to the Employee Assistance Society of North America, up to 40 percent of industrial fatalities and 47 percent of industrial injuries are associated with alcohol abuse and alcoholism.

One study that measured the association between the presence of marijuana and/or cocaine in a preemployment drug screen and employment outcomes confirmed that drug-using behavior was, indeed, linked with adverse results.[17] However, the risk was much less than previously estimated. Those with marijuana-positive urine samples had 55 percent more on-the-job accidents, 85 percent more injuries, and a 78 percent increase in absenteeism. For those with cocaine-positive urine samples, there was a 145 percent increase in absenteeism and an 85 percent increase in injuries.

In terms of the economic burden on society, the annual cost of alcohol and other drug abuse in the United States is estimated to range from $200 to $400 billion. This amount reflects expenses associated with treatment, research, prevention programs, treatment of related health problems, crime, motor vehicle accidents, reduced productivity, and lost employment. In addition, businesses and industries are also concerned with increased on-the-job accidents and injuries,

box 13.8

Alcohol and Drug-Abuse Treatments

Many health authorities now view dependence on alcohol or other drugs as a chronic relapsing disease. As such, drug dependence is often marked by the return of disease symptoms after their apparent cessation. Therefore, to measure the effectiveness of treatment, it is necessary to use graded measures of change. It is more reasonable to think in terms of remissions (lessening or reduction of symptoms) rather than cures.

Because there are so many different types of drug-dependent people, with so many variables—presence or absence of psychiatric disorders, educational or occupational achievements, family/social support system, family history, and genetics—a wide range of treatments are available after appropriate diagnoses have been made.

A partial listing of drug-abuse treatments includes these:

Drug-Free Treatments

- Therapeutic community

- Self-help groups such as Alcoholics Anonymous, Narcotics Anonymous, and others

- Psychotherapy of various types, including supportive-expressive, cognitive/behavioral, family therapy, and others

- Behavioral therapy specifically aimed at prevention of relapse

Drug-Based Treatments

- Methadone maintenance

- Naltrexone (nonaddicting narcotic antagonist, also used in treating alcoholism)

- Antabuse (blocks alcohol metabolism)

- Psychoactive medication when indicated

Source: National Institute on Drug Abuse.

inappropriate decisions and actions that endanger human lives, and on-site thefts to finance employee addiction.

To reduce alcohol and other drug abuse on the job, the American business community, in compliance with the *Comprehensive Drug Free Workplace Act of 1988*, has developed a variety of countermeasures to lower the enormous costs associated with drug-impaired worker performance. These procedures and programs apply to employers with federal contracts and all federal grantees, and are described as follows.

Development of clear, drug-free workplace policies that state expectations of behavior, employee rights and responsibilities, and actions to be taken in response to employees found to be using illegal drugs.

Establishment of a comprehensive and continuing drug education and

awareness program covering the elements of the drug-free workplace program, the signs and symptoms of drug use, and the services available to help users.

Introduction of a detection program to help supervisors recognize and address alcohol and other drug use by employees, and to deter and discover the use of alcohol and other drugs through drug testing.

Implementation of employee assistance programs or other appropriate mechanisms that will enable those in violation of established policies to be evaluated prior to proper treatment and/or rehabilitation.

Reporting to the federal government any convictions stemming from drug crimes committed in the workplace.

Although neither testing nor treatment is required by the federal act, many businesses and agencies, as well as the private sector (in response to executive order, not law) have added several supplements to the federal initiative. In an attempt to demonstrate "good-faith effort" in maintaining a drug-free workplace, some companies now use random drug testing of employees' urine specimens to detect or screen for substance use and abuse in the workforce. Other supplemental measures involve observation of telltale signs of drug abuse, use of undercover agents and surveillance videocameras to detect drug trafficking operations on company property, and searches of employees and their possessions to locate illegal drugs and to discourage the use of drugs during work.

Drug Testing in the Workplace

Over the past several years, **drug testing** has become one of the most effective techniques in promoting a drug-free workplace in America. The procedure has also become controversial because drug testing has evolved into a major civil rights issue, complicated by numerous grievances, complaints, and law suits.

The detection of drug use and abuse through random screening of urine specimens is now required for specific employees of the federal government, such as the executive branch, the Nuclear Regulatory Commission, the military services, and millions of workers in safety-related jobs with the Department of Transportation, as well as railroad employees, airline pilots, flight attendants, and mechanics. In addition, many Fortune 500 companies—major corporations, manufacturers, public utilities, and transportation services—conduct drug screening by urinalysis during preemployment physicals. And, of course, random testing of college athletes is now mandated by the National Collegiate Athletic Association.

Types of Drug-Testing Programs

Several types of drug-testing programs are currently available in the United States.[18]

- Random and comprehensive testing of employees in sensitive positions

- Voluntary testing of any employee or appointee who wishes to participate in the drug-testing program

- Reasonable suspicion testing (based on specific and particular facts and reasonable inferences from those facts)

- Special condition testing (as part of an examination following an accident or unsafe practice)

- Follow-up testing (administered by an agency or company during or after counseling or rehabilitation through an employee assistance program)

- Testing applicants for any position or appointment

In American businesses regulated by the U.S. Department of Transportation, five types of testing are generally required, including, preemployment, periodic as part of required medical examinations, random, reasonable suspicion, and postaccident. However, most private companies with drug-testing programs utilize only the following three options:

1. *Reasonable suspicion testing.* Employers may require urinalysis in "for cause" testing of a particular employee who has been identified by observation, absenteeism, health problems, accidents, or any other means as having job-related problems possibly associated with substance abuse. With positive urine results, employees may either receive disciplinary action or be referred to an employee assistance program for counseling, referral, and treatment.

2. *Random testing.* Most effective in early detection and in its deterrent effect on drug usage, random testing requires all employees to submit to urine tests routinely, every six months or on an annual basis.

3. *Applicant testing.* Employers might use a urine test to screen all new job applicants. Those who test positive for drug usage might be refused employment, cautioned that the positive test will limit their eligibility for certain positions, or referred for evaluation and possibly treatment.

Large-scale drug testing is conducted on urine samples as a first test or screening technique for chemical substances such as marijuana and cocaine. Most frequently, the tests also check for heroin and other opioids, amphetamines, phencyclidine (PCP), barbiturates, methaqualone, methadone, and certain minor tranquilizers. Urine is used as a test specimen because it is a normal product of the body, is readily available, and is easily collected in a relatively nonintrusive manner, although the use of urine as the test medium imposes practical limitations on the frequency of collection.

Urinalysis Testing

Two common urine-testing procedures used for initial screening are these:[19,20]

- *Immunoassay tests,* specifically the *enzyme multiplier immunoassay test* (EMIT), used most often in industry, and the *radioactivity immunoassay* (RIA) favored by the military. Both procedures use drug-specific antibodies to distinguish positive and negative samples. These tests are relatively fast, inexpensive, and very sensitive for most drugs.

- *Thin-layer chromatography* (TLC) identifies drugs by color retention, distance of travel over a coated glass plate or plastic film, and appearance under ultraviolet light. This particular test is somewhat less sensitive than EMIT.

If a urine specimen tests positive, then a *confirmatory test* will be performed using the *gas chromatography/mass spectrometry* (GC/MS) *technique* as the method of choice. More complicated, more time-consuming, and much more expensive than other tests, GC/MS is the most accurate, sensitive, and reliable method of urine testing. This procedure detects specific drug classes as well as drug metabolites based on molecular structure following separation with a GC absorbent material.

It is significant that urine testing for psychoactive drugs merely differentiates between people who have exposed themselves to the drugs being tested and those who have not. Thus, results of such testing give no indication of the pattern of drug use, whether the user abuses or is dependent upon a drug, or whether an individual is impaired physically or mentally by the drug at the time the sample is taken. (An exception to this general limitation is testing for urinary ethyl alcohol, whose concentration can be correlated with blood-alcohol content, from which degrees of impairment can be determined. But ethyl alcohol is not frequently checked for in urinalysis because it is oxidized within a relatively short time after consumption. Thus, even chronic alcoholics could pass a urine test if they refrained from alcohol for twelve hours prior to the test.)

Drugs other than ethyl alcohol tend to leave the body more slowly (see box 13.9). Depending on the sensitivity of the test, unique characteristics of the particular drug, and the drug taker's own metabolism, some drugs, such as cocaine, codeine, and Valium can be detected for a period of 1 to 3 days. Heroin, amphetamines, and phencyclidine can usually be identified for as long as 2 to 4 days after use, and barbiturates can be detected for up to 14 days. Thus, an individual who uses one of these drugs on the weekend could test positive at work on Monday or Tuesday.

Marijuana metabolites (breakdown products of marijuana's active ingredient) may be detected in urine for up to 10 days after a single smoking session. However, marijuana metabolites, which are stored in the body's fatty tissues, can sometimes be detected for up to three weeks after a heavy chronic smoker (several marijuana cigarettes per day) has stopped smoking.

Common Concerns with Urine Testing

Although drug testing by urinalysis is used increasingly by federal, state, and local governments, and by businesses and industries, many social and legal questions have arisen. For instance, to maintain the integrity of specimen collection, a supervisor should watch the testee urinate to prevent substitution of another's urine, contamination, or dilution of the specimen. The collection procedure may indeed violate the individual's right of privacy. On the other

At Issue

Is drug testing in the workplace an appropriate weapon in the "war on drugs"?

Point: Absolutely not! Except in certain occupations that directly influence public safety or national security, drug testing is a violation of a worker's rights. Requiring individuals to urinate in the presence of supervising observers in order to get a job or keep a job is a gross invasion of privacy and a human indignity. Moreover, such a requirement often reflects a class and/or racial bias as it rarely affects management personnel, especially those who make or enforce such a regulation. However, there are important legal questions that have not been resolved. The Fourth Amendment to the U.S. Constitution guarantees individual freedom from unreasonable searches and seizures. Without probable cause for the test, it is difficult to describe drug testing as legal or constitutional. Furthermore, because drug testing is expensive, not reliable, often produces false results, and is frequently applied without relationship to job impairment, the testing procedures appear to violate the Constitution's Fifth Amendment, which assures due process and freedom from self-incrimination.

Counterpoint: Because there is now a consensus that drug problems threaten the nation's well-being, drug testing in the workplace, military, and even schools and colleges is justified, even at the expense of reduced personal freedom. We do not live in utopia! Drug testing is not a Constitutional issue; it is a public safety, management, and education issue. We need to deter illegal drug use, and drug testing is the best available weapon in the "war on drugs." In some instances, drug testing may be the last line of defense in combating the epidemic of drug abuse. Whether the person is an airline pilot, a production worker, or a professional or collegiate athlete, a drug-abusing employee or player costs money, threatens productivity, and endangers good business management. We simply cannot tolerate the expenses associated with drug abuse in the workplace.

hand, is not the assurance of public safety more important than maintaining one's privacy?

Despite claims of high rates of accuracy and reliability, initial urine tests are somewhat fallible, with demonstrated error ranges of 0 to 100 percent. Laboratory and testing errors can contribute to *false positive results* (erroneous indications that at least one drug is present) and *false negatives* (inaccurate indications that a drug is absent from the urine specimen). Therefore, a confirmatory test is always necessary when the initial screening test is positive.

False positive results are sometimes related to other substances in the urine.[21] For instance, ibuprofen preparations (Advil, Motrin IB, Nuprin, Medipren, and

Rufen) can cause a false positive when a specimen is being tested for marijuana; drinking certain herbal teas can produce a false positive when testing for cocaine; and nonprescription stimulants (phenylpropanolamine and ephedrine) may test positive for amphetamine.

There are also several ways of producing false negative results, such as accidental or intentional switching of specimens, using diuretics, changing urine acidity/alkalinity chemically, and adding large amounts of salt to the specimen. Specimen switching has become a major enterprise generating a profitable black market for drug-free urine. To reduce such manipulation and contamination, most test subjects are observed during collection of specimens.

The Length of Time Drugs can be Detected in Urine Varies by Drug

box 13.9

Type of Drug	Average Time Detectable After Ingestion*
Cocaine	
(metabolite)	2–3 days
Cannabinoids (marijuana)	
Single use	3 days
Moderate use (4 times per week)	5 days
Heavy use (daily smoking)	10 days
Chronic heavy use	21–27 days
Opiates (including heroin, morphine, codeine)	48 hours
Phencyclidine (PCP)	About 8 days
Amphetamines & methamphetamines	48 hours
Benzodiazepines (including Valium, Librium)	
Therapeutic dose	3 days
Barbiturates	
Short-acting (including secobarbital)	24 hours
Intermediate-acting	48–72 hours
Long-acting (including phenobarbital)	7 days or more
Propoxyphene (including Darvon)	
Unchanged	6 hours
Metabolite	6–48 hours

*Interpretation of the time detectable must take into account many variables such as drug metabolism and half-life, subject's physical condition, fluid balance and state of hydration, route and frequency of ingestion, and testing technique and cutoff level used. These are general guidelines only.

Source: Office of Justice Programs, Bureau of Justice Statistics, U.S. Department of Justice.

While urine screening is good at identifying most drug users, the procedure does so only at the cost of falsely implicating at least some nonusers. Since the tests show only drug use and not necessarily abuse, many workers are opposed on the grounds that this may lead to further invasion of one's privacy while not at the worksite. Some management opposition has also developed regarding the relatively high cost of drug testing for large numbers of employees and because of the likelihood of prolonged challenges to the tests in courts of law.

Alternatives to Urine Testing

Some of the objections to urine tests may be resolved when hair analysis is approved as a means of drug testing.[22] With a radioimmunoassay process, strands of hair can be tested for cocaine, heroin, marijuana, methaqualone, and phencyclidine. Because human hair gives a history of drug use, hair samples can differentiate between recreational and chronic use and can reveal what drug was in the body in what amount, how often, and at what time. However, the use of radioimmunoassay hair analysis to detect illegal drugs is not yet scientifically supported by forensic toxicologists.

Nevertheless, hair has several advantages over urine testing for drugs of abuse:

Hair analysis expands the "time window" for the detection of an illicit drug up to several months or more, depending on the length of the hair.

Brief periods of abstinence from drugs will not significantly change the outcome of hair analysis.

Hair is relatively inert and easy to handle, and it requires no special storage facilities or conditions. Compared with urine samples, hair presents fewer risks of disease transmission.

Having some hair snipped from the head is less invasive and embarrassing for most people than supplying a monitored urine specimen.

Collecting comparable samples for repeat testing is easier with hair than with urine.

Contaminating or altering a sample to distort or manipulate test results is much more difficult with hair than with urine.

Another method of drug testing that is difficult to subvert is FACTOR 1000, a computer-based test that measures hand-eye coordination and reaction time. This method will also measure other non-drug related impairments such as fatigue and failure to concentrate. Another potential alternative to urine testing may evolve with the hoped-for perfection of brain scan equipment that will check for drug effects—brain waves called drug-evoked potentials that correlate specific brain-wave patterns with specific chemicals.

Employee Assistance Programs

Employee assistance programs (EAPs) are formal employer-financed programs administered by a company or through an outside contractor.[23] An EAP is designed to help in the identification and resolution of productivity problems associated with employees impaired by personal concerns, which might include health, marital, family, financial, alcohol and other drugs, or stress.

There are now more than 300,000 EAPs in the United States. Originating as a special resource for employees, they attempt to maintain and improve the health of a company's workers while minimizing the negative impact of problematic behavior, such as alcohol and other drug abuse, on worker productivity and employers' profits. In countering ATOD users, EAPs have concentrated on detection, counseling, and referral to treatment programs. Several interrelated functions are emphasized, including identification of impaired employee performance due to alcohol and other drug abuse; confrontation of the employee by a supervisor; referral for treatment; restoration of job productivity through the rehabilitation process; and follow-up procedures to assure continued worker effectiveness in the workplace. Such efforts are an example of secondary prevention activities.

More recently, EAPs have been expanded to combat employee abuse of prescription and OTC drugs as well as illicit psychoactive substances. Other areas of concern are also considered, including marital and family crises, money management and financial difficulties, and health problems other than alcohol and drug abuse, all of which can have unfavorable consequences on the well-being of workers and managers, too.

Usually, the stated purpose of most EAPs has been to reduce problems associated with impaired job performance. However, helping employees to achieve personal, social, and professional growth on the job is becoming an important secondary and concurrent goal of such programs. Model programs of health promotion that not only help prevent or postpone disease but also enhance wellness are now being implemented in both large companies and small businesses.

An essential component of many EAPs are various *health-promotion activities* that promote employee wellness and contribute to worker productivity, increased self-esteem, and reduction of stress generated in certain jobs. Health-promotion activities include

1. *environmental reform:* efforts to improve the mental health of employees through better working conditions, such as less stressful management styles and work-area restructuring;

2. *dissemination of health information:* use of posters, mailings, and presentations on various health-promotion and disease-prevention activities related to therapeutic and recreational drugs, nutrition, mental health, family living, communicable and noncommunicable diseases, and personal health status;

3. *voluntary lifestyle changes:* company-sponsored projects that bring about smoking cessation, stress management, improved physical fitness, and weight reduction among employees;

4. *risk identification:* use of health-screening laboratory tests, risk appraisal, and physical examinations to identify potential physical and mental problems before symptoms appear and referral to treatment and rehabilitation are needed; and

5. *high-risk intervention:* detection, intervention, and referral options associated with the secondary level of prevention. Individuals identified with various health problems—such as diabetes, hypertension, or substance abuse—are referred for treatment, rehabilitation, and eventual return to the workplace.

Alcohol-, tobacco-, and other drug-free workplace policies and procedures, employee assistance programs, employee and family education, worksite wellness programs, and changes in workplace culture and norms effectively reduce costs to the employer. According to the Center for Substance Abuse Prevention,

- For every dollar employers invest in EAPs, they can save $5 to $16.

- Workplaces free of alcohol, tobacco, and other drugs have a competitive edge in maintaining productivity and quality, improving employee health, and reducing medical claims and absenteeism.[24]

Drug Law Enforcement

A major part of society's response to drug abuse is expressed in the numerous laws and governmental programs intended to reduce the availability of illegal drugs to the general public and to penalize the promoters of such drugs. Sometimes, even the victims of drug abuse have been punished for their social offenses. Drug laws and their enforcement are now considered important parts of any drug-abuse prevention program. The many laws are intended to reduce drug supplies and deter consumption, and although their enforcement is sometimes imperfect, they are nevertheless an example of primary prevention activities (see fig. 13.4).

Efforts to control illegal drug sales and use are conducted by federal, state, and local agencies. Increasingly, these different levels of government join forces in a coordinated system and work together smoothly. On occasion, however, they still act independently, jealously guarding both resources and sources from one another.

Routine Enforcement Techniques

Local, state, and federal agents use a variety of **enforcement techniques** in their prevention activities against illicit drug use.[25] The following are among those frequently employed.

> *Informants*—using a second party, sometimes a paid "underworld" figure, who becomes the eyes and ears of the drug enforcement officer, develops contacts, and obtains information that otherwise would be inaccessible to the investigating officer.

Surveillance—secret and usually continuous watching of suspected individuals, vehicles, places, or objects in order to obtain information about criminal activities.

Undercover operations—investigations conducted by a law officer who uses various identities, disguises, or pretexts to gain the confidence of criminal suspects. This technique is especially hazardous and time consuming, and it is undertaken to determine the nature and extent of any criminal action in which the suspects may be involved.

Drug raids—searches of specific places, based upon "probable cause," that is, the reasonable belief that a criminal offense is being committed and that evidence of illegal drugs can be found in a particular location.

Interdiction—confiscating illicit drugs at national borders or ports of entry or seizing contraband at sea to prevent them from entering the United States.

Intelligence gathering—acquiring and organizing information in a systematic way that would lead to better enforcement of laws.

In addition, there is the process of "carding," with which many college students are familiar. Carding is a technique in which local or state-level police officials inspect the identification cards of young-looking individuals who are present in a tavern. Such on-the-spot checking of IDs is an attempt to prevent underage individuals from buying and/or drinking alcoholic beverages in a public place.

Federal Law Enforcement Agencies

In order to implement a national drug control strategy as detailed in box 13.10, numerous cabinet departments, departmental agencies, and special action organizations at the federal level have been assigned various responsibilities for drug-abuse prevention. Currently, the principal agency for drug law enforcement, including drug trafficking, investigation, drug

intelligence, and regulatory control, is the **Drug Enforcement Administration (DEA).** However, the Federal Bureau of Investigation (FBI) recently has been assigned concurrent jurisdiction with the DEA to investigate drug offenses. This new expansion in the war on drugs has improved greatly the resources and personnel now available for drug enforcement activities. Both the DEA and the FBI are administered within the Department of Justice.

In addition to setting standards for quality and content in alcoholic beverages and establishing and collecting taxes on the production of beverage alcohol, the Bureau of Alcohol, Tobacco, and Firearms (BATF) pursues major drug violators who use or traffic in firearms to support and protect illegal drug activities. Established together with the BATF under the Department of the Treasury are two other agencies that contribute to the drug-abuse control efforts of the federal government: (1) the Internal Revenue Service (IRS), which gathers intelligence and conducts investigations dealing with the tremendous untaxed profits generated by the illegal drug traffic industry; and (2) the U.S. Customs Service, which conducts financial investigations directed at drug-smuggling organizations, border-control measures, and air interdiction of illicit drugs. Within the Justice Department, the Immigration and Naturalization Service now conducts advanced investigations of drug trafficking when focusing on other criminal activity associated with its regularly assigned functions.

Reversing a 100-year ban that had prohibited military intervention in civilian affairs, Congress recently passed legislation allowing the use of available military resources in providing information and equipment support to civilian law-enforcement agencies. This action has the potential for improving significantly the federal attack on drug smuggling and enhancing the effectiveness of the U.S. Coast Guard, the U.S. Customs Service, and the U.S. Border Patrol. At-sea interdictions by the U.S. Navy will also help implement the federal war against drugs.

Federal Control Mechanisms

The legal foundation for federal efforts in reducing the consumption of illicit drugs is the

Comprehensive Drug Abuse Prevention and Control Act of 1970 and its more recent amendments, including the Anti-Drug Abuse Acts of 1986 and 1988. The major control mechanisms imposed on the manufacture, purchase, and distribution of controlled substances, as specified in the **Controlled Substances Act** (CSA), are described below and summarized in table 13.1.[26]

Registration of handlers of controlled substances, as conducted by the Drug Enforcement Administration. This registration procedure reduces the opportunity for unauthorized transactions of controlled substances.

Record keeping of all quantities of controlled substances manufactured, purchased, and sold, and inventories of these drugs by each handler. From such records it is possible to trace the flow of any controlled drug, from the time it is imported or manufactured, through the entire wholesale level to the hospital or pharmacy that dispensed it, and then to the patient. Such record keeping tends to discourage the diversion of drugs from legitimate channels of distribution and serves to reinforce the registration requirement.

Quotas on manufacturing limits on the quantity of controlled substances in Schedules I and II, as established by the DEA. These yearly quotas help reduce the availability of such drugs.

Distribution controls involve required recording of the movements of Schedule I and II drugs from the manufacturer to wholesaler to dispenser. A reinforcement of the registration requirement, this distribution control procedure makes certain that only authorized individuals may obtain Schedule I and II controlled substances with the filing of specific order forms.

Dispensing control mechanisms govern the delivery of a controlled drug to the ultimate user, either patient or research subject. Dispensing limits vary according to five schedules, as described in box 1.3 and in chapter 12, and include the requirement of a prescription order, specification of giving prescription orders by either written or verbal format, restriction of the refilling of psychoactive drugs, and maintenance of a minimum age level and patient identification procedure.

International import and export controls are placed on transactions involving

Major Federal legislation and international conventions

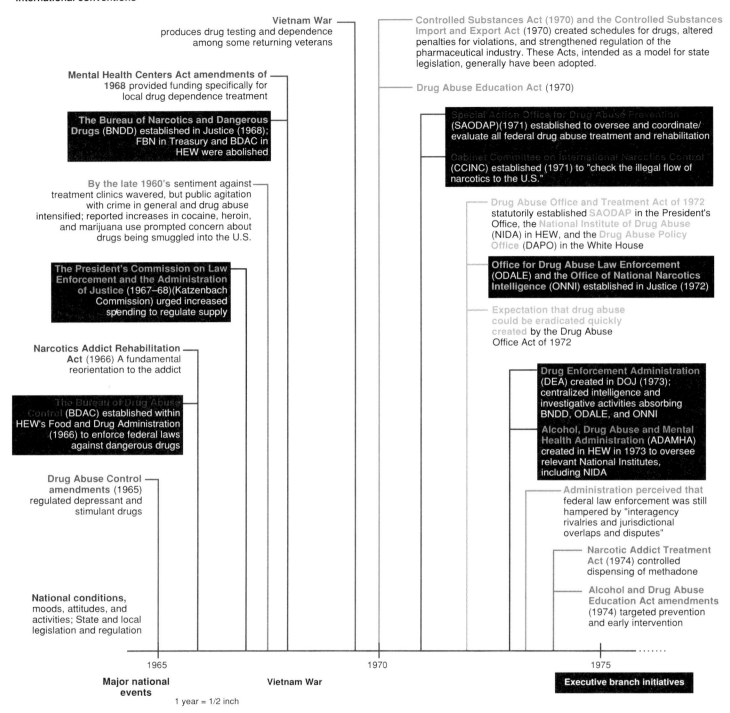

Vietnam War produces drug testing and dependence among some returning veterans

Controlled Substances Act (1970) and the **Controlled Substances Import and Export Act** (1970) created schedules for drugs, altered penalties for violations, and strengthened regulation of the pharmaceutical industry. These Acts, intended as a model for state legislation, generally have been adopted.

Mental Health Centers Act amendments of 1968 provided funding specifically for local drug dependence treatment

Drug Abuse Education Act (1970)

The Bureau of Narcotics and Dangerous Drugs (BNDD) established in Justice (1968); FBN in Treasury and BDAC in HEW were abolished

Special Action Office for Drug Abuse Prevention (SAODAP)(1971) established to oversee and coordinate/ evaluate all federal drug abuse treatment and rehabilitation

Cabinet Committee on International Narcotics Control (CCINC) established (1971) to "check the illegal flow of narcotics to the U.S."

By the late 1960's sentiment against treatment clinics wavered, but public agitation with crime in general and drug abuse intensified; reported increases in cocaine, heroin, and marijuana use prompted concern about drugs being smuggled into the U.S.

Drug Abuse Office and Treatment Act of 1972 statutorily established SAODAP in the President's Office, the National Institute of Drug Abuse (NIDA) in HEW, and the Drug Abuse Policy Office (DAPO) in the White House

The President's Commission on Law Enforcement and the Administration of Justice (1967–68)(Katzenbach Commission) urged increased spending to regulate supply

Office for Drug Abuse Law Enforcement (ODALE) and the Office of National Narcotics Intelligence (ONNI) established in Justice (1972)

Expectation that drug abuse could be eradicated quickly created by the Drug Abuse Office Act of 1972

Narcotics Addict Rehabilitation Act (1966) A fundamental reorientation to the addict

Drug Enforcement Administration (DEA) created in DOJ (1973); centralized intelligence and investigative activities absorbing BNDD, ODALE, and ONNI

The Bureau of Drug Abuse Control (BDAC) established within HEW's Food and Drug Administration (1966) to enforce federal laws against dangerous drugs

Alcohol, Drug Abuse and Mental Health Administration (ADAMHA) created in HEW in 1973 to oversee relevant National Institutes, including NIDA

Drug Abuse Control amendments (1965) regulated depressant and stimulant drugs

Administration perceived that federal law enforcement was still hampered by "interagency rivalries and jurisdictional overlaps and disputes"

Narcotic Addict Treatment Act (1974) controlled dispensing of methadone

National conditions, moods, attitudes, and activities; State and local legislation and regulation

Alcohol and Drug Abuse Education Act amendments (1974) targeted prevention and early intervention

1965   1970   1975

Major national events   Vietnam War   **Executive branch initiatives**

1 year = 1/2 inch

figure **13.4**

Over the past 30 years, the executive and legislative branches of the federal government have sought to control both the supply of and demand for drugs.

Source: Office of Justice Programs, Bureau of Justice Statistics, U.S. Department of Justice.

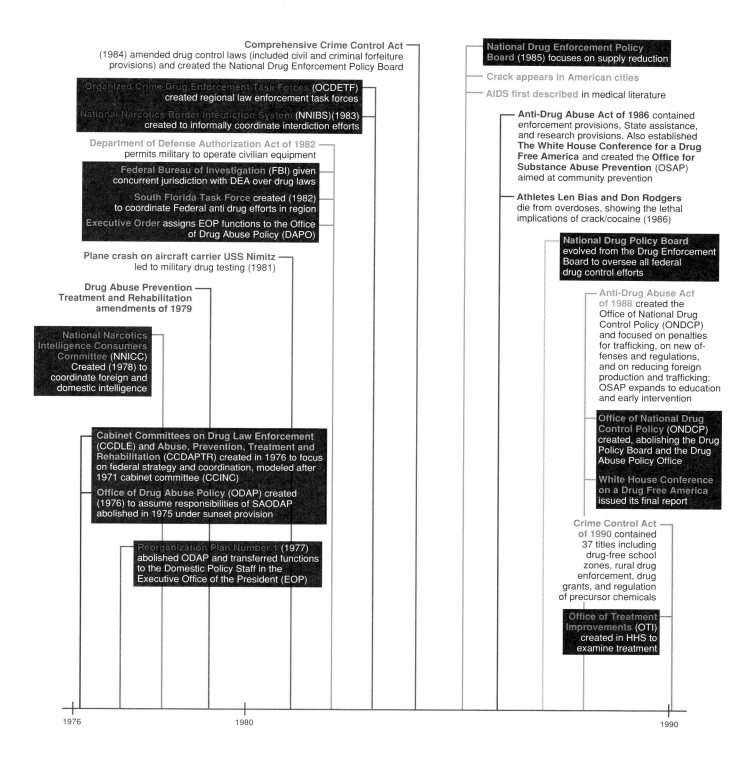

Comprehensive Crime Control Act —
(1984) amended drug control laws (included civil and criminal forfeiture
provisions) and created the National Drug Enforcement Policy Board

National Drug Enforcement Policy
Board (1985) focuses on supply reduction

Crack appears in American cities

AIDS first described in medical literature

Organized Crime Drug Enforcement Task Forces (OCDETF)
created regional law enforcement task forces

National Narcotics Border Interdiction System (NNIBS)(1983)
created to informally coordinate interdiction efforts

Department of Defense Authorization Act of 1982
permits military to operate civilian equipment

Federal Bureau of Investigation (FBI) given
concurrent jurisdiction with DEA over drug laws

South Florida Task Force created (1982)
to coordinate Federal anti drug efforts in region

Executive Order assigns EOP functions to the Office
of Drug Abuse Policy (DAPO)

Anti-Drug Abuse Act of 1986 contained
enforcement provisions, State assistance,
and research provisions. Also established
The White House Conference for a Drug
Free America and created the Office for
Substance Abuse Prevention (OSAP)
aimed at community prevention

Athletes Len Bias and Don Rodgers
die from overdoses, showing the lethal
implications of crack/cocaine (1986)

National Drug Policy Board
evolved from the Drug Enforcement
Board to oversee all federal
drug control efforts

Plane crash on aircraft carrier USS Nimitz —
led to military drug testing (1981)

Drug Abuse Prevention —
Treatment and Rehabilitation
amendments of 1979

National Narcotics
Intelligence Consumers
Committee (NNICC)
Created (1978) to
coordinate foreign and
domestic intelligence

Anti-Drug Abuse Act
of 1988 created the
Office of National Drug
Control Policy (ONDCP)
and focused on penalties
for trafficking, on new offenses and regulations,
and on reducing foreign
production and trafficking;
OSAP expands to education
and early intervention

Office of National Drug
Control Policy (ONDCP)
created, abolishing the Drug
Policy Board and the Drug
Abuse Policy Office

White House Conference
on a Drug Free America
issued its final report

Cabinet Committees on Drug Law Enforcement
(CCDLE) and Abuse, Prevention, Treatment and
Rehabilitation (CCDAPTR) created in 1976 to focus
on federal strategy and coordination, modeled after
1971 cabinet committee (CCINC)

Office of Drug Abuse Policy (ODAP) created
(1976) to assume responsibilities of SAODAP
abolished in 1975 under sunset provision

Crime Control Act —
of 1990 contained
37 titles including
drug-free school
zones, rural drug
enforcement, drug
grants, and regulation
of precursor chemicals

Reorganization Plan Number 1 (1977)
abolished ODAP and transferred functions
to the Domestic Policy Staff in the
Executive Office of the President (EOP)

Office of Treatment
Improvements (OTI)
created in HHS to
examine treatment

1976   1980   1990

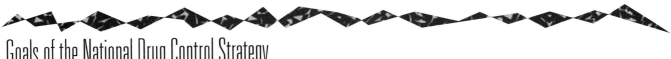

Goals of the National Drug Control Strategy

box 13.10

The National Drug Control Strategy has one overarching goal—the reduction of drug use. However, the major focus of the current strategy is on the most difficult and problematic drug-using population—hardcore drug users. In its implementation, the national strategy is a coordinated combination of both supply and demand reduction activities.

Goal 1: Reduce the number of drug users in America.

Goal 2: Expand treatment capacity and services and increase treatment effectiveness so that those who need treatment can receive it. Target intensive treatment services for hardcore drug-using populations and special populations, including adults and adolescents in custody or under the supervision of the criminal justice system, pregnant women, and women with dependent children.

Goal 3: Reduce the burden on the health care system by reducing the spread of infectious disease related to drug use.

Goal 4: Assist local communities in developing effective prevention programs.

Goal 5: Create safe and healthy environments in which children and adolescents can live, grow, learn, and develop.

Goal 6: Reduce the use of alcohol and tobacco products among underage youth.

Goal 7: Increase workplace safety and productivity by reducing drug use in the workplace.

Goal 8: Strengthen linkages among the prevention, treatment, and criminal justice communities and other supportive social services, such as employment and training services.

Goal 9: Reduce domestic drug-related crime and violence.

Goal 10: Reduce all domestic drug production and availability, and continue to target for investigation and prosecution those who illegally import, manufacture, and distribute dangerous drugs and who illegally divert pharmaceuticals and listed chemicals.

Goal 11: Improve the efficiency of federal drug law enforcement capabilities, including interdiction and intelligence programs.

Goal 12: Strengthen international cooperation against narcotics production, trafficking, and use.

Goal 13: Assist other nations to develop and implement comprehensive counternarcotics policies that strengthen democratic institutions, destroy narcotrafficking organizations, and interdict narcotrafficking in both the source and transit countries.

Goal 14: Support, implement, and lead more successful enforcement efforts to increase the costs and risks to narcotics producers and traffickers to reduce the supply of illicit drugs to the United States.

Source: From *National Drug Control Strategy: Reclaiming Our Communities from Drugs and Violence*, Office of National Drug Control Strategy, 1994.

Drug raids or "busts" are routine enforcement techniques in which searches uncover varying amounts of illegal drugs. Here a police official inventories a large amount of heroin, cocaine, and "drug money" seized in a raid in Chicago.

© *Mark Reinstein/Uniphoto Picture Agency*

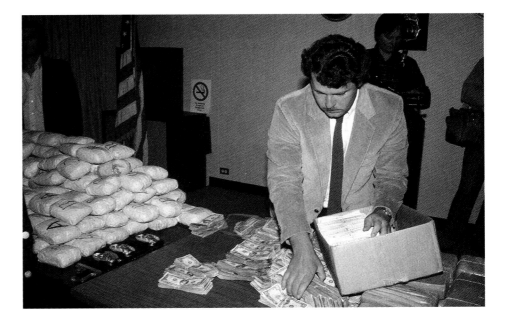

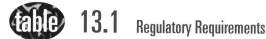

table 13.1 Regulatory Requirements

Controlled Substances	Schedule I	Schedule II	Schedule III	Schedule IV	Schedule V
Registration	required	required	required	required	required
Recordkeeping	separate	separate	readily retrievable	readily retrievable	readily retrievable
Distribution Restrictions	order forms	order forms	records required	records required	records required
Dispensing Limits	research use only	Rx: written; no refills	Rx: written or oral; refills[a]	Rx: written or oral; refills[a]	OTC (Rx drugs limited to M.D.'s order)
Manufacturing Security	vault/safe	vault/safe	secure storage area	secure storage area	secure storage area
Manufacturing Quotas	yes	yes	NO but some drugs limited by Schedule II	NO but some drugs limited by Schedule II	NO but some drugs limited by Schedule II
Import/Export *Narcotic*	permit	permit	permit	permit	permit to import; declaration to export
Import/Export *Nonnarcotic*	permit	permit	[b]	declaration	declaration
Reports to DEA by Manufacturer/ Distributor *Narcotic*	yes	yes	yes	manufacturer only	manufacturer only
Reports to DEA by Manufacturer/ Distributor *Nonnarcotic*	yes	yes	[c]	[c]	no

[a]With medical authorization, refills up to 5 in 6 months
[b]Permit for some drugs, declaration for others
[c]Manufacturer reports required for specific drugs

Source: U. S. Drug Enforcement Administration.

any Schedule I or II drugs or a narcotic drug in Schedule III. Such transactions must have the prior approval of the DEA before they are made. International transactions involving a nonnarcotic in Schedule III or any drug in Schedules IV or V must be made with prior notice or declaration (but not approval) to the DEA. Such controls limit the availability of domestic drugs and prevent exported drugs from reexportation from the original country of destination.

Security for storage of drugs is governed by rules of the DEA. High-security requirements (including vaults, alarm systems, and assigned security guards) are imposed for storage and apply to manufacturers, importers, exporters, and wholesalers of controlled drugs. Reduced security arrangements are imposed on researchers, physicians, pharmacies, and hospitals, corresponding to their smaller quantities of stored drugs.

Reports to the DEA regarding transactions in certain controlled drugs must be made on a periodic basis, and annual inventories must be filed with the same agency. The monitoring of all drugs in Schedules I and II and narcotics in Schedule III is carried out by the Automation of Reports and Consolidated Orders System (ARCOS). Manufacturers, wholesalers, importers, and exporters of any of these drugs must report all production activities, importations, exportations, and other distributions to the DEA.

Criminal penalties for trafficking are the most common and well-known control mechanisms. **Trafficking** is the unauthorized manufacture, distribution (delivery whether by sale, gift, or otherwise), or possession with intent to distribute any controlled substance. As noted in tables 13.2 and 13.3, the stiffer sanctions imposed by the Anti-Drug Abuse Act of 1986 (Narcotics Penalties and Enforcement Act) vary according to the CSA schedule, the weight of a mixture or substance containing a detectable amount of a CSA Schedule I or II controlled drug, whether the penalty is for a first or subsequent trafficking offense, and whether the defendant is an individual, a company, or a business association. In the latter instance, the fine imposed for "other

table 13.2 Federal Trafficking Penalties

CSA	PENALTY		Quantity	DRUG	Quantity	PENALTY	
	2nd Offense	1st Offense				1st Offense	2nd Offense
I and II	Not less than 10 years. Not more than life. If death or serious injury, not less than life. Fine of not more than $4 million individual, $10 million other than individual.	Not less than 5 years. Not more than 40 years. If death or serious injury, not less than 20 years. Not more than life. Fine of not more than $2 million individual, $5 million other than individual.	10–99 gm or 100 999 gm – mixture	METHAM-PHETAMINE	100 gm or more or 1 kg[a] or more mixture	Not less than 10 years. Not more than life. If death or serious injury, not less than 20 years. Not more than life. Fine of not more than $4 million individual, $10 million other than individual.	Not less than 20 years. Not more than life. If death or serious injury, not less than life. Fine of not more than $8 million individual, $20 million other than individual.
			100–999 gm mixture	HEROIN	1 kg or more mixture		
			500–4,999 gm mixture	COCAINE	5 kg or more mixture		
			5–49 gm mixture	COCAINE BASE	50 gm or more mixture		
			10–99 gm or 100–999 gm mixture	PCP	100 gm or more or 1 kg or more mixture		
			1–10 gm mixture	LSD	10 gm or more mixture		
			40–399 gm mixture	FENTANYL	400 gm or more mixture		
			10–99 gm mixture	FENTANYL ANALOGUE	100 gm or more mixture		

	Drug	Quantity	First Offense	Second Offense	
	Others[b]	Any	Not more than 20 years. If death or serious injury, not less than 20 years, not more than life. Fine $1 million individual, $5 million not individual.	Not more than 30 years. If death or serious injury, life. Fine $2 million individual, $10 million not individual.	
III	All	Any	Not more than 5 years. Fine not more than $250,000 individual, $1 million not individual.	Not more than 10 years. Fine not more than $500,000 individual, $2 million not individual.	
IV	All	Any	Not more than 3 years. Fine not more than $250,000 individual, $1 million not individual.	Not more than 6 years. Fine not more than $500,000 individual, $2 million not individual.	
V	All	Any	Not more than 1 year. Fine not more than $100,000 individual, $250,000 not individual.	Not more than 2 years. Fine not more than $200,000 individual, $500,000 not individual.	

[a] Law as originally enacted states 100 gm. Congress requested to make technical correction to 1 kg.

[b] Does not include marijuana, hashish, or hash oil.

Source: U. S. Drug Enforcement Administration.

table 13.3 Federal Trafficking Penalties—Marijuana

Quantity	Description	First Offense	Second Offense
1,000 kg or more; or 1,000 or more plants	Marijuana Mixture containing detectable quantity[a]	Not less than 10 years, not more than life. If death or serious injury, not less than 20 years, not more than life. Fine not more than $4 million individual, $10 million other than individual.	Not less than 20 years, not more than life. If death or serious injury, not less than life. Fine not more than $8 million individual, $20 million other than individual.
100 kg to 1,000 kg; or 100–999 plants	Marijuana Mixture containing detectable quantity[a]	Not less than 5 years, not more than 40 years. If death or serious injury, not less than 20 years, not more than life. Fine not more than $2 million individual, $5 million other than individual.	Not less than 10 years, not more than life. If death or serious injury, not less than life. Fine not more than $4 million individual, $10 million other than individual.
50 to 100 kg	Marijuana	Not more than 20 years. If death or serious injury, not less than 20 years, not more than life. Fine $1 million individual, $5 million other than individual.	Not more than 30 years. If death or serious injury, life. Fine $2 million individual, $10 million other than individual
10 to 100 kg	Hashish		
1 to 100 kg	Hashish Oil		
50–99 plants	Marijuana		
Less than 50 kg	Marijuana	Not more than 5 years. Fine not more than $250,000, $1 million other than individual.	Not more than 10 years. Fine $500,000 individual, $2 million other than individual.
Less than 10 kg	Hashish		
Less than 1 kg	Hashish Oil		

Includes Hashish and Hashish Oil

(Marijuana is a Schedule I Controlled Substance)

Source: U. S. Drug Enforcement Administration.

than an individual" is generally two and one-half times greater than for an individual offender.

The penalties for a *trafficking offense* can be rather complex, and most severe. For instance, in a first-time violation of trafficking in 5 kilograms or more of a substance containing a detectable amount of cocaine (its salts, optical and geometric isomers, and salts of isomers), an individual shall be sentenced to a term of imprisonment that may not be less than 10 years or more than life. However, if death or serious bodily injury results from the use of such substance, the sentence shall be not less than 20 years imprisonment or more than life. A fine not to exceed $4 million if the defendant is an individual, or $10 million if the defendant is other than an individual, will be imposed. In addition, a term of supervised release of at least 5 years of probation, in addition to any imprisonment, shall be imposed.

Simple possession of any illegal, nonprescribed controlled substance in any of the CSA schedules for one's own use is a violation of law punishable on the first offense by a maximum of 1 year imprisonment, a fine of not less than $1,000 but not more than $5,000, or both. Second-time offenders shall be sentenced to a minimum of 15 days imprisonment with a maximum of up to 2 years, and a fine of not more than $10,000.

If a person is found guilty of a first-time violation of simple possession after trial or upon a plea of guilty, the court may, without entering a judgment of guilty, defer further proceedings and place such person on probation up to 1 year. After the probation period, the court may discharge the individual without court adjudication and dismiss proceedings against him or her. If the offender was not over 21 years of age at the time of the offense, he or she may apply to the court for a complete removal of all pertinent official records.

In addition to the general federal statutes that make it a crime to deal in and illegally possess a controlled substance, there are special laws designed to protect children and schools from illegal drugs, as noted below.[27]

Selling drugs within 1,000 feet of a public or private elementary or secondary school is punishable by up to double the sentence that would apply if the sale occurred elsewhere. More severe mandatory penalties apply for repeat offenders.

When anyone over 21 years of age sells drugs to anyone under 18 years of age, the seller runs the risk of receiving up to double the sentence that would ordinarily apply to a sale to an adult. And if any person knowingly provides or distributes a controlled substance or controlled substance analogue to any person under 18 years of age, or if the individual employed, hired, or used in drug trafficking is 14 years of age or younger, the offender is subject to a term of imprisonment for not more than 5 years or a fine of not more than $50,000 or both.

State Legal Control Mechanisms

Along with the federal statutes dealing with trafficking and possession of controlled substances, there are numerous laws enacted by cities and states restricting the use or availability of certain drugs. For instance, at the state level, departments of alcohol beverage control (ABCs) or liquor control boards regulate alcoholic beverages, usually by controlling production, distribution, marketing, hours of sale, and by taxation.

All states also established minimum legal drinking ages. Between 1970 and 1981, twenty-nine states lowered the drinking age, usually from 20 or 21 to 18 or 19 years, as part of a national trend lowering the age of majority.[28] However, emerging research evidence and changes in the political and social climate of the nation prompted many states to return to higher drinking ages.

Though somewhat controversial, many studies indicated that raising the drinking age was an effective countermeasure for reducing alcohol-related automobile crashes involving property damage, injuries, and fatalities among teenagers and young adults. Uniform state drinking ages would also stop underage individuals from crossing one state line in order to purchase beverage alcohol legally in an adjoining state where the drinking age was lower. This practice of crossing state lines to purchase alcohol legally often resulted in numerous drunken driving accidents as the intoxicated young people attempted to drive back home across their own state line. This situation, in turn, led to the creation of "blood borders" between states—state lines having a high incidence of alcohol-related accidents, injuries, and deaths. Nevertheless, in 1984 nearly half of the states still maintained drinking ages lower than 21.

Then, over the next three years, at the urging of Mothers Against Drunk Driving (MADD) and with the support of the president, the U.S. Congress passed legislation that would persuade individual states to raise their minimum drinking age to 21 years. Under provisions of this law, if states did not adopt the 21-years standard, they risked losing a certain percent of federal highway funds. This congressional action represented a federal inducement to the states to act against alcohol-impaired driving. Such legislation was eventually found to be constitutional by the U.S. Supreme Court, after several states challenged the law. By 1988, all states had adopted the 21-year-old drinking age. Whether the imposition of a nationwide minimum drinking age will have the desired effects and anticipated benefits remains to be seen, although total yearly deaths related to alcohol-impaired operation of motor vehicles have been declining for the past several years.

Another moderate approach to drug law enforcement pertains to people having reached the age of 18 years but who are still underage in terms of the minimum legal drinking age. Where such individuals are found in violation of the state's alcoholic beverage laws, police officers in some states may issue a summons or warning instead of making an arrest. The summons is similar to a traffic ticket. It permits the underaged person to avoid arrest, jail, and the embarrassment of a criminal record and a court appearance with parents. (A court appearance, however, is still necessary.) As a substitute for arrest, the summons is used typically when drinking is the only charge. Possession of other drugs, disorderly conduct, and driving under the influence of an intoxicating drug would still result in arrest. While perceived as a lenient approach to underage alcohol users, the summons procedure enables police officers to catch more underage drinkers.

States also have numerous laws restricting the possession, sale, cultivation, and manufacture of illegal psychoactive drugs, as well as furnishing such substances to minors. Sometimes the penalties are harsher than those for corresponding federal offenses. The penalties tend to vary from state to state and with the specific drug or class of drugs (marijuana, hashish, hash oil, heroin and cocaine, LSD, amphetamines and barbiturates, and peyote, mescaline, and psilocybin), the relative amount of drug possessed, and the relative amount of the drug intended for sale.

The Antiparaphernalia Movement

The rapid growth of illicit drug use in the nation has prompted many community groups to seek legislation at the state and municipal levels of government to control the availability of drug-related paraphernalia. (This is known as the **antiparaphernalia movement.**)

The term *paraphernalia* refers to those articles used in administering, preparing, packaging, and storing drugs. Although it can refer to equipment for legal or illegal administration of legal or illegal substances, the term *paraphernalia* has been used more often with products intended for use with recreational drugs, especially marijuana and cocaine. Some common paraphernalia items sold at retail outlets include smoking papers, rolling machines, roach clips, lighters and matches, pipe/bowl screens, bowl loaders, bongs and water pipes, stash cleaners and containers, isomerizers, spoons, straws, snorters, screens, adulterants, drying devices, conversion/purification kits, nasal irrigators, cultivation kits, crack kits, freebasing kits, and diluents and adulterants designed for use in "cutting" controlled substances.

Presently, nearly all states and the District of Columbia attempt to control the sale of drug paraphernalia under state law or local ordinances. In most cases, such legislation is based on a model act proposed by the Drug Enforcement Administration.[29] Various legal options are used in controlling paraphernalia sales, including

> Forbidding the use of U.S. Postal Service, or any other interstate conveyance, as part of a scheme to sell drug paraphernalia.
>
> Prohibiting the importation and exportation of drug paraphernalia.
>
> Zoning and licensing regulations barring sales of paraphernalia to minors, limiting the type of advertising and display of such items, and controlling where "head shops" (retail outlets) can be located.
>
> Advertising restrictions banning the printed advertisement of the sale of paraphernalia.
>
> Prohibiting sales, including the gift or delivery of drug paraphernalia to minors, or permitting sales to minors only when they are accompanied by a parent or legal guardian.

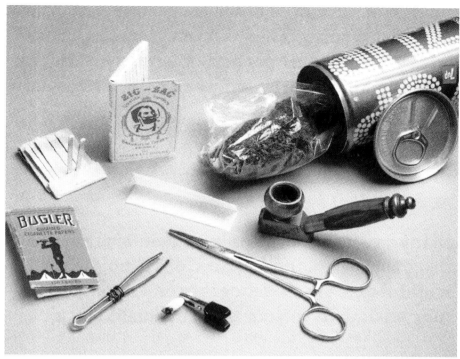

(a)

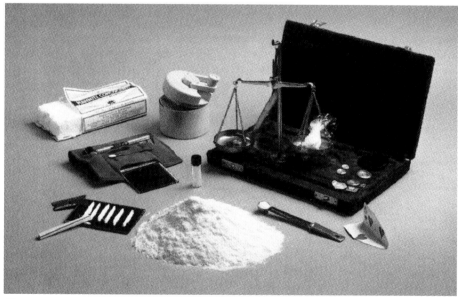

(b)

(a) Marijuana paraphernalia includes rolling papers, clips, and pipes. (b) Cocaine paraphernalia includes mirrors, razor blades, and scales used by drug dealers.

Source of photos: Office of the Attorney General, State of California and the U.S. Drug Enforcement Administration.

Banning drug paraphernalia, that is, a full-scale prohibition on the manufacture, sale, and possession of drug paraphernalia.

Civil forfeiture, a legal procedure that permits the seizure and destruction of paraphernalia items without arresting the retailer or the person possessing the paraphernalia object.

The effectiveness of such legal measures has not yet been established, although their constitutionality has been upheld by the U.S. Supreme Court.

Drug Laws of Other Nations

Penalties for violating drug laws vary considerably from one state to another within the United States. However, in comparison with drug laws of certain other nations, the United States is typically viewed as being easy on users of illicit psychoactives. "Draconian" is the best description for the drug laws of some countries in the Near East, Far East, Africa, and South America. Many nations impose long prison sentences—even life imprisonment—heavy fines, and permanent expulsion from the country for what Americans would probably consider relatively minor offenses. In some instances, illegal drug possession as well as drug use carries the death penalty.

Most Americans are uninformed about other nations' systems of justice. Many months of pretrial confinement can pose hardships of hunger, intimidation, torture, beatings from fellow prisoners, and extortion. In some countries, entrapment of foreigners in purchasing or smuggling illegal drugs is a national pastime. Neither the American ambassador nor the consul can get an American civilian out of a foreign jail. Consequently, travelers are encouraged to check out the drug laws of those nations to be visited. By leaving illegal drugs at home and by not purchasing them when abroad, Americans can avoid the degradation and pain of being imprisoned in another country.

Alternative Behaviors as Alcohol and Other Drug-Abuse Prevention

A very practical technique of abuse prevention, the **alternatives approach** is a way of helping young people respond to their real needs without using alcohol and other drugs. Emphasis is placed on expanding the individual's interests outward into life. Characterized as easy to implement yet requiring a long-term commitment, the alternatives program seeks to provide youths with attractive optional substitutes, not just to drugs but to drug-using lifestyles.

The alternatives approach to drug-abuse prevention is based on several principles of drug-using behavior:[30]

> People use drugs voluntarily—that is, because they want to.

> People are taught by example of others and by the media that drugs are an effective way to feel better.

> People take drugs to feel better, get high, or experience adventure. They also use drugs to deal with negative feelings and stressful situations.

> People do not usually stop using drugs until they discover something better.

> The same effects produced by drugs can usually be achieved through alternative means that are more constructive both personally and socially.

> Drug abuse can be prevented by helping people experience satisfying nonchemical behaviors.

Involvement in an alternative behavior should not be regarded merely as a substitute for using a drug, as in the case of a natural "high." Rather, an alternative to drug use should lead to a long-term constructive activity, and not just a short-term gratification. Some individuals, especially parents, have difficulty in distinguishing an alternative behavior undertaken as drug-abuse prevention from that intended simply as "going to camp" or "taking music lessons." The significant difference is that alternative behavior employed as drug-abuse prevention is begun, for instance, when parents become concerned about problems they see developing in their own children—problems of interaction with age-mates, decreased self-confidence, and increasing boredom and apathy. It is the underlying reason or motivation for starting the alternative behavior that characterizes it as a drug-abuse prevention technique.

Essential to the concept of alternatives are the several levels of experience, types of gratification, or satisfaction sought through taking drugs. These experience levels have been identified as *physical, sensory, emotional, interpersonal, social* (including sociocultural and environmental), *political, intellectual, creative-aesthetic, philosophical,* and *spiritual-mystical.*[31,32] For each level of experience, possible nondrug alternatives have been proposed, as seen in the examples in table 13.4.

Though there is considerable value in offering accurate information about the effects of drugs in a drug education program, education about the nonchemical alternatives themselves on each level of experience is frequently viewed as the best method of drug abuse prevention.

Responsible Use as Alcohol and Other Drug-Abuse Prevention

One of the more controversial aspects of drug-abuse prevention is the precise definition of what is to be prevented. This controversy is equaled in the prevention area by the complex definition of what is to be encouraged. Problems of preventing drug abuse, misuse, and use are as perplexing and debatable as is the goal of encouraging responsible drug use.

The various meanings associated with "abuse of drugs" and "responsible use of drugs" contribute to the competition and even contradictions found among prevention efforts. For instance, law enforcement officials typically view drug abuse as the use of any illicit drug. By contrast, medical authorities tend to define drug abuse as the failure of the patient to comply with directions for using prescribed medicines (drug misuse), engaging in dangerous self-medication, or the recreational use of psychoactive drugs. Except for Rx drugs used for therapeutic purposes, both legal and medical groups appear to foster total abstinence, or nonuse of illegal drugs, as the ultimate goal of drug abuse prevention.

This drug-free, zero-tolerance approach to prevention is precisely the stance taken by the federal government. According to the federal Center for Substance Abuse Prevention, "responsible use" efforts are not compatible with its philosophy that regards the use of alcohol or other drugs, in any amount, as unacceptable behavior for youth. Moreover, the term *responsible use* is not appropriate for adults either, since there is some risk for harm associated with all drug use.

By contrast, another definition offered by some social scientists may be more comprehensive, more acceptable for planning purposes, and more realistic in terms of the drug-using population. This group of professionals defines drug abuse as the use of any drug, including alcohol, that is harmful to the individual or to society. According to this definition, a new element of abuse prevention would have to be recognized: the reduction of negative consequences due to using drugs. Among the negative or adverse consequences to be lessened are illness and death, acute behavioral effects (e.g., paranoia), chronic behavioral impairment (e.g., apathy), intellectual impairment, injury, or death associated with conditions of use (e.g., malnutrition and AIDS—acquired immune deficiency syndrome), developmental difficulties (e.g., adolescent crises), barriers to social acceptance, and unfavorable social conditions (e.g., dissolution of marriages and families, unemployment, criminal behavior).

Prevention of such abuse, the negative or adverse consequences identified above, is a major shift in both thinking and planning efforts away from earlier attempts at imposing nonuse. This emphasis on personal and social aspects of

13.4 Nondrug Alternatives for Various Levels of Experience

Example 1

Levels of Experience: Type of Gratification	Corresponding Motives, Needs, Aspirations	Alternative Behaviors
Physical: pertaining to physical well-being and experience of the body	1. Physical relaxation 2. Relief from pain or anticipated illness 3. Increased physical energy, avoidance of fatigue	1. Relaxation exercises, hatha-yoga 2. Dance and movement training 3. Training in positive health habits 4. Dietary and nutritional training 5. Physical recreation, fun sports, and individual activities

Example 2

Social-Political: pertaining to identification or involvement with social causes or political movements and reaction to social and political inertia or change	1. Identification with antiestablishment forces 2. Rebellions against disliked laws 3. Overcoming discouragement or desperation with social-political future 4. Induced change in mass consciousness	1. Partisan political action, e.g., helping candidate campaigns 2. Nonpartisan lobbying fieldwork with politicians and public officials 3. Involvement in social service 4. Participation in Peace Corps, VISTA, etc.

Nondrug alternatives for other levels of experience include:

Sensory level: developing increased awareness of body position, balance, coordination, and small muscle control; massage; responsible expression of one's sexuality.

Emotional level: competent and empathetic individual counseling; instruction in the psychology of personal development; emotional awareness exercises, such as learning body language and the improvement of honest self-awareness.

Interpersonal level: competently managed peer and group discussion; sensitivity and encounter group activities; experiences in trusting and respecting others; participation in goal-directed groups, such as the Scouts, 4-H groups, church organizations, school clubs, and Big Brother and Big Sister programs.

Intellectual level: hobbies, games, puzzles, reading, and memory training.

Creative level: nongraded experiences in music, art, drama, crafts, sewing, and photography; development of communication skills, including writing, public speaking, and conversation.

Philosophical level: courses on values and ethics; counseling oriented toward meaning and values clarification; association with individuals committed to various personal philosophies; strengthening of ethnic, racial, and minority pride.

Spiritual-mystical level: study of spiritual literature; investigation of different belief systems; meditation; contemplation; prayer; spiritual dance and song.

Sources: Henry S. Resnik, "It Starts With People: Experiences in Drug Abuse Prevention," National Institute on Drug Abuse, DHEW Publication No. (ADM) 78-590, 1978; Allen Y. Cohen, "The Journey Beyond Trips: Alternatives to Drugs" in *Journal of Psychedelic Drugs,* vol. 3, no. 2, page 19, Spring 1971; Allen Y. Cohen, "Matching Alternatives to Specific Drug Behaviors, in Positive Alternatives: Perspectives and Directions" in *Alternative Pursuits for America's 3rd Century, A Resource Book on New Perceptions, Processes, and Programs,* pages 39–43, National Institute on Drug Abuse, 1975; and Dario McDarby, *Drug Abuse: A Realistic Primer for Parents,* page 7, Do It Now Foundation, Phoeniz, Arix., 1980.

abuse prevention includes all drugs— legal and illicit as well as therapeutic and recreational;

> acknowledges a distinction between the occasional or social use of a drug and the use of a substance that constitutes chemical dependency or significant personal and social impairment; and
>
> fosters *responsible* choices regarding the use of all drugs, that is, the choice to use only medically prescribed drugs or the choice to use readily available drugs, even those that are potentially more harmful.

The focus of such prevention activities would be **responsible drug use,** or "responsible decision making" that would eliminate, reduce, lessen, or minimize negative consequences from the use of any drug. Helping people of all ages in making responsible decisions about drug use and nonuse is not beyond criticism, however. In many instances, there are no safe procedures for using a particular drug. Only less-harmful procedures may be offered for consideration.

Certain "responsible use" actions might only reduce the negative consequences to the individual drug user and to society, but not

eliminate them altogether. As such, this non-abstinence approach that allows for responsible use as a viable option would meet strong opposition on ethical, religious, political, philosophical, legal, and medical grounds. Indeed, advocating responsible use of illicit recreational drugs appears to be contradictory to many prevention efforts. Moreover, such advocacy tends to encourage breaking drug laws for those who choose to engage in recreational use of illegal psychoactive substances. It is not likely that in the near future the "prevention of harm" will be substituted for the "prevention of use" as the explicitly stated goal of drug abuse prevention.

Yet, a similar prevention approach has been conducted for many years with regard to smoking cigarettes and drinking alcoholic beverages—drug-taking behaviors associated with very dangerous, potentially lethal though legal mind-altering chemicals. For example, to reduce the intake of harmful tars in smoke, the smoker is advised to smoke only halfway down on the cigarette; to avoid or minimize the effects of rapid intoxication, the drinker is cautioned never to consume ethyl alcohol on an empty stomach. In each case, the suggested action is part of a drug-abuse prevention program intended to lessen the adverse consequences of using a drug.

Applied to the social-recreational use of other psychoactive substances, primary prevention would stress responsible decision making, and the promotion of specific drug-taking skills that could contribute to non-problem-producing use of such drugs. The following lists of responsibilities to be considered *before* using psychoactive drugs have been modified from the *Final Report of the Task Force on Responsible Decisions About Alcohol.*[33] Recommendations of this task force (a creation of the Education Commission of the States) are presented here in three distinct, yet related, areas: situational responsibilities, health responsibilities, and safety responsibilities.

Situational Responsibilities

If recreational use of drugs is one of the acceptable behavioral options, it should not be the main purpose of the gathering.

If drug use is socially acceptable within the group, then nonuse should also be an acceptable option.

Recognize that the recreational use of psychoactive drugs need not be an essential ingredient of every social occasion.

Recognize that drug overdose or drug-induced intoxication is neither healthy, humorous, nor safe.

Never urge another person under the influence of a psychoactive drug to continue using more of that drug or to take yet another drug.

Realize that group norms influence drug-taking behavior and ought to include a reasonable time limit as well as a consumption limit.

Avoid severe drug-related intoxication and help others to do the same.

Make contingency plans for those who might overdose and become severely intoxicated, including accompanying them home, applying appropriate first-aid measures, or calling for medical assistance when needed.

Use recreational drugs only in settings that are conducive to pleasant and relaxing behavior.

Realize that it is usually preferred to use recreational drugs in a group, rather than alone, because the limitations and concern of group members are more likely to reduce the potential for harm.

Health Responsibilities

Remember that there are occasions on which using any recreational drug would be contraindicated, i.e., pregnancy, the existence of some particular health problem, and upon the advice of a physician.

Set a limit on the amount of any drug consumed in a recreational setting.

Exercise extreme caution about using one psychoactive drug in combination with any other drug.

Recognize that any of the so-called recreational drugs is a drug substance having specific effects on the body, brain, and thought processes of the drug user.

Follow the advice of a physician concerning the use or nonuse of any recreational drug.

Understand that using mind-altering drugs for purposes of coping with life's problems is an extremely high-risk behavior.

Recognize that one need not use drugs in a recreational setting in order to be liked or accepted by others.

Avoid injecting drugs into a blood vessel (vein) with borrowed or shared needles, because of the possibility of infection and of the transmission of the AIDS-causing virus.

Set definite limits on the amount of drugs used in order to avoid overdosing.

Safety Responsibilities

Avoid performing complex tasks, such as operating machinery, driving a car, or engaging in other physical activities with obvious safety hazards while using psychoactive drugs.

Refuse to ride with a driver who is using psychoactive drugs, and discourage such an individual from operating a motor vehicle.

Recognize that the changed behaviors and attitudes resulting from using drugs may affect and influence others through the power of example, especially children.

Confine the use of recreational drugs to those social situations that are relaxing, noncompetitive, and conducive to limited consumption.

Use recreational drugs in moderation, that is, limited to the smallest amount of a drug needed to produce the desired effects.

Be extremely cautious when experimenting with drugs from unknown sources.

The Role of the Family

Increasing interest has been given to the importance of the family in the origin, maintenance, and prevention of alcohol and other drug-related problems. Although experimental drug use by young people appears to be a social phenomenon of adolescence, more serious drug abuse is predominantly a family problem.[34] As indicated in chapter 2, the changing nature of the family—its mobility, loss of traditions, instability due to divorce, and blending of families following remarriage—is often related to the incidence of drug misuse and abuse.

Drug Abuse: A Family Affair

Despite the pro-alcohol and pro-drug influences of peers and the mass media, role modeling by parents is considered the foremost factor in the development of young people's attitudes toward drugs and the likelihood of abusing drugs. There appears to be a strong relationship between parents' use of alcohol and other drugs and the occurrence of drug use and abuse in their children. Thus the family can be considered as the origin or genesis of alcohol and other drug abuse in many instances.

Family dynamics (psychological forces and interactions), especially marked by poor communications, overinvolvement and overindulgence by parents, and punitive and psychologically distant relationships between parents and child, are also identified as supporting the continuation of a drug-abuse problem within the family. Frequently, family members unwittingly or intentionally enable the drug abuser to continue as a chemically dependent individual whose treatment is often delayed or sabotaged. The misbehavior of the drug abuser "feeds" the peculiar psychological needs of other family members.

Slowly, the drug user and the adverse consequences of drug abuse affect each member of the family. The nonabusers begin to display certain attitudes and behaviors in response to the disturbance. In an attempt to cover up the "problem," parents as well as brothers and sisters often begin to make excuses for the drug abuser's actions. Lying to protect the abuser serves to protect other family members from social embarrassment. In time, the entire family begins to rearrange its daily routines in order to accommodate the abnormal drug use or drinking. Idle threats, blaming the drug abuser for all family problems, seeking revenge on the "family destroyer," fears, feelings of shame, and even guilt are commonly experienced. Totally involved and endangered, the family is held captive by the drug abuser, whose basic problem is still denied.

Identification of Drug Use and Abuse

Detecting a drug problem in its earliest phase is considered the first line of defense parents have against their child's drug use and abuse. Unfortunately, parents often fail to do so, and typically, problems of serious abuse are often denied, even when a son or daughter overdoses or attempts suicide in front of the parents.

It is evident that parents need help in determining when drug involvement exists. Although there is no single criterion that would apply in all cases, there are several common signals or indicators of drug use. Box 13.11 lists twenty of these *warning signals* in the form of questions for parents. Taken as a whole, the questions represent the signs and symptoms of a drug problem.

Guidelines for Parental Intervention

When a young person becomes involved with drugs, the parents often panic, become angry, and invariably assume that their faulty rearing practices caused the drug use. Parents often fail to recognize that their only responsibility now is to assist their child in overcoming the drug problem. To accomplish such a goal, parents might consider the following guidelines for early drug-abuse intervention:[35,36]

Try Not to Panic

Drug experimentation is occurring at increasingly early age levels. Many young Americans try at least one drug before the age of 17. Remember that most experimentation does not progress to chemical dependence and that your child still loves you.

Attempt to Talk with Your Child

Find out as much as possible about the situation, and then bring the evidence to the child's attention, but do so without nagging or an outburst of anger. Try to understand why your child is taking drugs. Then tell your child that you still love him or her and want to maintain open communication.

Indicate to Your Child that You Do Not Consider Drug Use as an Acceptable Behavior in the Family

State firmly and very clearly the family rules on using drugs. For a junior-high-age child, a suggested ban on drugs should cover legal as well as illegal drugs. For older teenagers, the question of teaching "responsible" or "low-risk" drinking in the home is an issue for individual parental discretion. Whatever the rules may be, however, make sure they are clear and consistent.

Consider the Model That You Provide to Your Child Regarding Recreational and Therapeutic Drug Use

Parental misuse often sets a "double standard" for children who see mom and dad popping unneeded tranquilizers, drinking heavily, or using other mind-changing drugs more often than their own peers.

Be Prepared to Enforce the Rules of the House Regarding Drug Use and Its Behavioral Consequences

Assure your child that in the future he or she will indeed be punished if caught breaking a rule.

Become Informed about the Drug Scene

Become informed about the drug scene, the pressures to use drugs as experienced by children, the consequences of using drugs, aspects of drug safety, and the adventure and excitement of drugs as perceived by kids, and so on.

Questions for Parents

box 13.11

You may suspect that your child or teenager is having trouble with alcohol and other drugs, but short of smelling liquor on the breath or discovering pills in pockets, how do you tell? While symptoms vary, there are some common tip-offs. Your answers to the following questions will help you determine if a problem exists.

1. Has your youngster's personality changed dramatically? _____ Does he or she seem giddy, depressed, extremely irritable, hostile without reason? _____ Do his or her moods change suddenly, intensely, and without provocation? _____

2. Is your supply of liquor, mood or diet drugs dwindling? _____ (Unless you keep a close inventory, you may not detect diminished amounts for months.)

3. Is your youngster less responsible about doing chores? _____ About getting home on time? _____ About following instructions and household rules? _____

4. Has he or she lost interest in school? _____ In extracurricular activities, especially sports? _____ Are grades dropping? _____ Has the teacher complained that your youngster is sleeping or inattentive in class? _____ Is your youngster skipping school? _____ (Problems at school are frequent warning signs.)

5. Has your youngster changed friends and started hanging out with a drinking and drug-taking group? _____ Are there weekend-long parties? _____ (A youngster having problems with alcohol or other drugs will abandon old friends and seek out those with similar attitudes and behavior.)

6. Are you missing money or objects that are easily convertible into cash? _____ (A young abuser's need for alcohol or other drugs increases and becomes more expensive. Eventually, the need for drugs overcomes any guilt about stealing from family members or others.)

7. Have neighbors, friends, or others talked to you about your youngster's behavior or drug taking? _____ (These reports may have substance.)

8. Has your youngster been arrested for drunkenness? _____ Driving under the influence of alcohol or other drugs? _____ Disorderly conduct? _____ Delinquent acts? (Encounters with the legal system often indicate underlying problems with alcohol and other drugs. There is a strong correlation between alcohol and/or other drug abuse and delinquency.)

9. Does your youngster strongly defend his or her right to use alcohol and other drugs? _____ (People defend that which is most important to them.)

10. Does your youngster "turn off" to talks about alcohol and other drug addictions? _____ (Abusers would rather not hear anything that might interfere with their behavior, whereas the nonabuser will listen without becoming defensive.)

11. Does your youngster get into fights with other youngsters? _____ With other family members? _____

(More than 70% of all beatings, stabbings, and assaults have occurred when one or both participants have been drinking or abusing other drugs.)

12. Are there medical or emotional problems? _____ (Check for ulcers, bronchitis, high blood pressure, acute indigestion, liver and kidney ailments, hepatitis, nosebleeds, malnutrition, weight loss, depression, memory lapses, talk of suicide. Alcohol and other drugs take their toll. Youngsters on "uppers" or "downers" usually lose their appetite. The taking of PCP, "angel dust," leads to paranoia and hallucinations. Long-term marijuana users often develop bronchitis. Heavy drinkers experience problems with digestion, malnutrition, and depression.)

13. Do you detect physical signs—alcohol on the breath, change in pupil size in the eyes, hyperactivity, sluggishness, slurred or incoherent speech? _____ (These are all strong clues.)

14. Does your youngster lie to you and others often? _____ (For young abusers, lying becomes automatic. They fib without reason. There is a saying: "Young alcoholics and other drug abusers have two things in common—they have a terminal attack of the 'cool' and are stuck in 'sneak' gear.")

15. Does your youngster volunteer to clean up after adult cocktail parties? _____ (Draining half-empty glasses is a cheap high.)

16. Do you find bottles or drugs in the bedroom, garage, van? _____ (Parents of abusers are amazed to find stashes of alcohol or drugs under mattresses, in stereo speakers, behind insulation in garages.)

17. Is your youngster irresponsible in using the family car—taking it without permission, making excuses for not getting it home on time? _____ (Many teenagers drink in cars and then drive. They frequently cause motor vehicle accidents.)

18. Does your youngster stay alone in his or her bedroom most of the time, bursting forth only occasionally? _____ Does he or she resent questions about activities and destinations? _____ (Some secrecy, aloofness, and resentment on the part of teenagers is normal. But when carried to extremes, these may signal problems with alcohol or other drugs.)

19. Have your youngster's relationships with other family members deteriorated? _____ Does he or she avoid family gatherings that were once enjoyed? _____ (An abuser's ability to relate to others suffers. The primary family relationships are affected first.)

20. Has your youngster been caught dealing in drugs or giving them to friends? _____

Alcohol and other drug abuse can create "Mr. Hydes" out of once happy youngsters and isolate them from those who love them. The youngsters become strangers and sources of frustration, irritation, and disruption to the family.

From *Questions for Parents*. Copyright © Comprehensive Care Corporation, Minneapolis, Minnesota. Reprinted by permission.

Develop Life Experiences with Your Child

Work hard at developing life experiences with your child—experiences that are fun, meaningful, and constructive alternatives to drug and alcohol use. Use the supervised activities of other parents, churches, and youth groups, and make certain these individuals and organizations also know what is going on in the community about drug use.

Consult with Other Parents

Within the parent group, work out a common code of basic behavior rules—on drugs, drinking, dating, curfews, chaperoning, etc. Then present a unified parental front, a community set of standards. Acting together, a group of parents can break up the peer pressure that often fosters experimentation and regular drug use.

Now a nationwide movement, thousands of such parent groups have been formed to combat drug use among teens and preteens. Varying in size and using different approaches, the parent groups usually focus on stopping marijuana smoking and on promoting drug-free and alcohol-free parties for youth. Among these groups are the National Federation of Parents for a Drug-Free Youth (NFP) and the National Parents' Resource Institute for Drug Education (PRIDE). These and other groups, notably TOUGHLOVE, enable parents—with support—to begin confronting their child's intolerable behavior through unorthodox responses. Some parents, preferring to improve their communication and conflict-resolution skills, enroll in Parent Effectiveness Training (PET) or Communication and Parenting Skills (CAPS) programs.

Decide if Professional Treatment Is Needed When Regular or Frequent Drug Use Persists

Such intervention is usually advised if recommended by a school counselor or law enforcement officer, when the drug use causes other problems, such as truancy, poor school performance, or strained family relations, or when the parents doubt their own ability to cope with the child's drug use.[37]

But the most essential aspect of intervention is for the parents to stop enabling the drug abuser's involvement with mind-changing substances. And this step begins with learning "ignoring skills"—the series of disengagement activities that must be accomplished before successful intervention can occur. Several disengagement skills have been identified and often prove helpful:[38]

Do Not

take your drug-abusing child's anger personally;

nag your child or constantly remind him or her of the harmful effects of alcohol and other drug use, because nagging equals provoking, and provoking constitutes enabling; and

make excuses to other family members or friends about your child's drug abuse.

Never

confront your drug-abusing child when you are angry;

use physical or verbal violence toward your child; and

clean up your teenager's messes, such as paying fines, covering bad checks, or financing repair bills.

Avoid

saying things and making idle threats you do not really mean or cannot enforce.

Always

remind yourself, over and over again, that chemical dependence is a disease. Your son or daughter is sick, and you are not at fault!

Understanding the Stages in Adolescent Chemical Use

Many people fail to recognize that involvement with recreational drugs usually occurs in phases and may be progressive or level off at an early developmental stage.

In response to the adolescent drug-abuse epidemic, Dennis D. Nelson, a teacher-counselor in a large suburban high school, developed a program for identifying and helping young people who were abusing drugs. After two years of daily contact with students, Nelson formulated a chronology or pattern of adolescent chemical use that represented the students in his program. The resulting drug-use continuum of stages may be helpful to parents and students as well as to professional caregivers in promoting a better understanding of drug abuse.

In abbreviated form, the four stages frequently seen in adolescent chemical use are described below.[39]

1. *Experimental use*—Late grade school or junior high age students, especially boys, are great experimenters with various mood-altering substances. Some may never go beyond the experimental stage. . . . But a majority of them will continue to experiment and become regular users. They will use beer and pot in this stage, and will learn to seek and enjoy the mood swings that these substances will provide. A child who exhibits abuse at this stage may be establishing a lifelong pattern. Or the chemical use may level off and stay at the "social-recreational" level, causing no intrapersonal conflict or externally harmful consequences.

2. *More regular use*—Simply using more does not, by itself, indicate dependency. But a pattern of regular use, coupled with some adverse behavioral changes, can show a definite move toward possible dependency. . . . This may begin in late junior high or early senior high years. If teenagers have to lie to their parents about their savings account, about why they have dropped out of school sports or other activities, or about who their companions are, and have to maintain these fictions in order to continue using [alcohol or other] drugs, they will begin to experience real guilt. Unfortunately, this guilt produces feelings of intense self-hate, which results in increased drug use. A cycle of use-guilt-remorse-increased use begins.

3. *Daily preoccupation*—Although the user may accept preoccupation with [alcohol or other] drugs as normal, such behavior is one of the major indicators of a chemical problem. More and more of a student's time, energy, and money are spent on thinking about being high, and ensuring that a steady supply of drugs is available. . . . Questioning users at this stage reveals that very few of their daily activities do not include drug use. Although abusers may be able to cut down or quit using drugs altogether for a few weeks, these periods of abstinence generally will not last.

4. *Dependency*—In this stage, negative personal feelings have been building steadily until they require daily, even hourly medication with drugs. In this stage, abusers are unable to distinguish between normal and intoxicated behavior. To them, being high is normal, and no rationale or moral argument can break through their chemically maintained delusion. This delusion persists even in the face of overwhelming evidence that his or her abuse is out of control and is physically, mentally, and emotionally strangling him or her.

Because the pattern of stages described a large majority of students abusing alcohol and other drugs, it has been used in assessment interviews to show both young people and their families where the students are on the drug-use continuum.

The Family and Primary Prevention

Although parents can engage effectively in secondary prevention by identifying chemical use in children and making appropriate interventions, the primary prevention of drug abuse demands a more positive and even more prolonged parental effort.

Admittedly, there is no single method of preventing young people's involvement with drugs. However, there is considerable agreement that children who develop certain life skills or attributes within a healthy family will have little need of drug use, as they learn to manage their own lives effectively in a drug-using society. Characterized by the wholeness of each member, the healthy family is one that can

---

At Issue

How Should We Fight the Drug War?

Point: Let there be no mistake. Despite encouraging news about the recent overall decline in illegal drug use among Americans, the level of alcohol and other drug abuse among all age groups remains unacceptably high. Recent data indicate that the use of marijuana is actually increasing once again among our youth. However, the epidemic of illegal-drug abuse is now becoming endemic—a permanent condition often concentrating in young and older adults and in inner-city minorities. To fight a war on drugs, we must increase our efforts to limit the supply of drugs and penalize more harshly the drug pushers and users in our communities. We must interdict illegal drugs coming into this country, and stamp out the domestic drug crop and illegally manufactured drug substances here in America. Use the United States military in such a war. If we can fight and win wars halfway around the world, why can't our armed forces be involved in restoring law and order in our own neighborhoods? Additionally, we should punish more harshly those who traffic in drugs and use drugs in order to deter use in the future. Jailing the "drug scum" will, at the very least, keep them from returning to their lifestyle of addiction!

Counterpoint: It should be quite evident that reducing the supply of drugs will never result in more than temporary victories on the battlefield of the drug war. We need to place more emphasis on reducing the demand for drugs. This is no small task, because it involves changing the minds and hearts of our people. Such a war strategy involves awareness and educational programs that encourage people to refuse drug use, as well as nondrug diversionary activities that substitute for the pleasure obtained from drugs. More importantly, drug users and abusers, especially those addicted to cocaine and heroin, need treatment and rehabilitation, not imprisonment. Perhaps the ultimate victory will not be found in a war on drugs, but rather in a "drug peace" that would legalize all mind-changing drugs, control drug production, enable police to concentrate on real crime, empty our overcrowded jails and prisons, and deprive organized crime of its most profitable commodity.

---

develop in children clear ideas about themselves, about others, and about family boundaries or limits, and the recognition of and respect for differences as well as sameness.[40]

Children who grow up with love and security, who can express themselves freely, who can make sound decisions, and who are realistic, yet optimistic about their own abilities, will likely not become dependent on drugs.

Among the life skills or tools needed so desperately by children are these:[41]

The *ability to exercise self-discipline and self-control*—necessary to resist peer pressure and to say no regarding drug use.

Feelings of love and affection—demonstrated by parental attitudes and actions of concern, support, appreciation, consideration, and assigning value and significance.

Clearly defined limits—establishing an acceptable and expected framework of behavior that imparts a sense of dependability in the environment, which is maintained through fair and consistent discipline.

Open channels of communication—enhancing the mutual expression of needs, feelings, problems, and exchange of information through listening, hearing, understanding, and responding by both parents and children.

It is increasingly apparent that to prevent drug abuse, nothing can be more important than for parents to spend both "quality" time and "quantity" time with their children. Moreover, drug-abuse prevention within the family is based upon strengthening the personal and social skills of youths—skills of personal competency in clarifying values, making responsible decisions in relation to interrelationships and career choices, processing feelings, establishing positive behaviors, maintaining and enhancing mood via natural "highs," and refusing the allure of chemical "highs."

Strong relationships, therefore, serve as the best though often underutilized ammunition in the war on alcohol and other drug abuse.[42]

Chapter Summary

1. The prevention of drug abuse involves activities undertaken to avoid, reduce, or eliminate the adverse consequences of misusing and abusing drugs, especially those identified as psychoactive.

2. General drug-abuse prevention strategies include (a) reducing the supply of drugs; (b) reducing the demand for drugs; and (c) inoculating drug users against unhealthy, irresponsible drug-taking behavior.

3. The public health model of abuse prevention assumes the existence of a host-agent-environment relationship in which the host is the drug taker, the agent is the drug itself, and the environment is the setting or context in which drug use occurs.

4. The macro approach to drug-abuse prevention involves the promotion of a drug-free atmosphere as well as a community-wide effort to reduce substance abuse and chemical dependency.

5. There are primary, secondary, and tertiary intervention levels of abuse prevention activities. Primary prevention takes place before drug use or abuse occurs; secondary prevention efforts are applied during the early stages of drug use or abuse; and tertiary prevention activities are begun during the later or advanced stages of drug abuse.

6. Among various countermeasures to substance abuse in the workplace are drug testing by urinalysis and the implementation of employee assistance programs.

7. Drug law enforcement techniques include use of informants, surveillance, undercover operations, drug raids, interdiction, and intelligence gathering.

8. The federal strategy of drug law enforcement reflects a major supply reduction effort, although demand reduction activities are also emphasized.

9. The Drug Enforcement Administration is the principal federal agency responsible for drug law enforcement. Related enforcement activities are also conducted by the Federal Bureau of Investigation, the Bureau of Alcohol, Tobacco and Firearms, the Internal Revenue Service, the U.S. Customs Service, the U.S. Coast Guard, and the U.S. Border Patrol.

10. State, county, and city law enforcement agencies also make important contributions in restricting and/or penalizing possession, use, trafficking, manufacture, distribution, and sale of legal and illegal psychoactive drugs.

11. The legal basis of federal efforts to reduce the consumption of illicit drugs is the Comprehensive Drug Abuse Prevention and Control Act of 1970, Title II of which is known as the Controlled Substances Act.

12. Attempts to control and/or restrict the availability of articles used in administering, preparing, packaging, and storing psychoactive drugs intended for personal use are focused in the antiparaphernalia movement.

13. The alternative behaviors technique is a drug abuse prevention approach designed to provide individuals with attractive, optional substitutes to using drugs as well as to drug-using lifestyles. Alternative behaviors may be found in various levels of experience, ranging from the physical to the spiritual-mystical.

14. Drug-abuse prevention may also be described in terms of responsible drug use that considers situational, health, and safety responsibilities.

15. The family often plays a significant role in the origin, maintenance, and prevention of drug-related problems among family members, especially youth.

16. There are numerous common indicators of drug use and drug abuse among young people.

17. Frequently seen stages in adolescent chemical use are (a) experimental; (b) more regular use; (c) daily preoccupation; and (d) chemical dependency.

18. By using a variety of techniques, parents can assist children in overcoming drug problems.

19. Parents can function in the primary prevention of drug use and abuse by helping children develop basic life-skills, such as self-discipline, decision making, and benefiting from mistakes, and by providing models of strong and thoughtful adults, a sense of belongingness, feelings of love and affection, and open channels of communication.

Review Questions and Activities

1. Explain why there is a growing interest in drug-abuse prevention activities.

2. Compare and contrast the following general strategies of preventing drug abuse: supply reduction, demand reduction, and inoculation.

3. Survey your local community to determine the various components of a drug-abuse prevention program. Then determine whether each component or activity reflects a supply reduction, demand reduction, or inoculation strategy.

4. Define the following in relation to the public health model of drug-abuse prevention: host, agent, and environment.

5. Propose a drug-abuse prevention program for your local community using the host-agent-environment as a model. Which of the three parts of the model would you emphasize?

6. What efforts, organizations, and procedures would have to be coordinated in a macro approach to drug-abuse prevention?

7. How do the following intervention levels of drug-abuse prevention differ from one another: primary, secondary, and tertiary?

8. List several activities or procedures that could be used to reduce substance abuse in the workplace.

9. In addition to making "drug raids" or "drug busts," what are some other routine enforcement techniques used by law enforcement agents?

10. Describe the various components of the federal strategy to reduce drug abuse through drug law enforcement.

11. Describe the roles of the following federal agencies in drug law enforcement: Drug Enforcement Administration, Federal Bureau of Investigation, Bureau of Alcohol, Tobacco and Firearms, Internal Revenue Service, U.S. Customs Service, and the U.S. Border Patrol.

12. Identify several federal control mechanisms imposed on the manufacture, purchase, and distribution of controlled substances as authorized by the Controlled Substances Act.

13. Determine the various laws of your state that restrict the use or availability of both legal and illegal drugs. Do you think the minimum drinking age of 21 years is effective in reducing alcohol-impaired accidents in your community?

14. Do you believe the issuance of a summons instead of making an arrest is a better way of preventing drug abuse? Give two reasons to support your stand.

15. Explain why you would support or oppose the antiparaphernalia movement in your community.

16. Describe in detail the alternative behaviors approach as a drug abuse prevention technique. List at least ten individual or group activities that might replace, reduce, or prevent drug abuse.

17. Define the concept of "responsible use" as a drug-abuse prevention technique.

18. What types of responsibilities should be contemplated in any consideration of responsible drug use?

19. Do you believe that responsible drug use is an appropriate technique to prevent drug abuse? On what do you base your response?

20. In what ways might a family contribute to originating, maintaining, and preventing drug-related problems?

21. What are some common warning signals of drug use and abuse among young people?

22. If you were a parent, how might you assist your child if she or he were to have a drug problem?

23. What are some of the common indicators that describe the four stages in adolescent chemical use?

24. In what precise ways might a family function on the primary intervention level to prevent drug abuse? In your opinion, what is the most important thing a family can do to prevent drug or chemical abuse?

References

1. Institute for Health Policy of Brandeis University, *Substance Abuse: The Nation's Number One Health Problem* (Princeton, N.J.: Robert Wood Johnson Foundation, 1993), 31.

2. Lester Grinspoon and James Bakalar, "The War on Drugs—A Peace Proposal," *New England Journal of Medicine* 330, no. 5 (3 February 1994): 356–60.

3. Office of Justice Programs, Bureau of Justice Statistics, *Drugs, Crime, and the Justice System* (Washington, D.C.: U.S. Government Printing Office, 1992), 36.

4. Center for Substance Abuse Prevention, Substance Abuse and Mental Health Services Administration, *Prevention Works: A Discussion Paper on Preventing Alcohol, Tobacco, and Other Drug Problems,* DHHS Publication No. SAM–93–2046 (Washington, D.C.: U.S. Government Printing Office, 1993), 9.

5. Jack Durell and William Bukoski, "Preventing Substance Abuse: The State of the Art," *Public Health Reports* 99, no. 1 (January–February 1984): 23–31.

6. Office of Justice Programs, *Drugs, Crime, and the Justice System,* 74–75.

7. Office of National Drug Control Policy, *National Drug Control Strategy: Reclaiming Our Communities from Drugs and Violence* (Washington, D.C.: Executive Office of the President, 1994).

8. Center for Substance Abuse Prevention, *Prevention Works* 12–13.

9. Center for Substance Abuse Prevention, Substance Abuse and Mental Health Services Administration, *Prevention Plus II: Tools for Creating and Sustaining Drug-Free Communities,* DHHS Publication No. ADM–89–1649 (Washington, D.C.: U.S. Government Printing Office, 1993), 181–84.

10. Center for Substance Abuse Prevention, Substance Abuse and Mental Health Services Administration, *Signs of Effectiveness II— Preventing Alcohol, Tobacco, and Other Drug Use: A Risk Factor/Resiliency-Based Approach,* DHHS Publication No. SAM–94–2098 (Washington, D.C.: U.S. Government Printing Office, 1993).

11. This section is based, in part, on a publication of the Drug Enforcement Administration, *Controlled Substances: Use, Abuse, and Effects* (Washington, D.C.: Department of Justice, n.d.), 1, 4.

12. Ed Storti and Janet Keller, *Crisis Intervention: Acting against Addiction* (New York: Crown, 1988), 5.

13. Sharon Wegscheider, *Another Chance: Hope and Health for the Alcoholic Family* (Palo Alto, Calif.: Science and Behavior Books, 1981), 153—57.

14. Al Mooney, Arlene Eisenberg, and Howard Eisenberg, *The Recovery Book* (New York: Workman, 1992), 512.

15. Governor's Commission for a Drug-Free Indiana, *Putting Drugs Out of Work* (Indianapolis: Governor's Commission for a Drug-Free Indiana, 1993), section 1.

16. Center for Substance Abuse Prevention, *Making the Link: Alcohol, Tobacco, and Other Drugs in the Workplace*, CSAP Publication No. ML006 (Rockville, Md.: Center for Substance Abuse Prevention, 1994).

17. Craig Zwerling, James Ryan, and Endel Orva, "The Efficacy of Preemployment Drug Screening for Marijuana and Cocaine in Predicting Employment Outcome," *Journal of the American Medical Association* 264, no. 20 (28 November 1990): 2639–43.

18. Office of Justice Programs, *Drugs, Crime, and the Justice System,* 118.

19. Barry Stimmel and the Editors of Consumer Reports Books, *The Facts about Drug Use* (New York: Haworth Medical Press, 1993), 324–25.

20. Norman Miller, *The Pharmacology of Alcohol and Drugs of Abuse and Addiction* (New York: Springer-Verlag, 1991), 301–3.

21. Stimmel and others, *The Facts about Drug Use,* 329.

22. Tom Mieczkowski and others, "Testing Hair for Illicit Drug Use," *National Institute of Justice Research in Brief* (January 1993): 1–5.

23. Governor's Commission for a Drug-Free Indiana, *Putting Drugs Out of Work,* section 5.

24. Center for Substance Abuse Prevention, *Making the Link.*

25. Office of Justice Programs, *Drugs, Crime, and the Justice System,* 144–53.

26. Drug Enforcement Administration, U.S. Department of Justice, *Drugs of Abuse* (Washington, D.C.: U.S. Government Printing Office, 1989), 6–8.

27. Modified from the U.S. Department of Education, *What Works: Schools without Drugs* (Washington, D.C.: U.S. Department of Education, 1986), 49.

28. Alexander Wagenaar, "Legal Minimum Drinking Age Changes in the United States: 1970–1981," *Alcohol Health and Research World* 6, no. 2 (winter 1981/82): 21–26.

29. Kerry Healey, *State and Local Experience with Drug Paraphernalia Laws* (Washington, D.C.: U.S. Government Printing Office, 1988), 69–73.

30. Allan Y. Cohen, "The Journey beyond Trips: Alternatives to Drugs," *Journal of Psychedelic Drugs* 3, no. 2 (spring 1971): 7.

31. Dario McDarby, *Drug Abuse: A Realistic Primer for Parents* (Phoenix: Do It Now Foundation, 1980), 7.

32. Allan Y. Cohen, "Matching Alternatives to Specific Drug Behaviors," in *Alternative Pursuits for America's Third Century: A Resource Book on New Perceptions, Processes, and Programs,* NIDA (Washington, D.C.: U.S. Government Printing Office, 1975), 39–43.

33. Task Force on Responsible Decisions about Alcohol, Education Commission of the States, *Final Report: Booklet 2* (Denver: Education Commission of the States, 1975), 8–9 (summary). The task force project was supported by the National Institute on Alcohol Abuse and Alcoholism.

34. M. Duncan Staton, "Some Overlooked Aspects of the Family and Drug Abuse," in *Drug Abuse from the Family Perspective,* DHHS Publication No. ADM–80–910, ed. Barbara Gray Ellis (Washington, D.C.: U.S. Government Printing Office, 1980), 3.

35. National Institute on Drug Abuse, *Drug-Abuse Prevention for Your Family,* DHHS Publication No. ADM–81–584 (Washington, D.C.: U.S. Government Printing Office, 1980), 4–5.

36. Marsha K. Schuchard, "Celebrating Parent Power in Georgia," *NIDA Prevention Resources* 2, nos. 3–4 (winter 1978): 3–4.

37. Dorothy Cretcher, *Steering Clear: Helping Your Child through the High-Risk Drug Years* (Minneapolis: Winston Press, 1982), 95.

38. Dick Schaefer, *Choices and Consequences: What to Do when a Teenager Uses Alcohol/Drugs* (Minneapolis: Johnson Institute Books, 1987), 82–84.

39. Dennis D. Nelson, *Frequently-Seen Stages in Adolescent Chemical Use* (Minneapolis: CompCare, 1978).

40. Barbara Gray Ellis, "Report of a Workshop on Reinforcing the Family System As the Major Resource in the Primary Prevention of Drug Abuse," chapter 12 in *Drug Abuse from the Family Perspective,* 135.

41. Based in part on National Institute on Drug Abuse, *Drug-Abuse Prevention for Your Family,* 4–5.

42. David Wilmes, *Parenting for Prevention: How to Raise a Child to Say No to Alcohol/Drugs* (Minneapolis: Johnson Institute Books, 1988), 95–160.

chapter

14 | alcohol, tobacco, and other drug prevention education

Comprehensive Approaches to Drug
   Prevention Education
Comprehensive Policy Against Alcohol
   and Other Drug Use
Curriculum
Decision Making
Evaluation
Goals
Instructional Objectives
Life Skills
Methods
Normative Beliefs
Personal Commitment
RADAR Network
Resistance Skills
Resources
Strategies
Student Assistance Programs
Subject Matter
Systematic Planning Process
Values Clarification

chapter objectives

After you have studied this chapter, you should be able to do the following:

1. Define the key terms.

2. Compare the more traditional approach to school-based alcohol and other drug prevention education programs with an expanded, modern, comprehensive approach.

3. State at least three major goals of school-based alcohol, tobacco, and other drug prevention education.

4. List at least three *Healthy People 2000* objectives for each of the following areas: alcohol use and/or abuse, tobacco use, and other drug use and/or abuse.

5. Identify the basic steps in the recommended systematic planning process that can be used in alcohol, tobacco, and other drug education programs.

6. Distinguish among the several program or curricular strategies that are often used separately or in some combination in school-based alcohol and drug education.

7. Demonstrate several techniques for "just saying no" to the use of alcoholic beverages, tobacco products, and other drugs.

8. Identify several general principles that can be used in guiding the design and implementation of school-based alcohol and drug prevention programs.

9. Name three federal government sources of alcohol and other drug-related information.

10. Explain the nature and function of the RADAR Network.

11. Describe the basic elements of a comprehensive school policy against the use of alcohol and other drugs.

12. Discuss the several functions of a student assistance program.

Introduction

Most people think that alcohol, tobacco, and other drug prevention education—the major concern of this chapter—is an educational experience targeted largely to young people in school. However, an expanded view of this process involves several community-wide endeavors as well as a variety of nonclassroom school activities focused on students, parents, and school personnel offering pupil-support services.

Both national and local goals of alcohol, tobacco, and other drug education are directly related to the prevention of the use of all illegal mind-changing drugs by underage individuals and the prevention of the potentially harmful and life-threatening consequences of using alcohol, tobacco, and other drugs among the general population.

For effective psychoactive drug prevention education in the school, a systematic planning process is described for designing and implementing an appropriate curriculum—all the formal, structured learning experiences provided by the school regarding alcohol, tobacco, and other drug use and abuse. Several curricular strategies for use in schools are also identified, including those involving normative beliefs, personal commitment, resistance skills, alternatives, goal-setting, decision making, self-esteem enhancement, stress skills, and life skills.

A major portion of this chapter lists numerous resources for alcohol, tobacco, and other drug education programs, specifically prepackaged curricula, government agencies, the RADAR Network, private and voluntary agencies and companies, self-help groups, local community organizations

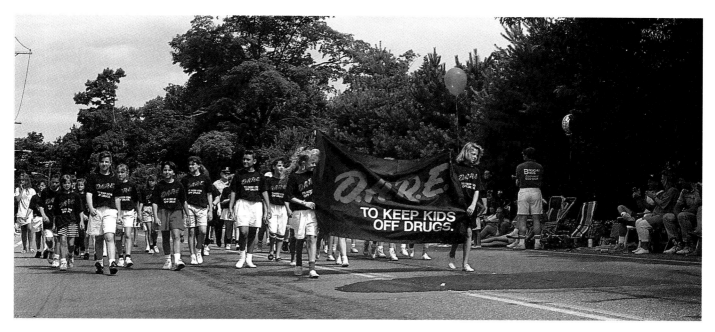

School-based programs to prevent ATOD use and abuse often involve students in out-of-classroom activities. Here youths in Natick, Massachusetts, march through city streets as part of a DARE program to keep kids off drugs.

© Rick Berkowitz/The Picture Cube, Inc.

and individuals, and periodicals related to alcohol and other drugs. The chapter concludes with a section on a comprehensive school policy against alcohol and other drug use, and a description of student assistance programs—a common mechanism for intervention and prevention activities reflecting school policies.

Basic Considerations: The What and Why of Alcohol, Tobacco, and Other Drug Prevention Education

Alcohol, tobacco, and other drug education takes place in many locations and situations other than the classroom. Although school-age youth are the traditional target for alcohol, tobacco, and other drug (ATOD) education, various prevention programs dealing with these mind-changing substances also reach both general and specific populations through other nonschool educational approaches, including these:

- Mass-media campaigns (such as public service announcements emphasizing that "Friends don't let friends drive drunk").

- Publicized community-wide strategies to reduce the supply of or demand for alcoholic beverages and illegal drugs (for instance, strict enforcement of the minimum drinking age and tobacco purchasing age).

- Worksite employee efforts (such as alcohol and other drug awareness projects and employee assistance programs).

- Policy and legislative initiatives (such as laws and regulations that reflect society's attitudes and values about availability, purchase, taxation, and use of alcoholic beverages, tobacco products, and illegal drugs of abuse).

- Training health care professionals and community leaders about alcohol- and other drug-related problems.

Such community-wide **comprehensive approaches to alcohol and other drug prevention education** are essential, since research indicates that individual-directed

school-based programs are not as effective in preventing or reducing alcohol and other drug problems when used independently from these more comprehensive techniques.[1] As a consequence, in addition to providing information about alcohol, tobacco, and other drugs, and the consequences of their use, elementary and secondary schools are urged to consider the following elements of an expanded alcohol and drug prevention program:

- Raise awareness and involvement in the local community (e.g., "red ribbon day").

- Increase the knowledge base of teachers and parents as well as students.

- Change students' norms and expectations about alcohol and drinking, about tobacco, smoking, and smokeless tobacco products, and about the actual number of those who use marijuana, cocaine, and other illegal drugs.

- Enhance parenting and positive family influences.

- Improve student coping, peer resistance, and decision-making skills.

- Increase involvement in school by parents and students.

- Expand student participation in healthy and legal alternatives to using alcohol and other drugs.

- Implement support services (such as peer counseling and student assistance programs).

- Deter use through regulatory and legal actions (e.g., strict enforcement of school policy on alcohol and other drug use, increased security near schools and other gathering places, strict enforcement of the minimum drinking age, and penalties for bringing other illegal drugs to school).

Now, that is some recipe for potential effectiveness! But all of these primary educational interventions are needed, in addition to a school curriculum about alcohol and other drug use. Each of the above efforts will affect youth alcohol and other drug use indirectly by changing one or more of the factors that appear to be related to the use of psychoactive drugs.[2]

Goals of ATOD Education in the Schools

As stated by the federal Center for Substance Abuse Prevention, ATOD education programs in schools are designed to reduce the extent of alcohol, tobacco, and other drug use and to prevent alcohol-, tobacco- and other drug-related problems from occurring in the future.[3] Such primary prevention is an attempt to lower the number of new users of psychoactive drugs, to delay an individual's first use of alcohol and tobacco products until at least the age of majority, and to improve individual (personal) strengths as an inoculant against using alcohol, tobacco, and other drugs. Additional goals of ATOD education include the promotion of healthy ways in choosing *not* to use these substances, and offering young people alternative social events free of alcohol and other drugs. On occasion, some ATOD education programs also seek to reduce the total number of drinkers, smokers, and other drug users among those youth who have already

At Issue

In ATOD education programs, should the concept of "responsible drug use" be included as part of the goals and objectives?

Point: In terms of school-based ATOD education programs, there should be no reference to the concept of "responsible drug use." Considering responsible use implies that some types of drug use are condoned or even encouraged, when all drug substances—even alcohol and tobacco—are illegal for school-age children, and their use is prohibited in most instances. If an educational program is to be preventive in nature, emphasis should be placed on abstinence or nonuse. Postponing the onset of drug use reduces both the likelihood of drug use in the future as well as the probability of developing drug problems. And these are proven facts! Saying no to drugs is not just the best policy; it is the only responsible policy.

Counterpoint: It is important for young people to know that most youths do not use drugs, except for alcohol, and that relatively few abuse illegal drugs. However, it is unrealistic to assume that all young people will remain abstinent from alcohol—a legal drug—in a society in which most individuals drink as adults. Should our schools prepare abstaining children to be responsible alcohol users as most adults are? Perhaps abstaining from drug use might be viewed as either a life-long choice or a temporary restraint until reaching the legal drinking age or applied to specific situations that have a high risk for developing problems. Then, the concept of responsible drug use could appropriately help people of all ages make informed, mature, and personally accountable decisions about drug use. As part of a prevention program, responsible drug use could encourage those people who use drugs to do so in ways that minimize overdosing, intoxication, transmission of the HIV-virus, and other conditions that could threaten health and safety. In reality, as Dr. Jean Mayer suggests, there are no toxic substances, only toxic concentrations of drug substances.

begun using these substances, by limiting either the duration or the scope of their drug use. (Such efforts may be labeled as secondary prevention, in some instances.) Note that these goals, expressed by alcohol and drug prevention experts, say nothing about promoting "responsible use of alcohol" or low-risk drug-using behaviors, since all underage use is considered unacceptable and illegal behavior.

Healthy People 2000 Objectives

The term *objectives* is often used in educational planning for specific statements of how students are supposed to be changed after a learning experience; the U.S. Public Health Service has formulated several specific ATOD-related objectives that now serve as measurable targets to be achieved by the year 2000. These objectives, part of an extensive national strategy to promote health and

prevent disease among Americans, can also serve as general goals of all ATOD prevention efforts. Listed below are modified objectives that pertain directly or indirectly to ATOD education in the schools:[4–6]

Objectives to reduce alcohol problems:

1. Reduce deaths by alcohol-related motor-vehicle crashes, by reducing "underage drinking."

2. Increase by at least one year the average age of first use of alcohol.

3. Reduce the proportion of young people who have used alcohol recently.

4. Reduce the proportion of high school seniors who have five or more drinks on one occasion in a recent two-week time period.

5. Increase the proportion of high school seniors who perceive social

disapproval and risk of physical or psychological harm associated with heavy use of alcohol (i.e., having five or more drinks once or twice each weekend).

Objectives to reduce tobacco use:

1. Reduce cigarette smoking to a prevalence of no more than 15 percent among people 20 years old and older.

2. Reduce the initiation of smoking by youths to no more than 15 percent as measured by the prevalence of smoking among people 20 through 24 years old.

3. Increase smoking cessation during pregnancy so that at least 60 percent of women who are cigarette smokers at the time they discover they are pregnant will quit smoking and maintain abstinence for the remainder of their pregnancy.

4. Reduce smokeless tobacco use to a prevalence of no more than 4 percent among men 18 through 24 years old.

5. Increase to at least 85 percent of the adolescent population, ages 12 through 17 years, who perceive great risk of harm to their health and social disapproval associated with smoking cigarettes.

Objectives to reduce other drug problems:

1. Increase by at least one year the average age of first use of marijuana by adolescents 12 through 17 years old.

2. Increase the proportion of high school seniors who perceive social disapproval associated with occasional use of marijuana and experimentation with cocaine.

3. Increase the proportion of high school seniors who associate risk of physical or psychological harm with regular use of marijuana and experimentation with cocaine.

4. Reduce to no more than 3 percent the proportion of male high school seniors who use anabolic steroids.

5. Reduce the proportion of young people who have used marijuana, cocaine, and other illegal drugs of abuse in the past month.

6. Reduce drug-abuse-related hospital emergency room visits.

Planning and Strategies: The How of Alcohol, Tobacco, and Other Drug Education

A major concern of ATOD education is how such a program is developed and introduced in a learning environment. The section focuses on the elements of educational planning, curricular strategies, and principles of curriculum design and implementation.

Educational Planning

An important feature of effective alcohol, tobacco, and other drug (ATOD) education is the process of planning. Whether it describes an entire curriculum or a small teaching unit, a plan usually consists of a written document stating what the learning experiences are designed to do, how the knowledge, attitudes, or skills will be taught, the resources needed for teaching, and the measures used to determine whether the plan achieved its objectives.

A systematic plan for teaching effectiveness considers both design and implementation of the **curriculum**—all the formal, structured learning experiences provided by the school on a particular topic—as well as a teaching unit. The several steps of the **systematic planning process** have been identified as these:[7,8]

Needs assessment—The process of determining what ATOD problems or concerns need to be included in the plan of instruction. Factors to be considered include surveys of needs, students' interests, district or state requirements, recommendations from authorities and concerned citizens, occurrence of problem behaviors (underage drinking parties, drinking and driving, pot puffing, etc.), persistence of myths about alcohol, other drugs and their effects, and society's needs and priorities.

Identification of strategies—Whether a purchased, state- or district-provided,

or local curriculum is used, identify and understand its basic philosophy. Several differing educational strategies, as detailed later in this section, are available for selection and provide the basic approaches to curriculum implementation.

Anticipation of instructional problems—Determine the amount of administrative and community support for the curriculum; consider the chances of realistically accomplishing the stated goals and objectives within the limitations of available resources, time, and teacher preparation; plan for possible controversies; and establish the degree to which the curriculum coordinates with other school and community activities relating to ATOD use by young people.

Development of goals—Establish **goals,** broad statements that give direction to instructional efforts and express the nature of change that the educative process will attempt to effect. In addition to "preventing underage smoking and drinking," other goals of ATOD education might include "promotion of responsible decision making regarding the use and nonuse of tobacco products and alcoholic beverages," "development of skills in resisting pressure to drink," "clarification of one's values regarding marijuana and intoxication," "increase in knowledge about alcohol, its effects, and laws regarding its purchase and use," and "reduction of commonly held myths and misconceptions about cocaine."

Selection of subject matter—Identification of **subject matter** or content areas to be included in the curriculum or teaching plan sets limits to what topics will be considered and at what grade level they will be introduced into learning opportunities. Once appropriate subject matter has been specified, instructional objectives can be formulated. Selected elements of subject matter are detailed in box 14.1.

box 14.1

Selected Content Elements of Subject Matter Related to ATOD Education

These content items can be used to formulate educational objectives and learning experiences for the grade levels indicated.

Lower Elementary Level

Nature of drugs and medicines

Wide availability of drugs

Difference between drugs and candy

Doctors and parents as sources of drugs

Drugs vs. poisons

Specific mind and behavior modifiers: alcoholic beverages, tobacco products, certain medicines

Activities of drinking, smoking, and drug taking vs. taking medicine

Difficulties in recognizing which substances are safe to eat or touch

Effects of poisons on the body

Occasions for using drugs: meals, family celebrations, communion wine, pain relief, curing illness, adult parties

Effects of smoking on the human body

Family differences in the use of beverage alcohol and tobacco products

Consequences of taking too many drugs at once

Good things about oneself

Social skill of helping others

Appropriateness of asking for help

Intermediate Level

Adult supervision in the use of drugs or medicines

Drug overdoses and poisonings

Hazards of self-medication and experimentation

Difference between over-the-counter drugs and prescription drugs

Variety of substances used to change feelings and behavior: alcohol, tobacco, marijuana, others

Reasons for using various drugs: relieve pain, cure illness, social, dietary, ceremony, pleasure, escape, tradition, curiosity

Reasons for nonuse of drugs, especially psychoactives: personal or family preference, cost, health, legal, religious or moral

Common and uncommon use of psychoactive substances

Saying no to peer pressure

Refusing offers to take drugs from friends and strangers

Legal and illegal use of pyschoactive drugs

Legal controls on purchase, possession, and use

Nature of habits and their development

Importance of rules

Nature of values as guides to behavior

Why it is wrong to take illegal drugs

Importance of helping others

Protective function of laws

Credible sources of information about drugs

Importance of retaining individuality while belonging to a peer group

Elements of healthy friendships

Junior High Level

Formation of attitudes regarding drug usage

Influence of peer pressure in relation to using drugs

How drugs work in the human body

Physical and mental changes resulting from use of various psychoactive drugs

Potential benefits vs. possible harmful effects of cigarette smoking

Manufacture and distribution of alcoholic beverages

Differences between beer, wine, and distilled spirits

Consequences of loss of inhibitions, intoxication

Nonuse of alcoholic beverages and cigarettes

Reasons associated with experimental and regular use of marijuana and other controlled substances

---

Formulation of instructional objectives—Developed to guide daily learning opportunities, **instructional objectives** are statements of specific, measurable outcomes and describe patterns of performance to be demonstrated by students upon completion of a particular lesson or series of learning situations. Accomplishment of related objectives should contribute to the realization of major goals. Examples of objectives include these: "After seeing the film *Spirits of America*, students will be able to describe three differing drinking customs in American society." "In a role-playing situation involving a nonsmoker who is being urged to try a cigarette, a student can demonstrate five different ways of saying no." "The student can explain why some people use tobacco despite its potential for harm and long-term health problems." "The student can analyze alcoholic beverage ads for various propaganda appeals used by sponsors."

Method selection—Planned learning procedures and activities that are used to help students accomplish specific objectives are known as **methods.**

continued

Risk taking in relation to living and drug taking

Propaganda appeals commonly used in advertising alcoholic beverages, cigarettes, and over-the-counter drugs

Medicines that cure or heal vs. medicines that control body functions

Development of drug dependencies through the use of psychoactive drugs, as well as laxatives and nose drops

Dangers of using medicines prescribed for another person

Use of outdated medications

Personal, sociocultural, family, and environmental factors that influence use, nonuse, and abuse of various psychoactive substances

Family drinking problems

Legal drinking age

Drug problems among teenagers, at school, and in society

Student responsibilities in promoting a drug-free school

Policies and laws regarding drug use

Pro-drug messages in music, videos, movies, and TV

Importance of the scientific method in making decisions

Senior High, College, and Adult Levels

Behavioral effects of psychoactive drugs

Recreational drugs vs. therapeutic drugs

Legal vs. illegal psychoactive drugs

Advantages and disadvantages of self-medication

Wise use of medications

Physical effects of cigarette smoking

Cigarette smoking and pregnancy; effects on the newborn

Alcohol's passage through the body

Phenomenon of intoxication

Legal drinking age

Moderate social drinking vs. problem-related drinking

Alcohol abuse and alcoholism

Drinking and driving; driving under the influence of drugs

Women and alcohol

Alcohol and pregnancy; fetal alcohol syndrome

Children of alcoholics and abusers of other drugs

Ways of helping problem drinkers and alcoholics

The appeal and potential for danger in using various psychoactive drugs

Situations in which dangerous drugs might be used socially or as therapeutic agents

Psychological and physical aspects of drug dependency

Drug use vs. drug abuse

Adverse drug reactions and side effects of using any drug; alcohol-drug interactions

Drug overdoses and emergency procedures

Warning signs of substance abuse, including problem drinking

Local, state, and federal laws on controlled substances

Infections related to nonsterile procedures of administering drugs

Treatment and rehabilitation programs for drug-dependent individuals

Stop-smoking programs

Community resources for helping drug-dependent people

Legal consequences of illegal drug use

Physical and mental effects of using steroids

Harmful effects of legal and illegal drugs on fetal development

Myths and stereotypes that seem to encourage drug use

Ways to cope with peers and social pressure to use drugs

Effects of drug use on personal financial resources

Parents' role in prevention of drug abuse

Influence of history and popular media on drug-taking practices

Information about the judicial system, policies, due process, court practices and penalties, and implications of conviction

---

Whether they promote individual student responses (assigned project, lecture, chalk talk, self-test, self-assessments, teacher demonstration, and guest speakers) or student interaction (debate, panel discussion, group projects, role playing, and skits), methods should support the anticipated student behaviors indicated in the educational objectives. Other methods, such as the use of various instructional media (videocassettes, films, slides, models, and puppets) may contribute to both individual response and student interaction.

Identification of resources—So-called tools of the trade, **resources** for alcohol education, include both personnel and materials that can be used to support the teaching function of the school. Frequently used resources include various instructional media (videocassettes, films, transparencies, etc.) and guest speakers from alcoholism treatment facilities, law enforcement officials, members of voluntary groups of recovering alcohol dependents, representatives of Mothers Against Drunk Drivers, and members and sponsors of Students Against Driving Drunk.

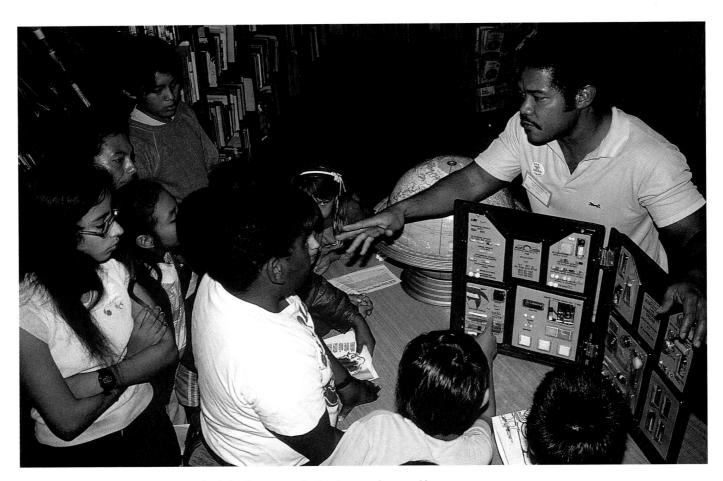

Effective ATOD prevention programs now begin in elementary schools where teachers provide information on the "gateway drugs" (alcohol, tobacco and marijuana), foster development of social skills, and promote a clear "no use" message.

© 1995 Len Berger/Picture Perfect

Development of evaluation procedures—The major concern of **evaluation** is to determine if the curriculum or teaching plan helped students accomplish specific instructional objectives. Various levels and types of evaluation procedures can be used. Process evaluation determines the adequacy of the curriculum design and its implementation in the school setting. Outcome evaluation tries to assess the students' accomplishments of the original objectives. Impact evaluation tries to gauge the total effects of an alcohol education prevention program within a certain community or over a specific period of time.

Revision of the instructional program—Based upon various evaluation procedures, make appropriate changes to either the design or implementation of the curriculum or teaching plan. Revisions should consider lack of student accomplishment of objectives, inadequacies of instruction, cost of the program, limitation of time, resistance of parents or school officials, and use of more efficient means of accomplishing the goals and objectives of the curriculum.

Curricular Strategies

In ATOD education activities, several basic **strategies** or underlying designs of the curriculum have emerged over the years.[9] Early educational efforts relied on scare tactics and moral persuasions that reflected the prohibitionist philosophy of the late nineteenth century, when instruction on the evil and harmful effects of alcohol, tobacco, and narcotics was mandated in many states. After many years of rather ineffective instruction, the scare strategy of instruction gave way to the "straight facts" approach to alcohol and narcotics education in the 1940s and 1950s. This information-based strategy assumed that young people would not use "dope" or drink or would stop drinking when they became informed about the physical and psychological effects of alcohol as well as the health hazards of drinking and the legal penalty for possession and intoxication.

Then, in the 1970s, the focus of alcohol and other drug education shifted away from the facts approach to a strategy that concentrated on the personality of the drug user. According to this new theory, young people used alcohol and other drugs because of low self-esteem, poor communication skills, and inadequate decision-making skills. The new curriculum designs featured affective education with strong doses of values clarification exercises, self-esteem building, decision making, and stress management techniques.

During the 1980s, yet another basic curriculum design emerged on the ATOD education scene. This current strategy assumes that drinking and drugging result from social influences of the environment, and that young people are vulnerable to social pressures to drink or use other illegal mind-changing drugs.

Presently, several program strategies are used separately or in some combination in school ATOD education programs.[10] These strategies or plans are the bases of the many prepackaged and locally developed curricula that are being used in the hope of preventing alcohol and other drug-related problems. Selected programmatic strategies are described on this page.

Normative Beliefs

The **normative beliefs** plan provides information to students about the actual rates of alcohol and other drug use from surveys, and thereby corrects exaggerations about near-universal drinking, smoking, and other drug use among their peers. By revealing and comparing personal attitudes and behaviors with others in a group, young people discover that not everyone is drinking, smoking, or taking other drugs, and that use of a psychoactive drug is not necessary to have a good time. Thus, students are freed from the common perception or "normative belief" that they must drink, smoke, or use another drug in order to be popular or socially acceptable.

Personal Commitment

Based on the theory that young people drink because they have a weak commitment to abstain from alcohol or other drug use, the **personal commitment** strategy encourages students to voluntarily make public or private pledges not to use or abuse alcohol, tobacco, or any other mind-changing drug. The act of pledging increases one's personal commitment not to engage in drinking, using tobacco, or drug taking.

Values

Use of the values plan assumes that young people who drink, use tobacco products, or take some other drug believe that the psychoactive substance is compatible with their personal values. Through various **values clarification** exercises, students are challenged to find conflicts between existing personal values and use of such substances. The intent of this approach is to increase the perception that drinking, smoking, or drug taking is inconsistent with one's personal lifestyle.

Information

The information plan is based on the assumption that drug-taking behavior is the result of one's unawareness of the consequences of alcohol and other drug use and abuse. By providing basic facts about the negative health and social consequences of using and abusing various psychoactive drugs, students increase their feelings of personal vulnerability to the hazards of drinking, smoking, and using other drugs, and thus continue to abstain or delay further use until a later time.

Resistance Skills

Peer pressure is thought to be a major reason why young people start using alcohol and other drugs. A curriculum featuring the development of **resistance skills** teaches students how to identify both peer and media pressures to drink, smoke, chew tobacco, or use some other drug, and how to cope with pressure situations (see box 14.2). By building a cognitive understanding of pro-alcohol influences and developing refusal (resistance) skills regarding the use of various drugs, students will strengthen their belief that they can effectively deal with such pressures.

Alternatives

The alternatives strategy, based on the idea that drug use is the result of a basic unawareness of alternatives to mind-changing drugs for enjoyment, provides young people with information about other, non-drug means for achieving excitement and having fun. Such a plan supposedly decreases the motivation to use alcohol, tobacco products, or other drugs to achieve desired mood states.

Goal Setting

Based on the theory that some young people use drugs because they lack basic goals in life, the goal-setting skills strategy teaches students a system for setting and achieving goals, and motivates them to set and then work on manageable goals and ambitions. In addition to increasing one's goal-setting ability, this strategy also attempts to increase one's feeling of achievement.

Decision Making

Because young people sometimes drink or take drugs due to their inability to make reasoned decisions, the **decision-making** curricular plan teaches students a system for organizing information and making choices among alternatives. The strategy's basic intention is to increase the frequency with which reason is used in making choices about using alcohol and other drugs or interacting with those who use these substances, such as deciding to ride (or refusing to ride) in a car with a drinking driver (see box 14.3).

Self-Esteem Enhancement

To increase their feelings of self-worth and better value their personal identity, the self-esteem-enhancement curricular plan encourages students to understand how internal and external events affect self-concept and feelings of self-worth. Students are helped to discover ways to deal with negative feelings toward themselves.

Stress Skills

Because drinking and other drug use are sometimes linked with poor coping skills, students are taught a variety of ways to relax under stress, to cope with pressure, and to resolve problems. With increased ability to cope with anxieties and tension, students can often reduce their stress levels.

Life Skills

The **life-skills** strategy teaches students how to be assertive, how to resolve interpersonal

Just Say No: A Peer Resistance Skill

In general, making decisions about using alcohol, tobacco, and other drugs will be easier for young people if they are familiar with the pressures that tempt them to try a drug. When people pressure others to start drinking, or smoking, or using another drug, they are really saying, "Don't think for yourself, just do what we do." Being independent means making one's own decisions. When the facts are known along with the risks of using various drugs, personal decisions will be easier. Remember, you always have the right to say no to a mind-changing drug.

Here are some suggestions on how to do it.

1. MAKE IT SIMPLE. Just say no. No explanations. If "No, thanks" doesn't work the first time, say it again or more strongly say, "No way!" Keep your refusal simple.

2. KNOW THE FACTS ABOUT DANGEROUS DRUGS. Then you can say, "No, I know it's bad for me. I'm not interested."

3. HAVE SOMETHING ELSE TO DO. In this way you can delay your decision. Say, "No thanks. I'm going to the movies. Do you want to go?"

4. WALK AWAY FROM THREATENING SITUATIONS. Be prepared for different forms of peer pressure. It can start out friendly or teasing; if so, you can respond the same way, but still say no. When the pressure seems threatening, just walk away.

5. AVOID THE SITUATION. If you know of places where people often use alcohol or other drugs, stay away. If you hear that people will be using alcoholic beverages or other drugs at a party, don't go.

6. CHANGE THE SUBJECT. If someone says, "Try this," in reply you might say, "No thanks. By the way, how did you do on the math test yesterday?"

7. HANG OUT WITH FRIENDS WHO DON'T DO DRUGS. You might already have friends who use alcoholic beverages or other drugs. Maybe, by saying no, you might make them think twice about doing drugs in the future. That's how peer pressure can be positive too.

8. BE A BROKEN RECORD. In a calm yet firm manner, state your position of not using drugs and then keep repeating it without showing anger or irritation and without giving reasons for not using alcohol or some other drug. Say, "No, no, no, no, no, no, no thanks! So long! No thanks! No, no, no, no, no, no, no thanks!"

9. USE THE "FOGGING TECHNIQUE" OF PASSIVE RESISTANCE. Simply agree with any criticism made about your nonuse, while not becoming defensive in any way. Even when your friends start calling you threatening names, continue to "stand your ground" and refuse to use the drug.

10. REFUSE TO CONTINUE THE DISCUSSION ABOUT DRUG USE. Tell your friends you are asserting your right to say no and that you are not going to talk about alcohol or other drugs anymore.

Source: Modified in part from the National Institute on Drug Abuse.

---

conflicts, and how to communicate more effectively with others. With these newly acquired life skills, students improve their ability to maintain social relations without the use of alcohol, tobacco, or other drugs.

Some Concluding Thoughts

It is now apparent that no single curriculum or teaching strategy is adequate to prevent alcohol use and abuse in all school populations. There is no one "magic instructional bullet"! Nevertheless, research now reveals that there is a tendency for successful alcohol and drug prevention education programs to include a combination of normative beliefs, personal commitment, information on various mind-changing drugs and their potential effects, and resistance skills strategies, as well as one or two other strategies, such as valuing and values clarification.[11] Another study indicates that drug-abuse prevention programs conducted in junior high school (fifteen classes in grade 7, with ten booster sessions in grade 8 and five additional booster sessions in grade 9) can produce meaningful and durable reductions in tobacco, alcohol, and marijuana use, if they (1) teach a combination of social resistance skills and general life skills, (2) are properly implemented, and (3) include at least two years of booster sessions.[12]

Based upon an analysis of current educational programs for the prevention of ATOD use and abuse, the following general principles emerge as important components in designing and implementing curricula:[13–16]

1. Kindergarten through grade 12 ATOD prevention education should

box 14.3

Making Decisions About Alcohol and Other Drugs

INTRODUCTION: This activity measures adolescent and preadolescent students' abilities to identify the steps in a systematic decision-making process. Although decision making may be described in many ways, this particular measure views the systematic process as involving five steps:

1. identifying or clarifying the decision to be made;
2. identifying possible decision options;
3. gathering/processing information;

4. making/implementing the decision; and
5. evaluating the decision.

This structured decision-making instrument evaluates this model only and should not be applied in evaluating general decision-making ability.

DIRECTIONS: Read each of the following stories about young people who are trying to make decisions. CIRCLE THE LETTER of the NEXT THING that the person should do in order to make the best decision. If you are unsure what the person should do, CIRCLE DON'T KNOW.

1. Jane has seen kids smoking in the restrooms at lunch and out on the playground after school. Some of Jane's friends have even tried smoking cigarettes. She figures that her friends may ask her to try a cigarette soon.

What should Jane do NEXT in order to make a good decision?
A. Ask her best friend what she should do.
B. Decide to try smoking just one cigarette.
#C. Know that she must decide whether to smoke cigarettes or not.
D. Don't know.

2. Mark tried smoking marijuana with some friends a few months ago. Since then he has started smoking more and more. He even smokes before school sometimes. Mark is not doing as well in school as he used to. He is worried that his grades will go down and his parents will get mad. He thinks it may have something to do with smoking marijuana too much. He wants to find a way to stop.

What should Mark do NEXT in order to make a good decision?
A. Decide to find new friends who do not smoke.
#B. Call a hotline for help about ways to stop smoking marijuana.
C. Know he must decide on a way to stop smoking marijuana.
D. Don't know.

3. Donna and her best friend want to go to the school dance Friday night, but they need a ride. Her friend's dad will be able to take them to the dance, but can't pick them up. Donna's older brother is going out with his friend the same night and said he would pick them up. Donna knows her brother likes to drink beer with his friends. She must decide whether or not to ride home with her brother. Donna and her friend think about what they could do. They could get a ride with Donna's brother or try to find another ride. If they can't find another ride they might not be able to go to the dance. Donna asks some questions in her health class about drinking and driving.

What should Donna do NEXT in order to make a good decision?
A. Know she must decide whether to get a ride from her brother.
B. Have her friend decide whether they should get a ride with her.
#C. Decide whether to get a ride home from the dance with her brother.
D. Don't know.

Source: Modified from *Program Evaluation Handbook: Alcohol Abuse Education*, pages 110–121, Center for Health Promotion and Education, Centers for Disease Control, and Prevention, 1988.
= the most appropriate response

be an integral part of a comprehensive school health education program.

2. In dealing with the adverse consequences of ATOD use in young people, concentrate on the immediate effects on the human being, and on the use of alcohol and drugs as a major obstacle to

responsible behavior, and reduce feelings that the risks of drug taking "cannot happen to me."

3. Provide accurate information on the effects of psychoactive drugs, especially in relation to one's inhibitions and drinking and driving, and on laws governing use

of alcohol and other drugs, as well as on the perceived benefits of ATOD use.

4. In both elementary and secondary school, provide educational programs on ATOD use with appropriate, planned, and sequential lessons and activities for all students

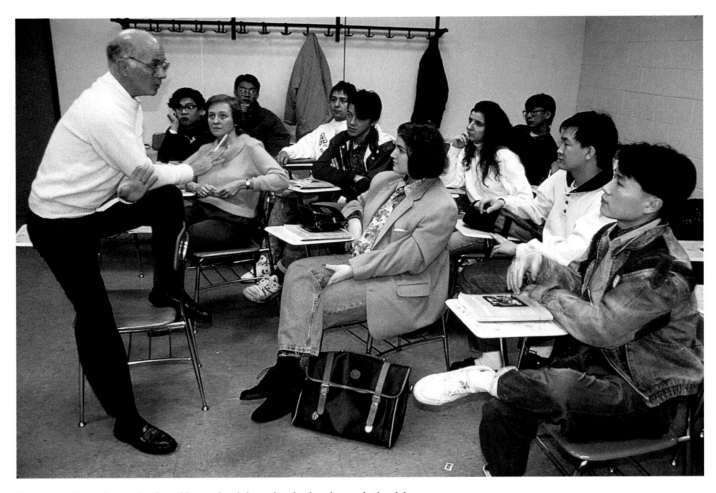

Small group discussions under the guidance of an informed, trained, and empathetic adult are among the most effective ATOD education methods. Here an adult counselor discusses ways for young people to cope with peers and social pressure to use alcohol, tobacco, and other drugs.

© Jeff Greenberg/The Picture Cube, Inc.

at every grade level. Instruction is especially effective when it begins early in life and is continuous.

5. Emphasize that the unlawful possession and use of alcoholic beverages and other drugs is wrong and potentially harmful.

6. In addition to school health education, ATOD education can also be correlated with other subject areas, including sciences, social studies, language arts, psychology, current events, home economics, and driver education.

7. Include information on family and peer norms regarding use,

acceptability, and unacceptability. Point out that most youths are not using alcohol or other drugs on a daily basis. Then use peers to make desirable norms more acceptable.

8. Reinforce peer resistance skills, decision making, problem solving, and social (life) competence skills.

9. Include plans and activities that involve parents and community members in supporting ATOD education in the school.

10. Determine if the learning experiences helped students achieve instructional objectives (see box 14.4).

Resources for ATOD Education

Resources are the "teaching tools" used by instructors to enrich and facilitate learning opportunities dealing with ATOD use and abuse prevention efforts in schools as well as in the community. Books, pamphlets, video tapes, films, projectors, chalkboards, government and private agencies, community groups, and specific individuals who can support an educational program are all examples of teaching resources.

Numerous organizations can provide valuable resource materials and information on various aspects of ATOD use and abuse as well as on ATOD education.

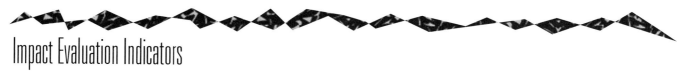

Impact Evaluation Indicators

box 14.4

The Department of Education's Regional Centers for Drug-Free Schools and Communities are responsible for assisting state and local agencies, schools and educators in developing effective prevention programs. They use, and recommend, the following checklist of indicators for evaluating the impact of prevention programs in reducing the use of drugs in schools and in educating students about the dangers of drug use.

Extent to Which Student Body Exhibits Positive Changes in Personal Attitudes, Knowledge, Characteristics and Behavioral Choices Listed Below

- demonstrate positive self-esteem*
- demonstrate refusal skills*
- don't use alcohol/drugs
- engage in self-protective behavior* (e.g., use seat belts)
- have networks of nonusing friends*
- know alcohol/drug use is harmful
- know effect of peer influence*
- show change in attitudes toward peer usage*
- show change in attitudes toward using alcohol/drugs*

Extent to Which Student Body Participates in Alternative Activities

- access to prevention and intervention programs
- are involved in peer leadership programs
- are involved in volunteerism
- participate in drug-free activities, events, and parties (e.g., Project Graduation)
- participate in teen clubs
- take part in peer counseling activities

Extent to Which Student Body Exhibits Positive Changes in the Following Education/Schooling Behaviors

- academic achievement
- high school graduation rates

- participation in sports and extracurricular activities at school
- school attendance
- serving as peer tutors

Positive Changes in Youth-Related Statistics

- admissions for detoxification
- alcohol/drug referrals
- alcohol/drug-related hospital admissions
- arrests
- deaths among children and youth
- DUI/DWI
- liquor law violations
- suicides and attempted suicides
- traffic fatalities
- use/abuse of alcohol/drugs*
- use of tobacco products*

Positive Changes in School-Related Statistics

- alcohol/drug related disciplinary referrals
- dropouts
- expulsions
- suspensions
- tardiness
- truancy/school absenteeism

*Typically ascertained via student surveys
Source: Office of Educational Research and Improvement, U.S. Department of Education.

Some materials are free; others are available for loan, rent, or purchase. There is no shortage of instructional media, although only representative sources have been listed.

Prepackaged ATOD Curricula

Project DARE—A comprehensive curriculum delivered by uniformed police officers and focused on fifth-, sixth-, and seventh-grade students. This drug-abuse resistance education program emphasizes providing

accurate alcohol and other drug information, teaching students decision-making skills, showing them how to resist peer pressure, and giving them ideas for positive alternatives to taking alcohol and other drugs. (See box 14.5.)

BABES—This primary prevention program is designed to give young children, $2\frac{1}{2}$ to 8 years of age, a lifetime of protection from substance abuse. Beginning Alcohol and Addictions Basic Education Studies assists young people to develop

positive living skills and provides them with accurate, nonjudgmental information about the use and abuse of alcohol and other drugs.

Paper People—Intended for elementary students, K–3, this program offers an alcohol and other drug use information base for the general student population and helps school personnel identify high-risk students (such as children of alcoholics) for enhanced early intervention.

An Introduction to DARE: Drug Abuse Resistance Education

box 14.5

The DARE curriculum is organized into 17 classroom sessions conducted by the police officer, coupled with suggested activities taught by the regular classroom teacher. A wide range of teaching activities are used: question-and-answer, group discussion, and role-play and workbook exercises, all designed to encourage student participation and response.

Each lesson is briefly summarized below, giving a sense of the scope of the DARE curriculum and the care taken in its preparation. All of these lessons were pilot tested and revised before widespread use began.

1. **Practices for Personal Safety.** The DARE officer reviews common safety practices to protect students from harm at home, on the way to and from school, and in the neighborhood.
2. **Drug Use and Misuse.** Students learn the harmful effects of drugs if they are misused as depicted in the film *Drugs and Your Amazing Mind*.
3. **Consequences.** Focus is on the consequences of using and not using alcohol and marijuana. If students are aware of those consequences, they can make better informed decisions regarding their own behavior.
4. **Resisting Pressures to Use Drugs.** The DARE officer explains different types of pressure—ranging from friendly persuasion and teasing to threats—that friends and others exert on students to try tobacco, alcohol, or drugs.
5. **Resistance Techniques: Ways to Say No.** Students rehearse the many ways of refusing offers to try tobacco, alcohol, or drugs–simply saying no and repeating it as often as necessary, changing the subject, walking away, or ignoring the person. They learn that they can avoid situations in which they might be subjected to such pressures and can "hang around" with nonusers.
6. **Building Self-Esteem.** Poor self-esteem is one of the factors associated with drug misuse. How students feel about themselves results from positive and negative feelings and experiences. In this session students learn about their own positive qualities and how to compliment other students.
7. **Assertiveness: A Response Style.** Students have certain rights—to be themselves, to say what they think, to say no to offers of drugs. The session teaches them to assert those rights confidently and without interfering with others' rights.
8. **Managing Stress Without Taking Drugs.** Students learn to recognize sources of stress in their lives and techniques for avoiding or relieving stress, including exercise, deep breathing, and talking to others. They learn that using drugs or alcohol to relieve stress causes new problems.
9. **Media Influences on Drug Use.** The DARE officer reviews strategies used in the media to encourage tobacco and alcohol use, including testimonials from celebrities and social pressure.
10. **Decision Making and Risk Taking.** Students learn the difference between bad risks and responsible risks, how to recognize their choices, and how to make a decision that promotes their self-interests.
11. **Alternatives to Drug Abuse.** Students learn that to have fun, to be accepted by peers, or to deal with feelings of anger or hurt, there are a number of alternatives to using drugs and alcohol.
12. **Role Modeling.** A high school student selected by the DARE officer with the assistance of the high school staff visits the class, providing students with a positive role model. Students learn that drug users are in the minority.
13. **Forming a Support System.** Students learn that they need to develop positive relationships with many different people to form a support system.
14. **Ways to Deal With Pressures From Gangs.** Students discuss the kinds of pressures they may encounter from gang members and evaluate the consequences of the choices available to them.
15. **DARE Summary.** Students summarize and assess what they have learned.
16. **Taking a Stand.** Students compose and read aloud essays on how they can respond when they are pressured to use drugs and alcohol. The essay represents each student's "DARE Pledge."
17. **Culmination.** In a schoolwide assembly planned in concert with school administrators, all students who have participated in DARE receive certificates of achievement.

Source: Bureau of Justice Assistance, U.S. Department of Justice.

Picada: 1–5—An elementary program for grades 1 through 5 providing twelve to fifteen days of structured, sequential lessons at each grade level. Emphasis is placed on developing resistance to alcohol and other drugs of abuse, and on building social competencies, enhancing self-esteem, and increasing knowledge of mind-changing chemicals.

Life Skills Training Program—A self-improvement approach to substance-abuse prevention for middle/junior high school students. Emphasis is placed on acquiring skills to resist peer pressure to drink, smoke, or use other drugs, and on making informed decisions, forming healthy relationships, coping with anxiety, and successfully dealing with the challenges of adolescent life.

Project SMART—A self-management and resistance-training program for grades 6 through 9 that teaches students how to deal with pro-drug influences and pressures from commercial ads, public events, adults, and peers. Tobacco, alcohol, and marijuana—the "gateway" drugs—are examined directly, and resistance skills are developed at several levels.

McGruff's Drug Prevention and Child Protection Program—A K–6 curriculum designed to educate children on alcohol and other drug use prevention, safety, and crime prevention. Lessons are structured to develop self-esteem so that children may resist peer pressure.

The Discovery Kit: Positive Connections for Kids—A program built around a multicultural kit of materials to assist schools and communities to reach out to children 10 to 15 years old and provide them with challenging materials to help them live healthy, productive, and drug-free lives. Activities promote "resiliency" among Native American, Hispanic American, and African American children from alcoholic families, by introducing creativity, positive thinking, group participation, problem solving, games, and writing exercises.

Learning to Live Drug Free—A K–12 curriculum model for prevention of alcohol and other drug use, designed by the U.S. Department of Education. This model includes information on child development as related to alcohol and other drugs of abuse, facts about drugs and alcohol, suggested lesson plans, and tips on working with parents and the community. Rather than an example of a comprehensive course curriculum, this model is more of a master plan for including alcohol and other drug use prevention activities into existing courses.

Here's Looking at You, 2000—A K–12 curriculum comprised of more than

150 lessons with extensive instructional media. This program aims to reduce risk factors leading to alcohol and other drug abuse by providing information on "gateway drugs," and by fostering development of social skills, and encouraging the bonding to school and family, while promoting a clear "no use" message.

Decisions About Drinking—A curriculum for grades 3 through 12, formerly known as the CASPAR Alcohol Education Program, that emphasizes active student involvement and offers information and insight into the nature of alcohol, drinking, and drunkenness. Composed of sequential modules, the curriculum follows a spiral pattern and features alcohol use, decision making, and alcoholism by focusing on real-life issues and situations.

Talking With Your Students About Alcohol—A fully compatible parent-school program using the "lifestyle risk reduction" model of prevention. Available initially on three levels (fifth or sixth grade; seventh or eighth grade; and ninth or tenth grade), the school-based curriculum attempts to increase abstinence, delay the onset of drinking, reduce high-risk use among those who have already begun to use alcohol, and increase low-risk attitudes regarding use of alcohol. Communities interested in Talking With Your Students About Alcohol are expected to also implement the Talking With Your Kids About Alcohol program so maximum benefit can be achieved.

Government Agencies

National Clearinghouse for Alcohol and Drug Information
P.O. Box 2345
Rockville, MD 20847–2345
(800) 729–6686 or (301) 468–2600
(Sponsored by the federal Center for Substance Abuse Prevention, this clearinghouse is the single best source

of free and inexpensive print materials on alcohol, alcohol and drug abuse prevention, and AOD education.)

U.S. Department of Education
Drug Abuse Prevention Oversight Staff
Office of the Secretary
400 Maryland Avenue, SW
Room 4145, MS 6411
Washington, DC 20202

U.S. Department of Justice
Drugs & Crime Data Center & Clearinghouse
Bureau of Justice Statistics
1600 Research Boulevard
Rockville, MD 20850
(800) 666–3332

U.S. Department of Transportation
National Highway Traffic Safety Administration
Office of Traffic Safety Programs
400 Seventh Street, SW, Room 5130
Washington, DC 20590

State Department of Education

State Department of Health

State Drug Abuse Prevention Agency

State Prevention Resource Center
(See box 14.6 for a listing of the Regional Alcohol and Drug Awareness Resource [RADAR] Network, consisting of state clearinghouses and specialized information centers of national organizations.)

Private, Voluntary Agencies, Associations, and Companies

Al-Anon Family Groups
World Service Office
P.O. Box 862, Midtown Station
New York, NY 10018–0862

Alcoholics Anonymous (AA)
World Service Office
475 Riverside Drive
New York, NY 10115

American Council for Drug Education
204 Monroe Street
Suite 110
Rockville, MD 20850

The RADAR Network

box 14.6

A new communication resource was established in 1988 to provide communities with information, publications, and services for combating alcohol and other drug problems. Known as the Regional Alcohol and Drug Awareness Resource (**RADAR**) **Network,** this nationwide intercommunication system features an office in each state that has access to the federal Center for Substance Abuse Prevention (CSAP). This network allows the public and professional groups to obtain information and services previously available only from the federal government.

RADAR centers answer information requests, house a resource center, and facilitate networking among groups involved in prevention of alcohol and other drug problems. They also keep CSAP up to date by providing information about prevention activites, and local trends in alcohol and other drug use.

State RADAR Network Centers

Alaska Council on Prevention of
Alcohol and Drug Abuse, Inc.
3333 Denali Street, Suite 201
Anchorage, AK 99503
(907) 258–6021

Division of Substance Abuse Services
Alabama Department of Mental
Health/Mental Retardation
200 Interstate Park Drive
P.O Box 3710
Montgomery, AL 36193
(205) 270–4648

Bureau of Alcohol and Drug Abuse
Prevention
Freeway Medical Center
5800 West 10th Street, Suite 907
Little Rock, AR 72204
(501) 280–4506

Department of Human Resources,
Social Service Division
Drugs and Alcohol Program
Government of American Samoa
Pago Pago, AS 96799
(684) 633-4485

Arizona Prevention Resource Center
Arizona State University
Box 871708
Tempe, AZ 85287–1708
(520) 965–9666

State of California
Department of Alcohol and Drug
Programs
1700 K Street, 1st Floor
Sacramento, CA 95814–4022
(916) 327–3009

Colorado Department of Human
Services
ADAD-PI-A2
4300 Cherry Creek Drive, S.
Denver, CO 80222–1530
(303) 692–2930

Connecticut Clearinghouse
334 Farmington Avenue
Plainville, CT 06062
(203) 793–9791

D.C. Alcohol and Drug Abuse Services
Administration
Office of Information, Prevention and
Education
2146 24th Place, NE
Washington, DC 20018
(202) 576–7315

Office of Prevention
Department of Services for Children,
Youth, and Their Families
1825 Faulkland Road
Wilmington, DE 19805–1195
(302) 633–2682

Florida Alcohol and Drug Abuse
Association, Inc.
1030 E. Lafayette Street, Suite 100
Tallahassee, FL 32301–4547
(904) 878–2196

Georgia Prevention Resource Center
Substance Abuse Services
2 Peachtree Street
4th Floor, Suite 320
Atlanta, GA 30303
(404) 657–2296

Department of Mental Health and
Substance Abuse
709 Governor Carlos G. Camacho
Road
P.O. Box 9400
Tamuning, GU 96911
(671) 646-9260

Coalition for Drug-Free Hawaii
Prevention Resource Center
1218 Waimanu Street
Honolulu, HI 96814
(808) 593–2221

Iowa Substance Abuse Information
Center
Cedar Rapids Public Library
500 First Street, SE
Cedar Rapids, IA 52401
(319) 398–5133

Boise State University
Idaho RADAR Network Center
1910 University Drive
Boise, ID 83725
(208) 385–3471

Prevention Resource Center Library
822 South College
Springfield, IL 62704
(217) 525–3456

Indiana University
Indiana Prevention Resource Center
840 State Road, 46 Bypass
Room 110
Bloomington, IN 47405
(812) 855–1237

Kansas Alcohol and Drug Abuse
Services
Department of Social and
Rehabilitation Services
300 S. W. Oakley
Topeka, KS 66606
(913) 296–3925

continued

Drug Information Services for
Kentucky
Division of Substance Abuse
275 E. Main Street
Frankfort, KY 40621
(502) 564–2880

Louisiana Office of Alcohol and Drug
Abuse
P.O. Box 3868
Baton Rouge, LA 70821–3868
(504) 342–9352

Prevention Support Services
The Medical Foundation
95 Berkeley Street, Suite 201
Boston, MA 02116
(617) 451–0049

Alcohol and Drug Abuse
Administration
Department of Health and Mental
Hygiene
201 W. Preston Street, 4th Floor
Baltimore, MD 21201
(410) 225–6914

Office of Substance Abuse
Information Resource Center
State House Station #57
Augusta, ME 04333
(207) 624–6528

Michigan Substance Abuse and Traffic
Safety Information Center
2409 East Michigan
Lansing, MI 48912–4019
(517) 482–9902

Minnesota Prevention Resource
Center
2829 Verndale Avenue
Anoka, MN 55303
(612) 427–5310

Missouri Division of Alcohol and
Drug Abuse
1706 East Elm Street
P.O. Box 687
Jefferson City, MO 65102
(314) 751–4942

Mississippi Department of Mental
Health
Division of Alcoholism and Drug
Abuse
239 North Lamar Street
1101 Robert E. Lee Building, 9th Floor
Jackson, MS 39201
(601) 359–1288

Alcohol and Drug Abuse Division
Department of Corrections
1539 11th Avenue
Helena, MT 59620
(406) 444–1202

North Carolina Alcohol and Drug
Resource Center
3109-A University Drive
Durham, NC 27707–3703
(919) 493–2881

North Dakota Prevention Resource
Center
North Dakota Division of Alcohol and
Drug Abuse
1839 East Capital Avenue
Bismarck, ND 58501–2152
(701) 328–2769

Alcohol and Drug Information
Clearinghouse
650 J. Street, Suite 215
Lincoln, NE 68510
(402) 474–1992

New Hampshire Office of Alcohol and
Drug Abuse Prevention
State Office Park, South
105 Pleasant Street
Concord, NH 03301
(603) 271–6100

New Jersey State Department of
Health
Division of Alcoholism and Drug
Abuse and Addiction Services
129 East Hanover Street
Trenton, NJ 08625–0362
(609) 984–6961

Department of Health/BHSD-DSA
1190 St. Francis Drive, Room N3200
Santa Fe, NM 87502–6110
(505) 827–2601

Bureau of Alcohol and Drug Abuse
505 E. King Street, Suite 500
Carson City, NV 89710
(702) 687–6239

New York State Office of Alcoholism
and Substance Abuse Services
1450 Western Avenue
Albany, NY 12203–3526
(518) 473–3460

Ohio Department of Alcohol and
Drug Addiction Services
2 Nationwide Plaza
280 N. High Street, 12th Floor
Columbus, OH 43216–2537
(614) 466–6379

Oklahoma State Department of
Mental Health and Substance Abuse
Services
1200 N.E. 13th Street, 2nd Floor
P.O. Box 53277
Oklahoma City, OK 73117
(405) 522–3810

Oregon Prevention Resource Center
(OPRC)
Office of Alcohol and Drug Abuse
Programs
Oregon Department of Human
Resources
500 Summer Street, NE
Salem, OR 97310–1016
(503) 378–8000

Pennsylvania Substance Abuse
Information Center
Columbus Square
652 W. 17th Street
Erie, PA 16502
(814) 459–0245

Administracion de Servicios de Salud
Mental Y Contra a Addicion
414 Barbosa Avenue
Hato Rey, PR 00928
(809) 767–5990

Rhode Island Department of
Substance Abuse
P.O. Box 20363
Cranston, RI 02920
(401) 464–2191

South Carolina Commission on
Alcohol and Drug Abuse
The Drug Store Information
Clearinghouse
3700 Forest Drive, Suite 300
Columbia, SC 29204
(803) 734–9559

South Dakota Divison of Alcohol and
Substance Abuse
3800 E. Highway 34
C/O 500 E. Capitol
Pierre, SD 57501–5070
(605) 773–3123

Tennessee Alcohol and Drug
Association Statewide Clearinghouse
545 Mainstream Drive, Suite 404
Nashville, TN 37228
(615) 244–7066

Texas Commission on Alcohol and
Drug Abuse
Resource Library and Clearinghouse
710 Brazos Street
Austin, TX 78701–2576
(512) 867–8821

Utah State Division of Substance
Abuse
Department of Human Services
120 North 200 West, 4th Floor
Room 413
Salt Lake City, UT 84103
(801) 538–3939

Virginia Department of Mental Health
Office of Prevention
P.O. Box 1797
Richmond, VA 23214
(804) 371–7564

Division of Mental Health
Prevention Unit
#6 & 7 Estate Diamond Ruby
Charles Harwood Hospital
Richmond St. Croix, VI 00820
(809) 774–7700

Office of Alcohol and Drug Abuse
Programs
103 S. Main Street
Waterbury, VT 05671–1701
(802) 241–2178

Washington State Substance Abuse
Coalition
12729 N.E. 20th, Suite 18
Bellevue, WA 98005–1906
(206) 637–7011

Wisconsin Clearinghouse
1552 University Avenue
Madison, WI 53705
(608) 262–9157

West Virginia Library Commission
RADAR Network Clearinghouse
Cultural Center
Charleston, WV 25305
(304) 558–2041

Wyoming Care Program
University of Wyoming
McWhinnie Hall, Room 115
P.O. Box 3374
Laramie, WY 82071–3374
(307) 766–4119

American School Health Association
P.O. Box 708
Kent, OH 44240

ARIS (Alcohol Research Information
Service)
1106 E. Oakland Avenue
Lansing, MI 48906

ASH (Action on Smoking
and Health)
2013 H Street, NW
Washington, D.C. 20006

Association for the Advancement
of Health Education
1900 Association Drive
Reston, VA 22091

CompCare Publications
2415 Annapolis Lane
Minneapolis, MN 55441

Do It Now Foundation
P.O. Box 21126
Phoenix, AZ 85036

ETR Associates
P.O. Box 1830
Santa Cruz, CA 95061–1830

Films for the Humanities & Sciences
P.O. Box 2053
Princeton, NJ 08543–2053

Hazelden Foundation
Pleasant Valley Road
P.O. Box 176
Center City, MN 55012

Just Say No Foundation
1777 North California Boulevard
Walnut Creek, CA 94596

Mothers Against Drunk Driving
(MADD)
669 Air Port Freeway, Suite 310
Hurst, TX 76053

National Congress of Parents and
Teachers
700 North Rush Street
Chicago, Il 60611–2571

National Council on Alcoholism and
Drug Dependence, Inc.
12 West 21st Street
New York, NY 10010

Parents' Resource Institute for Drug
Education (PRIDE)
50 Hurt Plaza, Suite 210
Atlanta, GA 30303

Rutgers University Center of Alcohol
Studies
Publications Division
P.O. Box 969
Piscataway, NJ 08855

Students Against Driving Drunk
P.O. Box 800
277 Main Street
Marlboro, MA 01752

Sunburst Communications
39 Washington Avenue
P.O. Box 40
Pleasantville, NY 10570–0040

Self-Help Groups

Alcoholics Anonymous
World Service Office
475 Riverside Drive
New York, NY 10115
(see local telephone directory)

Al-Anon Family Groups
World Service Office
P.O. Box 862, Midtown Station
New York, NY 10018–0862
(see local telephone directory)

Cocaine Anonymous
World Service Office
3740 Overland Avenue, Suite H
Los Angeles, CA 90034

Families Anonymous
P.O. Box 528
Van Nuys, CA 91408

Nar-Anon Family Group
Headquarters
P.O. Box 2562
Palos Verdes Peninsula, CA 90274

Narcotics Anonymous
World Service Office
P.O. Box 9999
Van Nuys, CA 91409

National Association for Adult
Children of Alcoholics
P.O. Box 35623
Los Angeles, CA 90035

National Association for Children of
Alcoholics
11426 Rockville Pike
Rockville, MD 20852

Potsmokers Anonymous
316 E. Third Street
New York, NY 10009

Rational Recovery Systems
P.O. Box 100
Lotus, CA 95651

Secular Organizations for Sobriety
P.O. Box 5
Buffalo, NY 14215–0005

TOUGHLOVE
P.O. Box 1069
Doylestown, PA 18901

Women for Sobriety
P.O. Box 618
Quakertown, PA 18951

Local Community Organizations and Individuals

Alcohol and drug treatment agencies
Community mental health centers
Hospital clinics on chemical
    dependency
Intervention programs for alcohol-
    impaired drivers
Members of Alcoholics Anonymous,
Al-Anon, Alateen, Narcotics
Anonymous
National Council on Alcoholism and
Drug Dependence, Inc., local affiliate
Psychologists, social workers, and
    counselors

ATOD-Related Periodicals

Addiction & Recovery: The Alcohol
    & Drug Publication
Alcohol, Drugs and Driving
Alcohol Health & Research World
American Journal of Drug and
    Alcohol Abuse
The Bottom Line on Alcohol in Society
The Drinking and Drug Practices
    Surveyor
Journal of Adolescent Chemical
    Dependency
Journal of Alcohol and Drug
    Education
Journal of Drug Education
Journal of Drug Issues
Journal of Psychoactive Drugs: A
    Multidisciplinary Forum
Journal of Studies on Alcohol
Journal of Substance Abuse
Prevention File: Alcohol, Tobacco &
    Other Drugs
Prevention Pipeline: An Alcohol and
    Drug Awareness Service
Psychology of Addictive Behaviors
Social History of Alcohol Review: The
    Journal of the Alcohol and
    Temperance History Group
Substance Abuse: Official Publication
    of the Association for Medical
    Education and Research in
    Substance Abuse
Traffic Safety

School Policies on Alcohol and Other Drugs

Instructional planning is an important and necessary step in the successful implementation of an alcohol and other drug use prevention program. However, the planned learning experiences of the curriculum should be seen as only one phase in the school's overall approach to the prevention and management of alcohol and other drug problems.

Before schools can engage in alcohol and other drug education effectively, the community and the professionals involved in working with young people need to establish a **comprehensive policy against alcohol and other drug use** and abuse that is strong, "clearly articulated, consistently enforced, and broadly communicated."[17]

Elements of a Comprehensive Policy

An effective alcohol and drug prevention policy needs to address issues of school security, student access to and distribution and use of illegal substances, use of security police and undercover agents, alcohol and drug seizures by faculty, reporting of suspected alcohol- and other drug-related behavior, alcohol and drug overdoses and emergency actions, in-service training of school staff, due process for student violators, limits on confidentiality, and student involvement in policy development.[18] It is also necessary that such a policy and its implementing procedures addressing the several issues noted above be revised regularly and administered fairly.

Additional elements for inclusion in a comprehensive alcohol and other drug prevention policy include the following:[19]

1. A clear statement that alcohol and other drugs and their use are prohibited on the school campus, at school-sponsored functions, and while students are representing the school.

2. A description of the consequences to be expected upon violating the policy, as well as the conditions for reinstatement of students who are disciplined or in treatment programs.

3. Appropriate assistance for students when intervention or follow-up is required within the school due to alcohol and other drug use.

4. Reciprocal communication between school and service agencies that treat alcohol and other drug problems.

5. Lines of communication with the home concerning either suspected or known student alcohol or drug problems.

6. Assurance that school policies on alcohol and other drug use are widely distributed, understood, and made applicable to the needs of the entire school population—school personnel, students, parents, and school board members.

7. A confidential process for referral of identified students and/or their families to qualified human service agencies or treatment programs.

8. Additional resources, such as alternative school programs, for dealing with students who have alcohol and other drug problems.

Student Assistance Programs

School personnel are sometimes reluctant to intervene in cases of student alcohol and other drug use because of the perceived lack of administrative support, feelings of vulnerability to legal sanction, and fear of retaliation by parents and students. Faculty and staff may also be hesitant to get involved with students' drug-related problems unless there is some mechanism for implementing a school's policy on alcohol and other drugs. Such a mechanism has evolved as **student assistance programs**.[20]

Student assistance programs (SAPs) are a relatively new approach for intervening in and preventing alcohol and other drug problems among school-age youth. Modeled after the employee assistance programs found in business and industry, student assistance programs focus on behavior and performance at school and use a referral process that includes screening

by teachers and other school personnel for alcohol and other drug involvement. Student assistance programs also work with self-referred youth.

As a partnership between community health agencies and the schools, SAPs address a number of important concerns. First, they approach alcohol and other drug use as a problem that affects a student's entire development. Second, they offer a strategy for eliminating alcohol and other drug use both during and after school hours. Third, they give school staff a mechanism for helping youth with a wide range of problems that may contribute to alcohol and other drug use. Lastly, SAPs can offer assistance to students who are suffering adverse effects from parental alcohol or other drug use.

Although the components and people responsible for them vary widely, the following activities are found in nearly every school with a student assistance program:

Early detection of student problems

Referrals to designated "helpers" within the school

In-school services (support groups, individual counseling)

Referral to outside agencies (mental health centers or clinics, private physicians, psychologists, family service organizations, Alcoholics Anonymous)

Follow-up monitoring once the student has returned after counseling, treatment, or rehabilitation

Teachers and other school personnel are advised and trained to identify students experiencing problems that interfere with their functioning at school. However, they are not expected to specify the nature of the problem or to intervene personally. Students are referred to appropriate assessment and assistance resources. Regardless of the mix of responsibilities and personnel centered in a student assistance program, the endorsement of the school board, principals, and community leaders is critical to the success of the program.

Chapter Summary

1. Traditionally, school-based ATOD education has been confined to classroom activities in elementary and secondary schools. However, general and specific nonschool populations can now be reached by mass-media campaigns, community-wide supply or demand reduction programs, worksite employee efforts, policy and legislative initiatives, and the training of health care professionals.

2. In addition to providing information about alcohol and other drugs and the consequences of their use, expanded ATOD prevention education programs also try to raise awareness and involvement in the local community, increase the knowledge base of teachers and parents, change students' norms and expectations, enhance parenting and positive family influences, and improve student coping, peer resistance, and decision-making skills. Such programs can also increase parental involvement in schools, expand student participation in legal alternatives to ATOD use, and deter use through regulation and legal actions.

3. The major goals of ATOD education are to reduce the extent of alcohol, tobacco, and other drug use, and to prevent alcohol-, tobacco-, and other drug-related problems from occurring in the future.

4. Among the Healthy People 2000 objectives—measurable targets to be achieved by the year 2000—are the reduction of ATOD usage, especially underage drinking and heavy alcohol use, increasing the average age of first use of alcohol and marijuana among young people, increasing the proportion of youth who perceive great risk of harm and social disapproval associated with ATODs, and a reduction in the initiation of smoking by young people.

5. A systematic plan for designing and implementing alcohol education consists of the following steps: needs assessment, identification of strategies, anticipation of instructional problems, development of goals, selection of subject matter, formulation of instructional objectives, selection of methods, identification of resources, development of evaluation procedures, and revision of the instructional program.

6. Curriculum strategies used in ATOD education programs include strategies focusing on normative beliefs, personal commitment, values, information, resistance skills, alternatives, goal setting, decision making, self-esteem enhancement, and the development of stress skills and life skills.

7. Resources, the "teaching tools" of instructors, include various prepackaged curricula, government agencies (especially the National Clearinghouse for Alcohol and Drug Information and the state-level prevention resource centers in the RADAR Network), private, voluntary agencies and companies, self-help groups (including Alcoholics Anonymous), local community organizations, and periodicals related to alcohol and other drugs.

8. In addition to ATOD education, schools need a comprehensive policy against alcohol and other drug use that addresses such issues as school security, student access to and distribution and use of illegal substances, alcohol and drug seizures, reporting of suspected alcohol- and other drug-related behavior, in-service training of school staff, due process for student violators, and limits of confidentiality.

9. A relatively new approach for intervening in and preventing alcohol and other drug problems among school-age youth is the student assistance program, modeled after the relatively successful employee assistance programs in business and industry.

Review Questions and Activities

1. Identify examples of "nonschool" alcohol and other education activities in the local community by analyzing newspapers, magazines, and public service announcements on radio and television, by locating businesses and industries that sponsor employee assistance programs and wellness programs, and by interviewing directors of local alcohol and other drug treatment programs. Also determine if there is a local affiliate of the National Council on Alcoholism and Drug Dependence, Inc. How does this organization promote education on alcohol and other drugs?

2. Procure a copy of the laws in your state that pertain to underage drinking; possession of alcoholic beverages, tobacco products, and other illegal drugs; and requirements for alcohol, tobacco and other drug education in the schools. Share your findings with other class members.

3. How would a modern, comprehensive approach to alcohol and other drug prevention education differ from a traditional school-based program that focused on the evil and harmful effects of alcohol and drinking, and using tobacco and other illegal drugs?

4. Why do the goals of ATOD education in the elementary and secondary schools rarely, if ever, mention responsible use, responsible drinking, or low-risk ways of using marijuana or other illegal drugs as desirable outcomes?

5. List the ten steps in the systematic curriculum planning process described in this chapter. Then, consult other curriculum planning texts (such as Joyce Fetro's *Step by Step to Substance Use Prevention* [Santa Cruz, CA: Network Publications, 1991]) for a comparison of the steps of various planning processes. Identify both differences and similarities.

6. Distinguish among teaching strategies based on the following: normative beliefs, personal commitment, values, information, resistance skills, alternatives, goal setting, decision making, self-esteem enhancement, stress skills, and life skills.

7. After procuring copies of alcohol, tobacco, and other drug education curricula from local schools, determine what major strategies, designs, or methods are utilized more frequently. If a particular prepackaged curriculum has been adopted, ask the school's ATOD education coordinator or the school principal why such a curriculum was adopted.

8. State several general principles that can be used in guiding the design and implementation of a school-based ATOD education program.

9. What specific advice could you offer to a young person who asks for help in saying no to drinking alcoholic beverages, or using a tobacco product or some other illegal drug?

10. Contact your State Prevention Resource Center to determine what types of information and other resources are now available for individuals and schools conducting alcohol and other drug education programs.

11. Interview a local police officer who has been trained to conduct the Drug Abuse Resistance Education (DARE) program in the schools. Determine what emphasis is placed on preventing use of alcohol in comparison with other drug usage. What curriculum strategies, designs, and methods are featured in the DARE program?

12. The following activity is a proposed class project to be undertaken only with the permission and cooperation of local school administrators. Using the publication *Prevention Plus III: Assessing Alcohol and Other Drug Prevention Programs at the School and Community Level* (see this chapter's references), conduct an assessment of a local school district's program of alcohol and other drug education activities. Use some of the assessment procedures described in this publication.

13. Examine the following texts—among others—to identify at least ten recommended methods appropriate for ATOD education in various grade levels in both elementary and secondary schools:

Patricia Gerne and Timothy Gerne. 1991. *Substance Abuse Prevention Activities for Secondary Students.* Englewood Cliffs, N.J.: Prentice Hall.

Linda Meeks and Philip Heit. 1992. *Comprehensive School Health Education: Totally Awesome Strategies for Teaching Health.* Blacklick, Ohio: Meeks Heit.

Linda Meeks, Philip Heit, and Randy Page. 1994. *Drugs, Alcohol, and Tobacco: Totally Awesome Teaching Strategies.* Blacklick, Ohio: Meeks Heit.

14. Why do you think schools need a comprehensive policy against alcohol and other drug use?

15. What is the value of a student assistance program?

References

1. Judith Funkhouser, Eric Goplerud, and Rosalyn Bass, "Current Status of Prevention Strategies," chapter 2 in *A Promising Future, Alcohol and Other Drug Problem Prevention Services Improvement*, Office for Substance Abuse Prevention Monograph No. 10 (DHHS Publication No. ADM–92–1807), ed. Mary Jansen (Washington, D.C.: U.S. Government Printing Office, 1992), 42.

2. Jean Linney and Abraham Wandersman, *Prevention Plus III: Assessing Alcohol and Other Drug Prevention Programs at the School and Community Level*, an Office for Substance Abuse Prevention publication, DHHS Publication No. ADM–91–1817 (Washington, D.C.: U.S. Government Printing Office, 1991), 20.

3. Ibid., 19.

4. Public Health Service, *Healthy People 2000: National Health Promotion and Disease Prevention Objectives—Summary Report* (Boston: Jones & Bartlett, 1992), 95–97. (Reprinted from DHHS Publication No. PHS–91–50213.)

5. National Center for Health Statistics, *Healthy People 2000 Review 1992* (Hyattsville, Md.: Public Health Service, 1993), 36–39.

6. Antonia Novello, "Focus on Health: Preventing Underage Drinking," *Challenge* (Fall 1992): 2–4.

7. National Institute on Drug Abuse, *Prevention Planning Workbook*, vol. 1 (Washington, D.C.: U.S. Government Printing Office, 1981), 2–4.

8. Center for Substance Abuse Prevention, Substance Abuse and Mental Health Services Administration, *Prevention Plus II: Tools for Creating and Sustaining Drug-Free Communities*, DHHS Publication No. ADM–89–1649 (Washington, D.C.: U.S. Government Printing Office, 1993), 94–164.

9. Mathea Falco, *The Making of a Drug-Free America: Programs That Work* (New York: Times Books, 1992), 33–36.

10. William B. Hansen, "School-Based Alcohol Prevention Programs," *Alcohol Health & Research World* 17, no. 1 (1993): 54–60.

11. Ibid., 58.

12. Gilbert Botvin and others, "Long-Term Follow-Up Results of a Randomized Drug Abuse Prevention Trial in a White Middle-Class Population," *Journal of the American Medical Association* 273, no. 14 (12 April 1995): 1106–12.

13. Center for Substance Abuse Prevention, *Prevention Plus II*, 40–41.

14. Kevin Volkan and Joyce Fetro, "Substance Use Prevention: Implications of Theory and Practice," *Family Life Educator* 8, no. 4 (Summer 1990): 17–23.

15. U.S. Department of Education, *Success Stories from Drug-Free Schools: A Guide for Educators, Parents, and Policymakers* (Washington, D.C.: U.S. Department of Education, 1992), 30.

16. Liane M. Summerfield, "Drug and Alcohol Prevention Education," *ERIC Digest* (March 1991): 1–2.

17. Office of Educational Research and Improvement, *Drug Prevention Curricula: A Guide to Selection and Implementation* (Washington, D.C.: U.S. Department of Education, 1988), 7.

18. John H. Langer, *Problems of Drug Abuse in Schools: The Need for a Consistent Policy*, a paper presented to the Coalition of National Health Education Associations at the Center for Disease Control, Emory University Campus, Atlanta, 25 March 1982.

19. Drug Enforcement Administration, *School Drug Abuse Policy Guidelines*, 2d ed. (Washington, D.C.: U.S. Government Printing Office, and Office of Educational Research and Improvement, 1980), 4–5; and DEA, *Drug Prevention Curricula: A Guide to Selection and Implementation* (Washington, D.C.: U.S. Department of Education, 1988), 3, 7–8.

20. Center for Substance Abuse Prevention, *Prevention Plus II*, 59–61, modified.

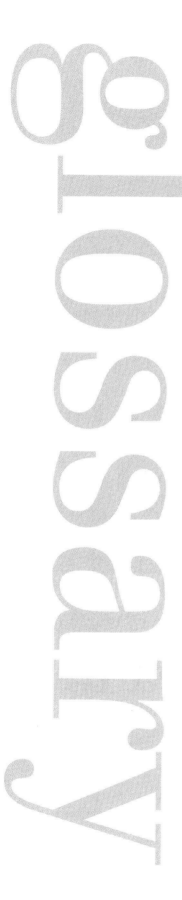

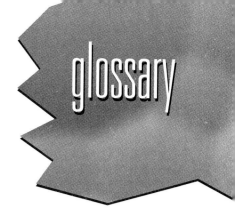

glossary

All terms in this glossary have been defined in relation to drug use, drug misuse, drug abuse and chemical dependency, prevention of substance abuse, or education about psychoactive and nonpsychoactive drugs and medicines.

Absorption passage of a substance from the stomach and intestine into the bloodstream, lymph, and cells.

Abstinence condition of not using a particular substance; refraining from using a drug, such as alcohol.

Acetaminophen an over-the-counter nonsalicylate analgesic and antipyretic drug derived from coal tar and marketed as Tylenol, Datril, and Panadol.

Acquired immune deficiency syndrome (AIDS) serious, life-threatening illness (for which there is no present cure), which involves a breakdown of the body's internal defense system.

Addiction a pattern of behavior characterized by an overwhelming involvement with using a drug and securing its supply, despite adverse consequences associated with use of the drug, and with a significant tendency to relapse after quitting or withdrawal. The term is used frequently to describe drug dependence, chemical dependence, substance abuse; state of psychological or physical need, or both, for a drug, characterized by compulsive use, tolerance, and physical dependence as manifest by withdrawal sickness (withdrawal or abstinence syndrome).

Additive drug reaction type of drug interaction in which two or more drugs that are similar in their general effects produce a cumulative net effect that is the sum of the effects of the individual substances.

Adulteration drug tampering in which cheaper, inferior, or hazardous substances are mixed with a particular drug.

Adverse drug reaction a drug effect other than the intended or anticipated one that is unusual, undesirable, discomforting, or life-threatening.

Agent one sector or element of the public health model of drug-abuse prevention, specifically relating to various drug substances, their content, formulation, distribution, prescription, and availability.

Agent-related etiology theory that relates drug abuse and drug dependence to a specific psychoactive drug, known as the agent.

Alcoholics Anonymous (AA) voluntary fellowship of problem drinkers who desire help in maintaining sobriety.

Alcoholism the disease of alcohol dependence in which an individual cannot consistently exert control over intake of alcohol; pathological pattern of alcohol use marked by impairment in one's social or occupational functioning due to alcohol and either tolerance or withdrawal symptoms.

Alcohol states of consciousness (ASC) various states of altered consciousness during the duration of alcohol's effects, depending on whether the blood-alcohol concentration is increasing or decreasing.

Alternatives approach technique of drug-abuse prevention that provides individuals with attractive, optional nondrug substitutes not only to drugs, but also to drug-using lifestyles.

Ambivalence perception of both positive and negative aspects occurring in the same thing at the same time.

Amotivational syndrome pattern of personality changes observed in some frequent users of marijuana and marked by apathy, lack of concern for the future, and loss of motivation, persisting beyond the period of intoxication.

Amphetamine synthetic central nervous system stimulant with cocainelike effects.

Anabolic-androgenic steroid formerly called anabolic steroids, these synthetic derivatives of testosterone are used to build lean muscle mass and to improve the strength and mechanical effectiveness of skeletal muscles.

Analgesia pain relief.

Analgesic drug taken internally to relieve or lessen pain.

Anorectic (anorexic) drug that tends to curb the appetite.

Antabuse disulfiram, a drug that interferes with alcohol oxidation and prolongs the presence of toxic acetaldehyde in the body, eventually causing severe physical effects. Consequently, Antabuse is used as a deterrent to discourage problem drinkers from resuming alcohol use.

Antagonistic drug reaction drug reaction that results when drugs that are taken together interact so that the effect of either or both agents is blocked or reduced.

Antianxiety agent a "controlled" drug, commonly referred to as a minor tranquilizer, that acts somewhat like a sedative-hypnotic and is useful in treating anxiety and neurotic conditions.

Antidepressant drug, such as an MAO inhibitor or a tricyclic compound, used to elevate mood and relieve certain types of mental depression.

Antihistamine drug that blocks the effects of the allergy chemical, histamine, and relieves sneezing, watery eyes, runny nose, and itching of the nose or throat.

Antihypertensive drug drug used to reduce high blood pressure.

Anti-infective drug drug that inactivates or eliminates invading, disease-causing microbes; antibiotic, antifungal preparation, sulfonamide, and antiseptic.

Antiparaphernalia law law or ordinance restricting or forbidding the sale and/or advertising of items related to use of illegal recreational drugs, such as pipes, bongs, roach clips, and roll-your-own cigarette papers.

Antiparaphernalia movement organized community-based attempt, often led by groups of concerned parents, to lobby for legislation or other governmental action to restrict or prohibit the availability of paraphernalia—articles used in administering, preparing, packaging, and storing drugs.

Antitussive drug preparation that relieves coughing.

Anxiety/panic reaction mental and emotional effects associated with use of drugs, such as marijuana and the psychedelics, that are perceived as unpleasant or undesirable, including panic, paranoid and/or dependency feelings, hallucinations, nonspecific fears, distortion of body image, and aggressive urges.

Aphrodisiac food or drug substance that is alleged to arouse sexual desire or improve sexual performance or response.

Appetite suppressant drug known as a diet aid (anorectic), which helps people curb their appetites, resulting in reduced food intake.

Appetitive drug use drug-taking behavior motivated by the desire for pleasurable responses and sensations.

Aspirin over-the-counter analgesic, antipyretic, and anti-inflammatory drug derived from acetylsalicylic acid and marketed as brand-name aspirin, such as Anacin, Bayer, Bufferin, and Cope.

Attention deficit-hyperactivity disorder brain disorder characterized by extreme motor restlessness, poor attention span, and impulsive and sometimes disorderly behavior. In children, this disorder is sometimes treated with amphetaminelike medications.

Automatism performance of an act, such as taking a medication, without awareness, thus accounting for consumption of multiple doses of a drug leading to an overdose, because an individual had forgotten the ingestion of each prior dose.

Autonomic nervous system a division of the peripheral nervous system that connects the central nervous system to the organs of the body cavity, such as the heart, stomach, and intestines, and whose nerves function automatically without conscious control.

Availability of drugs the physical presence of legal as well as illegal psychoactive drugs that allows people to engage in drug-taking behavior.

Axon nerve fiber that carries electrical impulses away from the cell body of a neuron.

Barbiturate sedative-hypnotic drug derived from barbituric acid and used in medical practice to calm nervous individuals and induce sleep.

Beer alcoholic beverage containing 2–6% alcohol by volume, derived from cereal grains through the brewing process.

Benefit-risk equation principle that in using a drug, the probability of good effects outweighs the possibility of adverse effects, based on the likelihood that absolute safety in drug reactions does not exist.

Benzodiazepine antianxiety drug, such as Librium or Valium, used in medical practice to treat anxiety and various neurotic conditions.

Bioavailability measure of a drug's activity within the body as determined by the quantified levels of that particular drug in the blood.

Bioequivalence characteristic or ability of one drug to produce the same therapeutic effect in the body as an apparently similar medication.

Blackout early warning sign of alcoholism characterized by alcohol-induced amnesia or memory blank-out, but not loss of consciousness.

Blood-alcohol concentration ratio of alcohol present in the blood to the total volume of blood, expressed as a percent; blood-alcohol level.

Blood-brain barrier selective movement of certain substances from the capillaries supplying the brain to nearby nerve cells in the brain. This selective barrier does not prevent psychoactive drugs from having their effects on the brain.

Bootlegging secret and unlawful transportation and sale of beverage alcohol.

Brand-name drug drug product whose generic name has been assigned a trademarked or patented name by a particular pharmaceutical company for advertising and sale.

Breathalyzer one of several instruments used to determine blood-alcohol concentration by measuring the concentration of alcohol in a sample of a drinker's breath.

Bromide first drug introduced as a sedative-hypnotic and used initially as a treatment for epileptic convulsions.

Bronchogenic carcinoma cancerous growth, malignant neoplasm, that arises in the lining of the bronchial tubes of the lungs.

Caffeine bitter tasting, odorless compound extracted from the fruit of the *Coffea arabica* plant, and one of the most widely used central nervous system stimulants.

Caffeinism stimulated condition of chronic poisoning due to overindulgence in caffeine, manifest by mood changes, anxiety, sleep disruption, tremulousness, headache, and ringing in the ears.

Cannabinoid chemical compound found only in cannabis products, particularly tetrahydrocannabinol, or THC.

Cannabis marijuana or any preparation derived from the hemp plant.

Cannabis sativa hemp plant from which marijuana is derived.

Carbon monoxide poisonous component of the gas phase of cigarette smoke that combines with the hemoglobin in red blood cells, thus reducing the oxygen-carrying capacity of the blood.

Carcinoma *in situ* noninvasive cancer; cancerous growth remaining at the site of its origin.

Cardiovascular disease disease of the heart and blood vessels, including coronary heart disease and atherosclerosis.

Cardiovascular drug drug that affects the function of the heart and the blood vessels of the body, including antianginal preparations, antiarrhythmics, digitalis, coronary vasodilators, and vasopressors.

Central nervous system that major part of the nervous system composed of the brain and the spinal cord.

Cerebellum part of the brain, below the cerebrum and behind the pons and medulla, that serves as a reflex center in coordinating and integrating skeletal muscle movements.

Cerebrum largest, most complex part of the brain, which coordinates and interprets internal and external stimuli; site of higher mental functions, i.e., memory and reasoning.

Chemically equivalent drug drug that contains the same amount of the same active ingredient in the same dosage form as contained in generic or brand-name drugs.

Chemotherapy use of drugs to kill or weaken organisms that invade the body or abnormal cells within the body.

Chewing tobacco form of "smokeless tobacco" that is chewed.

Chronic bronchitis chronic obstructive lung disease marked by recurring inflammation of the bronchial tubes with excessive mucus production, persistent cough, and reduced normal lung function.

Chronic obstructive lung disease slow, progressive interruption of the airflow within the lungs due to pulmonary emphysema and chronic bronchitis.

Cigarette a roll of finely cut tobacco or marijuana for smoking, typically enclosed in thin paper.

Ciliary function sweeping movements of cilia, tiny hairlike projections extending from the surface of the bronchial tubes, which sweep mucus and other debris out of the respiratory system into the mouth.

Co-alcoholism a form of co-dependence; the unusual coping mechanisms, attitudes, and behaviors that family members develop in response to a problem-drinking parent, spouse, child, or sibling.

Cocaine powerful central nervous system stimulant of natural origin, extracted from the leaves of the coca plant.

Cocaine psychosis severe, relatively rare psychotic reaction characterized by paranoia and hallucinations resulting from prolonged cocaine use.

Codeine naturally occurring narcotic widely used in medical practice, particularly as an antitussive, which is closely related to morphine but is less potent.

Co-dependence a disease or "subdisease" with various maladaptive behaviors that family members often develop in response to a drug-dependent parent, spouse, child, or sibling.

Cognitive experience psychedelic experience marked by clearness of thought.

Cold turkey process of suddenly quitting the use of a drug, particularly smoking cigarettes.

Combination oral contraceptive drug an oral contraceptive containing small amounts of both female sex hormones, estrogen and progestin.

Comprehensive approaches to drug prevention education community-wide efforts to prevent ATOD use and/or abuse that involve both schools and nonschool initiatives, including mass-media campaigns, law enforcement actions, worksite drug awareness programs, and policy and legislative restrictions.

Comprehensive Drug Abuse Prevention and Control Act legal foundation for reducing consumption of illicit narcotic and nonnarcotic drugs in the United States, enacted by Congress in 1970, in which most psychoactive drugs were categorized into five schedules according to their presumed potential for abuse and their current acceptability in medical practice.

Comprehensive policy against alcohol and other drug use established school policies, in addition to ATOD prevention education, that focus on school security, student access to and distribution and use of illegal substances, use of security police and undercover agents, alcohol and drug seizures by faculty, reporting of suspected alcohol and other drug-related behavior, and in-service training of school staff.

Congeners nonalcoholic substances, besides water, present in minute quantities in all alcoholic beverages.

Controlled drug psychoactive drug or medication having a significant potential for abuse and addiction, and therefore under the regulatory control of the Drug Enforcement Administration.

Controlled Substances Act public law enacted in 1970 that placed most psychoactive substances into one of five schedules according to their abuse potential, likelihood of causing psychic or physical dependence, and current acceptability for medical treatment.

Coping process of adjusting or accommodating to the demands of stress and daily living without being overwhelmed so that one's personal and social effectiveness is maintained.

Coronary heart disease buildup of cholesterol within the coronary arteries that supply the heart muscle.

Crack cocaine a smokable, intensified form of cocaine now considered one of the most addictive substances ever known.

Crashing disturbing period of mental depression occurring when a person stops taking a central nervous system stimulant after a period of chronic drug use.

Craving overwhelming desire to use a drug substance, usually to increase positive feelings and then to decrease negative experience of the withdrawal syndrome.

Cross-dependence condition in which one drug can prevent withdrawal symptoms associated with physical dependence on a different drug.

Cross-tolerance condition in which tolerance to one drug, *A*, results in a lessened pharmacological response to another, *B*, of the same drug class, even though the person never used drug *B* before.

Curriculum planned learning experiences provided by an educational institution.

Darvon synthetic narcotic (propoxyphene) closely related to methadone, which is used for relief of mild to moderate pain.

Decision making ATOD curriculum strategy that provides students with a system for organizing information about psychoactive drug use and then making choices among alternative behaviors or responses.

Decreased awareness condition of escaping from reality, problems, physical and emotional pain; desire for total narcosis or insensibility.

Decriminalization legal process of reducing the penalty for a particular behavior still restricted by law.

Delirium tremens severe form of the alcohol abstinence or withdrawal syndrome, characterized by hallucinations, mental disorientation, agitation with continuous motor activity, involuntary body tremors, and convulsions.

Demand reduction strategy for preventing drug abuse by reducing or eliminating the actual demand, desire, or need for various drug substances.

Demographics characteristics, such as age, gender, income, education, and occupation, that describe the human population's social and vital statistics.

Dendrite nerve fiber that sends electrical impulses toward the cell body of a neuron.

Depo-provera long-acting injectable contraceptive drug containing only progestin.

Depressant drug that slows down body functions; a sedative that depresses the central nervous system, relaxes, tranquilizes, or produces sleep.

Depression reduction in the rate of functional activity; a slowing down effect.

Designer drug synthetic substance produced by chemical alteration of an existing drug in order to make an "act-alike" psychoactive substance that would not be illegal upon its creation.

Detection identification of psychoactive substance use or drug abuse through observation of common signs and symptoms of drug-taking behavior or by other measures, including drug testing.

Detoxification process of making chemical substances nonpoisonous; removal of a toxic substance from the body.

Dextroamphetamine synthetic, central nervous system stimulant and one of three major amphetamine drugs.

Distilled spirits alcoholic beverages containing 40–50% alcohol by volume, made from fermented mixtures of cereal grains or fruits that are heated in a still.

Distribution circulation of an absorbed drug to all parts of the body by way of the bloodstream.

Distribution of consumption theory an alcohol and other drug-abuse prevention belief that links the prevalence of drug abuse problems with the per capita use of all drugs in a nation or society.

Diuretic drug that helps the body excrete excess water and salt, causing a sudden and copious flow of urine.

Doping use of ergogenic drugs to artificially improve athletic competition.

Dose quantity or amount of drug taken at any particular time.

Drug any substance that, upon entering a body, can change either the function or structure of the organism.

Drug abuse deliberate use of chemical substances for reasons other than their intended medical purposes and that results in physical, mental, emotional, or social impairment of the user.

Drug-abuse epidemic sudden increase in a disease condition (drug abuse) in a particular population or locality.

Drug Abuse Warning Network a large-scale drug-abuse data collection system sponsored by the National Institute on Drug Abuse.

Drug classes see *Drug families.*

Drug dependence state of psychological or physical need, or both, for a drug. Usually characterized by compulsive use, tolerance, and physical dependence manifest by withdrawal sickness; chemical dependence; condition often equated with addiction.

Drug Enforcement Administration (DEA) principal federal agency for enforcement of drug laws pertaining to drug trafficking, investigation, drug intelligence, and regulatory control, currently administered within the U.S. Department of Justice.

Drug families major categories or types of drugs that share important characteristics in terms of chemical composition or actions within the body.

Drug misuse unintentional or inappropriate use of prescribed or nonprescribed medicine, resulting in impaired physical, mental, emotional, or social well-being of the user.

Drug-receptor interaction drug reaction between specific drug molecules and unique, localized portions of or within particular human cells known as receptors.

Drug reinforcer any short-term effect of using a drug that is perceived as beneficial, which increases the likelihood of repeated drug use.

Drug testing technique used to detect drug use and abuse through screening or examination of urine, blood, and breath.

Dry-drunk phenomenon an alcoholic's typical state of mind when not drinking, marked by lack of insight, exaggeration of self-importance, overestimation of abilities, insensitivity to others' needs and feelings, rigid judgmental outlook, impatience, and dissatisfaction with life.

Ecstasy popular name for a designer drug, MDMA, that has psychedelic qualities and provides a euphoric "rush" of cocainelike, mind-expanding effects without scary visual distortions.

Enabling factors influences that make drug-taking behavior and/or substance abuse possible, such as the availability and accessibility of psychoactive drugs, actions of certain relatives or friends or agencies, and existence or lack of personal skills.

Endemic drug use continuing presence of a disease condition or behavioral practice (drug use) in a particular population or locality.

Endogenous opioid a natural, made-within-the-body substance that resembles morphine and produces opioid-like effects within the body; a booster of one's metabolic rate.

Endorphins   collective term describing any natural, internal body substance that has opioidlike activity.

Enforcement techniques   methods used by local, state, and federal law-enforcement agents to prevent illicit drug use, such as use of informants, surveillance, undercover operations, drug raids, interdiction, and intelligence gathering.

Enkephalins   first internal body substance, extracted from the brain and pituitary, identified as having a narcotic effect within the body.

Environment   one sector or element of the public health model of drug-abuse prevention, specifically relating to the setting or context in which drug use occurs, and the group or community customs, mores, or folkways that influence drug takers.

Environment-related etiology   theory that relates drug abuse and drug dependence to the sociocultural setting and all those external circumstances and interrelational settings (the environment) in which any psychoactive drug is used.

Environmental tobacco smoke   mixture of sidestream smoke, smoke from the nonburning ends of tobacco products, and exhaled mainstream smoke, along with air, in an enclosed space; the mixture of tobacco smoke and air inhaled by a nonsmoker in the process of involuntary or passive smoking.

Ephedrine   natural extract of a shrub that has a central nervous system stimulant effect; an FDA-approved drug for use as a decongestant, but widely advertised as a diet pill.

Ergogenic agent   a drug, such as a stimulant, narcotic analgesic, or steroid, used for purposes of artificially improving athletic competition.

Escape-avoidance drug use   drug-taking behavior motivated by the desire for relief from unpleasant sensations, tensions, disturbed interpersonal relationships, fears, and anxieties.

Esthetic experience   a psychedelic response related to a change in and intensification of sensory input, resulting in fascinating alterations in sensations and perceptions, such as synesthesias, beautiful mental images, and powerful music.

Etiology   study of the cause or causative factors of a disease condition or behavioral practice.

Evaluation   process that determines if the curriculum or teaching plan helps students accomplish specific instructional objectives.

Exempt narcotic   drug preparation containing a small amount of a narcotic substance that can be purchased legally in some states without a physician's written prescription.

Fail-safe medicine   medicine that supposedly works safely on all people at all times. Though many believe in such a medication, none exists.

Federal Food and Drug Act   first federal law in the United States, enacted in 1906, that prohibited interstate commerce in misbranded and adulterated drugs sold as medicines.

Fentanyl   a synthetic narcotic used as an intravenous analgesic-anesthetic.

Fetal alcohol syndrome (FAS)   common pattern of birth defects and mental retardation that occurs among some children born of alcoholic or alcohol-consuming mothers, and manifested by central nervous system dysfunction, growth deficiency, facial abnormalities, and other major and minor malformations.

Fixed-ratio combination product   drug preparation containing a combination of two or more drug ingredients intended to relieve multiple symptoms.

Flash   short, intense, generalized sensation of total well-being experienced soon after intravenous injection of cocaine or methamphetamine; the "rush" reaction.

Flashback   undesirable recurrence of a drug's effects with no recent drug consumption to explain changes in consciousness and experience of illusions and hallucinations.

Fluoxetine (Prozac)   a relatively new and frequently prescribed antidepressant drug that blocks the reabsorption of the neurotransmitter serotonin, resulting in continued stimulation of brain cells.

Flurazepam   nonbarbiturate sedative-hypnotic and minor tranquilizer prescribed under the brand name of Dalmane; a benzodiazepine promoted as a hypnotic.

Food and Drug Administration (FDA)   federal regulatory agency within the U.S. Department of Health and Human Services, with counterparts on the state level, responsible for assuring safety and effectiveness of drugs, protecting consumers against contaminants in food and against falsely represented, worthless, and dangerous drugs, medical devices, and cosmetics.

Food-drug interaction   interaction between certain foods eaten and drugs being taken, resulting in speeding up or slowing down drug effects, preventing drug effects, adversely affecting the body's use of food, and even life-threatening conditions.

Formication   hallucination associated with stimulant-induced psychosis in which an individual perceives imaginary ants, insects (crank bugs), or snakes crawling on or under his or her skin.

Freebasing   chemical process of changing common, white cocaine powder into a purer, more potent, smokable form of cocaine "base," which the user then smokes in a glass water pipe that is heated by a butane lighter or small blowtorch.

Generic drug   drug product given an official or nonproprietary name, one that is not patented, trademarked, or owned by a private individual or company. The generic name is often a contraction of the drug's more complex chemical name.

Genetic predisposition   inherited influence that makes some individuals susceptible to certain physical conditions, such as possible increased responsiveness to certain drugs or sensitivity to particular drug effects.

Glaucoma   disease characterized by increased pressure within the eye, which can damage the optic nerve and eventually lead to blindness.

Goals   broad, general statements of intent that give direction to a plan, such as an educational program; long-range targets indicating ultimate outcomes of some endeavor.

Hallucination   groundless false perception having no real external cause.

Hallucinogen   drug substance that induces or produces hallucinations in a drug user.

Hangover   temporary, acute physical and psychological distress following excessive consumption of alcoholic beverages.

Harrison Narcotics Act   federal law enacted in 1914 that established a mechanism of record keeping for the importation, manufacture, distribution, sale, and prescription of narcotic drugs. This act outlawed the nonmedical use of heroin and forbade dispensing of narcotics to known addicts.

Hashish   cannabis preparation more potent than marijuana and derived from the resinous secretions of the cannabis plant's flowering tops.

Hashish oil   dark, viscous liquid produced by repeated extraction of cannabis plant materials with a THC concentration greater than that of hashish.

Hemp plant   leafy plant grown in temperate and tropical areas throughout the world; source of marijuana and other cannabis preparations; *Cannabis sativa*.

Heroin   a semisynthetic narcotic, one of the more powerful dependency-producing drugs, made by treating morphine with acetic anhydride.

HIV infection   invasion of the body by the virus that causes acquired immune deficiency syndrome (AIDS), the human immunodeficiency virus (HIV).

Homeostasis   an organism's internal state of constancy or equilibrium necessary for normal functioning.

Host   one sector or element of the public health model of drug-abuse prevention, specifically relating to individuals and their knowledge about psychoactive drugs, the personal attitudes that influence drug use and patterns of abuse, and drug-taking behavior itself.

Host-related etiology   theory that associates drug abuse and drug dependence with some predisposition or unusual condition that makes a person (the host) particularly susceptible to the effects of a psychoactive drug.

Hyperkinetic disorder   brain disorder characterized by extreme motor restlessness, poor attention span, and impulsive and sometimes disorderly behavior. In children, it is treated by prescribed amphetamines.

Hyperplasia   precancer change in the lungs characterized by an increase in the number of layers of basal cells that underlie the inner surface of the bronchial tubes.

Hypnotic   drug that induces sleep, such as a barbiturate, flurazepam, methy prylon, glutethimide, and chloral hydrate.

Hypothalamus   portion of the brain that is a prime site of action of many psychoactive

drugs, which maintains homeostasis by regulating activities of the body cavity, emotions, and behavior.

Ibuprofen   nonsalicylate analgesic, antipyretic, and anti-inflammatory drug sold originally as a prescription-only painkiller but now available in OTC-strength preparations, marketed as Advil, Nuprin, Motrin, and Medipren.

Ice   a highly addictive smokable form of methamphetamine that produces a euphoric high that lasts several hours.

Idiosyncratic response   special sensitivity or unanticipated adverse reaction to a specific chemical substance.

Illusion   a false or misinterpreted sensory impression of reality; distortion of something that really exists.

Immunosuppressive effect   decreased effectiveness of the body's structural, cellular, and chemical defense mechanisms that helps protect the human body against assault from disease-causing bacteria, viruses, molds, and toxins.

Increased awareness   condition of psychic stimulation allowing for changes in thought processes, ideas, and behaviors.

Inhalant   chemical that evaporates easily and whose vapors, when breathed in, produce mind-altering effects.

Inhalation   process of breathing in; absorption of volatile chemicals into the blood by passing through the lungs.

Injection   introduction of a drug into the bloodstream without having to be absorbed through the digestive tract.

Inoculation strategy   strategy for preventing drug abuse by protecting drug users against unhealthy, irresponsible drug-taking behavior, as promoted through education emphasizing responsible decision making, rational limits on use, and precautions when interacting with psychoactive drugs.

Instructional or educational objective   curricular component that directs instructional activities on a daily basis; statement of what learners are to be like after they have successfully completed a learning experience.

Insulin   hormone produced in the body's pancreas that regulates the metabolism of sugar; antidiabetic drug that helps maintain the diabetic's blood sugar at near normal levels and keeps the urine as free of sugar as possible.

Interdiction   prevention of illicit drugs from entering the United States through confiscation at national borders or ports of entry and through seizure of contraband at sea.

Intervention   a structured, confrontational technique used in helping drug abusers overcome their psychological denial and accept the reality of their drug problems.

Intoxication   temporary state of mental chaos and behavioral dysfunction resulting from the presence of a neurotoxin, such as ethyl alcohol, in the central nervous system.

Involuntary smoking   form of passive smoking in which the secondhand "sidestream" smoke from the burning tobacco products of others is inhaled by nonsmokers.

Khat   East African shrub containing cathinone, a natural amphetaminelike substance; abbreviated name for methcathinone ("cat").

LAAM   synthetic narcotic, chemically related to methadone, that has a duration of action lasting from 48 hours to 72 hours.

Legalization   legislative declaration approving or authorizing a particular action.

Life skills   ATOD curriculum strategy that teaches students how to be assertive, how to resolve interpersonal conflicts, and how to communicate more effectively with others in order not to use alcohol, tobacco, and other drugs.

Look-alike drug   a copy or simulation of a controlled psychoactive drug consisting of one or more legal, uncontrolled nonprescription drugs.

Loss of control   inability of an alcoholic to predict consistently the length of drinking or the amount consumed once use of beverage alcohol has begun.

Lower-yield cigarette   cigarette containing relatively low amounts of nicotine and tar (defined as yielding 15 mg of tar or less per cigarette).

Lung cancer   uncontrolled cellular growth in the lungs, known specifically as bronchogenic carcinoma.

Lysergic acid diethylamide (LSD)   one of the most powerful synthetic psychedelics derived from ergot fungus, LSD is the model against which other mind-expanding drugs are compared.

Macro approach all-inclusive, drug-abuse prevention strategy in which the focus of prevention efforts is on the entire environment (public information, use of motivational psychology, lobbying for movies and TV shows containing drug-abuse prevention themes, and parental cooperation to help restrict undesirable consequences of recreational drug use) in promotion of a no-drug climate.

Mainlining drug administration method in which a chemical substance is injected directly into a vein; intravenous injection.

Mainstream smoke cigarette smoke inhaled by the smoker.

Major tranquilizer an antipsychotic drug that relieves symptoms of a psychotic nature, such as schizophrenia and paranoia.

MAO inhibitors monoamine oxidase, a drug having a central nervous system stimulant effect, which blocks a specific enzyme, thereby increasing a neurotransmitter substance that helps to elevate mood and relieve mental depression; antidepressant drugs.

Mariani's wine beverage made from the coca leaf and introduced in Europe during the nineteenth century.

Marijuana any part of the cannabis plant or its extract that produces physical or psychic changes in the human.

Marijuana high various mind-altering effects resulting from use of marijuana, including a sense of well-being, feeling of relaxation, and a dreamlike state, perceived as favorable responses to cannabis.

Medication error unintentional inappropriate use of a medication (such as decreasing or increasing a recommended dosage) due to impaired vision, poor memory, or failure to hear or understand proper directions.

Medicine drug substance used in diagnosis, cure, treatment, or prevention of disease, or in the relief of pain or discomfort.

Medulla oblongata direct, upward continuation of the spinal cord within the skull.

Mescaline major psychoactive ingredient of the peyote cactus.

Metabolism complex chemical changes that alter drugs and convert them to substances that can be eliminated from the body.

Methadone synthetic narcotic that produces many of the same effects of heroin and morphine but whose duration of action lasts up to 24 hours, thus making the drug useful in the treatment of heroin addiction.

Methadone maintenance continuing use of minimal doses of methadone, given orally, to stabilize heroin-dependent patients by reducing their craving for a drug and eliminating the "rush" sensation following heroin injection.

Methamphetamine synthetic amphetamine, known as "meth" or "speed," commonly abused by intravenous injection for the rapid, intense euphoria of the "rush" or "flash" effect.

Methaqualone synthetic, nonbarbiturate sedative-hypnotic that became both a frequently prescribed and highly abused drug until its legal production was halted in 1983.

Methcathinone synthetic, powerful stimulant that resembles cocaine and amphetamines, and produces a burst of energy along with a prolonged euphoria.

Method planned, organized technique, activity, or experience that instructors use to help students achieve certain objectives.

Mind expansion psychedelic state characterized by heightened awareness of sensory input, enhanced sense of clarity, diminished control over experiences, distortion of objective reality, and general alteration of the conscious state.

Minipill type of oral contraceptive containing only progestin.

Minor tranquilizer antianxiety agent that functions somewhat like a sedative-hypnotic, including meprobamate and benzodiazepine.

Modeling adoption by one individual, often a child, of another's (usually a parent) practice or attitude.

Mood modification change in thinking, feeling, and/or behavior, as induced by a psychoactive drug.

Moonshining illegal production of distilled spirits.

Morphine naturally occurring narcotic drug, derived from opium and used medically as a sedative and analgesic.

MPTP an extremely nerve-damaging designer analogue of meperidine whose use has resulted in permanent symptoms of Parkinson's disease.

Multifactorial theories explanations based on two or more interacting factors or causative influences.

Multimodality therapeutic approach comprehensive treatment and rehabilitation program for narcotic-dependent individuals, based upon several components providing various services to meet the physical, mental, social, and spiritual needs of patients.

Mutagenic effect production of a sudden change from the parent that appears in an offspring due to a toxic or adverse force, such as a drug, on a gene or chromosome.

Mutation change, alteration, or damage to genes within cells of an organism.

Naproxen sodium relatively new over-the-counter analgesic, originally available only as a prescription drug for the treatment of arthritis.

Narcolepsy neurological disorder characterized by recurring attacks of sleep, often induced by emotional excitement.

Narcotic drug that has both a sleep-inducing and pain-relieving action; an opioid or opiate.

Narcotic antagonist drug that tends to block and even reverse the effects of narcotics, thus making the antagonist useful in treating opioid dependence.

Narcotics Anonymous a self-help group patterned after Alcoholics Anonymous in which recovering drug addicts offer help to others seeking recovery from drug dependence.

Natural "high" feeling of elation or temporary euphoria sometimes associated with regular, vigorous exercise over a sustained time, and possibly related to the increased production of endorphins.

Neuron nerve cell (the basic unit of the nervous system), that is capable of receiving stimuli and transmitting electrical messages.

Neurotransmitter chemical substance manufactured in the axon; conducts a nerve impulse from one nerve cell to the dendrites of another nerve cell.

Nicotiana tabacum the tobacco plant whose leaves are processed for smoking, chewing, or sniffing.

Nicotine   a major component of the particulate phase of tobacco cigarette smoke; colorless, oily compound in tobacco that has a central nervous system stimulant effect.

Nonsalicylates   nonaspirin over-the-counter analgesics, specifically acetaminophen and ibuprofen.

Nonsmokers' liberation movement   efforts of nonsmokers of tobacco products to prohibit cigarette advertising in the media and to restrict or segregate smokers in specific and public places, in order to promote a tobacco-free environment.

Normative beliefs   ATOD curriculum strategy that provides information to students about the actual rates of alcohol and other drug use, based on surveys, and thereby corrects the false belief that there is near-universal drinking, smoking, and other drug use among peers.

Norplant   surgically inserted subdermal implants of Silastic capsules containing slow-release progestin-only chemicals that exert a contraceptive effect for as long as five years.

NSAID   abbreviation for a nonsteroidal anti-inflammatory drug, such as aspirin, ibuprofen, or naproxen sodium, that produces desirable effects by blocking the action of specific prostaglandin chemicals in the body.

Opioid   narcotic drug so named because it is derived from the opium poppy plant or made synthetically to have the same drug actions of morphine, a major ingredient of opium.

Opium   naturally occurring narcotic drug derived from the opium poppy, *Papaver somniferum,* and considered as the "mother drug" or main source of nonsynthetic narcotics.

Oral gratification   satisfaction or need fulfillment obtained through the mouth, or by placing something in the mouth.

Over-the-counter (OTC) drug   drug substance sold as medicine without a physician's order or prescription.

Oxidation   process in which oxygen is combined with a chemical substance.

Panic   sudden overpowering terror marked by numerous fears, overexcitation, and uncontrollable behavior.

Papaver somniferum   the opium poppy plant from which opium is derived.

Paraquat   herbicide or plant killer that has been used to reduce the growth of cannabis plants; a marijuana contaminant associated with both temporary and permanent damage to specific body organs.

Particulates   extremely small solid particles found in tobacco smoke, primarily nicotine and tar.

Passive smoking   involuntary inhalation of secondary, unfiltered "sidestream smoke" from the burning tobacco products of others.

Patient medication instructions (PMIs)   printed information dealing with specific drugs and their effects, available to practicing physicians for distribution to their patients, in order to promote effectiveness of drug therapy and patient compliance with instructions for proper use.

Peer-group influences   any attitude, value, or practice of one's age-mates or companions that is perceived as significant, and which a person eventually adopts because of low self-esteem, concern with affiliation, need to be accepted by others, and willingness to conform.

Peripheral nervous system   major division of the nervous system consisting of all the nerves that branch out from the central nervous system and connect it to other parts of the body, including the extremities. The two subdivisions of the peripheral nervous system are the somatic system and the autonomic system.

Personal commitment   ATOD curriculum strategy that encourages students to voluntarily make public or private pledges not to use or abuse alcohol, tobacco, or other psychoactive drugs.

Peyote   fleshy green cactus tips or mescal buttons of the peyote cactus which, upon chewing, swallowing, or smoking, will cause stomach disorders, nausea, vomiting, and a variety of LSD-like effects.

Pharmacology   branch of science dealing with the interaction of chemical agents with living organisms.

Phencyclidine   unique psychoactive drug having psychedelic, stimulant, depressant, hallucinogenic, psychotomimetic, analgesic, and anesthetic properties, used today only in veterinary medical practice, because of its unpleasant side effects in humans; PCP.

Physical dependence   state of physical need for a drug; functional adaptation to a drug in which the presence of a foreign chemical becomes normal and necessary.

Physicians' Desk Reference   annual publication compiled by representatives of pharmaceutical companies and which provides detailed information on prescribed drugs.

Placebo effect   production of a specific drug action or effect resulting from use of an inert substance (placebo) that has no pharmacologic effect; fake medicine or nonmedicated item administered for psychological benefit.

Polycyclic aromatic hydrocarbons   cancer-producing chemicals found in tobacco tar.

Polydrug use   simultaneous use of two or more drugs (or medicines).

Polypharmacy   use of two or more drugs at the same time during the course of treatment for a particular illness.

Potentiating drug interaction or reaction   drug interaction in which one drug intensifies the action of another drug, resulting in an exaggerated effect on the central nervous system.

Potentiation effect   greatly exaggerated drug response obtained when two drugs, taken together, produce a joint effect that is much greater than the sum of the effects of the two drugs when taken separately.

Predisposing factors   influences that make certain people susceptible in advance to use and abuse psychoactive drugs, for example, level of existing knowledge about drugs, personal beliefs and attitudes, and human biological and/or psychological characteristics.

Prescription   physician's order to a pharmacist to dispense a specific drug product to a patient.

Prescription drug   medicine that can be obtained only by the direction (oral or written prescription) of a physician.

Primary prevention   first level of intervention; prevention activities begun before an individual becomes diseased or impaired.

Problem drinking   use of alcohol that results in damage to the drinker, the drinker's family, or to the drinker's community.

Prohibition   forbidding of a certain act; period in American history (1920–33) during which time the manufacture, sale, transportation, and importation of intoxicating liquors was forbidden by national law.

Pseudostimulation   false or deceptive stimulation manifest as increased activity, animated feelings, and noisy behavior, caused in fact by the disinhibition and depressant effects of alcohol.

Psilocybin   psychedelic drug derived originally from so-called sacred or magic mushrooms, having effects similar to but less intense than LSD.

Psychedelics   drugs that can affect one's perception, awareness, and emotions, which sometimes cause hallucinations and illusions.

Psychoactive drug   mind-altering drug that affects thinking, feeling, and behavior.

Psychodynamic experience   psychedelic experience marked by a revelation in which subconscious material is brought to the surface of one's consciousness.

Psychological dependence   condition marked by a strong desire and intense craving to repeat the use of a drug for various emotional reasons, i.e., feeling of well-being and reduction of tension.

Psychopathology   one or more severe mental disorders, such as major depression, schizophrenia, organic brain syndrome, and bipolar manic-depression.

Psychosis   severe mental disorder characterized by loss of contact with reality.

Psychotherapy   purposeful conversation between two or more individuals through which trained therapists attempt to help clients achieve greater self-understanding, objectivity, and maturity.

Psychotic experience   psychedelic experience marked by panic, paranoid feelings, confusion, isolation, and/or mental depression; bad trip or bummer.

Public health prevention model   prevention model that focuses on three major intervention points or targets, within a conceptual framework of a host-agent-environment relationship.

Pulmonary emphysema   disease in which the lungs' ability to exchange gases is impaired due to the loss of alveolar elasticity and the stretching, rupture, and destruction of the lungs' tiny air sacs.

RADAR Network   Regional Alcohol and Drug Awareness Resource (RADAR) Network; serves as an intercommunication system providing individuals and communities with information, publications, and services for combating alcohol and other drug problems.

Rapid eye movement (REM)   characteristic movement of the eye during the sleep phase marked by dreaming.

Rauwolfia serpentina   Indian snakeroot shrub from which was derived reserpine, the first major tranquilizer used as an antipsychotic drug in treating mental illness.

Receptor   specific site on or within the brain or other body organ or cell to which drug molecules must attach in order to produce the characteristic effect of the drug.

Referral process   directing, convincing, and encouraging a drug abuser to contact a drug and alcohol treatment program for assistance in resolving drug-related problems.

Reinforcing factors   influences that generally encourage the continuation of drug-taking behavior once it has begun, for example, experience of pleasure or relief of pain, and the impact of media. May also be important in the initiation of drug use in some instances.

Reserpine   one of the major tranquilizers used as an antipsychotic medication to relieve symptoms of schizophrenia and paranoia.

Resistance skills   general term describing refusal or avoidance behaviors that help an individual say no to drug use or prevent drug abuse by giving reasons for nonuse, leaving the scene, choosing nondrug alternative activities, and utilizing the "broken record" and "fogging technique" of passive resistance to various pro-drug influences.

Resources   instructional media, such as books, pamphlets, films, slides, projectors, videocassette tapes, and government and private agencies, community groups, and individuals that can support educational programs.

Responsible drug use   use of any drug in such a way so as to eliminate, reduce, lessen, or minimize the negative consequences often associated with such use.

Reye's syndrome   a rare, acute, brain-damaging and sometimes fatal condition, characterized by vomiting and lethargy that may progress to delirium and coma, that occurs in young people and teenagers recovering from certain viral infections, namely, chickenpox and flu.

Risk factor   condition or characteristic that increases the probability of some behavior or event.

Rush   short-lived jolt and tingling sensation of intense well-being or euphoria experienced soon after injecting heroin directly into a vein.

Rush reaction   see *Flash*.

Salicylates   a family of painkilling, fever-reducing, and anti-inflammatory drugs, such as aspirin, containing salicylic acid.

Salicylism   toxic condition resulting from excessive intake of acetysalicylic acid, marked by nausea, vomiting, ringing in the ear, deafness, and even severe headache.

Secondary prevention   second level of prevention; prevention activities applied during the early stages of a disease and aimed at restoring health to those who have become ill or impaired.

Sedative   drug that has a calming effect, relaxes muscles, and relieves feelings of tension, anxiety, and irritability.

Sedative-hypnotic   drug that induces sleep and has a calming effect.

Sedativism   chemical dependency on sedative-type psychoactive drugs, particularly barbiturates, minor tranquilizers, and ethyl alcohol.

Self-limiting condition   disease condition, usually of a minor nature, that tends to run its course to recovery without treatment, such as the common cold.

Self-medication   practice of treating oneself with nonprescription medicine for relief of symptoms associated with relatively minor diseases or disorders.

Side effect   drug effect other than the intended or anticipated one.

Sidestream smoke   smoke inhaled from the burning tobacco products of others and originating from the lighted tip of a cigarette between puffs.

Sinsemilla   seedless variety of high-potency marijuana, prepared from unpollinated female cannabis plants.

Skin-popping   subcutaneous injection of a drug just beneath the skin's surface.

Sleep aid   over-the-counter drug for the promotion of mild sedation and sleep, usually containing an antihistamine that may produce drowsiness as a side effect.

Smokeless tobacco   tobacco products, such as chewing tobacco and snuff, that are not burned as they are used.

Snorting   drug-taking method in which a substance, such as cocaine, is inhaled or sniffed, with the finely chopped cocaine powder being absorbed through the mucous membrane lining of the nose.

Snuff preparation of powdered tobacco introduced into the nostrils by inhalation.

Snuff dipping insertion of powdered tobacco between the gum and cheek, where it is absorbed through the mucous membrane.

Social drinking particular group's customary way of using beverage alcohol; drinking that promotes interpersonal relations and enhances feelings of camaraderie and solidarity.

Social drug any chemical substance, especially alcohol and marijuana, used to help people better enjoy the company of others.

Solubility the ability of a drug to dissolve in body tissue, i.e., to spread from an area of high concentration to an area of low concentration.

Speed methamphetamine.

Speedball mixture of cocaine and heroin; combination of any central nervous system stimulant and depressant.

Speed runs prolonged periods of heavy stimulant use in which an amphetamine solution is injected as often as every hour.

Stimulant chemical substance that tends to speed up central nervous system function, resulting in alertness and excitability.

Stimulation increase in the rate of functional activity; speeding up of central nervous system function.

Strategies basic underlying designs of educational curricula that reflect a particular reasoning or philosophy and guide approaches to curriculum development and implementation.

Student Assistance Program (SAP) organized approach for intervening in and preventing alcohol, tobacco, and other drug (ATOD) problems among school-age youth; focuses on behavior and performance at school and uses a referral process that includes screening by teachers and other school personnel for ATOD involvement.

Subdermal implants Silastic capsules that are inserted beneath the surface of the skin where, for example, a slow-release, progestin-only chemical exerts a prolonged contraceptive effect.

Subject matter topical content, such as facts, theories, controversies, projections,

and ideas appropriate to the needs, interests, and developmental levels of the target audience.

Supply reduction strategy for preventing drug abuse by lowering, restricting, or eliminating the availability of a drug.

Surveillance secret and usually continuous watching of suspected individuals, objects, places, or vehicles in order to obtain information about criminal activities.

Synapse junction or meeting place between two nerve cells.

Synergistic drug interaction drug interaction in which there is a cooperative, facilitative, supra-additive effect between two or more drugs, resulting in an exaggerated drug effect or a prolonged drug action.

Synesthesia drug-related effect in which there is a mingling of the senses, in which one sensation may be translated into another, e.g., sounds may be seen and smells may be felt.

Systematic planning process plan that considers both design and implementation of a curriculum; usually consists of a written document stating what the learning experiences are designed to accomplish, how the knowledge, attitudes, or skills will be taught, the resources needed for effective teaching, and the measures used to determine whether the plan achieved its objectives.

Tar particulate matter in cigarette smoke containing various polycyclic aromatic hydrocarbons, phenols, cresols, radioactive compounds, agricultural chemicals, additives, and flavoring agents, all of which appear as a yellow-brown sticky mass when condensed.

Temperance moderation or restraint in the practice of some behavior or use of some substance, such as an alcoholic beverage.

Teratogen agent that causes defects in a developing embryo.

Tertiary prevention third level of prevention; prevention activities initiated during the advanced stages of an illness or disease, aimed at stopping the reactivation of the disease process after recovery.

THC most active and principal psychoactive ingredient of marijuana; delta-9-tetrahydrocannabinol.

Therapeutic agent drug substance used for treating and preventing disease or in preserving health.

Therapeutic community treatment approach to chemically dependent individuals consisting of ex-addicts and other trained personnel who work with drug abusers through encounter group therapy, tutorial-learning sessions, remedial and formal education, and assignment of various housekeeping chores within a drug-free residential environment.

Therapeutic index index for assessing the relative safety of drugs for use in large populations; ratio between the median lethal dose (LD_{50}) and the median effective dose (ED_{50}) of a particular drug used for a specific effect; more realistically calculated as the ratio between the effective dose in nearly all patients (ED_{99}) and the lethal dose in practically no patients (LD_1).

Therapeutics use of drugs in treating and preventing disease and in preserving health status.

Tobacco leaves of the tobacco plant, *Nicotiana tabacum*, prepared for smoking, chewing, or sniffing.

Tobacco additives cellulose-based tobacco substitutes added to cigarettes during manufacture to enhance flavor or facilitate processing.

Tolerance reduction in the pharmacological response to a particular drug in which continued intake of the same dose has diminishing effects; reduced sensitivity resulting in the need for increased dosage to achieve the desired drug effect.

Toxic reaction disturbance of function in one or more body systems caused by a drug overdose; poisonous condition, such as intoxication.

Toxic syndrome undesirable physical and mental experiences ranging from tremors and agitation to hostility and panic, resulting from chronic use of high dose levels of central nervous system stimulants.

Trafficking unauthorized manufacture, distribution, or possession with intent to distribute any controlled drug substance.

Transcendental (mystical) experience a psychedelic response known as the "peak" or mystical experience and characterized by development of a sense of unity, lack of time and space limits, deeply felt moods, feelings of awesomeness and reverence, and meaningfulness of philosophic insight.

Triazolam a frequently prescribed benzodiazepine drug, marketed as Halcion and promoted for its hypnotic effect.

Tricyclic compounds potent drugs used as antidepressants to elevate mood and relieve certain types of mental depression.

Trip variety of mind-altering effects induced by a psychedelic drug and subjectively interpreted.

Valium a frequently prescribed brand name of diazepam that functions as an antianxiety drug or minor tranquilizer; a benzodiazepine derivative.

Values clarification use of teaching methods that foster decision making based upon the recognition of values; instructional techniques that promote choosing freely from alternatives, prizing, and acting on one's beliefs and choices consistently and regularly.

Wine alcoholic beverage containing 10–14% alcohol by volume and made from fermented juice of grapes or other fruits.

Withdrawal symptoms withdrawal sickness or abstinence syndrome consisting of drastic changes in physical functioning and behavior (insomnia, tremors, nausea, vomiting, cramps, elevation of heart rate and blood pressure, convulsions, anxiety, psychological depression) due to overactivity of the nervous system, which are observed or experienced after use of a drug by a physically dependent person has been stopped.

Xanax an intermediate-acting benzodiazepine frequently prescribed as an antianxiety drug.

Youth rebellion rejection of parental values and conflict between parents and children over independence and self-identity, as symbolized by the sudden increase in the use of illegal psychoactive drugs.

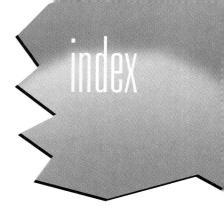

Index

Social drinking, 92, 93, 125
Social drugs, types of, 51
Solubility of drug, 62
Speed, 209
Speedball, 18, 205, 212
Speed runs, 201
Starch blockers, 279
Stimulants
  actions of, 8, 9
  amphetamines, 209–213
  betel nuts, 218–219
  caffeine, 199, 213–217
  cocaine, 201–209
  crashing from, 201
  and driving, 200
  effects of, 199–201
  ephedrine, 218
  medical uses, 213, 299–300
  methcathinone, 218
  nicotine, 199
  over-the-counter, 273, 282
  types of, 9
  yohimbe, 219
Stimulation, drug action, 64
Stoll, Dr. W. A., 228
STP. See DOM (STP)
Stress, and alcoholism, 119–120
Student assistance programs, 376
Subdermal implants, 303
Subthalamus, 71
Sudden infant death syndrome (SIDS), and
    cigarette smoking, 183
Suicide, 15–16
  and age, 15
  relationship to drug use, 15–16
Supply reduction strategy, drug abuse
    prevention, 319–320
Surveillance, 337
Synanon, 145
Synapse, 68
Synergistic effect
  drug interaction, 81
  sedative-hypnotics, 155
Synesthesia, 226
Systematic planning, drug prevention
    education, 361–364

Temazepam, 160
Temperance, 89
Teratogens, marijuana as, 259
Tertiary prevention, 331
Testes, 72

Testosterone, 72, 73
Thai sticks, 246
Thalamus, 71
THC, of marijuana, 250–252
Thebaine, 135
Therapeutic agents, 27
Therapeutic communities, narcotics
    treatment, 145
Therapeutic index, 65, 304
Therapeutics, definition of, 7
Thin-layer chromatography, 333
Time, and drug actions, 66
Toad licking, 238
Toad smoking, 238
Tobacco
  components of tobacco smoke, 180–181
  historical view, 173–174
  negative health effects, 182–183
  nicotine addiction, 181
  smokeless tobacco, 174, 188–191
  trends in use, 174
  See also Cigarette smoking
Tolerance
  acute tolerance, 79
  cross-tolerance, 79
  nature of, 79, 256
  reverse tolerance, 79
Toxic reaction, meaning of, 11
Toxic syndrome, to stimulants, 201
Trafficking, 341–343
  federal penalties for, 342–343
  meaning of, 341
Tranquilizers
  actions of, 153
  antianxiety agents, 161–165
  major, 153, 300
  meprobamate, 161–162
  minor, 153, 300
  types of, 153
Transactional analysis, alcoholism
    treatment, 123
Transcendental experience, and
    psychedelics, 226
Transdermal drug administration, 62
Triazolam, 160
Tricyclic compounds, 214

Urinalysis drug testing, 333–335
  alternatives to, 335
  drugs/average time detectable, 335
  false positives/false negatives, 334
  tests used, 333

Valium, facts about, 162
Values clarification strategy, drug prevention
    education, 365
Violence, and alcohol abuse, 111
Vitamins, over-the-counter, 273

Weight-control products, 277–280
  benzocaine, 278
  bulk-formers, 278
  diet foods/meal replacements/food
    supplements, 279
  diuretics, 279
  and eating disorders, 279
  fraudulent products, 279
  over-the-counter, 272, 277–280
  phenylpropanolamine, 277–278
  prescription, 298
Wernicke's syndrome, and alcohol abuse, 102
Wine, 94–95
Withdrawal syndrome
  in alcoholism, 121
  in barbiturates, 158
  and caffeine, 215
  and methadone, 138
  process of, 80
Women and drug use/abuse, 25–27
  alcohol effects, 27, 97
  and female athletes, 27
  and pregnancy, 25
  rationale for, 25
  and tranquilizer use, 164
  unique drug effects, 26–27
Workplace and drug abuse, 331–336
  costs related to, 332
  drug testing, 333–335
  employee assistance programs, 336
  facts about, 331–332
  workplace policies, 332–333

Xanax, 162

Yohimbe, 219
Youth rebellion, and drug use, 41